ANNUAL PROGRESS IN CHILD PSYCHIATRY AND CHILD DEVELOPMENT 1995

ANNUAL PROGRESS IN CHILD PSYCHIATRY AND CHILD DEVELOPMENT 1995

Edited by

MARGARET E. HERTZIG, M.D.

Professor of Psychiatry
Cornell University Medical College

and

ELLEN A. FARBER, Ph.D.

Assistant Professor of Psychology in Psychiatry
Cornell University Medical College

BRUNNER/MAZEL *Publishers* ● New York

Library of Congress Card No. 68-23452
ISBN 0-87630-793-4
ISSN 0066-4030

Published by
BRUNNER/MAZEL, INC.
19 Union Square West
New York, New York 10003

Manufactured in the United States of America
10 9 8 7 6 5 4 3 2 1

CONTENTS

ANNUAL PROGRESS IN CHILD PSYCHIATRY AND CHILD DEVELOPMENT 1995

Part I

DEVELOPMENTAL ISSUES

The five papers in Part I cover a variety of caretaking issues. The topics include parent-child relations, discipline, the developmental impact of multiple caretaking arrangements in kibbutzim, and the impact of deviations, such as parental depression and abuse, in parenting.

Chapter 1 is an interesting application of the use of an existing data base to examine new questions. Longitudinal studies are critical to understanding growth and development. However, given the constraints on obtaining longitudinal data, secondary analysis becomes an important vehicle for hypothesis testing. There are numerous data bases that have been made available to the scientific community for secondary analysis.

The data base for this paper is The New York Longitudinal Study (NYLS). The NYLS followed 133 middle-class children from 3 months of life to age 25. To date, many studies using the sample have assessed stability of temperamental variables and the ability to predict from temperamental dimensions to later functioning. Tubman and Lerner chose to address questions of continuity in parent-child relationships during adolescence and young adulthood and to investigate the impact of temperament variables on those relationships. Many studies of parent-child relationships in adolescence have focused on conflict. They chose to evaluate the broader relationship.

Interviews with the subjects during adolescence, college age, and young adulthood were used to rate the Emotional Quality and Interactional Quality of the parent-child relationship. Based on a semi-structured two- to three-hour interview with a psychiatrist, 9 dimensions of temperament were scored at the same three points in time. Young adult psychiatric symptoms were obtained by a psychiatrist asking the person to self-report on symptoms. One of the early childhood measures is psychological adjustment as rated in childhood by project psychiatrists. For middle childhood, a variable called "negative emotional or behavioral states" (NEBS) has been coded from the interviews with parents and teachers. Parents, teachers, and children were interviewed in the early years. As the subjects approached young adulthood, parents and teachers were no longer interviewed.

The authors use the multivariate technique of canonical correlation, a measure of the degree of association between sets of variables. Quality of parent-child relationships was fairly stable over the adolescent to young

1

adult years. Temperament characteristics, specifically adaptability and mood quality, were associated with concurrent relationship quality. Psychiatric symptoms, which were correlated with childhood ratings of mood disorders and aggressiveness, were also associated with concurrent ratings of parent-child relationships. NEBS ratings in early to middle childhood were associated with parent-child affective quality in later time periods.

The analyses also indicated that the association between temperament, symptomatology, and relationship quality was lower during adulthood than in adolescence. This supports the notion of discontinuity in relationships during the time of individuation. In sum, this report used longitudinal data to assess continuity in the perception of the quality of parent-child relations from adolescence to young adulthood.

In the second paper (Chapter 2) of Part I, Grusec and Goodnow reexamine the literature on discipline techniques and the effect of parental discipline methods on children's internalization. In their words, discipline is "one of the most emotional and significant interactions that occurs between parent and child." Discipline is considered effective if it leads to internalization; that is, intrinsic motivation leads the child to behave in socially acceptable ways. The authors review the numerous theories of discipline (e.g., psychoanalytic, social learning) and then present a model based on information processing that includes two main constructs—accurate perception of the message and acceptance of the message—required for internalization. The authors then specify the varied features of parental disciplinary actions that promote these two constructs.

Information-processing studies suggest that the frequency, consistency, clarity, and significance of a message is necessary for internalization. However, many parents use indirect methods of declaring rules and the reasons for them, such as "Hands off the table, were you born in a stable?" The efficacy of the types of reasoning that parents use would be an important area for future investigation.

The authors describe child characteristics, including temperament, mood, and developmental level, and parent characteristics, including warmth and characteristic disciplinary style, that moderate the efficacy of different types of discipline. In addition, types of reasoning are elaborated. Reasons will differ in their effectiveness based on whether they refer to the child or to the victim. Effectiveness may depend on the child's perspective-taking ability, interpretation of the statement, and the intensity of affect aroused. Parental reprimands may be more or less general, invoking a rule about a specific situation or about the more general rules of conduct.

Although this is a technical paper, practical issues can be extracted. The authors note that other parental goals of socialization, such as having the child develop flexibility and initiative, and maintaining self-esteem and a positive parent-child relationship, may at times take precedence over internalization. Some techniques, such as humor and drama, may offer ways of maintaining the relationship and avoiding confrontations rather than leading to internalization of the underlying values. One important point from this paper is that blanket statements about the most appropriate discipline techniques (e.g., reasoning versus power assertion) cannot easily be made. Rather, parents need to be flexible in each situation and with regard to the child's age and state. This paper reiterates the notion that cookbook approaches to parenting, however desirable, are rarely effective, because they do not allow for the complexities of human interaction.

Chapter 3 is a review of kibbutz care for infants and young children. The kibbutz, a communal living arrangement in Israel, provided a natural experiment for comparing the consequences of collective child-rearing methods with the "traditional" family approach used in the West. In " 'Children of the Dream' Revisited: 70 Years of Collective Early Child Care in Israeli Kibbutzim," the authors describe the historical roots of the kibbutz movement and changes in child care that have occurred there over time. They also review studies assessing the impact of collective child rearing on attachment relationships, social competence, and peer relationships.

Bettelheim coined the term "children of the dream" to refer to kibbutz children. The kibbutzim were originally planned as egalitarian communities where women would participate in equal ways with men in the work force and men would share in child rearing. Collective education was viewed as the way to accomplish these goals and to raise children lacking in individualistic tendencies who would foster the goals of the kibbutz. Of note, kibbutz founders used psychoanalytic theory to justify separating children from their parents and creating children's houses. In these houses, large numbers of infants were cared for by a small number of medically trained women. This was an attempt to protect children from the pathological consequences of conflicts in parent-child relationships. From social learning theory came the idea of the parents providing for emotional needs and the *metaplot* (caregivers) providing for instrumental and educational needs. Eventually Bowlby's theory, which highlighted children's preference for exploration and mastery in the context of security, and Piaget's theory of cognitive development and the need for a stimulating environment began to influence the kibbutzim. By the 1990s, most kibbutzim had abandoned collective sleeping. However, the infant houses have been retained for daytime care and socialization. Currently kibbutz child care is viewed as of high quality, characterized by a good physical environment, small group size, and a good caregiver-child ratio. However, caregiver instability is moderately high and may impact on the children's development.

Studies of the long-term effects of kibbutz child rearing with communal sleeping arrangements found that the children grew up to be well-functioning adults, but less capable of establishing intimate friendships. One speculation is that this resulted from the failure to achieve secure relationships in infancy when parents were not consistently available, particularly during times of stress, such as night wakings. Recent studies found that communal sleeping was significantly associated with anxious attachments, and that family-based sleeping was associated with a high rate of secure attachment. Quality of attachment with the *metaplot*, and not with the parents, predicted the children's later socioemotional functioning.

The authors' analysis of the existing data indicates that this sociological experiment has resulted in supporting father-child relationships, but has had a more ambiguous impact on mother-child relationships. That the extended network and the family network in kibbutzim have more predictive power than the mother-child relationship may be explained by the greater involvement of fathers and *metaplot* in child care. Studies of the kibbutz children's peer relations find the children to be socially skillful at very young ages. Children show advanced group-oriented skills and lower social problem-solving skills, leading to the findings in adults of high sociability and low intimacy.

This paper provides an interesting discussion of the nature of child rearing and how changes in its structure, such as communal sleeping arrangements and collective child rearing, have a variety of documented consequences. This paper also addresses the current controversy regarding out-of-home care for infants. The difficulty of providing sensitive, responsive care in a group setting is an issue of much contemporary interest. If high-quality care is available, nonparental daytime care does not inhibit the development of secure child-parent attachments.

The next two papers assess normal development in the context of risk factors including depression and abuse. Chapter 4 explores how emotional sensitivity and caring for others is affected by variations in parenting. Radke-Yarrow, Zahn-Waxler, and colleagues have longitudinal data on the children of depressed and nondepressed mothers. The authors address the following questions: (1) Does ongoing exposure to maternal disregulated affect and distress lead to elevated or depressed rates of caring behavior? (2) How do the mother-child relationship and child characteristics "modify" children's caring behavior?

The participants were 90 two- to four-year-old children. Fifty-two of the mothers were diagnosed with unipolar depression or bipolar illness. Children's caring behavior was observed in a simulated naturalistic environment allowing multiple opportunities for parent-child interaction. In addition, the mother was instructed to simulate feeling sad in response to a picture of a crying baby. Coded child responses included verbal sympathy, physical comfort, and helping behavior. Other risk factors evaluated were security of attachment relationship and the presence of child psychiatric problems including anxiety and oppositional behavior.

Overall, when mothers simulated sadness, children of depressed moms intervened more than did children of well moms. However, there is no simple association between parent diagnosis and children's caring behavior. Boys who are exposed to severe parental depression show more caring behavior than boys of well or less severely depressed mothers. Girls, on the other hand, show caring behavior regardless of maternal diagnosis. Among boys, attachment was not associated with helping behavior; among girls, secure attachment was associated with more helping behavior. In the naturalistic setting, high degrees of child helping were associated with severe maternal depression, secure attachment, and child psychiatric problems. This result raises the age-old question of whether some or all of the caring behavior is self-motivated (that is, to relieve anxiety).

The results also raise questions about the development of secure attachment under the care of a parent with affect regulation difficulties. The child may receive little help in understanding his or her own feelings or in learning to regulate his or her own emotions. Although secure attachment is viewed as a protective factor, some of the securely attached children were diagnosed with psychiatric problems. Further investigation may tease apart the elements of caretaking in depressed mothers whose children are securely attached to them.

Chapter 5 also covers normative development in children exposed to a deviant parenting environment. In this case, the parenting environment is maltreatment, and the development is the ability to talk about internal states, which typically occurs during the third year of life.

Beeghly and Cicchetti compared the internal-state language of low-income, maltreated 30-month-olds with children from similar socioeconomic backgrounds who were not maltreated. This enabled them to assess the cumulative effect of abuse over and above the general risk factor of low SES. Another risk factor assessed in this study was insecure attachment. Internal-state language is believed to reflect a toddler's emerging understanding of self and other, and to be important for regulating social interaction. Maltreated toddlers are known to have deviant early development of self and of the capacity for empathy.

The ability to talk about internal states in oneself and others emerges early in the second year of life and then increases dramatically the following year. Internal-state categories assessed in this study using maternal interview and laboratory observations include the following: sensory perception (e.g., sight, smell), physiology (hunger, fatigue), positive affect (love, joy), negative affect (hate, anger), affective behavior (hug, cry), moral judgment (good person), obligation (permission), volition (desire, need), ability (mastery), and cognition (knowledge, memory).

Internal-state language is related to children's general level of linguistic maturity (both receptive and expressive language). Maltreated toddlers received poorer scores than nonmaltreated toddlers on measures of expressive language. The scores of both groups were slightly lower than those of middle-class toddlers assessed in other studies. As hypothesized, maltreated toddlers had significantly fewer internal-state words than nonmaltreated toddlers. In particular, maltreated toddlers used fewer internal-state words for physiological state, negative affect, and moral obligation. On more task-oriented categories, such as perception, cognition, and volition, both groups were similar. Maltreated toddlers also used their internal-state words in a more restricted way, usually referring to only one person.

Of note, maltreating mothers were not good informants about their children's internal-state language, whereas middle-class and nonmaltreating lower-class mothers are good reporters. Interviews can be used with the latter two groups rather than observations of the child. As with the study on caring (Chapter 4), attachment appeared to play a moderating role. Toddlers at highest risk (maltreated and insecure) showed the most compromised internal-state language. Maltreated girls were least likely to use words about negative affect. The authors speculate that this may reflect the development of an internalizing pattern of coping with stress—a pattern seen more frequently in females. A tendency to repress negative emotions may lead to future difficulties with social relationships. The study indicates that both the quality of attachment and the capacity to talk about feelings are affected by maltreatment. In sum, this paper presents an interesting discussion of internal-state language as it relates to early self-development and self-other understanding.

1

Continuity and Discontinuity in the Affective Experiences of Parents and Children: Evidence From the New York Longitudinal Study

Jonathan G. Tubman
Florida International University, Miami

Richard M. Lerner
Institute for Children, Youth, and Families
Michigan State University, East Lansing

Canonical correlation described continuity and discontinuity in salient covariates of emotional and interactional components in parent-child relationships among NYLS participants from middle adolescence to young adulthood. The results underscore the importance of multiple indicators of parent-child relationship quality, and their implications for assessment and intervention efforts are discussed.

An extensive body of research has sought, across a wide variety of disciplinary orientations and investigative methodologies, to examine systematically the quality of parent-child relations in adolescence (Montemayor, 1983; Steinberg, 1989). Many have equated relationship quality with parent-adolescent conflict. Descriptive studies of the course or content of parent-adolescent conflict have examined facets of the same phenomenon via such methods as large-scale social surveys of attitudes (Bengtson & Black, 1973; Kandel & Lesser, 1969; Offer, Ostrov, & Howard, 1981), questionnaires regarding sources of conflict (Caplow, Bahr, Chadwick, Hill, & Williamson, 1982; Eyberg & Robinson, 1983; Harris & Howard, 1984),

Reprinted with permission from *American Journal of Orthopsychiatry*, 1994, Vol. 64, 112–125. Copyright © 1994 by The American Orthopsychiatric Association, Inc.

A revised version of a paper submitted to the *Journal* in November 1992. Research was supported in part by grant MH39957 from the National Institute of Mental Health.

observation of connections among sequences of behavior and conflict (Forehand, 1990; Patterson, 1982; Steinberg, 1981), and observation of processes of communication and negotiation in conflict situations (Grotevant & Cooper, 1985; Hauser et al., 1984; Kendall, 1991). Thus, parent-adolescent conflict has been measured via a variety of methods and levels of analysis.

Normative developmental transformations in parent-child relationships as children attempt to develop their own identities or "individuate" from their parents in late adolescence have been portrayed as sources of conflict. Traditional psychodynamic formulations of the development of autonomy among adolescents have emphasized the importance of establishing independent emotional relationships with parents after puberty and the intensification of relationships with peers, especially those of the opposite sex (Blos, 1967; Freud, 1958; Murphy, Silber, Coelho, Hamburg, & Greenberg, 1963). In contrast, Stierlin (1981) developed a more balanced formula that integrated parents' desires for continuity in relationships with adolescents' desires for separation. Other investigators have sought formulations of normative developmental processes that would accommodate both growing psychological and physical separation between parents and children and continuity in processes of mutual influence, affection, association, and respect (Grotevant & Cooper, 1986; Hill & Holmbeck, 1986; Smollar & Youniss, 1989). These formulations took into account continuity and discontinuity in various aspects of social relations as they are renegotiated, as well as reciprocal relations between parents and children.

Research regarding continuity-discontinuity in the process of individuation of adolescents from parents has considered the functional significance of conflict in parent-child relations (Cooper, 1988; Steinberg, 1989). Some studies have suggested that family communication processes, e.g., expression of viewpoints and disagreements, predict adolescent identity formation, perspective-taking, and conflict-resolution skills (Cooper, 1988; Grotevant & Cooper, 1985, 1986). Other research has documented associations between progressive discourse change among family members and adolescents' levels of ego development (Hauser et al., 1984), links between parenting styles and adolescent social competence (Baumrind, 1978), and relationships between the renegotiation of parent-child relations and adolescents' cognitive development and level of reasoning (Smetana, 1988). In addition, Steinberg (1989) has speculated that parent-child conflict in adolescence may have an evolutionary basis in that it forces adolescents to seek sexual partners outside of the family of origin and encourages autonomy among adolescent males. While conceptualizations of individuation and its functional significance may differ among these researchers, adolescent development is typically seen as occurring in the context of ongoing parent-child relations within which "individuality and connectedness" are negotiated (Grotevant & Cooper, 1986; Smollar & Youniss, 1989).

To the extent that contemporary research on parent-adolescent relations has focused on conflict between parents and children, it has given greater priority to the developmental course of parent-adolescent conflict and to categorizing families in terms of their level of conflict. Assessing the quality of parent-child relationships as a whole has been given less priority. However, as Montemayor (1986) has argued, families cannot simply be dichotomized on the dimension of parent-child conflict because parent-child dyads vary in the amount of conflict expressed. Parent-adolescent conflict has been found to vary systematically with family social context and structure, parent and child characteristics, and styles of parent-child interaction (Montemayor, 1986; Smetana, Yau, Restrepo, & Braeges, 1991). In contrast, the issues about which parents and children generally experience conflict have remained essentially the same for decades (Montemayor, 1983). Therefore, while distinctions on the basis of conflict may be useful in contrasting clinical and nonclinical samples, they accord too much importance to conflict as a component of the normative developmental course of parent-adolescent relations. This observation may be particularly pertinent if parent-child relations are to be studied into young adulthood when the likelihood of conflict over "normal, everyday, mundane family matters" (Montemayor, 1983) decreases due to the increasing physical and psychological separation between parents and children.

Thus, in describing the normative developmental course of parent-child relations from adolescence to young adulthood, it may be more fruitful to assess parent and child perceptions of relationships than to classify families by preexisting monolithic definitions. Frank, Avery, and Laman (1988) employed in-depth interviewing techniques to obtain multivariate assessments of autonomy and relatedness in relationships between young adults and their parents. This study derived several dimensions of relationship experiences in reports by the young adults; significant associations between these dimensions and children's age, sex, and marital status; and the identification of several theoretically relevant types of parent-child relationships. This study is an excellent example of how participants' own perceptions can be used to explore individual differences in multiple dimensions of parent-child relationships.

Unfortunately, most extant studies of self-perceptions of parent-child relationships in middle to late adolescence are cross-sectional or short-term longitudinal in design. This may limit the description of continuity-discontinuity in relationship ratings, the identification of concurrent or antecedent covariates of these ratings, and the description of parent or child characteristics associated with relationship quality. By further exploring individual differences in parents' and adolescent children's ratings of their relationships, using the resources of the New York Longitudinal Study (NYLS), the present report seeks to provide initial long-term longitudinal data about the continuity-discontinuity of parent and child perceptions, concurrent-antecedent covariates, and the clinical relevance of identified covariates. Variables used in this report were identified as relevant to the quality of parent-child relationships in earlier qualitative treatments of NYLS data; they include child temperament, childhood negative emotional-behavioral states, early parent-child relationship problems, and young adult psychiatric symptoms (Chess & Thomas, 1984; 1986; Thomas & Chess, 1977).

METHOD

Participants

Participants were the 133 middle-class children from the NYLS sample (Thomas & Chess, 1977). The sample is over 99% white and predominantly (78%) Jewish. All participants were initially studied in their first weeks of life, and have been followed at regular intervals since (Chess & Thomas, 1984). The NYLS employs a sample of convience, as all participant families were previously acquainted with the study's founders or with their professional colleagues. Of importance to the present report are the adolescent interviews at 16–17 years, the college-age interviews at 18–23 years, and the young-adult interviews at 25–31 years. Sample recruitment began in 1956 and ended in 1962. By 1984, 24 of the original 84 families had experienced divorce, affecting 34 of the 133 target children (25.6%). The sample has remained intact throughout the study, with a participation rate among target children of 97% ($N = 129$) in the latest wave of data collection, completed in 1987.

Measures

Affective experience ratings. Ratings of parent-child relationships were constructed for mothers and fathers separately, and for both parents combined (see below) at the adolescent and college-age interviews; parents were not systematically interviewed at the time of the young-adult interviews. Children's relationship ratings were constructed at the adolescent, college-age, and young-adult interviews. Ratings of or by both parents differ from those of or by mothers and fathers separately in that they were constructed from statements attributed to both parents in an interview or from statements made by a child about both parents. Emotional Quality was rated on a three-point scale: positive (3); mixed, variable, ambivalent, or neutral (2); and negative (1). Interaction Quantity was also rated on a three-point scale: high (3), medium (2), and low (1).

Data were generated following a method employed by Thomas, Chess, Birch, Hertzig, and Korn (1963). At each time of testing, statements were excerpted as thematic units from interviews if they contained any text that referred either to emotional aspects of parent-child relations (e.g., closeness or distance, love or hate, conflict and tension, or evaluations of the other person that included an emotional component) or to the interactional aspects of these relationships (e.g., giving advice, sharing problems, expressing feelings, making decisions, and the performance of joint activities). Other than those referring to a change in a relationship between past and present, all statements pertained to the present, or to the past month. All generated statements were rendered anonymous and gender-non-specific in references to NYLS children.

Reliability estimates of the thematic statement generation process were based on a randomly selected 15% of the five waves of transcripts, as measured by the number of times two individuals generated the same thematic statements; estimates ranged from 86% to 94%. A total of 7,912 thematic statements were generated and were then rated randomly by three of five raters. If two of the three raters did not rate a statement for at least one dimension, as happened with 2.2% of statements, it was discarded. Inter-rater reliability, the number of times at least two of the three raters agreed for each dimension, was 89.6% for emotional quality and 88.2% for interaction quantity for a randomly selected sample of 20% of the statements. Summary scores for each dimension were constructed by averaging across statements the modal ratings (by the three raters) for each child and parent at each time of data collection.

Missing data from parent and child ratings, which stemmed primarily from the process of statement generation (i.e., participants' lack of elaboration about parent-child relations) rather than from missing subjects, were estimated using least-squares estimates (Little & Rubin, 1987; Rovine & Delaney, 1990). The amount of data estimated varied by time of measurement and by source of rated statements, ranging from 3.6% to 35.4%, with an average of 16.2%. Emotional quality and interaction quantity rating means, standard deviations, and intercorrelations did not differ statistically before and after data estimation.

Temperament. Through scores derived from coded interview responses, each participant's temperament, or behavioral style, was measured in middle adolescence, at college age, and in young adulthood. Nine dimensions of temperament were assessed at each point, following Thomas and Chess (1977). The temperament domains and their definitions from Chess and Thomas (1984) were: *1)* Activity Level, the motor component present in functioning and the diurnal proportion of active and inactive periods; *2)* Rhythmicity, the predictability of biological functioning; *3)* Adaptability, responses to new or altered situations, and the ease with which those responses are modified; *4)* Approach/Withdrawal, the nature of an initial response to a new stimulus, be it a person, place, or thing; *5)* Threshold of Responsiveness, the intensity level of stimulation that is necessary to evoke a discernible response; *6)* Intensity of Reaction, the energy level of response, regardless of its quality or direction; *7)* Quality of Mood, the amount of pleasant versus unpleasant behavior; *8)* Distractibility, the effectiveness of extraneous environmental stimuli in interfering with or altering ongoing behavior; and *9)* Persistence, the continuation of an activity direction in the face of obstacles to its continuation.

At each time of testing relevant to this report, temperament scores were obtained for each participant from responses to standard questions posed in face-to-face interviews with an NYLS psychiatrist (e.g., Thomas, Chess, or others). The interviews were standard across the three points of measurement and followed a semistructured, two- to three-hour protocol, generally conducted in a participant's home or the interviewer's office. Temperament scores ranged from low (1) to high (7), and reflected clinicians' ratings of participants' temperament determined from their responses to questions in the face-to-face interview. The exact procedures for these interviews and the techniques used for coding and for establishing reliability have been reported in numerous publications (Chess & Thomas, 1984; Lerner, Hertzog, Hooker, Hassibi, & Thomas, 1988; Thomas & Chess, 1977). For the college-age interviews, an analysis of pooled interrater reliabilities (within time correlations) for 24 randomly selected interviews found moderate reliabilities (range .54 to .76) for eight of the nine temperament dimensions. One attribute (intensity), however, had a low (.33) pooled reliability (Chess & Thomas, 1984). In young adulthood, an analysis of 24 randomly selected interviews found simple (i.e., uncorrected) interrater reliabilities in the moderate range (.42 to .78) for seven temperament attributes and low uncorrected interrater reliabilities for Activity Level (.30) and Distractibility (.26) (Thomas, Chess, Lerner, & Lerner, 1989).

Adjustment in childhood. Evidence of poor psychological adjustment of the sample was rated by NYLS psychiatrists on a five-point scale for 11 dimensions at age three, from insignificant (1) to severe (5). The 11 dimensions from the age-three parent interviews were: sleeping; eating; elimination; fears, tics, and rituals; speech and communication; motor activity; relationship with parents; discipline; relationship with siblings; relationship with nonfamily persons; and coping and task mastery. Relationship to school was added as a twelfth dimension at the age-five parent interview. Each dimension was composed of a series of items rated individually and then averaged. Global adjustment scores at ages three and five were derived by adding the average score for each dimension and dividing by the number of dimensions. Therefore, the scores for global adjustment at ages three and five may be decomposed into scores for more specific domains of adjustment. Scores generated for the 11 adjustment dimensions at age three had interrater reliabilities (within time correlations) above .80 for seven of the dimensions, and reliabilities of .75 for sleep; .68 for fears, tics, and rituals; .64 for sleeping; and .32 for coping. At age five, all 12 adjustment dimensions had interrater reliabilities above .88 (Chess & Thomas, 1984).

Negative emotional or behavioral states. Negative emotional or behavioral states (NEBS) for the childhood years were coded by an independent psychiatrist employing an inductive content analysis of the NYLS childhood interviews with parents and teachers; for details of procedure and scoring see Chess and Thomas (1984), Lerner et al. (1988), and Thomas and Chess (1977). These interviews contained detailed descriptions of the child's behavior in the home and in school. For ages one through six, ratings were made for anxiety, aggressiveness, undercompliance, dissatisfaction, and problematic peer relations. For ages seven through 12, ratings were assigned for anxiety, depressive mood, aggressiveness, disobedience in the home, academic difficulties, and excessive parental physical punishment. Each behavior was scored as not present (0), mild (1), moderate (2), or severe (3). When a negative emotional or behavioral state was indicated in two interviews over a six-month interval by parents, it was given a score of one. When, in addition to reports by parents, teachers also indicated the presence of a negative state, the intensity was given a score of two. Finally, when both parents and teachers reported negative emotional behavioral states in interviews from two consecutive years, the intensity was given a score of three (Lerner et al., 1988). These NEBS ratings have shown considerable internal predictive validity in prior analyses. For example, the NEBS categories of anxiety and aggression have stability coefficients of .97 and .91, respectively, for ages one through six and seven through 12. In terms of external validity, childhood problems such as high anxiety and high aggressiveness were predictive of adjustment problems in adolescence (Lerner et al., 1988).

Young adult psychiatric symptoms. In the young-adult interview, participants were asked to describe any psychological symptoms, psychosomatic symptoms, or thought disturbances they were currently experiencing. Reported symptoms were placed by a psychiatrist in the following categories: anxiety, depression, thought disorders, passive-dependency, aggressiveness, mood disorders, motor disturbances, speech disorders, psychosomatic symptoms, and other symptoms. Like the childhood NEBS ratings, psychiatric symptom ratings in young adulthood were meant to index serious underlying adjustment problems. Symptom categories were rated on a four-point scale as not present (0), mild (1), moderate (2), or severe (3). Motor disturbances were not included in this study because none of the participants reported them in young adulthood.

Analyses

Canonical correlation was used to assess multivariate associations among sets of *a)* affective experience ratings and *b)* clinically relevant variables at occasions of measurement from early childhood to young adulthood. This technique was selected to identify features of parents and children that were linked to specific relationship ratings by mothers, fathers, or children both within and across times of measurement (Tatsuoka, 1988). Canonical correlation determines linear combinations (underlying dimensions, or canonical variates) in each of two sets of variables that are most highly correlated with one another without being correlated with additional, smaller linear combinations within either set of variables. The meaning of each canonical variate can be indirectly interpreted by examining the degree to which the original observed variables are correlated with their canonical variates, i.e., via canonical structure (Levine, 1977).

Tables 3 through 6 summarize canonical correlations between sets of relationship ratings during adolescence and sets of parent or child characteristics. These tables show canonical correlations and all variables correlated .40 or greater with their canonical variates; for each significant canonical correlation analysis, only one canonical correlation was significant. These tables also contain summary data from redundancy analyses of each canonical correlation. Total redundancy coefficients indicate the amount of variance in each set of variables that may be accounted for by all canonical variates, significant and insignificant, of the opposite set of variables (Levine, 1977). Therefore, for each of two variable sets, each table contains the structure of an underlying dimension, the correlation between these underlying dimensions, and the amount of variance in each dimension that may be accounted for by the other.

RESULTS

Relationship Ratings

Content. Tables 1 and Table 2 summarize the means and standard deviations in relationship ratings of mothers, fathers, parents, and children from middle adolescence to college age. In general, the means of these ratings may be characterized as stable. Between the adolescent and the college-age interviews none of the mean ratings of mothers, fathers, or parents fluctuated more than 0.14 on a scale of 1 to 3. Differences of this magnitude did not appear to be psychosocially significant. In addition, within times of measurement, mean ratings of emotional quality and interaction quantity of mothers, fathers, and parents did not vary by more than 0.20. Across target parent(s) within occasions of measurement, mean ratings by children ranged between 0.04 and 0.29. Across times of measurement, mean ratings did not range widely. The greatest difference across time was 0.35 for emotional quality ratings of children's statements about parents. However, differences were generally 0.20 or less. Few (two out of ten) significant gender differences were found in parents' ratings of children or in children's ratings of parents (two out of 18) (Tubman, 1990). Therefore, additional analyses were conducted using the total sample rather than by child's gender.

TABLE 1

Child and Parent Affective Experience Ratings: Emotional Quality

EMOTIONAL QUALITY	CHILD RATINGS			PARENT RATINGS		
	N	*M*	*SD*	*N*	*M*	*SD*
Mothers						
Adolescence	101	1.99	0.59	101	1.98	0.45
College age	131	1.96	0.61	131	1.98	0.55
Young adulthood	119	2.10	0.60			
Fathers						
Adolescence	96	2.05	0.65	96	2.03	0.59
College age	122	1.95	0.60	122	2.06	0.56
Young adulthood	110	2.02	0.69			
Parents						
Adolescence	96	2.16	0.45	96	1.99	0.46
College age	121	1.99	0.52	120	1.86	0.50
Young adulthood	107	1.81	0.42			

Note. Emotional Quality statements related 1 (negative), 2 (mixed, variable, ambivalent, or neutral), or 3 (positive).

TABLE 2
Child and Parent Affective Experience Ratings: Interaction Quantity

EMOTIONAL	CHILD RATINGS			PARENT RATINGS		
QUALITY	N	M	SD	N	M	SD
Mothers						
Adolescence	101	1.74	0.50	101	1.73	0.39
College age	131	1.68	0.53	131	1.73	0.50
Young adulthood	119	1.84	0.56			
Fathers						
Adolescence	95	1.60	0.45	96	1.76	0.59
College age	122	1.58	0.47	122	1.90	0.59
Young adulthood	110	1.71	0.60			
Parents						
Adolescence	96	1.90	0.36	96	1.82	0.43
College age	121	1.70	0.50	120	1.73	0.48
Young adulthood	71	1.75	0.48			

Note. Interactional Quality statements related 1 (low), 2 (medium), or 3 (high).

Covariates. Table 3 summarizes information about significant associations among children's temperamental characteristics and parent and child relationship ratings in adolescence and at college age. Several temperamental characteristics, in particular adaptability and mood quality, were associated with emotional quality and interaction quantity ratings. Positive mood quality and higher adaptability were consistently associated with higher relationship ratings. Canonical variates representing emotional quality in adolescence and at young adulthood and interaction quantity in adolescence were most highly correlated with fathers' and parents' ratings of children and with children's ratings of fathers in adolescence, as well as with nearly all relationships ratings at college age. Therefore, two dimensions of temperament can be identified as significant covariates in adolescence and at college age of child and parent reports, especially those of fathers, of the emotional and interactional components of parent-child relationships.

Significant relationships among childhood NEBS ratings and parent-child relationship ratings in adolescence and at college age are summarized in Table 4. NEBS ratings for anxiety, aggressiveness, disobedience, and academic difficulties for years seven through 12 were significantly intercorrelated. A similar cluster of preschool emotional and behavioral

TABLE 3

Significant Canonical Correlations (CC) of Temperament
and Concurrent Relationship Ratings:
Original Variables and Canonical Variates

TEMPERAMENT	PEARSON'S *r*		CC	RELATIONSHIP	PEARSON'S *r*
Adolescence			0.68**	Emotional Quality	
Adaptability	0.75			Child/Mother	0.48
Approach/Withdrawal	0.41			Child/Father	0.70
Intensity	−0.45			Child/Parents	0.59
Mood quality	0.91			Mother/Child	0.46
Persistence	0.44			Father/Child	0.67
Distractibility	−0.40			Parents/Child	0.93
Factor redundancy,	0.13			Factor redundancy,	0.20
Total redundancy,	0.17			Total redundancy,	0.26
Adolescence			0.69**	Interaction Quantity	
Adaptability	0.63			Child/Father	0.50
Approach/Withdrawal	0.55			Child/Parents	0.47
Intensity	−0.53			Father/Child	0.71
Mood quality	0.82			Parents/Child	0.87
Persistence	0.42				
Distractibility	−0.42				
Factor redundancy,	0.12			Factor redundancy,	0.14
Total redundancy,	0.19			Total redundancy,	0.22
College Age			0.52*	Emotional Quality	
Adaptability	0.63			Child/Mother	0.56
Intensity	−0.40			Child/Father	0.59
Mood quality	0.84			Child/Parents	0.69
				Father/Child	0.63
				Parents/Child	0.71
Factor redundancy,	0.05			Factor redundancy,	0.10
Total redundancy,	0.08			Total redundancy,	0.14

Note. Labels for emotion and interaction ratings refer to person making statement/person to whom statement refers. *$p<.05$; **$p<.001$.

symptoms was identified among NEBS ratings for years one to six (i.e., anxiety, aggressiveness, peer relations, and under-compliance). These clusters of problem behavior were consistently related to negative ratings of parent-child relationships, in particular, parents' ratings of children in adolescence and fathers' ratings at college age. Therefore, NEBS ratings of preschool and school-age children were significant distal covariates of ratings of affective experiences of parents and children in adolescence and at college age. Parental reactions to types of child behavior associated with NEBS ratings may have reinforced child behavior patterns, resulting in negative reciprocal patterns of parent-child interaction (Patterson, 1982). Alternatively, as suggested by Lerner et al. (1988), NEBS ratings may have been early indicators of adjustment problems in adolescence and at college

TABLE 4
Significant Canonical Correlations (CC) among Negative Emotional/Behavioral
States (NEBS) Ratings and Relationship Ratings:
Original Variables and Canonical Variates

NEBS RATING	PEARSON'S r	CC	RELATIONSHIP	PEARSON'S r
Years 7–12		0.49*	Emotional Quality	Adolescence
Anxiety	−0.54		Child/Mother	0.52
Aggressiveness	−0.75		Child/Father	0.49
Disobedience	−0.66		Child/Parents	0.56
Academic difficulties	−0.66		Mother/Child	0.65
Parental punishment	−0.66		Parents/Child	0.96
Factor redundancy,	0.09		Factor redundancy,	0.09
Total redundancy,	0.14		Total redundancy,	0.14
Years 7–12		0.55*	Interaction Quantity	Adolescence
Anxiety	−0.78		Child/Parents	0.40
Aggressiveness	−0.68		Mother/Child	0.50
Disobedience	−0.68		Parents/Child	0.94
Academic difficulties	−0.61			
Factor redundancy,	0.11		Factory redundancy,	0.08
Total redundancy,	0.15		Total redundancy,	0.13
Years 1–6		0.58*	Interaction Quantity	Adolescence
Anxiety	−0.56		Child/Mother	0.42
Aggressiveness	−0.69		Child/Parents	0.56
Undercompliance	−0.73		Parents/Child	0.91
Peer relations	−0.54			
Factor redundancy,	0.11		Factor redundancy,	0.09
Total redundancy,	0.14		Total redundancy,	0.11
Years 1–6		0.56**	Emotional Quality	College Age
Anxiety	−0.89		Child/Mother	0.58
Aggressiveness	−0.52		Child/Father	0.50
Peer relations	−0.72		Father/Child	0.82
			Parents/Child	0.46
Factor redundancy,	0.11		Factor redundancy,	0.09
Total redundancy,	0.14		Total redundancy,	0.11

Note. Labels for emotion and interaction ratings refer to person making statement/person to whom statement refers. $*p<.05$; $**p<.01$.

age that would be concurrent correlates of ratings or parent-child relationship quality.

Associations among indices of early childhood adjustment and relationship ratings at college age are summarized in Table 5. Several childhood adjustment problems were significantly correlated with their canonical variates, including discipline problems, parental attitudes, parent-child relationship quality, and global adjustment. Ratings of statements by mothers, fathers, and parents about their children were consistently correlated with the relationship variates at college age. Ratings of early childhood relationship and adjustment problems were negatively associated

TABLE 5

Significant Canonical Correlations (CC) among
Early Childhood Parent-Child Problems and Relationship Ratings:
Original Variables and Canonical Variates

CHILD PROBLEMS		PEARSON'S *r*	CC	RELATIONSHIP		PEARSON'S *r*
Age 3			0.40*	Emotional Quality		College Age
Discipline		0.45		Mother/Child		−0.79
Parental attitude		0.66		Father/Child		−0.63
Global problems		0.83		Parents/Child		−0.49
Factor redundancy,	0.06			Factor redundancy,	0.04	
Total redundancy,	0.09			Total redundancy,	0.06	
Age 3 and Age 5			0.47*	Interaction Quantity		College Age
Relationship: Age 5		0.78		Mother/Child		−0.48
Discipline: Age 5		0.50		Father/Child		−0.66
Parent attitude: Age 3		0.57		Parents/Child		−0.46
Global problems: Age 3		0.60				
Global problems: Age 5		0.68				
Factor redundancy,	0.06			Factor redundancy,	0.04	
Total redundancy,	0.10			Total redundancy,	0.12	

Note. Labels for emotion and interaction ratings refer to person making statement/person to whom statement refers. *$p < .05$.

with parent reports of the emotional quality of and the amount of interaction in parent-child relationships at college age. These data may reflect associations between indices of early parent-child conflict and correlates of conflict at college age. Conflict in early parent-child relationships may have initiated negative reciprocal interaction patterns between parents and children, a mechanism potentially capable of maintaining maladaptive levels of emotional quality and interaction quantity over long periods. These findings suggest that, although parent-child relationships undergo a process of renegotiation in middle to late adolescence, there may be substantial continuity in the affective experiences of both parents and children based on indicators of adjustment and behavior problems in early childhood. These distal influences appear to be more salient for parents than for children as parental, but not children's, relationship ratings at college age are significantly associated with the early childhood behavior and adjustment ratings in canonical correlation analyses.

Significant associations among psychiatric symptoms and young adult ratings of relationships with mothers, fathers, and parents are summarized in Table 6. The psychiatric symptoms of young adults were one of the few variable sets demonstrating significant associations with children's ratings of concurrent parent-child relationships. The psychiatric symptom variate was significantly correlated with several original variables, including mood disorders and aggressiveness, that were conceptually similar to several of

TABLE 6

Significant Canonical Correlations (CC) of Young Adult Psychiatric Symptoms
and Concurrent Relationship Ratings: Original Variables and Canonical Variables

SYMPTOMS	PEARSON'S r	CC	RELATIONSHIP	PEARSON'S r
Psychiatric		0.53*	Emotional Quality	
Thought disorders	0.48		Child/Father	−0.45
Passive-dependency	0.53		Child/Parents	−0.93
Aggressiveness	0.47			
Mood disorders	0.87			
Other symptoms	0.54			
Factor redundancy, 0.06			Factor redundancy, 0.06	
Total redundancy, 0.10			Total redundancy, 0.14	

Note. Labels for emotion and interaction ratings refer to person making statement/person to whom statement refers. *$p<.05$.

the childhood NEBS ratings. The young adult psychiatric symptom ratings may have indexed problem behavior that was negatively associated with relationship ratings, much as the NEBS ratings did. This significant association in young adulthood was another example of coexisting continuity and discontinuity in the affective experiences of parents and children through adolescence into young adulthood. First, this association in young adulthood paralleled associations between NEBS ratings and affective experience ratings in adolescence and at college age. Second, by young adulthood their lives had sufficiently individuated from those of their parents that only indicators of severe intrapersonal and interpersonal dysfunction were associated with the emotional quality of their parent-child relationships.

DISCUSSION

This report employed NYLS data to assess continuity and discontinuity in covariates of emotional quality and interaction quantity ratings of parent-child relations from adolescence to young adulthood. The findings allowed several conclusions. First, the mean levels of the relationship ratings were moderately high and did not fluctuate markedly between occasions of measurement. Second, canonical correlation analyses revealed significant associations between parent and child ratings of affective experiences and a range of clinically relevant variables including concurrent temperament ratings, NEBS ratings from early and middle childhood, early childhood adjustment ratings, and young adult psychiatric symptoms. Third, the number and magnitude of significant canonical correlations was highest in adolescence and dropped steadily to young adulthood, suggesting increasing individuation of adolescents from their parents across this period. Fourth, certain associations in canonical correlation analyses indicated significant degrees of substantive continuity in covariates of parent and child ratings of affective experiences.

These findings support those of contemporary research literature in locating associations among ratings of parent and child affective experiences and variables that appeared to be clinically relevant in earlier qualitative analyses of NYLS data (Chess & Thomas, 1984, 1986). For example, mood quality and adaptability have been cited previously as temperamental risk factors for poor fit between infants or children and their social environments, with implications for parent-child relationships (Bates, 1989; Carey, 1989; Hubert & Wachs, 1985). In addition, aggressive, antisocial, or non-compliant behavior by children and adolescents has been shown to elicit coercive parental behavior. Repeated experiences of high rates of coercive exchanges between parents and children may function to instigate and maintain mutually reinforcing patterns of negative interactions (Forehand, 1990; Forehand & Long, 1988; Patterson, 1986). In the NYLS sample, these temperamental and behavioral characteristics from early childhood to young adulthood were consistently associated with the emotional quality of and the amount of interaction in parent-child relationships throughout adolescence.

Data presented in this report support the notion of discontinuity in affective relationships between parents and children from middle adolescence to young adulthood. Declining numbers and magnitudes of significant canonical correlations between relationship ratings and child or parent variable sets across this period suggested ongoing individuation, i.e., the physical and psychological separation of parents and children (Grotevant & Cooper, 1986; Smollar & Youniss, 1989). Temporal decreases in significant associations between parent or child variable sets and relationship ratings were noted for canonical correlation analyses presented in this report. They have also been noted for other analyses that linked relationship ratings to concurrent ratings of child adjustment, substance use, and demographic variables (Tubman, 1990).

The majority (eight out of 14) of the canonical correlation analyses were statistically significant at adolescence, and the proportion dropped at college age (six out of 14) and again in young adulthood (three out of eight). The decreasing number and magnitude of significant canonical correlations underscored two points. First, as children separated both psychologically and geographically from parents, the emotional quality and the amount of interaction between parents and children were less likely to be influenced by "normal, everyday, mundane family matters" than by serious adjustment problems (Montemayor, 1983). Second, classifying parent-child relationships as conflicted or nonconflicted is less useful than is identifying characteristics of parents, children, or families that are associated with the quality of parent-child relationships (Montemayor, 1986).

These data also document significant degrees of continuity in several aspects of the affective relationships of parents and children. Indices of mood quality, adaptability, and aggressive or antisocial behavior were consistently associated with poorer-quality parent-child relationships from middle adolescence to young adulthood. These affective and behavioral covariates of relationship ratings were assessed both concurrently and in early to middle childhood. Of particular interest were the associations between early childhood NEBS ratings or early adjustment ratings and relationship ratings 15 to 20 years later at college age. These findings suggest that interactions in early parent-child relationships remain a salient distal influence upon the affective experiences of parents and children beyond middle adolescence. However, the relative influence of several factors—including stability of children's personality traits, stability of specific antisocial behavior, or stability of parental reaction patterns—for continuity in the covariates of the quality of parent-child relationships is not clear. Each of these factors may contribute to the continuity of experiences within parent-child relationships as data suggest less adaptive life-course patterns of ill-tempered children (Caspi, Elder, & Bem, 1987; Caspi, Elder, & Herbener, 1990); the stability of children's conduct disorders and significant associations with adult psychiatric diagnoses (Farrington, Loeber, & van Kammen, 1990; Robins, 1978); and consistent associations between child and adolescent conduct disorders and parental warmth, support, or communication style (Hanson, Henggeler, Haefele, & Rodick, 1984; Loeber & Dishion, 1984).

For clinicians and clinical researchers, these data have several implications. First, they suggest the value of moving beyond the unidimensional assessment of parent-child conflict to the identification of multiple covariates of the quality of parent-child relationships. Second, it appears to be useful to include several constructs in assessment and intervention efforts with parent-child relationships, including temperament, antecedent and concurrent problem behavior, and antecedent relationship quality. Third, it may be more useful to assess the degree of coexisting continuity and discontinuity in elements of parent-child relationships during adolescence than to focus on global stability or change in these relationships.

While both the internal and external validity of the present report were limited because it analyzed archival data (Tubman & Lerner, in press), it was intended as an initial exploration of the covariates of parent-child relationship ratings from adolescence to young adulthood. The value of these NYLS data lies not in their representativeness, but in their illumination of the scope of efforts needed to investigate continuity-discontinuity in parent-child relationships as children move from adolescence into young adulthood.

REFERENCES

Bates, J. E. (1989). Concepts and measures of temperament. In G. A. Kohnstamm, J. E. Bates, & M. K. Rothbart (Eds.), *Temperament in childhood* (pp. 3–26). New York: John Wiley.

Baumrind, D. (1978). Parental disciplinary patterns and social competence in children. *Youth and Society, 9,* 239–276.

Bengtson, V. L., & Black, K. D. (1973). Intergenerational relations and continuities in socialization. In P. B. Baltes & K. W. Schaie (Eds.), *Life-span developmental psychology* (Vol. 1, pp. 207–234). New York: Academic Press.

Blos, P. (1967). The second individuation process of adolescence. *Psychoanalytic Study of the Child, 22,* 162–186.

Caplow, T., Bahr, H. M., Chadwick, B. A., Hill, R., & Williamson, M. H. (1982). *Middletown families.* Minneapolis: University of Minnesota Press.

Carey, W. B. (1989). Practical applications in pediatrics. In G. A. Kohnstamm, J. E. Bates, & M. K. Rothbart (Eds.), *Temperament in childhood* (pp. 405–419). New York: John Wiley.

Caspi, A., Elder, G. H. Jr., & Bem, D. J. (1987). Moving against the world: Life course patterns of explosive children. *Developmental Psychology, 23,* 308–313.

Caspi, A., Elder, G. H. Jr., & Herbener, E. S. (1990). Childhood personality and the prediction of life-course patterns. In L. Robbins & M. Rutter (Eds.), *Straight and devious pathways from childhood to adulthood* (pp. 13–35). New York: Cambridge University Press.

Chess, S., & Thomas, A. (1984). *Origins and evolution of behavior disorders from infancy to early adult life.* New York: Brunner/Mazel.

Chess, S., & Thomas, A. (1986). *Temperament in clinical practice.* New York: Guilford.

Cooper, C. R. (1988). Commentary: The role of conflict in adolescent-parent relationships. In M. R. Gunnar & W. A. Collins (Eds.), *Development during the transition to adolescence: 21st Minnesota Symposium on child psychology* (pp. 181–187). Hillsdale, NJ: Lawrence Erlbaum.

Eyberg, S. M., & Robinson, E. A. (1983). Conduct problem behavior: Standardization of a behavioral rating scale with adolescents. *Journal of Clinical Child Psychology, 12,* 347-354.

Farrington, D. P., Loeber, R., & van Kammen, W. B. (1990). Long-term criminal outcomes of hyperactivity-impulsivity-attention deficit and conduct problems in childhood. In L. Robins & M. Rutter (Eds.), *Straight and devious pathways from childhood to adulthood* (pp. 62-81). New York: Cambridge University Press.

Forehand, R. (1990). Families with a conduct problem child. In G. H. Brody & I. E. Sigel (Eds.), *Methods of family research: Biographies of research projects: Vol. 2. Clinical populations* (pp. 1-30). Hillsdale, NJ: Lawrence Erlbaum.

Forehand, R., & Long, N. (1988). Outpatient treatment of the acting out child: Procedures, long term follow-up data, and clinical problems. *Advances in Behaviour Therapy and Research, 10,* 129-178.

Frank, S. J., Avery, C. B., & Laman, M. S. (1988). Young adults' perceptions of their relationships with their parents: Individual differences in connectedness, competence, and emotional autonomy. *Developmental Psychology, 24,* 729-737.

Freud, A. (1958). Adolescence. *Psychoanalytic Study of the Child, 13,* 255-278.

Grotevant, H. D., & Cooper, C. R. (1985). Patterns of interaction in family relationships and the development of identity formation in adolescence. *Child Development, 56,* 415-428.

Grotevant, H. D., & Cooper, C. R. (1986). Individuation in family relationships. *Human Development, 29,* 82-100.

Hanson, C. L., Henggeler, S. W., Haefele, W. F., & Rodick, J. D. (1984). Demographic, individual, and family relationship correlates of serious and repeated crime among adolescents and their siblings. *Journal of Consulting and Clinical Psychology, 52,* 528-538.

Harris, I. D., & Howard, K. I. (1984). Parental criticism and the adolescent experience. *Journal of Youth and Adolescence, 13,* 113-121.

Hauser, S. T., Powers, S. I., Noam, G. G., Jacobson, A. M., Weiss, B., & Follansbee, D. J. (1984). Familial contexts of adolescent ego development. *Child Development, 55,* 195-213.

Hill, J. P., & Holmbeck, G. N. (1986). Attachment and autonomy during adolescence. In G. Whitehurst (Ed.), *Annals of child development* (Vol. 3, pp. 145-189). Greenwich, CT: JAI Press.

Hubert, N. C. & Wachs, T. D. (1985). Parental perception of the behavioral components of infant easiness/difficultness, *Child Development, 56,* 1525-1537.

Kandel, D., & Lesser, G. S. (1969). Parent-adolescent relationships and adolescent independence in the United States and Denmark. *Journal of Marriage and the Family, 31,* 348-358.

Kendall, P. C. (1991). *Child and adolescent therapy: Cognitive-behavioral procedures.* New York: Guilford.

Lerner, J. V., Hertzog, C., Hooker, K. A., Hassibi, M., & Thomas, A. (1988). A longitudinal study of negative emotional states and adjustment from early childhood through adolescence. *Child Development, 59,* 356–366.

Levine, M. S. (1977). *Canonical analysis and factor comparison.* Newbury Park, CA: Sage Publications.

Little, R. J. A., & Rubin, D. B. (1987). *Statistical analysis with missing data.* New York: John Wiley.

Loeber, R., & Dishion, T. J. (1984). Boys who fight at home and school: Family conditions influencing cross-setting consistency. *Journal of Consulting and Clinical Psychology, 52,* 759–768.

Montemayor, R. (1983). Parents and adolescents in conflict: All families some of the time and some families all of the time. *Journal of Early Adolescence, 3,* 83–103.

Montemayor, R. (1986). Family variation in parent-adolescent storm and stress. *Journal of Adolescent Research, 1,* 15–31.

Murphy, E. B., Silber, E., Coelho, G. V., Hamburg, D. A., & Greenberg, I. (1963). Development of autonomy and parent-child interaction in late adolescence. *American Journal of Orthopsychiatry, 33,* 643–652.

Offer, D., Ostrov, E., & Howard, K. I. (1981). *The adolescent: A psychological self-portrait.* New York: Basic Books.

Patterson, G. R. (1982). *Coercive family process.* Eugene, OR: Castalia.

Patterson, G. R. (1986). Performance models for anti-social boys. *American Psychologist, 41,* 432–444.

Robins, L. N. (1978). Sturdy childhood predictors of adult antisocial behavior: Replications from longitudinal studies. *Psychological Medicine, 8,* 611–622.

Rovine, M. J., & Delaney, M. (1990). Missing data estimation in developmental research. In A. von Eye (Ed.), *Statistical methods for longitudinal research* (Vol. 1, pp. 35–80). New York: Academic Press.

Smetana, J. G. (1988). Concepts of self and social convention: Adolescents' and parents' reasoning about hypothetical and actual family conflicts. In M. Gunnar & W. A. Collins (Eds.), *Development during the transition to adolescence: 21st Minnesota symposium on child psychology* (pp. 79–122). Hillsdale, NJ: Lawrence Erlbaum.

Smetana, J. G., Yau, J., Restrepo, A., & Braeges, J. (1991). Parent-adolescent conflict in married and divorced families. *Developmental Psychology, 27,* 1000–1010.

Smollar, J., & Youniss, J. (1989). Transformations in adolescents' perceptions of parents. *International Journal of Behavioral Development, 12,* 71–84.

Steinberg, L. D. (1981). Transformations in family relations at puberty. *Developmental Psychology, 17,* 833–840.

Steinberg, L. D. (1989). Pubertal maturation and parent-adolescent distance: An evolutionary perspective. In G. R. Adams, R. Montemayor, & T. P. Gullotta

(Eds.), *Advances in adolescent development: Vol. 1. Biology of adolescent behavior and development* (pp. 71–97). Newbury Park, CA: Sage Publications.

Stierlin, H. (1981). *Separating parents and adolescents.* Northvale, NJ: Aronson.

Tatsuoka, M. M. (1988). *Multivariate analysis* (2nd ed.). New York: Macmillan.

Thomas, A., & Chess, S. (1977). *Temperament and development.* New York: Brunner/Mazel.

Thomas, A., Chess, S., Birch, H.G., Hertzig, M., & Korn, S. (1963). *Behavioral individuality in early childhood.* New York: New York University Press.

Thomas, A., Chess, S., Lerner, R. M., & Lerner, J. V. (1989). *Behavioral individuality in adult life.* Unpublished manuscript, New York University Medical Center, New York.

Tubman, J. G. (1990). *Affective experiences of children and parents: Their stability and covariates.* Unpublished doctoral dissertation, Pennsylvania State University, University Park.

Tubman, J. G., & Lerner, R. M. (in press). Affective experiences of parents and their children from adolescence to young adulthood: Stability of affective experiences. *Journal of Adolescence.*

PART I: DEVELOPMENTAL ISSUES

2

Impact of Parental Discipline Methods on the Child's Internalization of Values: A Reconceptualization of Current Points of View

Joan E. Grusec

University of Toronto, Toronto, Canada

Jacqueline J. Goodnow

Macquarie University, Sydney, Australia

It is generally argued that parental use of specific discipline techniques (e.g., reasoning vs. power assertion) differentially affects a child's internalization. This article offers an expanded formulation. Internalization as a result of discipline is proposed to be based on a child's accurate perception of the parental message and acceptance or rejection of it. Mechanisms promoting acceptance are perceptions of the parent's actions as appropriate, motivation to accept the parental position, and perception that a value has been self-generated. Features of the misdeed, discipline technique, child, and parent that affect accurate perception and acceptance-rejection are outlined. Other goals besides internalization, such as movement beyond the parent's position, maintenance of the child's self-esteem, and maintenance of the parent-child relationship, are discussed.

In this article, we examine the widely accepted proposal that parental discipline effectiveness is strongly influenced by the particular method used, a proposal that typically contrasts the use of reasoning with the use of

Reprinted with permission from *Developmental Psychology*, 1994, Vol. 30, 4–19. Copyright © 1994 by the American Psychological Association, Inc.

The writing of this article was facilitated by grants from the Social Science and Humanities Research Council of Canada to Joan E. Grusec and from the Australian Research Council to Jacqueline J. Goodnow. The comments of several anonymous reviewers are acknowledged with gratitude.

restrictive power assertion. Effectiveness in this case refers to *internalization*, that is, taking over the values and attitudes of society as one's own so that socially acceptable behavior is motivated not by anticipation of external consequences but by intrinsic or internal factors. This article outlines limitations to this proposal and argues for a position that provides a more complete account of the existing data than is currently available and that prompts new research initiatives.

Our position is developed in five parts. The first provides a brief history of interest in the topic of discipline and internalization and outlines reservations both with respect to the evidence for, and the explanations of, contrasting effects for specific methods.

The second part of the analysis considers a number of variables that are deemed to be important for a more complete understanding of the discipline process. These are the nature of the misdeed, the specific form of discipline, the characteristics of the recipient of discipline, and the characteristics of the disciplinary agent. For each of these variables, we consider evidence for an impact on internalization and the possible bases—cognitive or affective—for that impact. The effect of a parent's action emerges from this analysis as dependent not so much on the disciplinary methods per se as on the situation or interaction within which the disciplinary actions take place.

The third part of the analysis adopts a different starting point. It commences, not from the beginning of the exchange (e.g., the nature of the misdeed) but from its endpoint—internalization. Internalization, it is suggested, involves both the child's perception of the parent's position (a perception that may be accurate or inaccurate) and the child's acceptance or rejection of what is perceived to be the parent's viewpoint. Failure to internalize may then come about either through inaccurate perception or through rejection. This two-step framework allows a synthesis of the several conditions and processes that emerged in the first part of the analysis, integrating them around their particular impact on perception or acceptance.

The next section of the article points to a problem that tends to be overlooked when the emphasis is solely on internalization as a consequence of parent discipline. Other consequences need to be considered as part of the picture. One is the child's ability to move beyond the parent's specific position to one of his or her own, a consideration that points to successful socialization as more than the unquestioning adoption of another's position. A second consequence is the significance of outcomes such as the child's happiness or self-esteem, outcomes that may outweigh internalization in a parent's view or that may ultimately facilitate the adoption of a parental position.

The final section provides a summary of the article's main arguments, together with suggestions for future research.

The reader will note throughout an emphasis on internalization in terms of prosocial behavior (consideration for the feelings or needs of others) and moral standards (assessed, for instance, by resistance to temptation, reparation after deviation, evidence of guilt, and level of moral reasoning). The values and attitudes that may be internalized are, of course, more diverse than this. Developmental psychologists, however, have given particular attention to prosocial or moral values, perhaps because of the assumption that these values are maintained at some cost to the individual and are thus particularly in need of being taken over as one's own.

One last point needs to be made before we turn to background. Our goal is not a complete reanalysis of the concept of internalization and of the conditions or methods that promote it. Internalization is fostered by many methods other than discipline, including teaching, example, social reinforcement of appropriate behavior, and arrangement of the environment so that desirable behavior is naturally elicited. Investigators interested in the foundations of internalization have also pointed to a variety of socialization factors that encourage responsivity to parental wishes, including facilitation of the child's early self-regulatory capacity (Kopp, 1982), promotion of the child's feelings of security and trust (Bretherton & Waters, 1985), and provision of an atmosphere of mutual cooperativeness (Maccoby & Martin, 1983). Discipline attracts special attention, however, because it is an important means by which values are acquired and because the analysis of discipline methods by developmental psychologists has been detailed. In addition, as noted at the start, proposals about the effects of disciplinary methods appear to be somewhat problematic, to a point in which reanalysis and a shift in these proposals seem warranted.

BACKGROUND: VIEWS OF DISCIPLINE AND INTERNALIZATION

Much of the early research on discipline was inspired by psychoanalytic theory. Although specific details vary, psychoanalytic theorists in general have argued that frustration by parents leads to feelings of hostility on the part of their children. The hostility is repressed, however, because children fear that its expression will lead to punishment, particularly in the form of loss of love or abandonment. To maintain the repression and to elicit continuing parental approval, children adopt parental rules and prohibitions as well as a generalized motive to emulate the parent and to adopt the parent's inner states. One of the parental behaviors incorporated is punishment after transgression, now transformed into self-punishment or guilt that resembles early anxiety about punishment and abandonment. It is, then, fear of guilt that motivates children to act in accord with what have now become internalized societal standards of behavior, standards maintained completely independently of external sanctions or rewards.

Psychoanalytic theory had found the major motivation for internalization in the concept of identification with the aggressor. In contrast, Sears, Maccoby, and Levin (1957) found it in the desire of the child to imitate positive features of the parent. Combining concepts from psychoanalytic and learning theory, they suggested (a) that parental attributes acquire secondary reinforcement value because they are paired with experiences of physical caretaking and (b) that the child can therefore recreate pleasant experiences by being like the parent. Sears et al. were the first to focus on specific techniques of training or discipline, thereby setting the stage for contemporary approaches to understanding discipline effectiveness. Their argument was that parents who rely on love-oriented techniques such as praise, social isolation, and withdrawal of affection will have children with higher levels of conscience development, that is, children who have internalized parental standards and values, than those who rely on object-oriented techniques such as tangible rewards, deprivation of material objects or privileges, and physical punishment. In the former case, children must reproduce parental standards and values to assure themselves of parental love and to provide secondary reinforcement for themselves as a replacement for withdrawn attention. In the latter case, they will hide, flee, or find other ways of avoiding punishment, reactions that do not foster adoption of parental standards. In support of their argument, Sears et al. found that when mothers used withdrawal of love, provided they were nurturant and warm, their children exhibited self-control, developed their own standards of conduct, applied sanctions to their own behavior, and confessed and accepted responsibility for their own deviant behavior.

Sears et al. (1957) placed reasoning together with withdrawal of love because the two techniques tended to co-occur. Hoffman (e.g., Hoffman, 1970a, 1970b), however, argued for differentiating them. On the basis of his own data as well as reanalysis of the data of others, Hoffman demonstrated that parents who relied solely on object-oriented or power assertive approaches such as withdrawal of privileges, force, physical punishment, and threat were less likely to be successful in promoting resistance to temptation, guilt over antisocial behavior, reparation after deviation, altruism, and high levels of moral reasoning—all regarded as indexes of the internalization of moral values—than were parents who withdrew love by ignoring, isolating, and indicating dislike of their children. The most successful parents, however, were those who tended toward a greater use of reasoning or induction (often in combination with power assertion). Of particular importance was *other-oriented induction*, reasoning that draws children's attention to the effects of their misdemeanors on others, thereby sensitizing them to events beyond the personal consequences of their actions.

Rather than considering specific discipline techniques, some researchers have focused on typologies of parenting. The general issue has been the same—the relationship between child rearing practices and child outcomes—but the initial concern has been more with styles than with specific parental actions. W. C. Becker (1964), for example, drawing from a variety of studies of parenting including that of Sears et al. (1957), proposed two major dimensions for parenting: warmth–hostility and restrictiveness–permissiveness. Parents high in warmt.ı and restrictiveness were seen as most likely to produce compliant, well-behaved children, whereas those high in warmth and permissiveness were regarded as most likely to promote socially outgoing, independent, and creative children.

In W. C. Becker's (1964) analysis, the production of socially acceptable behavior seemed to involve the sacrifice of spontaneity and originality. Earlier, Baldwin (1948) had faced the same problem. He had proposed three dimensions of child rearing: warm–cold, democratic–autocratic, and emotionally involved–uninvolved. Democratic parenting, defined as parenting in which children shared in decisions about rules of behavior and parents made noncoercive suggestions, was most successful in producing socially outgoing and intellectually curious children but less so in promoting conformity to parental demands. A solution to the problem arose in Baumrind's (1971) division of parents into three groups: authoritarian, authoritative, and permissive. Authoritarian parents demand strict obedience and discourage give-and-take. Authoritative parents also set firm controls on the behavior of their children and make strong demands for maturity, but they are willing to listen to their children's point of view and even to adjust their behavior accordingly. Permissive parents make few demands and engage in very little discipline. It is the authoritative parents who are most successful in producing children who are socially competent and responsible, that is, who have accepted parental dictates as their own without sacrificing curiosity, originality, and spontaneity. Although Baumrind's terminology and emphasis are somewhat different from Hoffman's, their two positions do, in fact, present a consistent picture of child rearing effects: namely, that parents who tend to be harshly and arbitrarily authoritarian or power assertive in their parenting practices are less likely to be successful than those who place substantial emphasis on induction or reasoning, presumably in an attempt to be responsive to and understanding of their child's point of view.

Accounting for Differential Effectiveness

Considerable effort has gone into trying to explain why approaches to discipline function as they appear to do. Explanations either have emphasized a mixture of cognitive and affective mechanisms or have emphasized cognitive ones alone.

The most detailed attention to cognitive and affective mechanisms in combination comes from Hoffman (e.g., 1970b, 1982). Power assertion, he proposed, is detrimental to the socialization process, because it arouses anger and hostility in the child with accompanying opposition or unwillingness to comply with the parent's wishes. Power assertion also provides a model of aggression that leads to antisocial or immoral conduct. In addition, it keeps the source of a moral message salient to the child and hence makes it less likely to be accepted as the child's own than if the source is forgotten. In contrast, reasoning or induction, particularly that which emphasizes the negative effects of the child's misdeed on others, is more effective, because it develops the child's empathic capacities and induces negative feelings from which the child cannot escape even when the socializing agent is no longer present. Other-oriented induction also suggests a possible means of reparation for deviant acts, and it includes cognitive material needed to heighten awareness of wrongdoing and facilitate accurate generalization to new situations. Withdrawal of love is regarded as intermediate in effectiveness, because it does not arouse anger and hostility, but it also does not foster awareness of or sensitivity to the feelings and needs of others.

Hoffman (1983) noted that a small amount of power assertion can be beneficial if used in combination with reasoning: It has the important function of capturing the child's attention so that the parent's message will be heard. (Baumrind, 1983, also argued that the addition to reasoning of a modest degree of power assertion is necessary: In her case, she suggested that it motivates the child to initiate self-controlling mechanisms to avoid negative outcomes and that these self-regulatory mechanisms lead to reliable habits of prosocial behavior.)

Proposals focused on cognitive mechanisms alone have come from several individuals. Attribution theorists such as Lepper (1983), for example, argued that authoritative parents are successful because they provide just enough pressure to induce conformity, a condition that fosters internalization by making it necessary for a child to attribute his or her compliance to internal motivation or personal desire rather than to external pressure. Higgins (1989) suggested that children of parents who reason or explain acquire relatively strong knowledge about the relationship between their behavior and parental reaction to that behavior, and they consequently have strong self-guides or clear representations of attributes that the self ought to possess. Higgins's explanation is a more sophisticated version of an early social learning view that regarded rationales as enhancing the effects of punishment by making contingencies clearer to the child (e.g., Cheyne & Walters, 1970). In Higgins's approach and in Lepper's, it should be noted, the nature of reasoning no longer appears to matter as it did in Hoffman's analysis of mechanisms. Whereas Hoffman stressed that reasoning must be other-oriented, Lepper and Higgins have tended not to differentiate among kinds of reasoning.

The same reduced attention to the kind of reason used by the agent of socialization is found in constructivist approaches to the effects of disciplinary methods. According to Applegate, Burke, Burleson, Delia, and Kline (1985), for example, power assertion discourages the child's reflection on moral issues, whereas extensive explanations and opportunities for dialogue facilitate the child's elaboration of schemas for differentiating the psychological experience of others, a condition presumably likely to encourage respect for their rights. In Mancuso and Handin's (1985) analysis of reprimand, the use of reasoning implies that parents recognize that the child's construction of an event may differ from the one they have and that they must take this into account when attempting to change the child's construction so it is more in line with their own. In effect, the type of reason now matters, but type has to do with the degree of fit with the child's schemas.

Problems with Current Views

Problems arise both with regard to the evidence for the differential effectiveness of particular methods and with regard to proposals for why effects take the form that they do.

Issues of evidence. An immediate difficulty with the proposal for differential effectiveness is that closer examination of the relevant evidence reveals a somewhat less compelling picture than one might have expected. For example, demonstrated relationships hold only for mothers but not for fathers, and for middle-class but not for lower-class families. In addition, relationships are often differentially affected as a function of age, sex, and temperament of child (Brody & Shaffer, 1982; Kochanska, 1991).

Explanations for effects. The reservations here are fourfold. The first is that the current explanations do not provide a sufficient explanation for the apparently inconsistent effects. The question then arises as to what forms modification should take.

The second reservation treats the evidence as sufficient but queries the direction of effects. Bell (1968), for example, argued that parental discipline techniques were determined by the temperament of the child, with difficult children forcing stronger interventions in the form of power assertion. Lewis (1981) has suggested that Baumrind's (1971) measures of firm control may simply parallel low levels of conflict in the parent-child dyad but not be a causal factor. At the least, these positions argue for the importance of the child's characteristics in any account of differential effectiveness.

The third reservation has to do with considering reasoning, withdrawal of love, and power assertion as single categories. Reasoning provides an example of why this is problematic. Hoffman (1970b) clearly distinguished other-oriented reasoning from other forms of reasoning. But reasoning has come to be, in Maccoby and Martin's (1983, p. 51) terms, an "amorphous category," with exemplars ranging from normative statements, discussion of consequences, discussion of the feelings of others, and information, to noninformative and superfluous verbalizations.

The fourth reservation is directed toward the implication that a given parent uses one predominant style of disciplinary intervention. Authoritarian parents would appear to use the same degree of punitiveness regardless of the situation, and authoritative parents use more reasoning and negotiation regardless of the situation. Results of a number of studies reported over the last decade indicate, however, that mothers do not use a single style when dealing with their children's misbehavior. Instead, they vary their discipline practices according to the nature of the particular social standard that the child has violated (Grusec & Kuczynski, 1980; Trickett & Kuczynski, 1986; Zahn-Waxler & Chapman, 1982). A combination of power assertion and reasoning is used, for instance, in response to antisocial acts such as lying and stealing, whereas reasoning alone is used in response to failures to show concern for others (Grusec, Dix, & Mills, 1982). Damage to physical objects or lapses in impulse control elicit physical punishment followed by withdrawal of love, but aggression does not (Zahn-Waxler & Chapman, 1982). High arousal behavior (e.g., rough-and-tumble play) is followed by power assertion alone, whereas violations of social conventions (e.g., bad table manners) are followed by reasoning alone (Trickett & Kuczynski, 1986). In addition to using reasoning and power assertion in different combinations, mothers also use different forms of reasoning depending on the misdeed. The evidence is from Smetana

(1989), who reported that mothers use explanations referring to the needs and rights of others when dealing with events that harm others but explanations that refer to social order and conformity with rules when responding to violations of social conventions. Interestingly, nonrandom pairings of discipline techniques and misdeed have also been reported in cross-cultural studies of child rearing practices in Japan and India (Conroy, Hess, Azuma, & Kashiwagi, 1980; Sinha, 1985).

The importance of these variations lies in the possibility that the methods per se may be less important than the flexibility of their use. Hoffman (1970a) made a relevant observation many years ago, finding that different situations seemed to "pull" a particular type of discipline from the parent and that this variation of discipline technique by the situation was particularly the case among mothers of children who had a strong moral orientation. The minimal implication is that one may need to look at the nature of the misdeed, and at the connection between misdeed and disciplinary technique, as a part of the answer to how and when differential effectiveness occurs. The large-scale implication is that explanations should be directed toward accounting for why flexibility is effective, rather than being directed only toward the differential effectiveness of the methods themselves.

Conclusion. On the basis of the empirical evidence alone, it would appear that a reexamination of conceptualizations of the discipline process is in order—one directed toward a clearer understanding of anomalies in the research findings and toward a framework that will account for the anomalies and raise new research questions. We now begin this reexamination.

EXPANDING THE DESCRIPTION OF VARIABLES RELEVANT TO DISCIPLINE EFFECTIVENESS

In this section, variables that need to be considered—over and above the discipline technique—are discussed as a way of building an effective account of the effects of disciplinary methods on internalization. Table 1 depicts these variables. According to Table 1, any discipline situation includes two sets of behavior—the child's misdeed and the parent's response—and two individuals—the child and the parent. Also included in Table 1 are variables that need to be considered within each of these four components. First, we turn our attention to the misdeed, focusing on the need to define its nature. Next to be considered is the significance of the particular form of reasoning, power assertion, or withdrawal of love that is used. Finally, the impact of characteristics of the two actors in the situa-

TABLE 1
Four Components of a Discipline Situation and Their Constituent Features

Variable	Features
Nature of misdeed	Moral, social conventional, failure of concern for others, personal issue.
Nature of parental reaction	
Content	Empathy arousal, evidence of truth-value, arousal of insecurity, threats to autonomy.
Structure	Clarity of meta-rules; relevance of message; observance of due process; clarity, redundancy, and consistency of message; indirectness and implicitness of message; importance signaled; attention captured; decoding required.
Nature of child	Temperament, mood, past history with respect to discipline, age.
Nature of parent	Warmth, responsivity to child's wishes, characteristic disciplinary style.

tion—child and parent—on discipline effectiveness is discussed. Throughout the analysis, there will be a concern with both cognitive and affective processes, with particular attention given to the child's interpretation and evaluation of the parent's actions.

Nature of the Misdeed in Relation to the Parent's Method

Already noted is the fact that mothers vary their discipline depending on the nature of their child's misdeed, as well as Hoffman's (1970a) observation that the most effective mothers appear to be those who are the most flexible in their choice of discipline techniques. His observation is taken further in a report by Trickett and Kuczynski (1986). They found that abusive mothers were more likely to use one discipline technique—power assertion—regardless of misdeed, whereas nonabusive mothers used different discipline techniques including reasoning and power assertion alone or in combination, depending on the domain of the misdeed. These reports raise the possibility that effective discipline is discipline matched to the misdeed. Types of misdeed offering a basis for differentiation are listed in Table 1.

If we assume that a particular pairing of discipline technique and misdeed is the essence of effective flexibility, then we need to ask how any impact on effectiveness might come about. The mediator, we propose, is the child's perception of the acceptability of different interventions in different situations. In essence, children are more likely to make long-term alterations in their behavior if the discipline they receive is judged by them to be appropriate to the misdeed. What evidence is there for the feasibility of this argument? First, we discuss the contributing data for the use of different forms of reasoning, because this is the method for which there is more information available.

Misdeeds in relation to reasoning. We argue that (a) children offer different kinds of reasons for why different transgressions are wrong, (b) children judge adult appropriateness on the basis of whether adults use the same reasons that the children use with respect to a particular misdeed, and (c) the judgment of appropriateness alters effectiveness.

CHILDREN'S REASONS IN RELATION TO MISDEED. Children produce different reasons for why particular misdeeds are wrong. In a social–cognitive domain approach to social reasoning (e.g., Turiel, 1983), Turiel and his students have argued that children, from a very early age, distinguish between moral violations (i.e., acts that intrinsically harm others either physically or psychologically) and violations of social conventions (i.e., acts that involve failure to comply with externally driven rules about social order). In the case of moral transgressions, children refer to the rights and welfare of others. In the case of social conventions, they refer to the maintenance of rules and of the social order. In related fashion, Grusec and Pedersen (1989) reported a difference between children's reasoning about events that involve violations of moral norms or antisocial acts, such as lying, stealing, and aggression, and events that entail a failure to show concern for others, such as not helping and not sharing. In the first case, children focus on the importance of internalized rules of right or wrong. In the second, their focus is on issues of niceness, correctness, and concern for others. (The source of these different reasons is unclear. Although the question is an important one, its answer is unnecessary for purposes of the present argument.)

CHILDREN'S JUDGMENTS OF APPROPRIATENESS. If children provide different reasons for why an act is bad that depend on the nature of the act, they could also find reasoning from a parent that is similar to their own more acceptable than parental reasoning that is dissimilar from their own. There are several indications that this is a reasonable argument. Nucci (1984) reported that children ranging in age from 8 to 14 years rate teachers' reactions to deviation as better if they are domain-appropriate than if they are domain-inappropriate. Children's ratings of teachers are also affected by the teacher's use of domain-appropriate reasoning, so that a teacher who refers to rules when reacting to stealing, or a teacher who talks about taking the other's point of view when responding to swearing, is rated less favorably than one who reasons more appropriately. Killen (1991) noted that preschoolers make similar distinctions when they are asked about peer conflicts, selecting as the best teacher response one that is appropriate for the domain.

APPROPRIATENESS AND DIRECT EFFECTS ON INTERNALIZATION. Does the child's judgment that a parent's reason is acceptable actually promote a change in behavior? There is little direct relevant data, but one study is supportive. Eisenberg-Berg and Geisheker (1979) compared the effectiveness of two kinds of reasoning in inducing a child to share with others. One was empathy-oriented ("sharing will make the other child happy and excited"). The other referred to norms ("it's good to share"). The empathy-oriented statement is closer to the kinds of reasons that children use to justify the importance of concern for others than is the normative statement (Grusec & Pedersen, 1989), and it is interesting to note that it was also more effective in promoting sharing in the absence of surveillance by adults.

Misdeeds in relation to power assertion or any kind of discipline intervention. In the previous section, we have considered the impact of reasoning in relation to the specific misdeed. We now ask what evidence there is that children make judgments about the appropriateness of various forms of power assertion or of any parental intervention at all.

For *power assertion* there are fewer leads than was the case for reasoning. It should be noted, however, that children see punishment, in the form of deprivation of privileges, as fairer in the case of moral transgressions (harmful acts) than in the case of failures to be prosocial (Grusec & Pedersen, 1989). Children also see adults as having more right to intervene in the case of moral transgressions than in the case of social-conventional transgressions (Tisak, 1986). They might thus be more willing to accept some forms of parental punishment in the former than in the latter case. We suspect that they might also see some forms of overt power (such as the statement, "Do it because I say so") as more honest in the case of social conventions than some elaborate reason, and that the inferred honesty might promote effectiveness.

The *acceptance of any kind of discipline intervention* is again an area in which the evidence to date is slight. There are some acts—behaviors such as watching television on a sunny day or playing the radio loudly when alone—that children see as solely in the realm of personal decision (Nucci, 1981; Smetana, 1988) and therefore as inappropriate for any parental intervention. If acceptability or perceived appropriateness is indeed a mechanism underlying discipline effectiveness, then one would expect that no intervention, regardless of kind, would be effective in these cases.

Varieties of reasoning and other forms of discipline. Considering the effects of the type of misdeed has provided a first possible way to clarify some anomalous results related to the effectiveness of disciplinary methods. It has also highlighted a particular aspect of process, namely, the possibility that the effectiveness of a particular method may depend on the child's judgment of its appropriateness to the domain of the misdeed.

Considering the nature of the misdeed has also introduced the need to differentiate among forms of reasoning. Indeed, there is a need to distinguish both among forms of reasoning and among other forms of discipline. Some of these distinctions (see Table 1) will be reviewed with an eye to how the more detailed picture helps both to clarify results and to indicate how impact comes about.

As in the previous section, more will be said about forms of reasoning than about forms of other discipline techniques. This is in part because reasons may be distinguished from one another on two bases: one of content (e.g., whether the reference is to the child or to the victim) and one of structure (e.g., the clarity of the reason offered). For other forms of discipline, the distinctions offered will be on the single basis of content.

Variations in reasoning

DISTINCTIONS BASED ON CONTENT. Research has drawn attention to a number of ways of distinguishing among the reasons that parents may offer to a child who has behaved in an unacceptable fashion. There is no intention to be comprehensive here. Rather, we offer some representative examples of the ways in which distinctions among kinds of reasons might suggest how effectiveness or ineffectiveness come about. Three possibilities are outlined. Effectiveness may depend on (a) the child's ability to take the perspective of another, (b) the child's interpretation of the parent's actions or statements, and (c) the kind and intensity of affect aroused in the child.

The first possible basis (perspective taking) arises in the course of comparing effectiveness when the other person, in other-oriented reasons, is a peer or an adult. Effectiveness is greater when the other person is a peer (Hoffman & Saltzstein, 1967; Saltzstein, 1976), presumably because it is easier to understand the perspective of someone who is more similar.

The second possible basis, the nature of the child's interpretation, returns to the type of issue that was highlighted in the analysis of the nature of the misdeed. The concern now, however, is not with perceived appropriateness in terms of domain but with the child's judgment that a reason has truth-value, based on the ease with which a parental statement may be verified. The issue arises in Kuczynski's (1982) analysis of why appeals referring to the consequences of antisocial behavior for the self are less effective than those referring to its consequences for others in promoting enduring resistance to temptation. He suggested that self-oriented rationales leave children in a better position to calculate the risks of noncompliance, possibly deciding that the benefits of deviation outweigh potential negative outcomes. Other-oriented rationales do not offer such an opportunity, because the child can never be sure what consequences the other would suffer and hence cannot discount the justification for good behavior. In effect, truth-value can be established for self-oriented rationales in a way it cannot for other-oriented rationales.

The third and last possible basis to the effectiveness of the specific form of reasoning has more to do with affect than with cognition. Kuczynski (1982) again provided an example. He found that the intensity of the appeal (manipulated by telling children that they, or the experimenter, would be "a little bit unhappy," "very unhappy," or "very, very unhappy") was also a determinant of internalization, in addition to the type of reason given. A full explanation of the results, Kuczynski proposed, calls for considering the possibility that the kind and the amount of motivation aroused are two separate determinants of the child's internalization (a possibility also pointed to by Hoffman, 1988). If particular forms of reasoning then differ on either the dimension of the kind of affect involved (e.g., empathy, fear, or guilt) or the amount of affect, their impact on effectiveness should be expected to differ.

DISTINCTIONS BASED ON STRUCTURAL QUALITIES. Suppose we regard reasons as "messages" or "communications" between parents and children. The rephrasing immediately brings to mind the variety of questions people have asked about other forms of message delivery or communication: questions, for instance, about the clarity of the message, the decoding skills and the schemas that the receiver brings to bear on the task, the extent to which some forms of "shorthand" have been established between the two parties, the goals behind any communication ("Am I mainly concerned with conveying content or with establishing a relationship between us?"), and the way each party allocates blame for an error or a misunderstanding ("Were you unclear or did I not listen?").

Mancuso and Lehrer (1986) offered two structural distinctions in their discussion of parental reprimands, one pertaining to the level of generality with which a reprimand is stated and the other to whether a reprimand is *tangential* or *relevant*. Differences in the level of generality may be illustrated by parental responses to a sibling dispute. When a child calls his or her sibling a "jerk," for instance, parents may respond with the reprimand, "Stop that," or with statements that are both more general and refer to an underlying rule such as, "We don't use that kind of language in this house" or, still further up the hierarchy, "Brothers and sisters should be nice to one another." Low-level statements, Mancuso and Lehrer suggested, are not likely to lead to the understanding of any general rule. The ideal outcome, in their view, is one in which children come to understand (and presumably take on as their own) not only a rule pertaining to the specific situation but also the parent's "implicative structure about the rule" (Mancuso & Lehrer, 1986, p. 75). The distinction is similar to one that Wertheim (1975) made among family rules. The most specific level of understanding, in her analysis, consists of *ground rules* (e.g., "If family member X is out, her job is done by Y"). At a more general level is the understanding of *meta-rules* (e.g., "How the house runs is everyone's responsibility") and *meta-meta rules* (e.g., "Your responsibilities are only to the family; you have no obligations to strangers").

The distinction between tangential and relevant reprimands is of a different order. Relevant reprimands, in Mancuso and Lehrer's (1986) definition, take account of the child's schemas and elaborate on them, diminishing the gap between the schemas of the child and those of the parent. Tangential demands do not have this quality. The more relevant the reprimand, Mancuso and Lehrer proposed, the more likely the child is to understand the reasoning behind it. Mancuso and Lehrer's interest in relevance might well be taken further, especially because it contributes to an additional way of specifying the bases for a child's judgment that a parent's action is "appropriate." Previously, it was proposed that the child's judgment of appropriateness is a response to the feeling that the form of discipline fits the domain of the misdeed and to the feeling that a reason has truth-value. We now add the possibility that the child's sense of appropriateness may depend on the judgment that the parent's response is relevant and appropriate in degree of response, and that the parent observes "due process" or "proper procedures." The sense of irrelevance, for instance, and of violations of due process, is likely to be especially strong on occasions when a parent refers to misdemeanors of a totally different kind (introduced perhaps by phrases such as, "While we're on the subject of things that could improve"), or when a parent brings in past history (e.g., "This is not the first time"), especially if the past action has already been brought into court, discussed, and paid for. In both cases, a child may be inclined to regard a parent's statements as irrelevant. Once this perception occurs (or the perception that the parent is being excessive or unfair), the chances of internalization seem likely to be low.

The level of generality of a reason and its relevance are two particular structural qualities. A larger set of structural qualities appears in the information-processing approaches adopted by Cashmore and Goodnow (1985) and by Higgins (1989). These have to do with the clarity or redundancy of a parental message (Cashmore & Goodnow) and with the frequency, consistency, clarity, and "significance" (indications of the importance to parents) of a statement (Higgins). These qualities are proposed as influencing the nature of the child's schemas and motivation (Higgins) and, in a more limited claim for outcomes, the accuracy with which the child perceives the parent's position (Cashmore & Goodnow). Supporting such proposals are correlations between the extent to which parents agree with one another—a form of redundancy—and the accuracy with which children can describe the viewpoints of parents (Cashmore & Goodnow).

At this point, one might be tempted to argue that the clearer the statement of reasons, the more likely it is that internalization will occur. What gives one pause, however, is evidence that parents often offer reasons to their children in ways that are far from being clear or explicit. For example, in their responses to children using pragmatic forms of language of which they disapprove, parents often use indirect ways of stating both the rules and the reasons for them (J. A. Becker, 1988, 1990). They say, for instance, "What's the magic word?," when children have not said "Please"; "I must be going deaf" or "Don't yell" when children have not answered a parent's question; or " 'She' stands in the stable" or " 'She' is the cat's mother" when children have referred to the mother, or to some other female, in that female's presence. In their responses to children's breaking rules related to household patterns or household tasks, the range of indirect statements, of implicit rather than explicit reasons, is even more striking (Goodnow, 1992; Goodnow & Warton, 1991). Mothers often use metaphorical ways of delivering their messages. They ask, for instance, "Were you born in a tent?" when what they want the child to do is to close the door. They ask, "Who was your servant last year?" or say, "This is a home, not a hotel" rather than "Don't behave like that, remember you're part of a family." Mothers turn also to theatrical performances or drama: in the mothers' terms, "going into my fishwife act," "throwing one of my mentals," or "having a rant and a rave." These techniques are a far cry from the delivery of clear and coherent information or from explicit appeals to the feelings of others. A parental message is certainly being delivered, but it is implicit rather than explicit.

At the moment, there are no data about the effectiveness of such indirect statements of a parent's position, just as there is no information about the effectiveness of combining humor—often used as another indirect way of making a point—with a reprimand. Like irony, the use of indirect statements may backfire with children, giving rise to anger and a rejection of a parent's view. Suppose one assumes, however, that parents are not completely off-course and that these indirect ways of providing reasons are effective in promoting internalization. What could be the bases to such an impact? One possibility is again affective. The indirectness marks for a child the presence of feeling on a parent's part but avoids the resentment and anger that direct confrontation, or a direct negative attribution, might provoke in the child. A further possibility is more cognitive. These arresting phrases may catch the attention of children, alerting them to the presence of feeling on the parent's part, forcing them to reflect on what the parent has said, and requiring them to do some "cognitive unpacking." The child's cognitive effort may ultimately lead to internalization of the parental view. It may also, as Hoffman (1988) had suggested, lead to children feeling that the parent's implied position is one that the children themselves have thought out.

Variations in other forms of discipline: Power assertion and withdrawal of love. Just as forms of reasoning need to be differentiated from one another, so also do forms of *power assertion.* Power assertion is a type of discipline with a wide variety of exemplars, including physical punishment, withdrawal of privileges or material resources, displays of anger, commands, disapproval, and shame and humiliation. One might add as well a distinction among power assertive actions in terms of severity (Lepper, 1973, for example, has shown that mild power assertion is less detrimental to internalization than strong power assertion) and in terms of whether the disciplinary action is public or private, a distinction that Reid and Valsiner (1986) reported as of considerable importance to parents and presumably to children. Like reasoning, power assertion is an amorphous category.

It is highly unlikely that all forms of power assertion would have similar effects on the child. On what bases could different effects come about? An important basis for distinction, we suggest, comes from the differential threat that forms of power assertion offer to either a child's sense of autonomy or a child's feelings of security. Consider, for example, physical punishment. It certainly limits a child's autonomy. But delivered by an out-of-control parent, it may have frightening qualities as well. A similar case may exist with respect to displays of anger. Parents speaking with raised voices emphasize the importance to them of their child's compliance. But those who go further to yell, scream, and physically chase their children also transmit the message that their behavior may no longer be predictable. These frightening features of a parent's behavior may foster insecurity as, indeed, would other forms of power assertion such as disapproval, humiliation, and sarcasm.

Differentiating what is threatened by power assertion provides a way to specify more precisely what negative affect may be involved or how it may arise. There is also the possibility that what is threatened may influence the impact of a particular method on internalization. Threats to autonomy may promote active rejection of a parent's point of view and a desire to behave counter to the values of the parent. Threats to security, however, may foster greater degrees of compliance, at least in the parent's presence. If the threats to security are strong enough to reduce the salience of parental pressure, it might even be that some forms of power assertion could contribute to greater internalization of parental values than others. In this case, compliance with parental demands might have to be attributed to intrinsic reasons and this would generate a feeling in the child of having conformed to a self-generated value.

Withdrawal of love is the final form of discipline to be noted. It combines separation or the threat of separation from the parent with the suggestion that the child is creating unhappiness in the parent that can be modified only through good behavior (Sears et al., 1957). Its particular effect, Hoffman (1970a) suggested, is likely to be the promotion of guilt as defined in psychoanalytic terms (i.e., an irrational response to one's own impulses), but not the kind of guilt that permits a conscious self-critical reaction to deviation. The suggestion has received little attention since 1970. However, it does prompt the proposal that the main impact of this method on internalization is by way of its effect on the child's sense of security.

Questions of sequence. It has been argued that there is a need to differentiate particularly among forms of reasoning and power assertion. In making the argument, we considered each discipline class separately. It would be incorrect to conclude, however, that the issue now is one of simply choosing the "best" form of a particular class of discipline. Consider reasoning and power assertion. The optimal impact on internalization may arise from some particular sequence of a particular form of reasoning and a particular form of power assertion. Some form of power assertion, for instance, might be needed first to gain the child's attention, with reasoning then used to make the parent's position clear (e.g., Hoffman, 1970a). In contrast, one might argue that parents should first make sure that the message is clear and understood, using power assertion only after this if it is needed to drive the message home. Certainly it would seem counterproductive to drive home a message other than the one intended. In an optimal sequence, one might even use some form of power assertion or some arresting form of reasoning to gain attention, some form of clear and explicit message to make sure the message is understood correctly, and then some further form of power assertion or appeal to reason in order to drive the message home. At the moment, the data and the differentiations among methods do not allow us to answer such questions about optimal sequences.

Discipline effectiveness and characteristics of the child. We move now from a discussion of the nature of the misdeed and of the parent's response to the characteristics of the two participants in the discipline situation. We discuss the child first.

Characteristics of the child affect his or her perception and evaluation of parental discipline. Obvious candidates, listed in Table 1, are the child's temperament, mood, previous history with respect to discipline, and developmental status. Children who are temperamentally imperturbable and low in anxiety may be less responsive to low-key or non-power-assertive discipline (Kochanska, 1991). Children who are feeling irritated may be more reactive to threats to autonomy than those who are feeling happy. Girls may differ from boys in their reactions to the same discipline event because they have had different histories with respect to discipline: They may, for example, be more responsive to other-oriented induction because they have more frequently been exposed to discussions of the effects of their actions on others.

The variable of developmental status will be used to show, in detail, how a particular characteristic of the child can modify reactions to discipline. Age effects have not gone unnoticed in the literature on discipline, although the data are limited and surprisingly little attention has been paid to the way in which age might have an effect. Maccoby (1984) has drawn attention to how developmental changes have an impact on parenting behavior in general. More specifically, Brody and Shaffer (1982), in their review of a large number of studies of disciplinary methods, concluded that while power assertion seems to have the same negative effect on moral development regardless of age, reasoning is more likely to be associated with advanced moral development only in children 7 years of age and older. However, a systematic explanation of relationships with age, other than Brody and Shaffer's comment that young children may lack the logical abilities and role-taking skills to fully comprehend reasoning, is missing.

What one needs to consider is how and why changes with age might affect a child's response to discipline of various kinds. We next discuss responses to reasoning, power assertion, and parental use of discipline in general.

Reasoning from a developmental perspective. The young child's inability to decenter means that certain forms of reasoning should be less easily comprehended than others. As Brody and Shaffer (1982) suggested, young children may have greater difficulty responding to other-oriented induction because they cannot take the other's perspective very easily. Research indicates that reference to the physical consequences of deviation produces greater suppression of behavior in 4-year-olds than does reference to the more abstract notion of respecting the property of others, whereas the two forms of reasoning are equally effective for 7-year-olds (Parke, 1974). Similar interactions with age appear when rationales referring to the consequences of deviation are compared with more complex rationales emphasizing the importance of a transgressor's intention (LaVoie, 1974). There is preliminary evidence, then, that the fit between the kind of reason offered and the child's age-related ways of thinking about the social world is important in an understanding of discipline effectiveness. The issue is still one of appropriateness, but this time it is appropriateness to the child's developmental status.

Power assertion from a developmental perspective. Changing cognitive abilities also provide a basis for understanding how the effects of power assertion might be modified over the course of development. Examples come from the young child's (a) difficulty in realizing that transgressions cannot always be detected, (b) failure to discount external causes for behavior when internal causes are also present, and (c) inability to understand cues indicating that a message is not to be taken at face value. In each case, the suggestion is that these limitations cause power assertion to function differently than it would in older children.

Some theoretical direction for the first example is provided in a critique by Perry and Perry (1983) of the attributional approach to discipline effectiveness, with particular attention to its denial of a positive role to strong power assertion or coercion. Perry and Perry argued that when children are at an early age, parents must establish strong habits of good behavior even if obvious external coercion is required to do so. They suggested that young children, because of their limited cognitive capacities, are never sure their deviations will be undetected, and so they conform even in the absence of apparent surveillance. As they mature, children now have a greater capacity to know when they are unlikely to be detected in a transgression but, because of strong habits they have acquired, they continue to conform. Now the conformity cannot be attributed to external causes, however, and so internal attributions are made.

The second example comes directly from attribution theory. The principle of discounting is central to an understanding of how individuals attribute behavior to self-generated rather than externally imposed events. It is used when an event is multiply determined: When a plausible cause is present in a situation, the role of another possible cause will be dismissed (Kelley, 1972). This principle allows attribution theorists to propose that the presence of an external motive of the kind produced by fear of punishment will lead the child to attribute behavior to that external motive because it is generally more salient than any internal motive. The phenomenon of discounting thereby lends further theoretical support to the limitations of power assertion as a discipline technique.

The evidence suggests, however, that children do not discount reliably until some time between second and fourth grades (Costanzo, Grumet, & Brehm, 1974; Karniol & Ross, 1976; Smith, 1975). The failure to discount is allegedly a reflection of their inability to decenter, that is, to consider internal and external motivators independently. In fact, not only do younger children fail to discount, they actually use an additive principle in which they infer greater desire the more possible causes are present. The more external pressures present in a socialization situation, then, the more likely they are to feel that an individual has acted out of personal desire.

Although this idea is different from Perry and Perry's (1983) view concerning the role of power assertion in early socialization, it also suggests that power assertion may have very different effects on the behavior of younger than of older children. Supportive data come from Siegal and Cowen's (1984) demonstration that young children evaluate physical punishment by mothers more favorably than do older children.

The last example of how cognitive limitations affect reactions to power assertion comes from Bugental, Kaswan, and Love (1970). They found that younger children, limited in their ability to decenter, had difficulty dealing with messages delivered in a "kidding" or sarcastic way. Because these children cannot reconcile managed positive affect that is not supported by verbal content, they take such messages at face value, rating them more negatively than do adults.

Parental intervention from a developmental perspective. There are developmental changes in children's perceptions of the rights of adults to impose any kind of discipline, be it power assertion, reasoning, or withdrawal of love. Drawing on information about children's perceptions of the rights of adults to exercise authority, Nucci (1981) suggested that an important feature of the child's developing autonomy or distinctiveness from others comes from changes in what children regard as personal issues, that is, events for which parental control is seen to be inappropriate. With increasing maturity, children view increasing numbers of events as inappropriate domains for parental direction and therefore are less willing to tolerate any form of parental authority exercised around these events.

Smetana (1988) made a further distinction, identifying as "multifaceted" issues such as not going on a picnic with the family, wearing punkish clothes, and not cleaning one's room. These are events having features of both personal issues and social conventions. Smetana reported that children and adolescents continue to see that parents have the authority to demand conformity in the area of morality and social convention. They change in their conception of the boundaries of legitimate parental authority in the case of multifaceted and personal issues, however, perceiving parents to have less authority in these domains over time. In essence, then, as children grow in autonomy and as schemas with respect to parental authority change, discipline of all kinds should become less acceptable in some, but not all, domains of behavior.

General effect of age. Age has been considered in terms of the way it might affect the child's response to reasoning, to power assertion, and to any form of parental intervention. To close this section, we first note that age may also have some general effects on a child's response, cutting across the responses to specific disciplinary actions. With increasing age, for instance, a child should be better able (a) to recognize the intention behind a parent's behavior and to respond to that intention, (b) to recognize departures from a parent's usual style as exceptions rather than as the collapse of an expected order, and (c) to interpret the affective cues that indicate, even without words or a specific disciplinary act, the significance of a transgression to a parent.

Discipline Effectiveness and Characteristics of the Parent

The final addition to analyses of discipline practices has to do with parent characteristics. Parents have attributes that mediate the meaning of their specific disciplinary actions. These are listed in Table 1. As previously noted, power assertion from a warm and nurturant parent is more effective than power assertion administered by a parent who is normally cold toward a child. Parents who are responsive to their children's needs and wishes increase the willingness of their children to comply in turn with parents' needs and wishes. Maccoby and Martin (1983) referred to this condition as one of reciprocal compliance. Characteristic disciplinary style is the third variable listed in Table 1. Consider, for example, the effects of social class. In a social class, or in a culture in which power assertion is used frequently, it may be more acceptable than in a Western middle-class culture from where most of the research on discipline has been conducted. Acceptability in this case is simply a function of expectation.

Another example of how characteristic disciplinary style may influence disciplinary effectiveness has to do with the sex of a parent. This example will be developed in detail. We begin with the observation that mothers and fathers who administer the same discipline appear to have different effects. Other-oriented induction, for instance, is correlated with internalization for middle-class mothers but not for middle-class fathers (Hoffman & Saltzstein, 1967). Maternal communicativeness about deviation is correlated with adolescent boys' resistance to temptation whereas paternal communicativeness is not (LaVoie & Looft, 1973). What might be the possible mediators of this differential responsivity? The suggestion is that mothers and fathers have different disciplinary styles and that this leads children to make different judgments about the acceptability of their actions. These differential judgments of acceptability then lead to different responses to parental actions.

With respect to different disciplinary styles, Lytton (1980) reported that mothers use more explanations than fathers with their 2-year-old boys, and LaVoie and Looft (1973) suggested that mothers are more communicative in the discipline situation than are fathers; that is, mothers report more frequently than fathers that they would first question their sons about the facts surrounding a transgression before imposing discipline. According to Vuchinich, Emery, and Cassidy (1988), fathers also have a different style from mothers when they intervene as third parties in disputes between other family members. Mothers are more likely to mediate between the disputants and to gather information, whereas fathers adopt a more authoritarian style characterized by statements such as "I don't want to listen to this, You two button it" or "Don't argue with your mother, you're going."

For evidence about differing perceptions, we turn to Dadds, Sheffield, and Holbeck (1990), who asked 8- to 13-year-olds to say what techniques of discipline—ranging from permissiveness through directed discussion, time out, and physical punishment—mothers and fathers would and should use when dealing with three different transgressions: refusing to pick up toys, punching and hurting another child, and engaging in a temper tantrum. Dadds et al. reported that both *would* and *should* ratings were higher for punishment for fathers than for mothers in the case of refusing to pick up toys; that is, children believed fathers would use more punitive techniques than mothers and that it was appropriate for them to do so. More positive evaluations of power assertive interventions for fathers than mothers also appear in the work of Siegal and Barclay (1985) and Siegal and Cowen (1984), who found that physical punishment is often approved of, at least by working-class children, as a primary disciplinary tool for fathers, whereas mothers' use of physical punishment may be seen as a secondary, although justifiable, option. From this evidence, we suggest that the greater acceptability of power assertion from fathers accounts for the fact that fathers' uses of induction and communicativeness are not predictors of internalization.

Again it has been argued that the impact of a particular discipline action is mediated by the child's judgment of acceptability and appropriateness. That judgment may now be based, however, on the extent to which a specific action is in keeping with an individual's past style and—going beyond the individual—perhaps the culturally determined expectation of what is suitable behavior for fathers and for mothers.

EXPANDING THE DESCRIPTION OF PROCESS AND OUTCOME: A MODEL OF DISCIPLINE EFFECTIVENESS

We have argued that closer attention to a variety of variables is needed for an understanding of how discipline affects internalization. We now turn our attention from those variables to internalization itself and a closer examination of that outcome. Some suggestions about process have already been alluded to in discussions of the impact of discipline variables on the child's knowledge of a parent's position, the child's judgments about the appropriateness or justice of a parent's actions or intentions, and the child's perception of a position as self-generated. By now making a more fine-grained analysis of internalization, we can bring together the effects of discipline variables in a framework that gives them coherence.

A major part of that framework consists of the proposal that internalization is not likely to be reached in a single bound. The question then arises as to what steps might be involved and how these steps might be differentially influenced by particular features of discipline.

Steps Toward Internalization

One way to identify steps to internalization is to place it within an information-processing framework. The relevant material comes from analyses of internalization in the form of cross-generational agreement on values. We shall take from this material three proposals sketched by Furstenberg (1971) and extended by Cashmore and Goodnow (1985). After describing these proposals, we then develop them, placing within them ideas presented in earlier sections of this article.

The first proposal is that the move toward similarity or dissimilarity in values across generations involves two steps. One of these is the child's perception of the parent's message, a perception that may be accurate or inaccurate. The other is the acceptance or rejection of the perceived message.

The second proposal is that different conditions affect the two steps. Accuracy of perception will depend on getting the child's attention and on the clarity or redundancy of the parent's message. Acceptance or rejection, in contrast, is seen to depend especially on the warmth of the relationship between parent and child. This proposal, Furstenberg (1971) argued, accounts for equivocal data about the effects of warmth on agreement between generations. Warmth, he suggested, should affect the occurrence of acceptance or rejection, but not the accuracy of perception. The researcher's yield would consist only of muddy data and inconsistent correlations unless effects on the two aspects were separated from one another. Similar possibilities for understanding, we suggest, are likely to apply to predictions from the use of reasoning or power assertion to the occurrence of internalization. To take one possibility, clarification is likely to be useful if a child's failure to internalize is the result of not having fully heard or understood the parental message, but not if the problem lies in rejection of an accurately heard message. One can well imagine also that a small amount of power assertion might, as Hoffman (1988) suggested, increase the likelihood of children not ignoring the parent and, in the process, promote accurate perception although not acceptance. In contrasting fashion, some forms of empathic reasoning might promote acceptance but, to the extent that they involve little in the way of explicit spelling-out of a position, do little to promote accurate perception.

The final proposal is that a lack of similarity across generations (and, by implication, a failure to internalize) may stem from two quite different sources: inaccurate perception or accurate perception, followed by rejection of the message. Some examples of the contrast are provided by Cashmore and Goodnow (1985), whose study yielded two kinds of situations leading to a common final result, namely, a difference in the positions of the two generations. In the first case, children were accurate in their perception of their parents' positions, for example, their perceptions of how highly their parents valued characteristics such as being neat or obedient. The children themselves, however, placed a lower value on these characteristics than their parents did. In effect, the difference between generations reflected accurate perception but not an acceptance of the parents' views. In the second case, children were not accurate in their perception of how highly their parents valued such characteristics as being interested in other people or being curious about how the world works. The values they attributed to their parents, however, were similar to the values they reported for themselves. In such cases, the basis to a lack of congruence across generations is inaccurate perception. Rejection of the parents' values does not seem to be involved. Rather, children appear to attribute to parents the values that they themselves hold.

These proposals, applied to an understanding of discipline and extended, provide a framework into which a number of variables can be fitted. One way of doing this is to group variables associated with discipline into those that affect accurate perception and those that affect acceptance-rejection. Figure 1 presents a summary of these variables.

PARENTAL DISCIPLINE METHODS

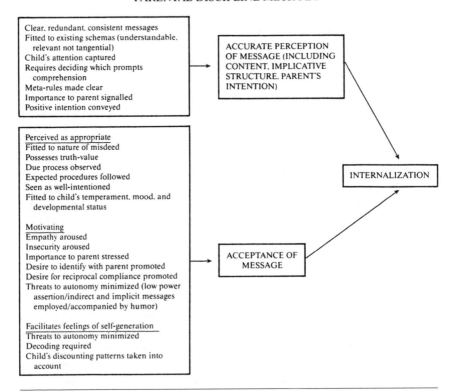

Figure 1. Features of parental disciplinary actions promoting accurate perception and acceptance (internalization) of a parent's message.

Variables affecting accurate perception. A number of variables proposed to influence accurate perception of the parent's message have been discussed in this article. They are listed at the top, left-hand side of Figure 1. Included are clarity, redundancy, and consistency of the message. Also included is the fit of a discipline technique to the child's existing schemas—such considerations as whether the child is able to take the perspective of the other and whether the parental response seems tangential or relevant to the child. Other variables are the use of power assertive interventions and dramatic modes of presentation that may help to draw the child's attention to the message the parent is trying to deliver. Implicit as opposed to explicit messages require the child to decode the parent's position and thereby lead to better comprehension. Finally, the extent to which the parent assists the child in acquiring not only an accurate grasp of a ground rule but also an accurate grasp of the meta-rule or implicative structure is also a determinant of accurate perception of the message.

Added to this list are other variables that go beyond the specific content of the message. For example, children may have differential awareness of the importance of a particular value or a particular misdeed to the parent. They may, in fact, know that an area is emotionally significant to parents ("They are really twitchy about this") before they know what a parent's position is (Goodnow, 1992). Recognizing importance, it is suggested, influences the likelihood of taking the trouble to listen.

A second addition has to do with the child's perception of the parent's intentions. A comment from Loevinger (1959) is helpful here. In Loevinger's view, the child's response to any parental method involves an estimate of the parent's intention. The most devastating generation gap (for the parent) occurs when the child interprets a parent's actions as expressing precisely the intention that is most at odds with the parent's perception of what he or she is trying to do. A parent engages, for instance, in the careful offering of reasons with the intention of avoiding power assertion, but the child perceives the words as punitive, as nagging, as "talking me to death." The child who perceives ill will, like the child who has little sense of how important a topic is to a parent, is unlikely to make the effort to tune in to the parental message. The child who perceives good-will, or importance, is more likely to pay attention, promoting the chances of accurate perception.

Variables affecting acceptance or rejection of the parent's message. Figure 1 lists variables relevant to acceptance of the parent's message. These variables are grouped according to their impact on (a) the extent to which the child perceives parental behavior to be appropriate, (b) the child's motivation, and (c) the degree to which the child sees a value or standard as self-generated.

The first group has to do with the child's evaluation of the acceptability of the parent's intervention—variables already discussed in some detail. Acceptance, it was argued, is especially likely to be influenced by the child's judgment that the parent's actions are appropriate to the nature of the misdeed, that the parent's intervention has truth-value and that due process has been observed, and that the parent's actions fit the child's expectations about what is an appropriate form of intervention for the disciplinary agent—expectations affected by the parent's sex and social class. Added to this is the child's judgment that the intervention is well-intentioned. Finally noted is the degree to which an intervention is appropriately matched to the child's temperament, mood state, and developmental status.

The second group deals with the extent to which the child is motivated to accept the parental message. High degrees of empathic arousal, threats to feelings of security, and the extent to which the value is perceived as important to the parent are important contributors here. Also important, of course, is the variable of parental warmth, which is frequently alleged to have its impact by way of increasing the child's desire to identify with or be like the parent. To warmth may be added parental responsivity or past willingness to comply with the child's wishes, which promotes the child's willingness to comply in turn with the parent's wishes. The final entry here is minimal threat to the child's autonomy, achieved by low levels of power assertion, humor, and indirect and implicit messages: Threats to autonomy increase motivation not to comply or even to act counter to parental wishes.

The last group of events involves variables that may lead to feelings on the child's part that a value is self-generated, with this feeling promoting acceptance. These variables include interventions in which the salience of external pressure is minimized and in which attributions to intrinsic motivation thereby become more likely. The use of implicit messages may also facilitate feelings of self-generation because of the cognitive effort involved in extracting the parental message. Another facilitator of feelings of self-generation of a value and hence of acceptance of the parental message is the extent to which agents of discipline take advantage of or are guided by knowledge of the extent to which a child actually discounts external pressure.

Cognition and affect in accurate perception and acceptance. A distinction between perception and acceptance might bring with it a temptation to regard cognition as primarily important for understanding or accurate perception and affect as primarily relevant to acceptance or rejection. It should already be clear, however, that this separation will not work. Cognition and affect must be expected to influence one another at all steps along the way. If we take as an example the step of accurate perception, then affect as well as factors such as the clarity of a parent's message or the child's decoding skills needs to be considered. "Too little power-assertion or love-withdrawal," to take one possibility from Hoffman (1988, p. 525), "may result in children ignoring the parent. Too much . . . may produce fear, anxiety, or resentment, which may interfere with the effective processing of the information." In related fashion, the affection a child feels for a parent must be expected to influence the degree of effort given to attempts at understanding what is expected and to monitoring whether or not one's actions are in fact pleasing to that parent.

Affect and cognition also need to be seen as influencing one another in ways that are not likely to be unidirectional or simple. According to Hoffman (1986), for instance, "affect may initiate, terminate, accelerate, or disrupt information-processing; it may determine which sector of the environment is processed and which processing modes operate; it may organize recall and influence category accessibility; it may contribute to the formation of emotionally charged schemata and categories; it may provide input for social cognition; and it may influence decision making" (p. 246). A similar array of effects could probably be generated for the influence of cognition on affect.

It is conceivable also that the nature and the direction of influences will vary with conditions such as type of misdeed or affect and the child's developmental status. It seems highly likely, for instance, that the impact of a component we have emphasized—the child's judgment of the appropriateness of a parent's action—would be less important below the age of, say, 3 years, than after that time; indeed, a great deal of the material documenting the particular importance of affective processes in the development of internalization comes from research with very young children. Such multiple possibilities of influence, it is proposed, will always need to be a part of our disentangling the ways in which internalization comes about.

GOALS OF SOCIALIZATION

The assumption to this point has been that internalization is the desired outcome of parental actions. We turn now to the possibility of other parental goals that might accompany and, on occasion, be preeminent over that of internalization. One is a goal of flexibility and initiative in the child's behavior rather than straightforward adoption of parental standards. The second is prevention of damage to the child's self-esteem or the parent-child relationship, even if this decreases the likelihood of adoption of values.

Internalization and Flexibility

Nonagreement with parents may be seen as a desirable outcome if it is accompanied by acceptable negotiation skills (Kuczynski & Kochanska, 1990; Kuczynski, Kochanska, Radke-Yarrow, & Girnius-Brown, 1987). Rather than regard noncompliance as dysfunctional, Kuczynski and his colleagues consider one would do well to see it as often offering opportunities to develop strategic negotiation skills, that is, to assert autonomy in an approved or tolerated fashion. The outcome measure to use would then consist of the acquisition, not of the parent's initial position, but of values and skills related to resistance and the negotiation of alternatives.

A similar point is made by Smetana (1988), reporting on families in which parents and their adolescent children did not agree on the issue of who should set the rules in areas such as cleaning up one's room. In families in which a lack of agreement was not accompanied by conflict (and presumably parental attempts at disciplinary control), parents and children were similar in their use of sophisticated reasoning about the issue. The lack of internalization of one value seems once again to be offset by the internalization of something else a parent values, namely, skill or thoughtfulness in the way one approaches an issue, communicates one's concerns, and attempts to persuade. Interestingly enough, both Kuczynski (Kuczynski & Kochanska, 1990; Kuczynski et al., 1987) and Smetana (1988) appear to be describing a socialization situation reminiscent of Baumrind's (1971) authoritative parenting, one in which the child's views and wishes are taken into account by the parent and in which the socially competent children are those whose skills at negotiation are encouraged.

The alternative values need not always be negotiation skills. That point comes from Goodnow (1992), who commented that most of the literature on agreement across generations is marked by the debatable assumption that this is the optimal outcome for society or in the eyes of parents. Parents, she argued, may often wish that their children will go beyond their parents or develop different strengths, provided that there is similarity on some core values. The radical activists studied by Block (1972), Goodnow suggested, had not internalized their parents' exact political positions, but they did appear to have internalized the value of commitment to whatever cause was undertaken, that is, the value of not being half-hearted in one's actions. It would again be of interest to know how children come to internalize the large message, disregarding the specific ways it might be acted on.

Internalization and Affective Outcomes

The preceding comments have all been to the effect that the lack of internalization of one value may be offset by the internalization of another. Internalization of any value, however, may be a less important outcome— to the researcher or to the parent—than the achievement of some affective state: a happy child, a harmonious relationship, and so on.

In the midst of concern with outcomes such as resistance to temptation, altruism, or level of moral reasoning, developmental psychologists have given relatively little attention to the child's affective responses to parents' methods. Exceptions are Coopersmith (1967) and Hazzard, Christensen, and Margolin (1983), who have focused on the long-term effects of parental discipline on the child's developing self-esteem.

Another form of attention comes from Goodnow (1992). Her primary focus was on the way that concern for protecting a relationship may give rise to the use of particular methods. Humor, drama, and theater, for instance, are methods she proposed as possibly not the most effective for the internalization of a parent's position but as often maintaining a relationship and avoiding confrontations. She offered a similar type of explanation for the use of negative attributions to oneself rather than to the transgressing other, for example, saying, "I'm fussy about (or "have a thing about") bathrooms or milk bottles on the table" rather than "Your standards are low" or "You really are a slob." The parent, in this analysis, may set aside the goal of internalization, hoping to win in the long run by fostering the child's goodwill and thereby increasing the chances of later acceptance of the parent's view. A similar point is made by Higgins (1981) in an analysis of what he has called the *communication game*. In communications between people who care about establishing or maintaining a relationship with one another, he reported, the goals of clarity and explicitness may be sacrificed in favor of the relationship goal. One can well imagine, in fact, that highly explicit messages, accompanied by detailed instructions on precisely what to do, could throw cold water on a close relationship or kill it entirely. If maintaining the relationship is the primary goal, and its achievement conflicts with achieving the internalization of some particular moral or prosocial standards, the latter outcome may well be treated as secondary.

Deferring or setting aside of the goal of internalization may be particularly likely to occur if the cost of internalization appears to be, as Higgins (1989) argued that it often is, an increase in the child's emotional vulnerability: a sharp rise in anxiety and guilt, for instance, or a loss in self-esteem. Indeed, loss of self-esteem could lead to a reduction on the child's part in standards for acceptable behavior and therefore work against an ultimate goal of internalization.

CONCLUSION AND DIRECTIONS FOR FUTURE RESEARCH

This article has offered a reconceptualization of the discipline process that draws from two literatures: developmental psychology's account of discipline and the internalization of parental standards and an information-processing account that focuses on intergenerational agreement about values. We have argued that an approach emphasizing the effects of specific forms of discipline on child outcomes needs to be replaced by one that considers interrelationships between the form of discipline and variables that include characteristics of the child's misdeed, the child, and the parent. The existence of these interrelationships means that a particular discipline intervention could have very different effects depending on the misdeed, child, and parent variables operating in the situation. The reformulation requires that parents be flexible in their disciplinary reactions, matching them to the child's perceptions of and reactions to the conflict situation: Effective parenting involves sensitivity to the child's emotional state and cognitions.

We have proposed a framework that incorporates variables affecting discipline effectiveness and offers explanations for their impact on internalization. The proposal is that internalization needs to be viewed as a two-pronged event. Children must accurately perceive the message parents intend to convey, and they must be willing to accept the message, that is, allow it to guide their behavior. Acceptance involves three components: The child must perceive the message as appropriate, the child must be motivated to comply with the message, and the child must feel the message has not been imposed but rather has been self-generated.

Finally, we have underlined the existence of goals other than internalization. Just as any specific disciplinary action needs to be considered as part of a situation or interaction, so also the goal of internalization needs to be considered as part of a set of parental goals.

What reorientation of research on discipline does this new framework suggest? We offer some possible directions in which investigators might proceed. First, research should address itself to the way in which different forms of discipline have an impact separately and together on the two stages of accurate perception and acceptance. What variables promote each of these stages, and how do they have their effect? How do cognitive and affective mechanisms interact in the production of accurate perception and acceptance? And how are these interactions affected by conditions such as the nature of the misdeed, the nature of the specific method, the characteristics of the parent and of the child, and the nature of the parent-child relationship?

Second, attention needs to be paid to how the child's age, temperament, mood, expectations, and past history have an impact on the effectiveness of any discipline intervention. Needed as well is elaboration of the factors that lead the child to see an intervention as appropriate: Do variables such as the match of the discipline to the misdeed—whether or not the parental intervention has truth-value, whether due process is followed, whether discipline matches the child's developmental status, and whether it is in line with the child's expectations—have the hypothesized effects on acceptance? And, of course, we need to determine the extent to which messages that are seen as appropriate are indeed more likely to be used as guides for behavior than those that are seen as inappropriate.

In this article, we have pointed to a number of discipline techniques that parents use that have received relatively little attention to date, techniques such as irony, humor, indirect statements, and drama. An adequate theory of discipline must address the function served by these techniques and how they have an impact on outcomes. Finally, researchers need to consider other outcomes than internalization in their investigations, including the encouragement of new values and ways of behaving that may differ to an extent from parental values and ways of behaving, the maintenance of a child's self-esteem, and the parent's ability to tolerate noncompliance when it serves a positive goal. Answers to such questions will provide the beginnings of a better understanding of one of the most emotional and significant interactions that occurs between parent and child.

REFERENCES

Applegate, J. L., Burke. J. A., Burleson, B. R., Delia, J. G., & Kline, S. L. (1985). Reflection-enhancing parental communication. In I. E. Sigel (Ed.), *Parental belief systems* (pp. 107–142). Hillsdale, NJ: Erlbaum.

Baldwin, A. L. (1948). Socialization and the parent-child relationship. *Child Development. 19,* 127–136.

Baumrind, D. (1971). Current patterns of parental authority. *Developmental Psychology Monographs, 4*(No. 1, Pt. 2).

Baumrind, D. (1983). Rejoinder to Lewis's reinterpretation of parental firm control effects: Are authoritative families really harmonious? *Psychological Bulletin, 94,* 132–142.

Becker, J. A. (1988). The success of parents' indirect techniques for teaching their preschoolers pragmatic skills. *First Language, 8,* 173–181.

Becker, J. A. (1990). Processes in the acquisition of pragmatic competence. In G. Conti-Ramsden & C. Snow (Eds.), *Children's language* (Vol. 7, pp. 7–24). Hillsdale. NJ: Erlbaum.

Becker, W. C. (1964). Consequences of different kinds of parental discipline. In M. L. Hoffman & L. W. Hoffman (Eds.), *Review of child development research* (Vol. 1, pp. 169–208). New York: Russell Sage Foundation.

Bell, R. Q. (1968). A reinterpretation of the direction of effects in studies of socialization. *Psychological Review, 75,* 81–95.

Block, J. H. (1972). Generational continuity and discontinuity in the understanding of societal rejection. *Journal of Personality and Social Psychology, 22*, 333–345.

Bretherton, I., & Waters, E. (Eds.). (1985). Growing points of attachment theory and research. *Monographs of the Society for Research in Child Development, 50*(1–2, Serial No. 209).

Brody, G. H., & Shaffer, D. R. (1982). Contributions of parents and peers to children's moral socialization. *Developmental Review, 2*, 31–75.

Bugental, D. B., Kaswan, J. W., & Love, L. R. (1970). Perceptions of contradictory meanings conveyed by verbal and nonverbal channels. *Journal of Personality and Social Psychology, 16*, 647–655.

Cashmore, J. A., & Goodnow, J. J. (1985). Agreement between generations: A two-process approach. *Child Development, 56*, 493–501.

Cheyne, J. A., & Walters, R. H. (1970). Punishment and prohibition: Some origins of self-control. In T. M. Newcomb (Ed.), *New directions in psychology* (Vol. 4, pp. 281–366). New York: Holt, Rinehart, & Winston.

Conroy, M., Hess, R. D., Azuma, H., & Kashiwagi, K. (1980). Maternal strategies for regulating children's behavior. *Journal of Cross-Cultural Psychology, 11*, 153–172.

Coopersmith, S. (1967). *The antecedents of self-esteem.* San Francisco: Freeman.

Costanzo, P., Grumet, J., & Brehm, S. (1974). The effects of choice and source of constraint on children's attribution of preference. *Journal of Experimental Social Psychology, 10*, 352–364.

Dadds, M. R., Sheffield, J. K., & Holbeck, J. F. (1990). An examination of the differential relationship of marital discord to parents' discipline strategies for boys and girls. *Journal of Abnormal Child Psychology, 18*, 121–129.

Eisenberg-Berg, N., & Geisheker, E. (1979). Content of preachings and power of the model/preacher: The effects on children's generosity. *Developmental Psychology, 15*, 168–175.

Furstenberg, F. F., Jr. (1971). The transmission of mobility orientation in the family. *Social Forces, 49*, 595–603.

Goodnow, J. J. (1992). Analyzing agreement between generations: Do parents' ideas have consequences for children's ideas? In I. E. Sigel, A. McGillicuddy-DeLisi, & J. J. Goodnow (Eds.), *Parental belief systems* (pp. 293–317). Hillsdale, NJ: Erlbaum.

Goodnow, J. J., & Warton, P. (1991). The social bases of social cognition: Interactions about work and their implications. *Merrill-Palmer Quarterly, 37*, 27–58.

Grusec, J. E., Dix, T., & Mills, R. (1982). The effects of type, severity and victim of children's transgressions on maternal discipline. *Canadian Journal of Behavioural Science, 14*, 276–289.

Grusec, J. E.. & Kuczynski, L. (1980). Direction of effect in socialization: A comparison of the parent vs. the child's behavior as determinants of disciplinary techniques. *Developmental Psychology, 16*, 1–9.

Grusec, J. E., & Pedersen, J. (1989, April). *Children's thinking about prosocial and moral behavior.* Paper presented at the Biennial Meeting of the Society for Research in Child Development, Kansas City, KS.

Hazzard, A., Christensen, A., & Margolin, G. (1983). Children's perceptions of parental behaviors. *Journal of Abnormal Child Psychology, 11*, 49–59.

Higgins, E. T. (1981). The "communication game": Implications for social cognition and persuasion. In E. T. Higgins, C. P. Herman, & M. P. Zanna (Eds.), *Social cognition: Vol 1. The Ontario symposium* (pp. 343–392). Hillsdale, NJ: Erlbaum.

Higgins, E. T. (1989). Continuities and discontinuities in self-regulatory and self-evaluative processes: A developmental theory relating self and affect. *Journal of Personality, 57*, 407–444.

Hoffman, M. L. (1970a). Conscience, personality, and socialization techniques. *Human Development, 13*, 90–126.

Hoffman, M. L. (1970b). Moral development. In P. H. Mussen (Ed.), *Carmichael's manual of child psychology* (Vol. 2, pp. 261–360). New York: Wiley.

Hoffman, M. L. (1982). Development of prosocial motivation: Empathy and guilt. In N. Eisenberg (Ed.), *The development of prosocial behavior* (pp. 281–313). San Diego, CA: Academic Press.

Hoffman, M. L. (1983). Affective and cognitive processes in moral internalization: An information processing approach. In E. T. Higgins, D. Ruble, & W. Hartup (Eds.), *Social cognition and social development: A sociocultural perspective* (pp. 236–274). Cambridge, England: Cambridge University Press.

Hoffman, M. L. (1986). Affect, motivation, and cognition. In R. M. Sorrentino & E. T Higgins (Eds.), *Handbook of motivation and cognition: Foundations of social behavior* (pp. 244–280). New York: Guildford Press.

Hoffman, M. L. (1988). Moral development. In M. Bornstein & M. Lamb (Eds.), *Developmental psychology: An advanced textbook* (pp. 497–548). Hillsdale, NJ: Erlbaum.

Hoffman, M. L., & Saltzstein, H. D. (1967). Parent discipline and the child's moral development. *Journal of Personality and Social Psychology, 5*, 45–57.

Karniol, R., & Ross, M. (1976). The development of causal attributions in social perception. *Journal of Personality and Social Psychology, 34*, 455–464.

Kelley, H. H. (1972). Attribution in social interaction. In E. E. Jones, D. E. Kanouse, H. H. Kelley, R. E. Nisbett, S. Valins, & B. Weiner (Eds.), *Attribution: Perceiving the causes of behavior* (pp. 151–174). Morristown, NJ: General Learning Press.

Killen, M. (1991). Social and moral development in early childhood. In W. M. Kurtines & J. L. Gewirtz (Eds.), *Handbook of moral behavior and development: Research* (Vol. 2, pp. 115–138). Hillsdale, NJ: Erlbaum.

Kochanska, G. (1991). Socialization and temperament in the development of guilt and conscience. *Child Development, 62*, 1379–1392.

Kopp, C. B. (1982). Antecedents of self-regulation: A developmental perspective. *Developmental Psychology, 18*, 199–204.

Kuczynski, L. (1982). Intensity and orientation of reasoning: Motivational determinants of children's compliance to verbal rationales. *Journal of Experimental Child Psychology, 34*, 357–370.

Kuczynski, L., & Kochanska, G. (1990). The development of children's noncompliance strategies from toddlerhood to age 5. *Developmental Psychology, 26*, 398–408.

Kuczynski, L., Kochanska, G., Radke-Yarrow, M., & Girnius-Brown, O. (1987). A developmental interpretation of young children's noncompliance. *Developmental Psychology, 23*, 799–806.

LaVoie, J. C. (1974). Cognitive determinants of resistance to deviation in seven-, nine-, and eleven-year-old children of low and high maturity of moral judgment. *Developmental Psychology, 10*, 393–403.

LaVoie, J. C., & Looft, W. R. (1973). Parental antecedents of resistance-to-temptation behavior in adolescents. *Merrill-Palmer Quarterly, 19*, 107–116.

Lepper, M. (1973). Dissonance, self-perception, and honesty in children. *Journal of Personality and Social Psychology, 25*, 65–74.

Lepper, M. (1983). Social control processes, attributions of motivation, and the internalization of social values. In E. T. Higgins, D. N. Ruble, & W. W. Hartup (Eds.), *Social cognition and social development: A sociocultural perspective* (pp. 294–330). Cambridge, England: Cambridge University Press.

Lewis, C. C. (1981). The effects of parental firm control: A reinterpretation of findings. *Psychological Bulletin, 90*, 547–563.

Loevinger, J. (1959). Patterns of parenthood as theories of learning. *Journal of Abnormal and Social Psychology, 59*, 148–150.

Lytton, H. (1980). *Parent-child interaction: The socialization process observed in twin and singleton families.* New York: Plenum Press.

Maccoby, E. E. (1984). Socialization and developmental change. *Child Development, 55*, 317–328.

Maccoby, E. E., & Martin, J. A. (1983). Socialization in the context of the family: Parent-child interaction. In P. H. Mussen (Series Ed.) & E. M. Hetherington (Vol. Ed.), *Handbook of child psychology: Vol. 4. Socialization, personality, and social development* (pp. 1–102). New York: Wiley.

Mancuso, J. C., & Handin, K. H. (1985). Reprimanding: Acting on one's implicit theory of behavior change. In I. E. Sigel (Ed.), *Parental belief systems* (pp. 143–176). Hillsdale, NJ: Erlbaum.

Mancuso, J. C., & Lehrer, R. (1986). Cognitive processes during reactions to rule violation. In R. D. Ashmore & D. M. Brodzinsky (Eds.), *Thinking about the family: Views of parents and children* (pp. 67–93). Hillsdale, NJ: Erlbaum.

Nucci, L. (1981). The development of personal concepts: A domain distinct from moral or societal concepts. *Child Development, 52*, 114–121.

Nucci. L. (1984). Evaluating teachers as social agents: Students' ratings of domain appropriate and domain inappropriate teacher responses to transgression. *American Educational Research Journal, 21,* 367–378.

Parke, R. D. (1974). Rules, roles, and resistance to deviation: Recent advances in punishment, discipline, and self-control. In A. Pick (Ed.), *Minnesota symposia on child psychology* (Vol. 8, pp. 111–143). Minneapolis, MN: University of Minnesota Press.

Perry, D. G., & Perry, L. C. (1983). Social learning, causal attribution, and moral internalization. In J. Bisanz, G. L. Bisanz, & R. Kail (Eds.), *Learning in children: Progress in cognitive development research* (pp. 105–136). New York: Springer-Verlag.

Reid, B. V., & Valsiner, J. (1986). Consistency, praise, and love: Folk theories of American parents. *Ethos, 14,* 282–304.

Saltzstein, H. D. (1976). Social influence and moral development: A perspective on the role of parents and peers. In T. Lickona (Ed.), *Moral development and behavior* (pp. 253–265). New York: Holt, Rinehart, & Winston.

Sears, R. R., Maccoby, E. E., & Levin, H. (1957). *Patterns of child-rearing.* Evanston, IL: Row, Peterson.

Siegal, M., & Barclay, M. S. (1985). Children's evaluations of fathers' socialization behavior. *Developmental Psychology, 21,* 1090–1096.

Siegal, M., & Cowen, J. (1984). Appraisals of intervention: The mother's versus the culprit's behavior as determinants of children's evaluations of discipline techniques. *Child Development, 55,* 1760–1766.

Sinha, S. R. (1985). Maternal strategies for regulating children's behavior. *Journal of Cross-Cultural Psychology, 16,* 27–40.

Smetana, J. (1988). Adolescents' and parents' conceptions of parental authority. *Child Development, 59,* 321–335.

Smetana, J. G. (1989). Toddlers' social interactions in the context of moral and conventional transgressions in the home context. *Developmental Psychology, 25,* 499–508.

Smith, M. C. (1975). Children's use of the multiple sufficient cause schema in social perception. *Journal of Personality and Social Psychology, 32,* 737–747.

Tisak, M. (1986). Children's conceptions of parental authority. *Child Development, 57,* 166–176.

Trickett, P. K., & Kuczynski, L. (1986). Children's misbehavior and parental discipline in abusive and non-abusive families. *Developmental Psychology, 22,* 115–123.

Turiel, E. (1983). *The development of social knowledge: Morality and convention.* Cambridge, England: Cambridge University Press.

Vuchinich, S., Emery, R. E., & Cassidy, J. (1988). Family members as third parties in dyadic family conflict: Strategies, alliances, and outcomes. *Child Development, 59,* 1293–1302.

Wertheim, E. S. (1975). The science and typology of family systems: Further theoreti-
    cal and practical considerations. *Family Process, 14*, 285–309.

Zahn-Waxler, C., & Chapman, M. (1982). Immediate antecedents of caretakers'
    methods of discipline. *Child Psychiatry and Human Development, 12*, 179–192.

Zahn-Waxler, C., Radke-Yarrow, M., & King, R. A. (1979). Child rearing and chil-
    dren's prosocial initiations toward victims of distress. *Child Development, 50*,
    319–330.

3

"Children of the Dream" Revisited: 70 Years of Collective Early Child Care in Israeli Kibbutzim

Ora Aviezer

University of Haifa, Haifa, Israel

Marinus H. Van IJzendoorn

Leiden University, Leiden, The Netherlands

Abraham Sagi

University of Haifa

Carlo Schuengel

Leiden University

This article focuses on kibbutz care for infants and young children. It reviews (a) past and present practices of collective education within the context of its historical background and guiding principles and (b) the results of developmental research regarding the impact of multiple caregiving and group care on children's socioemotional development within the framework of attachment theory. The research results indicate that, from a psychological point of view, collective sleeping is a problematic aspect of kibbutz child rearing. However, group care and multiple caregiving of high quality do not necessarily interfere with the formation of close relationships between parents and children or with the development of social skills.

An Israeli kibbutz (pl., kibbutzim) is a cooperative, democratically governed, multigenerational community with an average population of 400–

Reprinted with permission from *Psychological Bulletin*, Vol. 116, 99–116. Copyright © 1994 by the American Psychological Association, Inc.

Writing of this article was facilitated by a PIONEER grant (PG5 59-256) awarded to Marinus H. Van IJzendoorn by the Netherlands' Organization for Scientific Research.

900 people. Each kibbutz is economically and socially autonomous but is also affiliated with one of three kibbutz organizations called "kibbutz movements" that offer support and guidance to individual kibbutzim. In the past, the kibbutz movements were deeply divided by political and ideological differences that were expressed even on the level of child-care practices. With the passage of time, however, most of these differences have lost their significance, and many kibbutz members today favor the idea of establishing a single united kibbutz movement. Every kibbutz member works for the kibbutz economy and is in turn provided by the community with housing, food, clothing, health and educational services, recreation, and other living needs. In the past, kibbutzim had been fairly isolated agricultural communities in which living conditions were exceedingly hard. Today kibbutz economies are based on a diversity of industries and agricultural activities and are able to provide members with a satisfying standard of living.

The kibbutz is known as being one of the very few utopian experiments that have succeeded in establishing a radically different way of living and of raising children. As many as four generations have been brought up in kibbutzim since the first such communities were founded at the turn of the century. The kibbutz child-rearing system, also called collective education, has been treated in the literature as furnishing a "natural laboratory" for testing the consequences of child-rearing methods that derived from a unique philosophy and from practices markedly different from those used in the West (Beit-Hallahmi & Rabin, 1977; Bettelheim, 1969; Rapaport, 1958; Spiro, 1958).

Our goal in this article is to evaluate the positive and negative aspects of collective child rearing, particularly in regard to the socioemotional consequences for young children. We begin with a short review of the historical roots of the kibbutz movement and the guiding principles of collective education. This is followed with a description of educational practices in the past and of the changes that brought kibbutz child care to its present form. Then, in the second part of the article, the results of studies on kibbutz children are reviewed within the context of dynamic changes in kibbutz life both recently and in the past and with reference to developmental research. Particular emphasis is given to attachment relationships and their consequences. Finally, the development of social competence and relationships with peers is reviewed and discussed.

HISTORICAL BACKGROUND

The early pioneers of the kibbutz movement were idealistic young people who rejected the culture of the *shtetl* that had dominated the life of Eastern European Jews for centuries and sought to create instead a new society founded on socialist and Zionist principles (Melzer, 1988; Selier, 1977). The task they set for themselves was in no way minor. They proposed to create a collective society that emphasized production and physical labor, striving at the same time to achieve both national and personal independence under conditions of perfect equality. The Marxian precept "from each according to his ability, to each according to his needs" was established as the primary and essential principle of kibbutz life. The political aspirations of kibbutzniks dictated their settlement in remote locations, where they were constrained to cultivate barren land in a harsh climate and a hostile environment. In these circumstances, the decision to raise children collectively contributed to the protection and well-being of the young. Children were thus housed in the only brick building on kibbutz grounds and never went hungry, whereas the adults of the community lived in tents and their food was rationed. Early in kibbutz history, this reality interacted with an awareness of the role of child rearing in furthering the goals of the collective by discouraging individualism, abolishing inequalities between the sexes, and bringing up a person who was better socialized to communal life (Gerson, 1978).

One of the principal goals of early kibbutzim was to alter the patriarchal organization of the family that was typical of Eastern European Jewish culture; in this culture, women were economically dependent on men and parental authority over children was absolute. Collective education was assigned an important place in achieving this goal. It was instituted so as to free women from the burdens of child care, thereby allowing them to participate in the socioeconomic life of the community on an equal footing with men. Men, on the other hand, would share in the duties of child care and become nurturing rather than authoritarian figures in the lives of their children. Moreover, bringing children up collectively was regarded as essential in fostering the solidarity of the group and restraining individualistic tendencies in both children and adults. Educational practices in kibbutzim were accordingly established so as to reflect the egalitarian and democratic philosophy of the kibbutz community (Gerson, 1978).

The kibbutz community therefore assumed total responsibility for all of the material needs of its children in the way of food, clothing, and medical care and for seeing to their spiritual well-being, the latter including mental health, developmental progress, and parental counseling (Gerson, 1978). This responsibility extended to each child individually, who was in a sense regarded as being a "kibbutz' child"; and it also created an informal communal socialization network (Rabin & Beit-Hallahmi, 1982). Thus, child care and education were, first and foremost, conceived of as being social mechanisms. It was only later that the needs of children became a central concern in the consciousness of the community (Alon, 1976) and that kibbutzim tended to assume the character of a "child-centered community" (Lewin, 1990; Rabin & Beit-Hallahmi, 1982) in which psychological theory came to influence educational conceptualizations and practices (Kaffman, Elizur, & Rabinowitz, 1990).

THE GUIDING PRINCIPLES OF COLLECTIVE EDUCATION

During the formative years of collective education, psychoanalytic theory was eagerly adopted as an educational guide. A token of this influence is already apparent in the work of Bernfeld, a reforming pedagogue whose utopian visions were widely accepted among young German Jews who immigrated to Palestine and joined the kibbutz movement (Melzer 1988). Given that one of the principal goals of the kibbutz founders was to change family relations, it is not surprising that psychoanalytic views about the pathological consequences of conflicts in parent-child relations should have had a special appeal for them (Lavi, 1984, 1990a). Kibbutz educators interpreted these views as furnishing support for the ideas of dividing the task of socialization between parents and educators (caregivers and teachers) and of nonreliance on parents alone in educating infants and young children. Maintenance of two emotional centers for kibbutz children—the parental home and the children's house—was thought to protect children against their parents' shortcomings while preserving the benefits of parental love (Golan, 1959). The practice of having children sleep away from the parental home was justified on the grounds that it spared them from the trauma of exposure to the so-called "primal scene" and from the conflicts with parents that are imminent in the Oedipus complex (Golan, 1959).

Observers of the kibbutz have characterized parental involvement as emotional and directed toward need gratification, whereas caregivers have been described as being goal directed and instrumental (Bar-Yosef 1959; Rabin & Beit-Hallahmi, 1982). This role division was considered to be beneficial for children because the objective attitudes and professional approach of caregivers were conducive to the children's mastery of autonomous behavior and social learning without in any way compromising their parents' love (Gerson, 1978; Golan, 1958). In addition, living among peers from an early age was regarded as being an inseparable part of bringing up future kibbutz members because it presented children with a supportive environment for dealing with the kind of human values perceived to be at the core of kibbutz life, such as sharing and consideration for others (Hazan, 1973).

COLLECTIVE EDUCATION IN PRACTICE: PAST AND PRESENT

There has never been a simple one-to-one correspondence between child-rearing practices on kibbutzim and the beliefs of adult members. Socioeconomic and physical conditions, as well as new psychoeducational theories, have always had an impact on how kibbutz children are brought up, and ideological differences have existed between the different kibbutz organizations since their foundation. Individual kibbutzim, moreover, adopted day-to-day practices that accommodated their particular needs and the prevailing emotional atmosphere of the community (Lavi, 1990a). It is nevertheless possible to describe the practices that are typical of a collective kibbutz upbringing and to present these practices from a dynamic perspective of historical changes.

Past Trends

Before the 1940s, the medical model dominated approaches to child care both inside and outside the kibbutz (Gerson, 1978; Lewin, 1986). Cleanliness was maintained in infant houses to the point of sterility, infant feeding was rigorously scheduled, parental visits were restricted, and caregivers (Hebrew: s. *metapelet*, pl. *metaplot*) were trained in hospitals (Lewin, 1986). Caregivers were regarded as the experts and the ultimate authority in kibbutz children's care (Gerson, 1978). Characteristically, a very small staff of two or three caregivers took care of a large group of between 12 and 18 children. Some of these early practices can be better understood when one takes into account the ecological context of kibbutzim at the time; these were isolated communities far from medical facilities. Moreover, because of the prevalence of serious diseases in this pioneering period, the major concern was to keep babies alive, which was indeed managed quite successfully by the kibbutzim (Gerson, 1978). These years were naturally difficult for many families, some of whom left the kibbutz.

After World War II and Israel's War of Independence, the emphasis shifted from physical health to the emotional needs of children and mothers. This change was supported by a gradual improvement in economic conditions and the increasing influence of the conceptualizations of Bowlby (1951) and Spitz (1946) in regard to "maternal deprivation," which replaced both the medical model and classical psychoanalysis (Lavi, 1984). Parental participation in child care through the infant's 1st year, particularly on the part of mothers, was also allowed to increase. Mothers were granted maternity leave, which over the years was expanded from 6 weeks to a period of 3 or 4 months. In addition, demand feeding replaced schedule feeding, and breast-feeding was encouraged. As a result of changes that evolved in the 1970s, infants no longer live in the infant house on arrival from the hospital but remain at home with their mothers for the duration of maternity leave (Kaffman et al., 1990). Daily visits of mothers were instituted in the early 1960s for the purpose of allowing mothers to spend time with their children (this period was humorously referred to as the "love hour"). The growing awareness in kibbutzim that children need intimacy for their emotional growth, as well as space and stimulation for activity, has been translated into improvements of the physical environment in the children's houses, a reduction of the size of groups to 4–7 children, and an improvement in the caregiver to children ratio. Training of caregivers has shifted its emphasis to developmental knowledge, educational practices, and the caregiver's role in supporting children's emotional development as it is expressed in tasks such as weaning, toilet training, and nocturnal fears (Lewin, 1985).

In the late 1960s, under the influence of Piaget's theory, children's cognitive development was emphasized (Lewin, 1985). Piaget's views of development as a product of interactions between children and their environment were easily accommodated by the egalitarian philosophy of collective education. The nature of children's activity, creativity, and play became the center of attention, as well as age-related curricula (e.g., Haas, 1986; Lewin, 1983).

COLLECTIVE SLEEPING ARRANGEMENTS

Collective sleeping arrangements for children away from their parents constitute probably the most distinctive characteristic of kibbutz practices in collective child raising. Many cultures practice multiple caregiving (e.g., Barry & Paxton, 1971; Konner, 1977; Morelli & Tronick, 1991; Tronick, Winn, & Morelli, 1985), and the pattern is in many ways similar to the practice in kibbutzim (Rabin & Beit-Hallahmi, 1982). However, a worldwide sample of 183 societies showed that none of them maintained a system of having infants sleep away from their parents (Barry & Paxton, 1971). The major reasons for instituting collective sleeping for children in the early years of kibbutzim were (a) the concern for children's safety, and (b) women's equality and training children for communal life (Fölling-Albers, 1988b; Lavi, 1984). These aims were later interpreted by kibbutz educators as concordant with fundamental psychoanalytic ideas. Thus, kibbutzim had created a psychological ideology that was used to justify collective sleeping arrangements as contributing to the children's well-being as well as mental health.

The children's house on a kibbutz in fact functions as the children's home in almost every respect. Only a few kibbutzim still maintain communal sleeping arrangements for children; in those where the custom continues, however, this facility serves as the place in which children spend most of their time, eat their meals, are bathed, and sleep at night, in much the same way as they might do at home—hence the term "children's house." The children's house is designed to fulfill all such functions. It consists of a number of bedrooms that are each shared by three or four children, a dining area, showers, and a large space for play activities and learning. Children have private corners in their bedrooms where they keep their personal things, and these corners are decorated according to the child's preference. Family time is in the afternoon and evening, when both parents try to be available. Children are returned to the children's house for the night by their parents, who put them to bed; a caregiver or a parent then remains with them until the night watchwomen take over.

Two night watchwomen are responsible for all children in the kibbutz under 12 years of age. The women are assigned on a weekly rotation basis, and they monitor the children's houses from a central location, usually the infant house, by making rounds and through the use of intercoms. In most cases, night watchwomen are not complete strangers to the children (Ben-Yaakov, 1972). However, the weekly rotation system makes sensitive response to the infants' needs nearly impossible. Moreover, intervention by an unfamiliar adult when infants experience distress may elicit a response of stranger anxiety (Bronson, 1968; Spitz, 1965). Thus, although collective sleeping may allow for sufficient monitoring of children's safety, it leaves children with only a precarious and limited sense of security. Independent support for this view was recently offered in a study that found that the longest period of uninterrupted sleep (defined as the longest continuous period scored as sleep without any identified awakening) was more extended for children sleeping at home than for children in communal dormitories (Ophir-Cohen, Epstein, Tzischinsky, Tirosh, & Lavie, in press). It should be noted that this measure of sleep was derived from the recently developed Automatic Scoring Analysis Program conducted on actigraphic data (Sadeh, Lavie, Scher, Tirosh, & Epstein, 1991). On the basis of the same actigraphic technique of data collection and analysis, Epstein (1992) recently compared sleeping patterns in 1–6-year-old kibbutz children when they slept collectively with their sleeping patterns at home 1 year later. The findings showed that sleep efficiency (defined as the ratio of sleep to total sleep time) in collective sleeping is low and that it improved when children were moved to sleep at home to a level of efficiency similar to that of family-reared children. This improvement occurred despite overcrowding in kibbutz family homes that had not yet been adapted to accommodate the children on a permanent basis. A more detailed discussion of this topic follows in a later section.

Most kibbutzim had abandoned collective sleeping by the beginning of the 1990s (this practice is currently in effect in only 3 of the country's 260 kibbutzim). Doubts about children's collective sleeping had been voiced as early as in the 1950s, and a small number of kibbutzim have always maintained home-based sleeping arrangements (Lavi, 1984). The movement to change children's sleeping arrangements gained momentum in the 1960s and 1970s, along with an upsurge in familistic tendencies (Fölling-Albers, 1988b; Tiger & Shepher, 1975). This trend was reinforced by the growing prosperity of kibbutz economies, which resulted in the building of better family homes for members on the one hand and the weakening of ideological identifications of young kibbutz members on the other (Lavi, 1990b). Familistic trends accelerated significantly in the 1980s, as had been predicted by some researchers (e.g., Beit-Hallahmi, 1981; Rabin & Beit-Hallahmi, 1982). Moreover, these trends have continued, notwithstanding serious economic problems that required many kibbutzim to commit themselves to heavy financial obligations to be able to make the necessary modifications for family housing (Melzer & Neubauer, 1988).

The success of familism in kibbutzim reduced women's participation in community life (Gerson, 1978; Lavi, 1984), pushing their struggle for equality into the background. Collective education failed to free kibbutz women from child care as their primary responsibility or from leading a dual-career life combining motherhood and work. Frustrated by their work options, many kibbutz women invested in motherhood (Keller, 1983), and women were the leading proponents for changing the practice of collective sleeping for children. Thus, along with the men, they helped to preserve the sex-typed occupational structure of kibbutzim (e.g., the absence of men in the caregiver's role), rather than attempting to change it (Fölling-Albers, 1988a).

Present Practices

Kibbutz infants are exposed to multiple caregiving very early in their lives (Lavi, 1990a). In their first 3 months, kibbutz infants receive exclusive maternal care in the family's residence. They are brought to the infant house as soon as their mothers return to work part time. During the initial period of their stay in the infant house, they are cared for jointly by the mother and the metapelet. Mothers are almost exclusively in charge of feeding, and they arrange their work schedule accordingly; caregivers are responsible for the infants between maternal visits. During the second half of the infants' 1st year, caregivers gradually assume responsibility for the children's various needs as the mothers increase their work load. Thus, by the infants' 2nd year, they come under the full care of the caregivers, who play an increasingly larger role in their socialization with respect to issues such as table manners, sharing, play habits, and knowledge of the environment.

Table 1 contains an overview of the caregiving responsibilities during early childhood in the kibbutz. This description represents a summary of various periods; the delegation of responsibilities may change further.

Children join the toddler group, which is larger than the infant group (10–12 children), at about the middle of their 2nd year, but the 1:3 ratio of adults to children is maintained. At this stage, caregivers are responsible for a wide range of the children's needs (e.g., administering of medication, toilet training, appropriate nutrition, and growth and age-appropriate activities of individual children). When children approach 3 years of age, they move to the nursery class, which is somewhat larger and where the ratio of adults to children is reduced to 1:4. Parents are welcome to spend time in the children's house; they visit whenever they can, and caregivers try to accommodate them.

Home-based sleeping has changed the proportion of time spent by kibbutz children in the children's house to a pattern similar to that of nonkibbutz day-care settings. Children come to the children's house in the morning and go home during late afternoon. Maternal responsibilities for infants' care throughout the 1st year have remained the same, but the love hour practice is no longer officially observed. Most parents, even among those originally opposed to home-based sleeping, are now satisfied with the change in sleeping arrangements (Lavi, 1984). Children's sleeping at home has clearly changed the balance between the two emotional centers of the family and the community. The family has become the principal authority and has assumed additional caregiving functions, whereas the caregivers' influence has declined and become secondary. Thus, a process is taking

TABLE 1
Overview of the Distribution of Caregiving Responsibilities During Early Childhood

Caregiving Responsibility	Age Period						
	0–6 Weeks	6 Weeks–6 Months	6–9 Months	9–14 Months	14 Months–Kindergarten	Postkindergarten
Feeding	Parent(s): on demand	Parent(s): if possible, every 3–4 hr	Parent(s): weaning, caregiver begins to take over	Caregiver (3 meals per day)	Caregiver	Caregiver
Washing/diapering	Parent(s): between feedings	Parent(s), caregiver	Parent(s), caregiver	Caregiver	Caregiver	Caregiver
Play	Parent(s)	Parent(s), caregiver, love hour	Parent(s), caregiver, love hour	Parent(s), caregiver, love hour	Parent(s), caregiver, peers, love hour	Parent(s), caregiver, peers, love hour
Socialization	Not available	Parent(s)	Parent(s), caregiver	Parent(s), caregiver	Parent(s), caregiver	Parent(s), caregiver, peers
Education	Not available	Not available	Not available	Caregiver	Caregiver	Caregiver
Night care[a]	Caregiver, watchwomen	Caregiver, watchwomen	Caregiver, watchwomen	Caregiver, watchwomen	Caregiver, watchwomen	Caregiver, watchwomen

Note. The information included here is based on data from Ben-Yaakov (1972) and Rabin and Beit-Hallahmi (1982). The picture of the kibbutz child-rearing system is continuously changing. For this reason, the information provided here may not be adequate in light of recent developments. However, it represents the system in its most characteristic form.

[a] In home-based sleeping provided by parents. In collective sleeping, parents wake up children in the morning up until 9–14 months of age.

place in which responsibilities are being redefined, although the sense of the community's commitment to its children has been preserved.

Collective education in the 1990s is therefore faced with the need of negotiating new ways of expressing the influence of the collective without infringing on the autonomy and privacy of families. This is not an easy task, considering the heterogeneous nature of multigenerational kibbutz populations. Also, recent economic difficulties and difficulties in providing adequate professional manpower have resulted in demands to reduce the costs of early care by restructuring it to resemble nonkibbutz day care in Israel (Sagi & Koren-Karie, 1993). Clearly, early child care in kibbutzim is changing. As in the past, the changes are taking place within the context of general processes in which collective responsibility is being reduced and new ideas for the accountability of the community for the actions of individual members and the resultant consequences are being negotiated. This topic is, however, beyond the scope of the present article.

SUMMARY OF THE HISTORICAL REVIEW

The kibbutz approach to child rearing established a radically different method of raising children that was legitimized by both socialist and psychoanalytic ideas. Its original conceptualization as a social mechanism for promoting the goals of a new society led to the institution of unique childcare practices. More specifically, the practices of nonmaternal care for infants and toddlers, children dwelling with their peers in children's houses instead of with their families, and the division of the tasks of socialization between parents and caregivers (teachers) differed markedly from the educational practices common in Western societies (see Lamb, Sternberg, Hwang, & Broberg, 1992; Melhuish & Moss, 1991).

The course of the evolution of early care in kibbutzim reflects the changes occurring in the physical and socioeconomic conditions of these communities, as well as changes in ideology, educational conceptualizations, and knowledge. During the early period of kibbutzim, collective education was, in part, determined by the difficult conditions of existence; thus, children's health and physical development were regarded as the primary criteria for child care. The rigors of the environment, adherence to the medical model, inexperience and lack of knowledge, and ideological zeal all contributed to the strict practices involving kibbutz children and their parents. Growing knowledge about young children's emotional and cognitive development and improved economic conditions later led to a shift in emphasis to emotional needs and to a restructuring of early care in kibbutz education. The definition of children's well-being thus came to include more than mere physical health and resulted in an emphasis on caregiving practices and furnishing children with a stimulating environment.

A historical overview of early child care in the kibbutz reveals an important shift in the relative weights assigned to the two major agents of socialization: the family and the community. In the beginning, the influence of the community was preeminent. Thus, its representatives—the caregivers—were granted ultimate authority over educational practices. In later years, there has been a gradual ascendancy of familism, expressed by more intense parental involvement. The institution of home-based sleeping has finalized the process by transferring most caregiving functions to the family. The practice of collective sleeping arrangements for children, which is rapidly disappearing, has become a historically unique phenomenon that deserves an evaluation in terms of its socioemotional consequences.

THE KIBBUTZ SYSTEM OF EARLY CARE: A RESEARCH REVIEW

As noted earlier, child rearing in kibbutzim has attracted a fair amount of attention motivated by interest in the developmental outcomes of its unique practices. Any comprehensive system such as kibbutz child care can be evaluated from a variety of points of view. In what follows, we briefly consider studies of parental attitudes, caregivers' roles, and the quality of care offered by collective education. We then evaluate in depth the developmental consequences of kibbutz child rearing, with an emphasis on socioemotional development.

Parental Attitudes

A hypothesis frequently proposed about kibbutz mothers is that their lower than usual participation in the care of their children may result in guilt feelings that lead to insecure mother-child relationships (e.g., Fölling-Albers, 1988b; Liegle, 1974). According to Bettelheim (1969), however, kibbutz women suffer from maternal guilt feelings because of their subconscious rejection of their own mothers. No empirical evidence corroborates either of these claims. Lewin (1990) found that most kibbutz mothers regard the infant house and metapelet as assisting them in their motherhood. However, women's prominent support of familistic trends suggests that recent generations of mothers lay claim to a larger share in the caregiving role than did mothers in the founding generations of the kibbutzim (Kaffman et al., 1990; Lavi, 1984; Spiro, 1979; Tiger & Shepher, 1975). Kibbutz mothers entertain specific notions about themselves in the role of educators. They perceive themselves as being more nurturant and influential in the development of interpersonal behavior in their children. They attribute to the metapelet a more demanding role and regard themselves as less influential than her in regard to such age-related behaviors as dressing and toilet training. In comparison, day-care mothers perceive themselves as being more nurturant and influential than caregivers in every domain of child development (Feldman & Yirmiya, 1986).

The Role of Caregivers

Caregivers are assigned a central role in kibbutz education. Their influence on children's development of autonomy and socialization to kibbutz life is considered paramount, and their constant and stable presence is thought to potentially compensate for poor maternal functioning (Gerson, 1978). Indeed, metaplot have been reported to perceive themselves as the most important influence in children's social development and physical care (Kaffman et al., 1990); however, they have also been reported to be uncertain about their professional role when mother-infant relations require intervention (M. Harel, 1986). The trust kibbutz mothers have expressed in their infants' caregivers (Feldman & Yirmiya, 1986; Lewin, 1990) has been attributed to the sharing of responsibilities and the openness of kibbutz child-care services to parental and community supervision (Feldman & Yirmiya, 1986) and to the professional expertise of caregivers (M. Harel, 1986). Like kibbutz mothers, most metaplot (who are often mothers themselves) have been supportive of home-based sleeping and of infants remaining with their mothers for more extensive periods after their birth (Kaffman et al., 1990).

Systematic observations of caregivers' interactions with toddlers have shown that the approach of metaplot toward children is positive but is adversely affected by poor physical conditions and caregivers' fatigue (Gerson & Schnabel-Brandes, 1990). Gerson and Schnabel-Brandes suggested that the metaplot's strong commitment to the ideological and pedagogical values of the kibbutz and their strong involvement with the children contributed to their positive approach. However, Rosenthal (1991) found that superior training and experience rather than ideological commitment distinguished kibbutz metaplot from caregivers in other Israeli day-care settings.

Quality of Early Care in the Kibbutz

In a recent overview of Israeli day-care centers by Sagi and Koren-Karie (1993), the quality of kibbutz child care was rated as being the best in the country. The specific advantages indicated by these authors were the high quality of the physical and educational environment in the kibbutz system, the small group size (8–12 children), a good caregiver to child ratio (1:3–1:4), and the high level of caretakers' commitment. Note that these standards of care had developed in the kibbutz long before the quality of nonmaternal care had become an issue of professional concern, and their advantage had already become evident. For instance, Gewirtz (1965) attributed the decline of smiling he found among infants from institutions and day nurseries, as compared with infants reared in families and kibbutzim, to less stimulation and availability of caregivers in those child-care settings in which custodial care and poor children to adult ratios prevailed.

Rosenthal (1991) examined three Israeli child-care settings in regard to the educational quality of the physical environment, the content and emotional tone of each program, and the characteristics of the daily interactions of the children with their caregivers. Her findings corroborated Sagi and Koren-Karie's (1993) assessment. The kibbutz environment was significantly better than the environment of both center care and family day care. Emotional atmosphere and children's daily interactions in the kibbutz resembled those in family day care, in which group size and adult-child ratio are similar. However, kibbutzim scored significantly better in these respects than did center care. In addition, children's social orientation and active learning are determined by developmentally appropriate activities, which are another aspect of quality caregiving (Howes, Phillips, & Whitebook, 1992; Rosenthal, 1991). Rosenthal (1991) also measured the extent to which toddlers in the various settings engaged in active learning and social interaction as an indication of the quality of their experience. She found that kibbutz children were more active in both learning and social exchanges and attributed this finding to their experience in an environment that combined structural aspects and processes of better quality care as delineated by Phillips and Howes (1987).

Yet, caregivers' stability, which is another important aspect of quality care, seems to be a relative weakness in the kibbutz child-care system. Gerson and Nathan (1969) surveyed the entire caregiver population of the kibbutz movement and found a 25%–33% annual turnover rate. Caregiver turnover rates were highest for toddler groups and lowest for infant groups. Although no current data are available on the topic, Lewin (1982) reported that caregiver turnover has always been a problem and has not decreased over the years. Turnover rates are related to the quality of a caregivers' work environment, the position often being characterized by low salaries and low prestige (Whitebook, Howes, & Phillips, 1989). It is interesting to note that caregiving does not have much prestige in kibbutzim either, despite proclaimed convictions concerning its importance (Gerson & Nathan, 1969). A possible reason is that early care is often regarded as a task that women can perform instinctually without formal training (Gerson, 1976). Although turnover rates reported for kibbutzim are somewhat lower than those in the United States (Whitebook et al., 1989), they are nevertheless high enough to suggest substantial instability. In a comprehensive system of care—such as that found in kibbutzim—that delegates many parental tasks to caregivers, the consequences of such instability may be even more severe. Yet, the cohesive, intimate nature of the kibbutz community, with its high degree of familiarity and involvement among people, may contribute to a sense of consistency and predictability for both children and parents. The sharing of caregiving responsibilities may be viewed as a source of instability in the children's house. However, unlike other child-care environments, kibbutz caregiving takes place within the context of enduring relationships. These relationships, in turn, can sustain adults' mutual trust (Feldman & Yirmiya, 1986) and support children's sense of living in a stable, secure environment (see Rabin, 1965). One can conclude that the quality of kibbutz care has been excellent in regard to its structural dimensions and basic caregiving characteristics; at the same time, however, caregiver stability has been relatively weak and may therefore have had adverse effects on children's socioemotional development (Howes et al., 1992).

The Developmental Consequences of Kibbutz Child Rearing

In this section, we consider the research on the developmental consequences of kibbutz child rearing, which has been in force for more than 4 decades. Classical evaluations of kibbutz child rearing were based on participant observation techniques and clinical impressions that focused on nonmaternal care for small children. Succeeding research efforts concentrated on comparing kibbutz children with their counterparts outside the kibbutz on measures that have often furnished global assessments of development, with implications for future personality characteristics. Exposure to multiple relationships in early childhood, which is inherent in group care, became the main issue in this regard. The current wave of research has been concerned with the socioemotional development of kibbutz children and has focused on attachment theory. Within the context of a growing worldwide prevalence of nonmaternal and group care in early childhood, studies have concentrated on the effects of the unique characteristics of collective upbringing on interpersonal relations and personality formation.

Classical Evaluations of Kibbutz Child Rearing

The general impression of most early observers of kibbutz children was that their relations with their parents were warm and affectionate; however, the delegation of child-care functions to caregivers was judged to be a potential obstacle to the formation of exclusive relationships between mothers and infants and a potential impediment for future personality development (Bettelheim, 1969; Irvine, 1952; Spiro, 1958; Winograd, 1958). However, both Spiro (1958) and Bettelheim (1969) concluded that kibbutz children appeared to grow into well-functioning and adapted adults, despite early indications of emotional insecurity (Spiro, 1958) and some interference with the development of personal identity, emotional intimacy, and individual achievement (Bettelheim, 1969).

Spiro (1958) observed, in an anthropological study, that kibbutz children often felt rejected by their caregivers and had to face aggression from their peers. Their emotional pain resulted in introversion and resistance in their interpersonal contacts with kibbutz members and outsiders. However, Spiro did not perceive the reality of kibbutz children as similar to institutions in which emotional deprivation prevails (Bowlby, 1951). Bettelheim (1969) believed that the "children of the dream," as he called kibbutz children, would experience early in their childhood a balanced mixture of trust and distrust of the environment. The relatively large number of caregivers would be a source of distrust, but the availability of caregivers in all situations and the continuous presence of the peer group would prevent the development of separation anxiety. According to Bettelheim, the absence of extremely positive or negative emotions in the experience of kibbutz children underlies an "emotional flatness" that he observed in their personalities. Unfortunately, many of the early observations were unsystematic (some were even based on secondhand reports) and often relied on small unrepresentative samples without control groups. Hence, they have been criticized as anecdotal and speculative (Lavi, 1990a; Rabin & Beit-Hallahmi, 1982).

The Early Studies

The first systematic empirical investigation of the effects of collective child rearing was conducted by Rabin (1958, 1965). Rabin compared the performance of kibbutz children of various ages with that of children from a rural semicommunal setting (moshav) on a battery of tests of mental and social development to assess the hypothesis that kibbutz children suffer from partial psychological deprivation because of their repeated transitions between the parental home and the children's house. His results indicated a significant developmental lag in the socioemotional and verbal learning of kibbutz infants, although it was not considered to be pathogenic. This lag was found to have disappeared by 10 years of age, when there was evidence of early independence and less problematic puberty (Rabin, 1965). These results highlighted the differential effects of group environment in regard to multiple interpersonal relations at different ages. Although the presence of multiple "significant others" in infancy may be overwhelming to the tender personality, it may be supportive of ego development later in middle childhood and adolescence.

Rabin's work was, however, faced with various criticisms. Golan (1958) argued that the developmental delay found in kibbutz infants did not result from maternal deprivation. He attributed it to the caregivers' focus on satisfying infants' physical needs at the expense of providing them with personal contact and arranging adequate environment for play. Furthermore, Kohen-Raz (1968) criticized Rabin's sample as small and unrepresentative. He studied a larger sample of infants and found that the developmental level of kibbutz infants was equal to that of family-raised Israeli infants and to that of an American normative sample. In addition, contradictory findings of new studies challenged Rabin's conclusions about kibbutz infants. Gewirtz (1965) found that the smiling response of kibbutz infants through the first 18 months was similar to that of family-raised infants. Greenbaum and Landau (1977) found that kibbutz infants possessed advanced linguistic skills comparable to those of family-reared infants in spite of less time spent with their mothers; Holdstein and Borus (1976) found the same for kibbutz preschoolers. It was therefore concluded that collective education had no adverse effects on infant development (Kohen-Raz, 1968), and the nurturing, stimulating character of the kibbutz environment was underscored (Holdstein & Borus, 1976).

Rabin's (1965) findings represented the development of kibbutz infants as observed during the 1950s, when his study had been conducted. Because Rabin did not assess the quality of child care as a variable separate from interpersonal relationships, it would be difficult to argue that one or the other was an exclusive cause. Moreover, it is important to note that most of the early studies used developmental measures that evaluated social-verbal learning rather than socioemotional experience. Thus, given the wide consensus that the quality of day care is an important factor in children's development (Clarke-Stewart, 1989; Fein & Fox, 1988; Howes, 1988b), it is not surprising that improvements in the quality of early child care in the kibbutz were associated with improved performance on developmental measures; these measures do not, however, allow for direct assessment of emotional development.

Long-Term Effects of Collective Early Care

Long-term effects are an important aspect of the consequences of early care. Kibbutz children, adolescents, and young adults have been judged to be emotionally healthy, constructive, and successful. Rabin (1965) based these conclusions on projective psychological tests (e.g., Rorschach, Draw a Person, Sentence Completion, and Thematic Apperception Test) in which he found indications of intellectual achievements, greater personality maturity, and ego strength. Also, Zellermayer and Marcus (1971) noted the scarcity of delinquency and drug abuse. In one of the few longitudinal studies of kibbutz-raised individuals, Rabin and Beit-Hallahmi (1982) interviewed Rabin's (1965) subjects 20 years after they had originally been studied. They found that collective-raised and moshav-raised adults were very similar in terms of their level of education and achievements. Furthermore, they were found to be similar in their functioning as spouses and in their identification with their parents. However, Rabin and Beit-Hallahmi also found some empirical support for a lower capability among kibbutz-reared adults to establish intimate friendships. This was attributed to the differential effect of the early experiences of the two groups. Similarly, a reduced need for affective involvement and emotional intimacy, as assessed by the Family Relations Test (Anthony & Bene, 1957), was found by Regev Beit-Hallahmi, and Sharabany (1980) among school-aged children and by Weinbaum (1990) among kindergartners who lived in kibbutzim with communal sleeping arrangements. Berman (1988) summarized a number of studies that investigated the effects of traditional collective upbringing (including communal sleeping) and concluded that such an upbringing had an impact on personality development by causing "a consistent interference with emotional experience, creativity, and the quality of object relations as expressed especially in intimate relationships" (p. 327). Thus, although it is generally agreed that kibbutz children grow up to become well-functioning adults, the findings indicate that they experience less emotional intensity in interpersonal relations, possibly as a result of their experiences in infancy. However, a direct assessment of the emotional experience of infants in collective child care and its consequences had to await new theoretical formulations and research procedures of the kind offered by attachment theory.

ATTACHMENT RESEARCH: INFANTS' RELATIONSHIPS AND THEIR CONSEQUENCES

Bowlby's (1951) publication on maternal deprivation, as well as the work of researchers such as Spiro, Rabin, and Bettelheim, inspired changes in kibbutz child-care practices (Lavi, 1984). Still, the primary research orientation was that of classical psychoanalytic theory, and it was not until the 1970s and 1980s that attachment theory became one of the leading paradigms. The conceptual framework and research procedures of attachment theory, particularly, the strange situation paradigm (Ainsworth, Blehar, Waters, & Wall, 1978), opened new avenues for investigating issues that have concerned kibbutz research since the 1950s, including the effects on infant development of early exposure to multiple caregivers in the context of group care.

According to attachment theory, the security of infants' attachment to their caregivers is determined by the quality of the care they receive (Bowlby, 1969/1982). Sensitive responses to infants' signals and needs are associated with secure attachments, whereas rejection of infants' communications and inconsistent care are related to insecure attachments (Ainsworth et al., 1978). A multiple caregiving arrangement exposes infants to repeated separations from their primary caregivers as well as to new relationships. When nonmaternal care involves group care, the feasibility of providing sensitive care to individual children within a group and the nature of relationships with additional caregivers become important issues for examination. The increasing numbers of children who are exposed to various multiple caregiving arrangements lend additional importance to the study of these issues. Therefore, our review of attachment research in kibbutzim examines the relationships of kibbutz infants and the consequences of these relationships in terms of socioemotional development.

Infants' Relations with Parents

The first studies focused on children's relations to their mothers and concluded that collective upbringing does not interfere with the intensity of attachment relations. In a stressful situation very similar to the strange situation paradigm, 2–4-year-old kibbutz children (Maccoby & Feldman, 1972) and 8–24-month-old kibbutz infants (Fox, 1977) used their mothers as a secure base. However, neither Maccoby and Feldman nor Fox were able to apply the extensive classification system of attachment behavior in the strange situation (Ainsworth et al., 1978). This is probably the reason why they chose to measure the intensity of attachment as if it were a personality trait. In current conceptualizations, attachment is viewed as a strategy of dealing with the emotions elicited by stressful events and with the status of the attachment figure in this process. Three fundamental strategies have been identified: (a) denial of negative emotions and avoidance of the attachment figure, who is not expected to provide relief (A); (b) open communication with the attachment figure about negative emotions (B); and (c) preoccupation with negative emotions and ambivalence toward the attachment figure, who for the child is both a source of stress and a potential "haven of security" (C; Main, 1990). The classification of attachment behavior in the strange situation paradigm is based on several strategies. A child's attachment to the primary caregiver can be classified as insecure–avoidant (A), secure (B), or insecure–resistant (C). The view of attachment as a relational organization underlies much of the later research.

Sagi, Lamb, Lewkowicz, et al. (1985) used the strange situation paradigm (Ainsworth et al., 1978) and its classification system to study the relationships of 85 communally sleeping kibbutz infants with their parents and caregivers. They also examined the relationships with their mothers of 36 Israeli infants attending city day-care facilities. They found that only 59% of kibbutz infants were securely attached to their mothers, as compared with 75% of Israeli day-care infants and the 65%–70% levels found in most studies. Among children with insecure attachments in both Israeli samples, anxious–ambivalent relationships were overrepresented. Skewed distributions of attachment relationships, including that found by Sagi and his colleagues, have raised concern that the strange situation may not be cross-culturally valid (Grossmann, Grossmann, Spangler, Suess, & Unzner, 1985; Sagi, Lamb, Lewkowicz, et al., 1985). However, recent secondary analyses and meta-analyses (Sagi, Van IJzendoorn, & Koren-Karie, 1991; Van IJzendoorn & Kroonenberg, 1988), as well as analyses of cross-national data (Lamb, Thompson, & Gardner, 1985; Sagi, 1990; Van IJzendoorn, 1990), have indicated that this procedure is valid for assessing universal communicative patterns between adults and infants that may be affected by stress (Van IJzendoorn & Kroonenberg, 1988) or by cultural preferences (Sagi, 1990). Clearly, more research was needed to find precursors of attachment relationships in kibbutz children so as to understand the unusual rates of insecure relationships.

Communal sleeping in children's houses—the unique characteristic of a collective upbringing—was postulated by Sagi and his colleagues to be a possible antecedent for the development of insecure attachments, and a new study was designed to investigate this assumption. Before we describe this study, it should be noted that, until the mid-1980s, decisions about sleeping arrangements were closely related to ideological differences among the major kibbutz movements. The traditional, more politically socialist movement advocated communal sleeping and emphasized conservative interpretations of kibbutz ideology. Moreover, the transition to home-based sleeping brought further changes. The relative weight of the children's house and the influence of the metapelet were reduced in home-based sleeping, whereas the educational practices of both caregivers and parents were characterized as more permissive than in communal sleeping (Lavi, 1990b). Thus, it can be argued that sleeping arrangements were associated with a host of other important variations. However, the influence of these variations on developmental outcomes was not assessed separately from sleeping arrangements. Nathan (1984), in his summary of the relevant research, concluded that children who were raised in different sleeping arrangements were very similar on outcome variables including behavior disorders, social adjustment, self-image, and adolescents' autonomy from parents.

In a new quasi-experimental study, 23 mother-infant dyads from traditional kibbutzim (with communal sleeping arrangements) and 25 dyads from nontraditional kibbutzim (where family-based sleeping was instituted) were observed in the strange situation paradigm (Sagi, Van IJzendoorn, Aviezer, Donnell, & Mayseless, in press). The distribution of attachment relationships for communally sleeping infants was confirmed and was even more extreme than in the earlier study: Only 48% of the infants were securely attached to their mothers. However, the distribution for infants in family-based sleeping arrangements was completely different. Eighty percent of these infants were securely attached to their mothers, a rate similar to that found among urban Israeli infants (Sagi, Lamb, Lewkowicz, et al., 1985).

To rule out alternative explanations for the effect of communal sleeping arrangements, assessments were also made of the ecology of the children's house during the day, maternal separation anxiety, infants' temperament, and mother-infant play interactions. The two groups (i.e., family-based and communal sleepers) were found comparable on all of these variables. Thus, it was concluded that collective sleeping, experienced by infants as a time during which mothers were largely unavailable and inaccessible, was responsible for the greater insecurity found in this group. Inconsistent responsiveness was inherent in the reality of these infants, because sensitive responding by mother or caregiver during the day sharply contrasted with the presence of an unfamiliar person at night. Inconsistent responsiveness has previously been considered to be an important antecedent condition of insecure, ambivalent attachment (Ainsworth et al., 1978).

Figure 1 represents the distribution of attachment classifications with mothers and illustrates how the collective kibbutz samples differ from other groups in Israel and elsewhere in the world. The plot is based on an earlier correspondence analysis of the then-known studies of attachment (see Van IJzendoorn & Kroonenberg, 1988). In addition, we calculated the relative positions of the subgroups of kibbutzim both with and without collective sleeping from Sagi et al. (in press). The first dimension in Figure 1 shows a progression of an overrepresentation of the A classification on the left to an overrepresentation of the C classification on the right, the second dimension indicates a B versus A plus C overrepresentation. The plot clearly shows that the collective kibbutz samples are very much at variance with other Israeli samples and samples from other countries. The anomalous position of the collective kibbutz samples is accounted for by the overrepresentation of insecure and, particularly, ambivalent attachments. Thus, Sagi et al.'s (in press) recent findings underscore the sensitivity of the strange situation paradigm to the nature of infants' emotional communications with their caregivers, even though they are derived from experiences in variable rearing conditions embedded in various cultural contexts.

More evidence about problematic aspects of communal sleeping can be derived from the Adult Attachment Interview (AAI; Main & Goldwyn, 1991), which assesses adults' current mental representations with regard to their early childhood attachment relationships. Sagi et al. (1992) presented the AAI to 20 mothers from kibbutzim maintaining collective sleeping arrangements and to 25 mothers from home-sleeping kibbutzim. Parent-child concordance in attachment classifications was relatively low for the communally sleeping group (40%) and relatively high for the home-sleeping group (76%). Possibly, caring for infants within the ecology of collective sleeping may have disrupted the transmission of parents' internal model of relationships into their parenting style.

Sagi, Lamb, Lewkowicz, et al. (1985) also observed communally sleeping kibbutz infants with their fathers in the strange situation paradigm; they

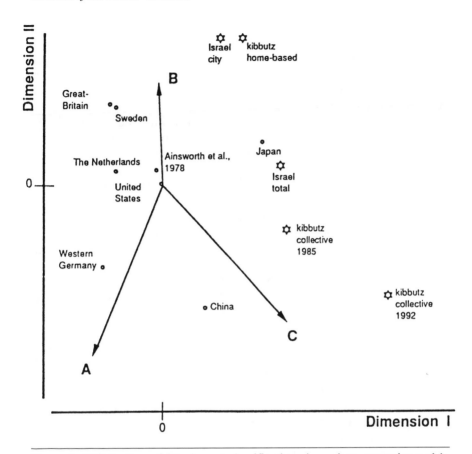

Figure 1. Distribution of attachment classifications in various countries and in various Israeli samples (based on Van IJzendoorn & Kroonenberg, 1988). This plot is based on the meta-analysis by Van IJzendoorn and Kroonenberg of almost 2,000 worldwide attachment classifications. The distribution of the attachment classifications is plotted for each country by use of correspondence analysis. The origin of the plot represents the global distributions. The distance between points represents discrepancy; the direction of the discrepancy is indicated by the three vectors. Van IJzendoorn and Kroonenberg provided locations of the data points. Only Ainsworth, Blehar, Waters, and Wall's (1978) sample and the Israeli samples have individual data points in this figure. Added to Van IJzendoorn and Kroonenberg's plot is the sample of Sagi, Van IJzendoorn, Aviezer, Donnell, and Mayseless (in press). This sample is indicated by kibbutz home-based and kibbutz collective 1992. This information is also accounted for in Israel total.

found that independent of the infants' attachment to mothers, the rates of secure attachments to fathers (67%) were no lower than those commonly found in other populations. This suggests that communal sleeping has presented no particular problem for infants' relationships with their fathers. Moreover, an examination of the behavior patterns of mothers and fathers at home with communally sleeping infants aged 8–16 months revealed that kibbutz mothers and fathers behave differently toward their infants during natural interactions, in a manner similar to mothers and fathers in other cultures. However, unlike other cultures, kibbutz infants showed no preference for one parent over the other (Sagi, Lamb, Shoham, Dvir, & Lewkowicz, 1985). The infants' lack of preference was interpreted as an indication that neither parent was functioning as the primary caregiver because kibbutz infants were being cared for in the children's house. It is possible, however, that the infants' behavior reflects their experience with parents who do not regard any part of child care as being the exclusive responsibility of only one parent (Shamai, 1992). In addition, kibbutz fathers tend to spend more time with their infants than do their urban counterparts (Sagi, Koren, & Weinberg, 1987); thus, it is possible that the time infants spend together with their parents may in itself be an important contribution to the relationships between parents and children (Clarke-Stewart, 1988).

Research on children in day care (Farran & Ramey, 1977; Goossens & Van IJzendoorn, 1990; Howes et al., 1992; Howes, Rodning, Galluzzo, & Meyers, 1988), and on kibbutz children (Fox, 1977; Sagi, Lamb, Lewkowicz, et al., 1985) has suggested that caregivers and teachers function as attachment figures in addition to the parents. Sagi, Lamb, Lewkowicz, et al. (1985) observed 84 kibbutz infants with their caregivers (metaplot) in the strange situation. They classified 53% of the infant-metaplot relationships as secure, independently of the classifications of these infants' relationships with their mothers and fathers. Goossens and Van IJzendoorn (1990), in a Dutch sample, and Howes et al. (1992), in an American sample, found similar rates of secure relationships between children and their caregivers (57% and 51%, respectively). Although these rates of security were somewhat lower than those commonly found between infants and parents, Sagi and Van IJzendoorn (in press) and Van IJzendoorn, Sagi, and Lambermon (1992) concluded, from an evaluation of two data sets (Goossens & Van IJzendoorn, 1990; Oppenheim, Sagi, & Lamb, 1988), that it is justified to argue that infants indeed develop attachment relationships to their professional caregivers and that these relationships reflect the interactive history of the caregiver-infant dyad. Note that the rates of secure relationships with mothers found in kibbutzim where communal sleeping is in force (59%) actually resemble rates found for secure relationships with caregivers

(51%–57%). One can conclude that in an environment of multiple caregivers, children form multiple attachment relationships that are independent of each other.

Note that the traditional argument favored by attachment theory (Main & Weston, 1981; Sroufe, 1985) about the lack of concordance in the attachment relationships of a single infant to its mother and father has been recently challenged by Fox, Kimmerly, and Schafer (1991). Their meta-analytic study on the concordance of infant-mother and infant-father attachment showed a significant—albeit small—degree of similarity between these two relationships. One might speculate that the concordance of attachment between parental and nonparental caregivers is weak or absent because assortative mating is much less likely to play a role. Steele, Steele, and Fonagy (1993) proposed that the concordance between infant-mother and infant-father attachment quality exists because of the concordance between maternal and paternal attachment representations. In a combination of studies on the concordance of attachment representations in husbands and wives, Van IJzendoorn and Bakermans-Kranenburg (in press) found a modest association: Secure wives are more often married to secure husbands than might be expected by chance. If attachment is transmitted across generations, this association would lead to a correspondence between infant attachment to father and infant attachment to mother. Although pertinent data are lacking, the same association seems unlikely between parental and nonparental attachment representations. In the same vein, maternal modeling of caregiving behaviors that might determine the quality of infant attachment is more likely between a child's mother and father than between the child's parents and nonparental caregivers. In an environment of multiple caregivers, therefore, attachment relationships might be independent, at least for parental and nonparental caregivers. More data on attachment networks and attachment representations in the kibbutz are needed to confirm these speculations.

Consequences of Attachment Relationships

These recent findings of attachment research in a sense support Rabin's (1965) argument that kibbutz infants suffer from a partial psychological deprivation; they also suggest that collective sleeping is an important contributing factor to this effect. Such a conclusion would be in accord with the findings of earlier research that collective sleeping has a long-lasting moderating impact on socioemotional needs and styles (Berman, 1988; Regev et al., 1980). Rabin conjectured that partial deprivation of this kind in infancy has a very limited long-term effect on development. Additional data must be examined to whether the quality of early relationships, as assessed in the strange situation paradigm, has a long-term developmental effect.

Oppenheim et al. (1988) assessed a broad spectrum of socioemotional competencies of most of the subjects in the sample of Sagi, Lamb, Lewkowicz, et al. (1985) when they were 5 years old in an attempt to understand the consequences of early relationships. They found that secure attachment to the caregiver during infancy was the strongest predictor of children being empathic, dominant, independent, achievement oriented, and behaviorally purposive in kindergarten; on the other hand, no significant relationships were found between these socioemotional developments and the quality of children's attachment to their parents. These results suggest that the influence of attachment relationships may be viewed as domain specific. Because the infants' relations with caregivers had been formed in the context of the infant house, they are the best predictor of children's socioemotional behavior in similar contexts.

However, one can expect attachment relationships in a multiple caregiver environment to interact in such a way that the predictive power of individual relationships is weaker than that of their combination (Howes et al., 1988; Tavecchio & Van IJzendoorn, 1987). Van IJzendoorn, Sagi, and Lambermon (1992) examined a sample of kibbutz children and a sample of Dutch children for the predictive power of the extended network of infants' relationships (mother, father, and professional caregiver) in comparison with the family network (mother and father) and the mother-infant relationship. They found that secure extended-network relationships were the best predictor of later advanced socioemotional functioning, although this finding was much stronger for kibbutz children. In the Dutch sample, the security of the extended network was related to children's higher developmental quotient and autonomous behavior in preschool. However, in the kibbutz sample, security of the extended network was related to a higher IQ and more independent behavior in kindergarten, as well as to higher ego resilience, ego control, field independence, dominance, goal-directed behavior, and empathy. Security of the family network in the kibbutz was also related to some of these variables, whereas infant-mother relationships were, by themselves, unrelated to any of the children's outcome variables. Thus, one can conclude that the quality of early relationships does predict future development. However, the ecology of infant care in regard to the extent of the child's exposure to multiple relationships determines the relative contribution of individual relationships to developmental outcome.

Moreover, there is evidence here, as well as in Howes et al. (1988), that within a matrix of multiple relationships, secure relationships with professional caregivers are not only feasible but also contribute to the child's well-being by either adding to a network of secure attachments or, possibly, compensating for their absence. Relationships between professional caregivers and children thus have the potential of adding a significant dimension to children's socioemotional development without interfering with the parent-child relationship, as was strongly believed by kibbutz educators (Gerson, 1978).

Summary and Discussion

The study of kibbutz child rearing from the perspective of attachment theory has allowed a direct assessment of the impact of multiple caregiving in infancy both on children's experience as infants and on their future development. Investigations of collective child rearing, with its unique philosophy and practices, highlight issues that may be pertinent to other multiple-care arrangements but tend to be overlooked or underrated. On the basis of data available from studies of kibbutz children, one can conclude that early extensive day care and the repeated separation from parents inherent to such care do not necessarily interfere with the formation of close relationships between parents and children. The similarly high rates of secure attachments found in kibbutzim practicing family-based sleeping and in Israeli day care centers, and their difference from both samples of communal sleeping (see Figure 1), suggest that neither day care nor kibbutz care can in itself explain the unusual rates of insecure attachments found in kibbutzim with collective sleeping arrangements. Rather, the increase in infants' insecurity probably reflects a child-care environment in which infants experience inconsistent care as a result of parental absence during the night without an adequate replacement.

Nevertheless, understanding the effects of collective sleeping, which is an extreme practice, may highlight the effects of the repeated separations from mothers that are inherent in any multiple caregiving arrangements, Two variables have been proposed to attenuate the effects of separations on the quality of infant attachment: high-quality alternative caregiving (Goossens, 1987; Howes et al., 1988), which may alleviate the stress that infants experience in situations of maternal absence, and maternal compensating efforts, which may moderate the effects of temporary traumatic separations (e.g., those occurring as a result of hospitalizations) so as not to result in long-term insecurity (Van IJzendoorn, Goldberg, Kroonenberg, & Frenkel, 1992). Collective sleeping arrangements have been problematic in both respects. Although kibbutzim have provided high-quality child care during the day, the quality of night care in the infant house has been poor because it has most often been provided by strangers who can offer only a precarious sense of security to the infants. On the other hand, maternal compensation is not very likely, because even sensitive parents may not feel an urgency to compensate for their absence during the night in a situation in which routinely implemented separations are the norm for all of the children in the community. This circumstance points to the dangers inherent in maintaining multiple care arrangements for infants without also guaranteeing alternative caregiving of adequate quality.

A number of studies have shown that quality caregiving (Droege & Howes, 1991; Howes et al., 1992; Rosenthal, 1991) is relevant to children's socioemotional development in that it determines the quality of children's experience in day care and affects parent-child relations (Goossens, 1987; Howes et al., 1988). In this regard, therefore, one should consider the discrepancy between the quality of collective child care during the day and during the night. More specifically, the low-quality aspect of kibbutz child care, which is associated with collective sleeping, must be controlled for when dealing with the broader controversy about the impact of extensive day-care experience in infancy on socioemotional development (Belsky 1988; Clarke-Stewart, 1988, 1989; Gamble & Zigler, 1986). Indeed, the finding of normal rates of secure attachment among kibbutz infants, who experience early and extensive care of high quality during the day and who sleep at home at night, is consistent with studies that suggest that high quality of care is an important determinant of children's socioemotional experience (e.g., Howes, 1990; Howes et al., 1992).

We have until now emphasized the increased rates of insecure attachment in situations of collective sleeping. However, one should not overlook the fact that almost 50% of the mothers of communally sleeping infants have been able to provide their infants with a sense of a consistent, secure relationship. This group underscores the need to understand resiliency in the face of adverse conditions (Belsky, 1990).

The finding that both the extended network and the family network in kibbutzim have more predictive power than does the mother-child relationship may be explained by the greater involvement of kibbutz fathers and caregivers in child care. Recall that the increased involvement of others in child care was regarded as beneficial to both women and children and had an important ideological value. In Israel, kibbutz fathers tend to spend more time with their infants than do nonkibbutz fathers (Sagi et al., 1987), possibly because the organization of kibbutz life allows both parents equal time to spend with their children. More time for leisure and availability of Israeli fathers have been found to determine the extent of their play and affiliative behaviors, whereas their attitudes and perceptions regarding fatherhood have predicted caregiving and play (Levy-Shiff & Israelashvili, 1988).

As a result of the high value placed by kibbutz culture on parental involvement (Shamal, 1992), no aspects of child care have been viewed by parents of either sex as being the exclusive responsibility of one parent or the other. Yet, the duties of professional caregiving have never been assumed by kibbutz men. Thus, it would seem that kibbutz fathers are relatively privileged because they have more leisure time with their children within a culture that values paternal involvement in child care but does not regard the father as having primary responsibility. However, in the name of women's equality, which used masculine criteria for achievements (Palgi, Blasi, Rosner, & Safir, 1983), maternal involvement in child care has been reduced. It would appear, then, that in comparison with other child-rearing environments, collective education has supported father-child relationships while being ambiguous toward mother-child relationships. This may explain the differential influence exerted by collective education combined with communal sleeping on infants' relationships with their mothers and fathers and the similarity in rates of security between mothers and caregivers (Sagi, Lamb, Lewkowicz, et al., 1985). Recently published autobiographical recollections of kibbutz-raised women (Leshem, 1991) support this conclusion.

The kibbutz data suggest that as women increase their involvement in out-of-home employment and increasingly share the duties of caring for their children with other caregivers (professionals or family members), the relative influence of the mother-child relationship may also change. Role changes within families, as they translate into daily functioning, may affect parental relationships with infants, and different child-rearing conditions may increase or decrease the influence of these relationships on children's development (Belsky, 1990). Given the processes of change experienced by many families, there is a need for more information about the attitudes of parents toward child care and parenting roles; such information will provide a better understanding of the interrelationships among child-care ecology, parental functioning, and children's relations with parents. The consequences of these changes for children's development in different ecologies and cultures remain an empirically open question. We have thus far focused on children's relations with various adults, but the collective orientation of the kibbutz has also been manifested in the role assigned to the peer group in the socialization of children. Therefore, our review would be incomplete without a discussion of the relations of kibbutz children with their peers.

RELATIONS WITH PEERS

In the educational conceptualization of collective education, the peer group was viewed as offering a natural environment for children's activity because it both directs their behavior and protects their independence (Golan, 1961). Group activities and sharing, as well as respect for the rights of others, were emphasized by adults from an early age (Rabin & Beit-Hallahmi, 1982). At the time, this view was at odds with the prevailing belief that young children were unable to benefit from group life because of their competition for the attention and love of adults (Freud, 1973; Isaacs, 1948) and their egocentric and non-communicative thinking (Piaget, 1959). Group living among children from the time of infancy, as practiced in kibbutzim, has intrigued some observers who have been impressed by the unexpected presence of emotional ties between infants and toddlers. Bettelheim (1969) and Kaffman (1965) described close relations between such infants and detected distress when one of the infants was absent. Zaslow (1980) found that individual group members were sought out as early as the end of the 1st year, and such closeness was influenced by sharing a room in the infants' house, mutual responsiveness, and close relations between parents. Spiro (1958) observed 10-month-old infants playing together so often that they seemed to be a subgroup within the large group and described the peer group as a constant source of stimulation as well as security. Winograd (1958) observed mutuality and empathy in the behavior of children much younger than the age at which such behaviors were assumed to be meaningful.

Recent research on infants and toddlers together (Eckerman & Didow, 1988) suggests that the observations just reported have captured a natural social capacity readily displayed by kibbutz children because of the intensive social character of their environment. Although infant sociability is viewed as a natural capacity, it must be distinguished from social competence, which refers to effectiveness with peers through coordinated interactions and reciprocal actions within a relevant affective context. Early peer encounters have been thought to provide children with the social experience necessary to support the development of social competence (Eckerman & Didow, 1988; Howes, 1988a). Moreover, it has been suggested that peer familiarity facilitates social interaction and the development of specific relationships based on the continued presence of the partner (Doyle, Connolly, & Rivest, 1980; Howes, 1988a). Kibbutz infants and toddlers are exposed to peers very early, the peer group is stable, and peer familiarity is very high. In addition, adults value the role of peers in children's lives. These features of peer experience have been found to facilitate social competence in young children (Howes, 1988a); thus, one can expect social competence to be well developed among kibbutz children.

Two kinds of studies have assessed social competence in kibbutz infants, toddlers, and preschoolers: investigations of group processes and peer relationship formation and assessments of play quality as a demonstration of social skills. The data indicate that kibbutz children are competent in both respects. Faigin (1958) found that 2-year-old toddlers had already developed a strong identity with the group, expressed in concepts such as "we" and "ours" and by mutual defense of group members in between-groups competitions and rivalries. Although leadership belongs to the metapelet, the group functions as a socializing agent in terms of controlling the behavior of its members. Laikin, Laikin, and Constanzo (1979), as well as Y. Harel (1979), explored group processes in toddler groups and identified group behaviors at very young ages; however, role taking, following group "rules," and negotiations in regard to objects and toys were found to be behaviors that develop with age. Play in groups formed according to children's choice, which increased in frequency between the ages of 24 and 30 months, involved more mature and intensive social interactions than parallel play or whole-group activities not involving choice (Y. Harel, 1979).

Ross, Conant, Cheyne, and Alevizos (1992) recently published a study that investigated toddlers' relationships and conflict interventions in two kibbutz groups whose members' average age was 20 months. They found that unique adjustments were made by children in their interactions with specific partners and observed conflicts as well as positive interactions. These adjustments tended to be mutual and spanned broad periods of time, thus taking the form of reciprocal relationships in which conflicts and positive interactions were integrated. Considerations of rights and fairness seemed to guide third-party conflict interventions, which sometimes involved attempts to mediate, compensate, or reprimand; however, alliances more than fairness determined the outcome of a conflict. These behaviors were taken as an indication that very young children are able to sort out the nature of social exchanges in which they were not initially involved. The nature of peer relations in these groups, with their siblinglike familiarity that afforded members a comfortable context for acquiring social experience, may have made such sophisticated behaviors possible.

Studies that have evaluated play quality and social behavior among kibbutz and urban Israeli children reveal that kibbutz children are very skilled social players. Toddlers from kibbutzim were found to be more likely to engage in positive social interaction with peers than family day-care and center day-care children (Rosenthal, 1991). Kibbutz toddlers were more involved in associative–dramatic play and showed less unoccupied behavior and parallel play. Functional play appeared earlier in kibbutz nursery school children, but it was more frequently observed among urban kindergarten children (Meerovitch, 1990). Finally, kibbutz children displayed coordinated play more frequently and were less competitive in group encounters and less involved in object exchange and struggle over toys; however, they were also less affectively involved with their peers and more verbally aggressive than were urban nursery school children. When kibbutz children were not interacting with peers, they spent more time in solitary play and interaction with the caregivers and less time watching their peers (Levy-Shiff & Hoffman, 1985). However, communally sleeping preschoolers exhibited lower levels of effective problem solving but higher autonomy in daily routine tasks, despite parents' reports that did not indicate that kibbutz children were less attached to them (Levy-Shiff, 1983).

The data suggest that although social competence is developmental, the social environment that provides the context for its acquisition has a strong impact. The attitudes of adults toward early peer interaction influence the social environment of children and thus may play an important role in children's social experience (Howes, 1988a). Indeed, kibbutz caregivers emphasize group behaviors at a very early stage (Faigin, 1958; Rabin & Beit-Hallahmi, 1982). In interviews, caregivers have reported that they encourage children to help one another and to share (Laikin et al., 1979), as well as to engage in social rather than individualistic achievements (Meerovitch, 1990). In addition, adult actions and attitudes have been observed to have an impact on children's behaviors. Y. Harel (1979) reported that children used initiations and rule-setting behaviors to which they had previously been introduced by their caregivers, and Zaslow (1980) identified close relationships between parents as a variable related to closeness between infants. Richman's (1990) findings supported the hypothesis that kibbutz children will behave more prosocially than nonkibbutz children because prosocial behavior reflects children's experience with expectations in their environment. Moreover, he found that kibbutz kindergarten children whose parents and caregivers were themselves kibbutz born helped more and that kibbutz children whose metaplot were kibbutz born shared more. Richman thus concluded that the expectations of kibbutz-born adults concerning prosocial behavior have had an impact on the children they bring up.

The research reported thus far suggests that peers are emotionally important to kibbutz infants and toddlers and that prosocial behaviors are found at a very early age among kibbutz children. However, social behaviors are developmental, and adults play an important part in the learning of such behaviors. It seems reasonable to assume that the influence of the peer group derives from its stable presence and from the continuity of interpersonal relationships that it allows, as well as from adult emphasis on the importance of the group and of group rules and values. The pervasiveness of the early peer group may also be illustrated with studies that have shown that early peers do not tend to marry each other in adulthood because they seem to consider themselves more like siblings (Shepher, 1971).

However, a complex picture regarding the development of social competence emerges from this review. It seems that young kibbutz children display advanced group-oriented skills and sophisticated behaviors in peer interactions together with indications of greater affective distancing and lower levels of affective problem-solving skills. Affective behavior and problem-solving skills—neither of which are group-oriented skills—are involved in social competence and have been predicted on the basis of the quality of attachment relationships (Sroufe & Fleeson, 1986), which also determine children's social competence in interactions with peers (Easterbrooks & Lamb, 1979; Sroufe & Fleeson, 1986). Within this framework of attachment theory, both lower problem skills and lower capacity for intimacy can be related to the higher rates of insecurity found among communally sleeping infants (Sagi, Lamb, Lewkowicz, et al., 1985; Sagi et al., in press), thereby explaining the coexistence of high sociability and low intimacy.

Thus, the intensive social nature of the environment of kibbutz children could support their acquisition of advanced social skills, whereas the complicated socioemotional nature of their experience in communal sleeping underlies their affective behaviors and style. This theoretical basis allows one to predict that home-based kibbutz toddlers will be more competent than their collectively sleeping counterparts. Indeed, Laikin et al. (1979) found more mature social interaction in groups of home-based sleeping toddlers than in communally sleeping groups, which they explained in terms of different interactive needs. Alternatively, the higher competence of home-based toddlers may be attributed to the more extensive nature of their interpersonal experience in their families. Unfortunately, these conclusions are only tentative because no research, to the best of our knowledge, has directly explored the association between family interactions and social competence among kibbutz children from the two ecologies. Moreover, because the studies of social competence in kibbutz children represent a variety of theoretical formulations, operational definitions, and measurements, it is difficult to derive a single conclusive interpretation. The various facets of social development in very young children who experience an intensive social environment, as increasing numbers of children do, and the specific conditions that shape social development are topics for further research, which may be especially interesting to pursue with kibbutz children.

SUMMARY AND CONCLUSIONS

Collective child-rearing represents a special case of group care because children's exposure to multiple significant others and to peer-group living, although serving adults' goals, was put into practice as a result of the belief of adults that it was beneficial to children. The present review shows that collective kibbutz education has undergone tremendous changes in the course of the 70 years of its existence. Initially, an extreme form of collectivism, motivated by economic needs and ideological convictions, was instituted. Its intended goal was to nourish a "new type" of human being that would be untainted by the shortcomings that those who instituted the practice had observed in their own upbringing.

Judged strictly in terms of this ambition alone, collective education can be regarded as a failure. The family as the basic social unit has not been abolished in kibbutzim. On the contrary, familistic trends have become stronger than ever, and kibbutz parents have reclaimed their rights to care for their own children. Collective education has not produced a new type of human being, and any differences found between adults raised on and off the kibbutz have been minimal. Moreover, research results indicate that collective sleeping arrangements for children negatively affect socioemotional development in the direction of a more anxious and restrained personality. Collective sleeping, which may have been justified in early periods in the history of kibbutzim, was abolished as it became clear that it did not serve the emotional needs of most kibbutz members. Its disappearance demonstrates the limits of adaptability of parents and children to inappropriate child-care arrangements.

However, setting aside communal sleeping as too radical a practice, collective child rearing seen from a broader perspective has to its credit remarkable achievements unprecedented in other cultures. It has furnished high-quality care for all of the children in the community without exception and long before multiple caregiving was contemplated for the population at large. Only in Eastern Europe have such attempts been made, at the cost of providing mediocre care (Weigl & Weber, 1991). Collective education has developed a long-term practice of normal multiple caregiving that is supported by caregivers and parents, as well as the community.

Thus, with the discontinuance of collective sleeping, secure relationships have come to prevail to an extent similar to that found among nonkibbutz children. Collective education affords children the benefit of a network of relationships in a supportive environment.

The kibbutz practice of raising children in peer groups from infancy highlights the role of peers in children's social experiences and the contribution of these experiences to the development of social competence. However, social competence is a multifaceted construct that includes group-oriented skills as well as intimacy, affective behavior, and emotional style. Group oriented skills can be facilitated by a social environment of familiar peers in which group behaviors are supported by adults' guidance. The affective dimension seems to require secure relationships with sensitive and responsive adults; these relationships may provide the foundation for the capacity to enter intimate relations with others. Further research is needed to understand the complexities of children's social competence.

The kibbutz, as a unique experiment in nature (Beit-Hallahmi & Rabin, 1977), has contributed to theories of early socioemotional development while reiterating the detrimental effects of poor-quality care in institutional settings (Bowlby, 1951; Spitz, 1946). Nevertheless, leaving aside the practice of communal sleeping arrangements, the kibbutz child-care system demonstrates the potentials of sharing tasks and responsibilities of child rearing with nonparental caregivers—without detrimental effects for either the children or the parents involved—and underscores some of the conditions that have to be taken into account in the current day-care debate regarding the influence of extensive day-care experiences during infancy on later socioemotional development.

REFERENCES

Ainsworth, M. D. S., Blehar M., Waters, E., & Wall, S. (1978). *Patterns of attachment.* Hillsdale, NJ: Erlbaum.

Alon, M. (1976). Mishnato hachinuchit shel Shmuel Golan [The educational thought of Shmuel Golan]. In Y. Arnon (Ed.), *Hachinuch hameshutaf* (pp. 11–24). Tel Aviv, Israel: Sifriyat Poalim.

Anthony, E. J., & Bene, E. (1957). A technique from the objective assessment of the child's family relationships. *Journal of Mental Science, 103,* 541–555.

Barry, H., & Paxton, L. M. (1971). Infancy and early childhood: Cross-cultural codes 2. *Ethnology, 10,* 466–508.

Bar-Yosef, R. (1959). The pattern of early socialization in the collective settlements of Israel. *Human Relations, 12,* 345–360.

Beck, S. J. (1950). *Rorschach's test* (Vol. 1). New York: Grune & Stratton.

Beit-Hallahmi, B. (1981). The kibbutz family revival or survival. *Journal of Family Issues, 2,* 259–274.

Beit-Hallahmi, B., & Rabin, A. (1977). The kibbutz as a social experiment and as a child-rearing laboratory. *American Psychologist, 12,* 57–69.

Belsky, J. (1988). The effects of infant day-care reconsidered. *Early Childhood Research Quarterly, 3,* 235–272.

Belsky, J. (1990). Parental and nonparental child care and children's socio-emotional development: A decade in review. *Journal of Marriage and the Family, 52,* 885–903.

Ben-Yaakov, Y. (1972). Methods of kibbutz collective education during early childhood. In J. Marcus (Ed.), *Growing up in groups* (pp. 197–295). London: Gordon & Beach.

Berman, E. (1988). Communal upbringing in the kibbutz. *Psychoanalytic Study of the Child, 43,* 319–335.

Bettelheim, B. (1969). *The children of the dream.* London: Collier-Macmillan.

Bowlby, J. (1951). *Maternal care and mental health.* Geneva: World Health Organization.

Bowlby, J. (1982). *Attachment and loss: Vol 1. Attachment.* New York: Basic Books. (Original work published 1969).

Bronson, G. W. (1968). The development of fear in man and other animals. *Child Development, 39,* 409–432.

Clarke-Stewart, K. A. (1988). "The effects of infant day-care reconsidered" reconsidered: Risks for parents, children, and researchers. *Early Childhood Research Quarterly, 3,* 292–318.

Clarke-Stewart, K. A. (1989). Infant day care: Maligned or malignant? *American Psychologist, 44,* 266–273.

Doyle, A., Connolly, J., & Rivest, L. (1980). The effect of playmate familiarity on the social interaction of young children. *Child Development, 51,* 217–223.

Droege, K. L., & Howes, C. (1991, July). *The influence of caregiver behavior on children's affective displays.* Paper presented at the biennial meeting of the International Society for the Study of Behavioral Development, Minneapolis, MN.

Easterbrooks, M. A., & Lamb, M. (1979). The relationship between quality of infant-mother attachment and infant competence in initial encounters with peers. *Child Development, 50,* 380–387.

Eckerman, C.O., & Didow, S. M.(1988). Lessons drawn from observing young peers together. *Acta Padiatrica Scandinavica, 77*(Suppl. 344), 55–70.

Epstein, R. (1992, March). *Sheina bakibbutz—Lina meshutefet mul lina mishpachtit* [Sleep in the kibbutz—collective versus home-base sleeping]. Paper presented at the Technion Workshop on Studies of Sleep in Children. Haifa, Israel.

Faigin, H. (1958). Social behavior of young children in the kibbutz. *Journal of Abnormal and Social Psychology, 56*, 117–129.

Farran, D. C., & Ramey, C. T. (1977). Infant day care and attachment behaviors toward mothers and teachers. *Child Development, 48*, 1112–1116.

Fein, G. G., & Fox, N. (1988). Infant day care: A special issue. *Early Childhood Research Quarterly, 3*, 227–234.

Feldman, S. S., & Yirmiya, N. (1986). Perception of socialization roles: A study of Israeli mothers in town and kibbutz. *International Journal of Psychology, 21*, 153–165.

Fölling-Albers, M. (1988a, July). *Education in the kibbutz as "women's business": Emancipation of women between idea and reality.* Paper presented at Utopian Thought and Communal Experience, New Lanark, Scotland.

Fölling-Albers, M. (1988b). Erziehung und frauenfrage im kibbutz [Child rearing and women's emancipation in the kibbutz]. In W. Melzer & G. Neubauer (Eds.) *Der kibbutz als utopie* (pp. 88–120). Basel, Switzerland: Beltz.

Fox, N. (1977). Attachment of kibbutz infants to mother and metapelet. *Child Development, 48*, 1228–1239.

Fox, N., Kimmerly, N. L., & Schafer, W. D. (1991). Attachment to mother/attachment to father: A meta-analysis. *Child Development, 62*, 210–225.

Freud, A. (1973). *Normality and pathology in childhood.* London: Hogarth Press.

Gamble, T. J., & Zigler, E. (1986). Effects of infant daycare: Another look at the evidence. *American Journal of Orthopsychiatry, 56*, 26–42.

Gerson, M. (1976). Hitnahaguta hachinuchit shel metapelet bapeuton [The educational behavior of a caregiver in the toddlers' house]. In Y. Arnon (Ed.), *Hachinuch hameshutaf* (pp. 123–144). Tel Aviv, Israel: Sifriyat Hapoalim.

Gerson, M. (1978). *Family women, and socialization in the kibbutz.* Lexington, MA: Heath.

Gerson, M., & Nathan, M. (1969). Seker hametaplot bagil harach batnua hakibutzit [A survey of caregivers in early education in the kibbutz movement]. *Yediot (3).* Oranim, Israel: Institute for Research on Collective Education.

Gerson, M., & Schnabel-Brandes, A. (1990). The educational approach of the metapelet of young children in the kibbutz. In Z. Lavi (Ed.), *Kibbutz members study kibbutz children* (pp. 40–49). New York: Greenwood Press.

Gewirtz, J. (1965). The course of infant smiling in four child-rearing environments in Israel. In B. M. Foss (Ed.), *Determinants of infant behavior III* (pp. 205–260), New York: Wiley.

Golan, S. (1958). Collective education in the kibbutz. *American Journal of Orthopsychiatry, 28*, 549–556.

Golan, S. (1959). Collective education in the kibbutz. *Psychiatry, 22*, 167–177.

Golan, S. (1961). *Hachinuch hameshutaf* [Collective education]. Tel Aviv, Israel: Sifriat Poalim.

Goossens, F. A. (1987). Maternal employment and day care: Effects on attachment. In L. W. C. Tavecchio & M. H. van IJzandoorn (Eds.), *Attachment in social networks* (pp. 135–183). Amsterdam: Elsevier.

Goossens, F. A., & Van IJzendoorn, M. H. (1990). Quality of infants' attachment to professional caregivers: Relations to infant-parent attachment and day-care characteristics. *Child Development, 61,* 832–837.

Greenbaum, C. W., & Landau, R. (1977). Mothers' speech and the early development of vocal behavior: Findings from a cross-cultural observation study in Israel. In P. H. Leiderman, S. R. Tulkin, & A. Rosenfeld (Eds.), *Culture and infancy: Variations in the human experience* (pp. 245–270). San Diego, CA: Academic Press.

Grossmann, K., Grossmann, K. E., Spangler, G., Suess, G., & Unzner, L. (1985). Maternal sensitivity and newborns' orientation responses as related to quality of attachment in northern Germany. *Monographs of the Society for Research in Child Development, 50* (1–2, Serial No. 209).

Hass, M. (1986). *Peutim poalim umitnasim beargaz hagrutaot ubeteivot peilut* [Toddlers acting and experiencing the junk and activity boxes]. Oranim, Israel: Institute for the Teaching of Science and the Improvement of Teaching Methods.

Harel, M. (1986, September). *Dialogues at risk.* Paper presented at the International Conference for Infant Mental Health, Chicago.

Harel, Y. (1979). *Hitnahagut chevratit bikvutsat peutot bakibbutz* [Social behavior in toddlers' groups in the kibbutz]. Unpublished master's thesis, University of Haifa, Haifa, Israel.

Hazan, B. (1973). Introduction. In A. I. Rabin & B. Hazan (Eds.), *Collective education in the kibbutz* (pp. 1–10). New York: Springer.

Holdstein, I., & Borus, J. F. (1976). Kibbutz and city children: A comparative study of syntactic and articulatory abilities. *Journal of Speech and Hearing Disorders, 4,* 10–15.

Howes, C. (1988a). Peer interaction of young children. *Monographs of the Society for Research in Child Development, 53* (1, Serial No. 217).

Howes, C. (1988b). Relations between early child care and schooling. *Developmental Psychology, 24,* 53–57.

Howes, C. (1990). Can age of entry into child care and the quality of child care predict adjustment in kindergarten? *Developmental Psychology, 26,* 292–303.

Howes, C., Phillips, D. A., & Whitebook, M. (1992). Thresholds of quality: Implications for the social development of children in center-based child care. *Child Development, 63,* 449–460.

Howes, C., Rodning, C., Galluzzo, D. C., & Meyers, L. (1988). Attachment and child care: Relationships with mother and caregiver. *Early Childhood Research Quarterly, 3*, 403–416.

Irvine, E. E. (1952). Observations on the aims and methods of child rearing in communal settlements in Israel. *Human Relations, 5*, 247–275.

Isaacs, S. (1948). *Social development in young children.* London: Paul, Trench, & Trubner.

Kaffman, M. (1965). A comparison of psychopathology: Israeli children from kibbutz and from urban surroundings. *American Journal of Orthopsychiatry, 35*, 509–520.

Kaffman, M., Elizur, E., & Rabinowitz, M. (1990). Early childhood in the kibbutz: The 1980s. In Z. Lavi (Ed.), Kibbutz members study kibbutz children (pp. 17–33). New York: Greenwood Press.

Keller, S. (1983). The family in the kibbutz: What lessons for us? In M. Palgi, J, R. Blasi, M. Rosner, & M. Safir (Eds.), *Sexual equality: The Israeli kibbutz tests the theories* (pp. 227–251). Norwood, PA: Norwood.

Kohen-Raz, R. (1968). Mental and motor development of kibbutz, institutionalized and home-reared infants in Israel. *Child Development, 39*, 489–504.

Konner, M. (1977). Infancy among the Kalahari desert San. In P. H. Leiderman, S. R. Tulkin, & A. H. Rosenfeld (Eds.), *Culture and infancy* (pp. 287–328). San Diego, CA: Academic Press.

Laikin, N. G., Laikin, M., & Constanzo, P. R. (1979). Group processes in early childhood: A dimension of human development. *International Journal of Behavioral Development, 2*, 171–183.

Lamb, M. E., Sternberg, K. J., Hwang, C. P., & Broberg, A. G. (Eds.). (1992). *Child care in context: Cross cultural perspectives.* Hillsdale, NJ: Erlbaum.

Lamb, M. E., Thompson, R. A., & Gardner: W. (1985). Measuring individual differences in strange situation behavior. In M. E. Lamb, R. A. Thompson, W. Gardner, & E. L. Charnov (Eds.), *Infant-mother attachment* (pp. 203–222). Hillsdale, NJ: Erlbaum.

Lavi, Z. (1984, April). *Correlates of sleeping arrangements of infants in kibbutzim.* Paper presented at the International Conference for Infant Studies, New York.

Lavi, Z. (1990a). Introduction. In Z. Lavi (Ed.), *Kibbutz members study kibbutz children* (pp. 1–16). New York: Greenwood Press.

Lavi, Z. (1990b). Transition from communal to family sleeping arrangement of children in kibbutzim: Causes and outcome. In Z. Lavi (Ed.), *Kibbutz members study kibbutz children* (pp. 51–55). New York: Greenwood Press.

Leshem, N. (1991). *Shirat hadeshe* [The song of the grass: Conversations with women of the kibbutz first generation]. Ramat Efal, Israel: Yad Tabenkin.

Levy-Shiff, R. (1983). Adaptation and competence in early childhood: Communally raised kibbutz children versus family raised children in the city. *Child Development, 54*, 1606–1614.

Levy-Shiff, R., & Hoffman, M. A. (1985). Social behavior of urban and kibbutz preschool children in Israel. *Developmental Psychology, 21*, 1204–1205.

Levy-Shiff, R., & Israelashvili, R. (1988). Antecedents of fathering: Some further exploration. *Developmental Psychology, 24*, 434–440.

Lewin, G. (1982). Megamot bachinuch bagil harach [Trends in early education]. *Hachinuch Hameshataf, 105*, 29–35.

Lewin, G. (1983). Kvutsat hapeutim vehametapelot—Ma kore lema'ase? [The toddlers' group and the caregivers—What happens in practice?]. *Hachinuch Hameshutaf, 108*, 4–24.

Lewin, G. (1985). *Tahalichei shinui bachinuch hameshutaf bagil harach* [Processes of change in early care in collective education]. Oranim, Israel: Institute for the Teaching of Science and the Improvement of Teaching Methods.

Lewin, G. (1986). Hachinuch hameshutaf leor hazichronot [Collective education as reflected in memories]. *Hachinuch Hameshutaf, 122*, 4–83.

Lewin, G. (1990). Motherhood in the kibbutz. In Z. Lavi (Ed.), *Kibbutz members study kibbutz children* (pp. 34–39). New York: Greenwood Press.

Liegle, L. (1974). *Gezin en gemeenschap in de kibboetz* [Family and community in the kibbutz]. Utrecht, The Netherlands: Spectrum.

Maccoby, E., & Feldman, S. (1972). Mother attachment and stranger reactions in the third year of life. *Monographs of the Society for Research in Child Development, 37*(1, Serial No. 146).

Machover, K. (1949). *Personality projection in the drawing of the human figure.* Springfield, IL: Charles C Thomas.

Main, M. (1990). Cross-cultural studies of attachment organization: Recent studies, changing methodologies, and the concept of conditional strategies. *Human Development, 33*, 48–61.

Main, M., & Goldwyn, R. (1991). *Adult attachment rating and classification systems.* Unpublished manuscript, University of California, Berkeley.

Main, M., & Weston, D. R. (1981). The quality of toddler's relationship to mother and to father: Related to conflict behavior and the readiness to establish new relationships. *Child Development, 52*, 932–940.

Meerovitch, A. (1990). *Hitpatchut hamischak bagil harach bair ubakibbutz—Hashpa'at hasviva al hitpatchut hahebetim hakognitivi vehachevrati shel hamischak bagil harach* [Early childhood play development in the kibbutz and in the city—Influence of the environment on development of the cognitive and social aspects of play in early childhood]. Unpublished master's thesis, Bar Ilan University, Ramat Gan, Israel.

Melhuish, E. C., & Moss, P. (1991). *Day care for young children: International perspectives.* London: Tavistock.

Melzer, W. (1988). Die bedeutung von utopien fur die genese der kibbutzim und ihres erziehungsarrangements [The importance of utopias for the creation of kibbutzim and their educational practices]. In W. Melzer & G. Neubauer (Eds.), *Der kibbutz als utopie* (pp. 38–69). Basel, Switzerland: Beltz.

Melzer, W., & Neubauer. G. (1988). Was ist ein kibbutz? Theoretischer anspruch und wirklichkeit-erfahren in kibbutz Ayeleth Hashahar [What is a kibbutz? Theory and practice in kibbutz Ayeleth-Hashahar]. In W. Melzer & G. Neubauer (Eds.), *Der kibbutz als utopie* (pp. 24–37). Basel, Switzerland: Beltz.

Morelli, G. A., & Tronick, E. Z. (1991). Efe multiple caretaking and attachment. In J. L. Gewirtz & W. M. Kurtines (Eds.), *Intersections with attachment* (pp. 41–51). Hillsdale, NJ: Erlbaum.

Murray, H. A. (1943). *Thematic Apperception Test manual.* Cambridge, MA: Harvard University Press.

Nathan, M. (1984). *Lina meshutefet—Lina mishpahtit, takzirei vesikoumei mechkarim* [Communal versus familial children's sleeping arrangement: Abstract and summaries of studies]. *Yediot (15).* Oranim, Israel: Institute for Research on Collective Education.

Ophir-Cohen, M., Epstein, R., Tzisehinsky, O., Tirosh, E., & Lavie, P. (in press). Sleep patterns of children sleeping in residential care, in kibbutz dormitories and at home—A comparative study. *Sleep.*

Oppenheim, D., Sagi, A., & Lamb, M. E. (1988). Infant-adult attachments on the kibbutz and their relation to socioemotional development 4 years later. *Developmental Psychology, 24,* 427–433.

Palgi, M., Blasi, J. R., Rosner, M., & Sahr, M. (Eds.). (1983). *Sexual equality: The Israeli kibbutz tests the theories.* Norwood, PA: Norwood.

Phillips, D. A., & Howes, C. (1987). Indicators of quality in child care: Review of research. In D. A. Phillips (Ed.), *Quality in child care: What does research tell us?* (pp. 1–20). Washington, DC: National Association for the Education of Young Children.

Piaget, J. (1959). *The language and thought of the child.* London: Routledge & Kagan.

Rabin, A. I. (1958). Infants and children under conditions of "intermittent" mothering in the kibbutz. *American Journal of Orthopsychiatry, 28,* 576–586.

Rabin, A. I. (1965). *Growing up in the kibbutz.* New York: Springer:

Rabin, A. I., & Beit-Hallahmi, B. (1982). *Twenty years later.* New York: Springer.

Rapaport, D. (1958). The study of kibbutz education and its bearing on the theory of development. *American Journal of Orthopsychiatry, 28,* 587–597.

Regev, E., Beit-Hallhami, B., & Sharabany, R. (1980). Affective expression in kibbutz-communal, kibbutz-familial, and city-raised children in Israel. *Child Development, 51,* 223–237.

Richman, C. L. (1990, May). *Factors related to the prosocial development of kibbutz children.* Paper presented at the meeting of the American Psychological Society, Dallas, TX.

Rosenthal, M. (1991). Daily experiences of toddlers in three child care settings in Israel. *Child and Youth Care Forum, 20,* 37–58.

Ross, H. S., Conant, C., Cheyne, J. A., & Alevizos, E. (1992). Relationships and alliances in the social interaction of kibbutz toddler. *Social Development, 1,* 1–16.

Sacks, J. M., & Levy, S. (1950). The sentence completion test. In L. E. Abt & L. Bellak (Eds.), *Projective psychology* (pp. 357–402). New York: Knopf.

Sadeh, A., Lavie, P., Scher, A., Tirosh, E., & Epstein, R. (1991). Actigraphic home monitoring of sleep-disturbed and control infants and young children: A new method for pediatric assessment of sleep-wake patterns. *Pediatrics, 87,* 494–499.

Sagi, A. (1990). Attachment theory and research from a cross-cultural perspective. *Human Development, 33,* 10–22.

Sagi, A., Aviezer, O., Joels, T., Koren-Karie, N., Mayseless, O., Sharf, M., & Van IJzendoorn, M. H. (1992, July). *The correspondence of mother's adult attachment with infant-mother attachment relationship in traditional and non-traditional kibbutzim.* Paper presented at the XXV International Congress of Psychology, Brussels, Belgium.

Sagi, A., Koren, N., & Weinberg, M. (1987). Fathers in Israel. In M. E. Lamb (Ed.), *The father's role: Cross-cultural perspectives* (pp. 197–226). Hillsdale, NJ: Erlbaum.

Sagi, A., & Koren-Karie, N. (1993). Day-care centers in Israel: An overview. In M. Cochran (Ed.), *International handbook of day-care policies and programs* (pp. 269–290). New York: Greenwood Press.

Sagi, A., Lamb, M. E., Lewkowicz, K., Shoham, R., Dvir, R., & Estes, D. (1985). Security of infant-mother, -father, and -metapelet attachments among kibbutz-reared Israeli children. *Monographs of the Society for Research in Child Development, 50* (1–2, Serial No. 209).

Sagi, A., Lamb, M. E., Shoham, R., Dvir, R., & Lewkowicz, K. (1985). Parent-infant interaction in families on Israeli kibbutzim. *International Journal of Behavioral Development, 8,* 273–284.

Sagi, A., & Van IJzendoorn, M. H. (in press). Multiple caregiving environments: The kibbutz experience. In S. Harel & J. P. Shonkoff (Eds.), *Early childhood intervention and family support programs: Accomplishments and challenges.* Baltimore: Paul H. Brooks.

Sagi, A., Van IJzendoorn, M. H., Aviezer, O., Donnell, F., & Mayseless, O. (in press). Sleeping away from home in a kibbutz communal arrangement: It makes a difference for infant-mother attachment. *Child Development.*

Sagi, A., Van IJzendoorn, M. H., & Koren-Karie, N. (1991). Primary appraisal of the strange situation: A cross-cultural analysis of the pre-separation episodes. *Developmental Psychology, 27,* 587–596.

Selier: F. J. M. (1977). *Kibboetz, gezin en gelijkheidsideaal* [Kibbutz, family and the ideal of equality]. Assen, The Netherlands: Van Gorcum.

Shamai, S. (1992). *Patterns of paternal involvement in the kibbutz: The role of fathers in intact families in the education of their preadolescent children.* Unpublished master's thesis, Haifa University, Haifa, Israel.

Shepher, J. (1971). Mate selection among second generation kibbutz adolescents and adults: Incest avoidance and negative imprinting. *Archives of Sexual Behavior, 1,* 293–307.

Spiro, M. E. (1958). *Children of the kibbutz.* Cambridge, MA: Harvard University Press.

Spiro, M. E. (1979). *Gender and culture: Kibbutz women revisited.* Durham, NC: Duke University Press.

Spitz, R. A. (1946). Hospitalism: A follow-up report. In *The psychoanalytic study of the child* (Vol. 2, pp. 113–117). Madison, CT: International Universities Press.

Spitz, R. A. (1965). *The first year of life: A psychoanalytic study of deviant object relations.* Madison, CT: International Universities Press.

Sroufe, L. A. (1985). Attachment classification from the perspective of infant-caregiver relationships and infant temperament. *Child Development, 56,* 1–14.

Sroufe, L. A., & Fleeson, J. (1986). Attachment and the construction of relationships. In W. Hartup & Z. Rubin (Eds.), *Relationships and development* (pp. 51–71). Hillsdale, NJ: Erlbaum.

Steele, M., Steele, H., & Fonagy, P. (1993, August). *Associations among attachment classifications of mothers, fathers, and their infants: Evidence for a relationship-specific perspective.* Paper presented at the 4th European Conference on Developmental Psychology, Bonn.

Tavecchio, L. W. C., & Van IJzendoorn, M. H. (Eds.). (1987). *Attachment in social networks.* Amsterdam: Elsevier.

Tiger, L., & Shepher, J. (1975). *Women in the kibbutz.* San Diego, CA: Harcourt Brace Jovanovich.

Tronick, E. Z., Winn, S., & Morelli, G. A. (1985). Multiple caretaking in the context of human evolution: Why don't the Efe know the Western prescription for child care? In M. Reite & T. Field (Eds.), *The psychology of attachment and separation* (pp. 293–322). San Diego, CA: Academic Press.

Van IJzendoorn, M. H. (1990). Developments in cross-cultural research on attachment: Some methodological notes. *Human Development, 33,* 3–9.

Van IJzendoorn, M. H., & Bakermans-Kranenburg, M. J. (in press). Attachment representations in mothers, fathers, and clinical groups: A meta-analytic search for normative data. *Journal of Consulting and Clinical Psychology.*

Van IJzendoorn, M. H., Goldberg, S., Kroonenberg, P. M., & Frenkel, O. J. (1992). The relative effects of maternal and child problems on the quality of attachment: A meta-analysis of attachment in clinical samples. *Child Development, 63,* 840–858.

Van IJzendoorn, M. H., & Kroonenberg, P. M. (1988). Cross-cultural patterns of attachment: A meta-analysis of the strange situation. *Child Development, 59,* 147–156.

Van IJzendoorn, M. H., Sagi, A., & Lambermon, M. W. (1992). The multiple caretaker paradox: Some data from Holland and Israel. *New Directions in Child Development, 57,* 5–24.

Weigl, I., & Weber, C. (1991) Day care for young children in the German Democratic Republic. In E. C. Melhuish & P. Moss (Eds.), *Day care for young children* (pp. 46–55). London: Tavistock.

Weinbaum, E. (1990, August). *Family and kibbutz child-rearing effects on emotional moderation.* Paper presented at the 98th Annual Convention of the American Psychological Association, Boston, MA.

Whitebook, M., Howes, C., & Phillips, D. (1989). Who cares? *Child care teachers and the quality of care in America: The national child care staffing study.* Oakland, CA: Child Care Employee Project.

Winograd, M. (1958). The development of the young child in a collective settlement. *American Journal of Orthopsychiatry, 28,* 557–562.

Zaslow, M. (1980). Relationships among peers in kibbutz toddler groups. *Child Psychiatry and Human Development, 10,* 178–189.

Zellermayer, J., & Marcus, J. (1971). Kibbutz adolescents: Relevance to personality development theory. *Journal of Youth and Adolescence, 1,* 143–153.

4

Caring Behavior in Children of Clinically Depressed and Well Mothers

**Marian Radke-Yarrow, Carolyn Zahn-Waxler,
Dorothy T. Richardson, Amy Susman, and Pedro Martinez**
National Institute of Mental Health, Bethesda, Maryland

Young children's sensitivity and responsiveness to mothers' needs were investigated under conditions of high and low parenting risk (depressed and nondepressed mothers, SADS-L). Child characteristics of gender, affect, and impulse control problems and the mother-child attachment relationship were examined as they related to children's caring actions. Children's caring behavior was observed in an experimental situation in which their mothers simulated sadness and in a naturalistic setting. Attachment alone and child's problems alone were not predictors, and maternal diagnosis alone was not a strong predictor. Girls were significantly more caring than boys. Severe maternal depression was necessary to bring out high levels of responding in boys. Highest frequencies of caring were from children with severely depressed mothers, problems of affect regulation, and secure attachment. The importance of recognizing interacting influences and diverse underlying processes in the development of children's caring behavior is discussed.

This is a study of young children's sensitivity and positive responsiveness to their mothers' needs. It focuses on children's contributions to mother-child relationships. Mothers' contributions to the health of these

Reprinted with permission from *Child Development*, 1994, Vol. 65, 1405–1414.

This work was supported by the National Institute of Mental Health, Bethesda, MD; the John D. and Catherine T. MacArthur Foundation Research Network on Transition from Infancy to Early Childhood; and the Institute of Noetic Sciences. The authors wish to thank John Bartko, Theoretical Statistics Branch, NIMH, and Kathleen McCann, George Washington University, for consultation on statistical analyses, and Hattie Bingham for preparation of the manuscript.

relationships have long been emphasized in variables such as sensitive and supportive responding to the child's developmental and individual needs, but the child's contributions have rarely been the specific focus of inquiry. In this study, children's caring behavior directed to the mother was investigated. Preschool-age children of clinically depressed mothers and children of well mothers were compared.

Depressed mothers, by virtue of their illness, experience affective distress and psychological neediness, which may interfere with optimal parenting and may impose special emotional demands on the child. At a time when young children are learning to identify and regulate their own feelings and emotions, having to cope with mothers' emotional needs may compromise these children's social-emotional development. The prototypic depressed mother is characterized by anxious and depressive affect, irritability, helplessness, emotional unavailability, and absorption in self. If these characteristics carry over into the maternal role, as they have been shown to do (Gordon, Burge, Hammen, Adrian, & Jaenicke, 1989; Weissman & Paykel, 1974), they are likely to create stressful conditions for children. Although depression is an episodic illness, there is increasing evidence of a certain persistence and continuity in patterned depression-related behaviors in the intervals between episodes (Billings & Moos, 1985; Harder, Kokes, Fisher, & Strauss, 1980; Stein et al., 1991). The depressed mother may thereby build a coherent and relatively continuous history of disordered functioning in which the child is exposed to her emotional stress. Specific symptoms of depression are not uniform across mothers, however. Not all depressed mothers express all symptoms or express them with equal severity and intensity. However, the shared features of depression—disregulated affect and affective distress—are qualities of depressed mothers that variously enter into the rearing environment of their children.

Research on depressed mothers' functioning provides evidence of maternal impairments. High rates of dysphoric mood and low rates of happy affect are reported by Hops et al. (1987). Negative views of the child (Kochanska, Radke-Yarrow, Kuczynski, & Friedman, 1987), high rates of criticism (Jaenicke et al., 1987), and low involvement with the child as well as overinvolvement with the child (Davenport, Zahn-Waxler, Adland, & Mayfield, 1984) have been found. However, investigators acknowledge a wide variability among depressed mothers in type and extent of parenting patterns.

There are a number of potential risks to the child of a depressed mother. Foremost, as already noted, are possible interferences with the child's emotional development. The child may receive little help in understanding his or her own feelings or in learning to regulate his or her own emotions (Tronick, Ricks, & Cohn, 1982). When children's emotional needs are not met, the groundwork is laid for problems (Cicchetti & Schneider-Rosen, 1986). Moreover, in these circumstances, the child's expectations regarding adult caregivers are built on a dysfunctional affective model. On the other hand, children may be overwhelmed by mothers' needs and prematurely take on a caregiving role themselves, thereby forfeiting their own dependent role.

Although the idea of mother-child behavior as an interactive process is generally accepted, research has given less attention to the child's active participation in shaping the interactions of depressed mothers and their children. Examining children's responses to their mother's depressive illness remains an important area of investigation. Their response specifically to their mother's affective stress is a particularly critical element in their patterns of coping with the risks involved in depressed parenting. Does mother's distress elicit avoidance, rejection, or helping and comforting from the child?

The empirical studies of young children's prosocial behavior provide important anchors for the present study by indicating how aware and responsive young children are to the affective states and needs of others. Research during the 1970s by Rheingold and her associates (Hay, 1979; Rheingold, Hay, & West, 1976) demonstrated that children even before the age of 2 engage in behavior benefiting another person (e.g., helping, sharing, giving). Murphy's (1937) monumental study of preschool children's sympathetic behavior had many descendant studies showing children's reactions to the emotional distress of others in varied forms of helping, affection, and comforting (e.g., Dunn, 1988; Eisenberg-Berg & Lennon, 1980; Yarrow & Waxler, 1978). Reactions to others' distress were not without negative responses of crying, anger, and aggression. These studies established that the caring behaviors we are investigating in the present study are in the repertoires of young children.

Socialization variables have been investigated for their facilitating or hindering influences on the development of children's prosocial behavior. Studies of children in risk populations are of special interest. Caring behavior was rarely seen in physically abused preschool-age children (Klimes-Dougan & Kistner, 1990; Main & George, 1985). These studies raise the larger question of the vulnerability of young children's ability or motivation to respond supportively toward others when caregivers are dysfunctional.

Issues regarding the motives and mechanisms represented in prosocial behavior remain perplexing despite extensive research in this area. Empathy, a cognitive and affective construct, has been used to explain caring actions. It refers to the experience of others' emotional, psychological, or physical states, and also to the capacity to imagine and understand the other's state. While empathy does not necessarily result in prosocial behaviors, such behaviors have been shown to have accompaniments of affective concern and efforts to comprehend distress in others as early as the second year of life (Zahn-Waxler, Radke-Yarrow, Wagner, & Chapman, 1992; Zahn-Waxler, Robinson, & Emde, 1992). Such links between prosocial acts and expressions of affective concern have been demonstrated in older children as well (Eisenberg et al., 1989).

Empathy may also be part of an emotional reaction that includes guilt and inappropriate feelings of being responsible for the distress of others. Hoffman (1982) has hypothesized that empathy and guilt share a common affective core, beginning in the first years of life. Empathy occurs in response to distress in another person, whether the distress is caused or only witnessed by the child. Guilt results when the child assumes that she has caused the distress. But for young children, perceptions of "cause" are often blurred, and hence empathy and guilt may be indistinguishable under some circumstances. For example, preschool children of depressed mothers showed elevated levels of empathy and guilt, compared to children of well mothers, in their story themes interpreting hypothetical situations of interpersonal conflict and distress (Zahn-Waxler, Kochanska, Krupnick, & McKnew, 1990).

The Present Study

Our focus is on caring behavior of young children as it relates to the mother's depression or wellness. Our data are observed child behaviors directed to the mother. Does the disregulation in maternal affect elevate or diminish rates of caring by children? Interestingly, both predictions are theoretically reasonable. The prediction that children of depressed mothers are less likely than children of well mothers to show caring behavior rests on the probability that children's own needs are likely to go unattended when their mother is depressed, and therefore children may be less able to respond to others' needs. It is also reasonable to expect that maternal distress loses signal value for the young child because of its continued presence. An alternative prediction is that children's caring behavior will be increased by depressed mothers' recurring signals of distress. Children's sensitivities and anxieties may be heightened and behavior directed to relieving their mothers' distress may be increased. These predictions, however, fail to take into account varied child characteristics and varied mother-child relationships that may modify the child's ability or inclination to be positively responsive to the mother. Three potential modifiers are examined:

1. As the young child's primary context, the attachment relationship is a potentially significant modifier of the child's perceptions, expectations, and affect regarding the mother, as well as regarding feelings about self. The attachment relationship was, therefore, considered as it related to children's caring actions.

2. Gender of child was examined since, in many studies of children's prosocial behavior, females have been found to be more prosocial than males (see review by Eisenberg & Lennon, 1983). Also, there is evidence pointing to a gender difference in ability to interpret affective cues and states of others (Brody, 1985; Eisenberg & Lennon, 1983), with an advantage reported for females. Gender is of further relevance because of the significantly higher prevalence of unipolar depression among women than men (Weissman & Klerman, 1977). Early behavioral differences between girls and boys of depressed mothers in an affect-relevant dimension such as caring behavior are, therefore, of interest.

3. A second child characteristic deemed relevant in early caring responses is the child's own social-emotional well-being. A major developmental task for young children is to progress in affect regulation and impulse control. If they are having difficulties in these respects, how is positive behavior toward the mother affected?

The orientation of the study and the research questions can be summarized as: Maternal disregulated affect, inherent in clinical depression, places special demands on children. Do these conditions lead to elevated or depressed rates of caring behavior directed to the mother by their children? How is children's caring responding modified by the mother-child relationship and by child characteristics of gender and psychosocial well-being?

METHOD

Subjects

The participants were 90 preschool-age children and their mothers, a subsample (based on children's age, 24 to 48 months) of the NIMH longitudinal study of child development in families of depressed and well mothers (Radke-Yarrow, 1989). Thirty-two of the mothers had a diagnosis of major (unipolar) depression, 20 had a diagnosis of bipolar illness, and 38 had no current or past psychiatric disorders. Diagnoses were based on a standard psychiatric interview (SADS-L, RDC criteria; Spitzer & Endicott, 1977). The affectively ill mothers were without other Axis I diagnoses, except that anxiety might be secondary to depression. Ten interviews were assessed independently by the staff psychiatric nurse and a staff member of the New York Psychiatric Institute, with 100% agreement on assignment of diagnoses on all of the cases.

In addition to a diagnosis, mothers were evaluated on the severity of their illness. Research by Harder et al. (1980) and Keller et al. (1986) indicates that severity of mother's depression has a significant bearing on risk for the child. The more severe and chronic the depression, the greater the magnitude of impact on the child. Therefore, severity as well as diagnosis of depression were used to classify mothers. Criteria for severity were: early onset (25 years of age and under), at least three episodes of major depression, total time in episodes at least 6 months, and GAS score below 50 (an index of impairment in functioning based on information from the SADS; Spitzer, Gibbon, & Endicott, 1973). Twenty-five mothers (12 unipolar and 13 bipolar) were classified as severely depressed; 27 (20 unipolar and 7 bipolar) were classified as less severely depressed.

While these criteria of severity are a good basis for estimating how much maternal affect enters into parenting behavior, data from the larger longitudinal study provide further confirmation. Measures of frequencies of mothers' displayed negative affects were available from observations of mothers in 5 hours of interaction in seminaturalistic conditions (Radke-Yarrow, Nottelmann, Belmont, & Welsh, 1993). Negative affects were displayed significantly more often by unipolar and bipolar depressed mothers than by well mothers, but the unipolar and bipolar groups did not differ from each other. Further, displays of negative affects were significantly more frequent by severely depressed mothers than by less severely depressed and well mothers. Less severely depressed mothers and well mothers did *not* differ from each other. These data provided the empirical rationale for the classifications used in the present analyses: (*a*) depressed versus well mothers, and (*b*) severely depressed versus less severely depressed and well mothers combined.

The mothers in this study were the major caregivers of their children. The families were predominantly middle and upper- middle class (Hollingshead, 1975). All but two of the families were intact. Eighty-one families were Caucasian, one family was Asian, and eight were Black.

The children were between 24 and 48 months of age. Age and gender distributions were very similar in the diagnostic groups. As participants in the longitudinal study, each child had periodic psychiatric evaluations. At these ages, assessment was based on a videotaped psychiatric play inter-view consisting of a standard sequence of procedures planned to challenge the child in a number of ways: the child's ability to separate from mother and relate to an unfamiliar adult, explore and use the environment, and express and regulate affect appropriately. The first phase of the session involved interaction of mother, child, and psychiatrist, introductory to the child's accompanying the psychiatrist to the playroom. Ten minutes fol-lowed in which the child was invited to play with neutral toys (such as blocks and crayons). The clinician interacted nondirectively. For the next 10 min, the child had the opportunity to play with a number of materials relevant to the child's family (e.g., doll house, dolls identified as mother, father, sister). In the next 10 min, toys with aggressive potential were pro-vided (e.g., pounding blocks, punching bag). The child's behavior was assessed for separation anxiety, generalized anxiety, depressive affect, and disruptive or oppositional behavior. Behavior was labeled problematic if, in the psychiatrist's judgment, it was so deviant as to suggest the need for careful monitoring or posed a serious interference with the normal course of development. Although DSM-IIIR criteria were the basis of classifica-tion, at this early age, designation of a problem was not regarded as a diag-nosis but as behavior of clinical concern. (For details regarding procedures and classification, see Radke-Yarrow, Nottelmann, Martinez, Fox, & Bel-mont, 1992.) Mothers' reports of child problems were not included in the assessments used in the present analyses, but are part of the longitudinal assessments. Ten cases were blind-scored by a second psychiatrist; kappa on assigned problem areas was .77. The psychiatric evaluations were made within 2 weeks of the observations of caring behavior (see Table 1).

Procedure

Mothers and children were observed and videotaped on 3 days in a com-fortable research apartment. The sessions were composed so as to provide a reasonably natural series of situations that were representative of daily routines and rearing demands (eating, playing, talking together, encounter-ing problems, and interacting in unstructured situations). Mother and child were alone on 2 of the days. On the third day, a sibling (on average, 3 years older) was present. A sample of 50 min of interaction in the unstruc-tured times (10 5-min segments sampled over the 3 days) was the basis for assessment of children's empathic and prosocial behavior. Beginning of sessions, Strange Situation, and end of sessions were not included. *Naturalistic data.* The 5-min segments were viewed independently by two observers, blind to diagnostic data, to identify prosocial episodes, followed

TABLE 1
Description of Sample

| | Maternal Depression | | |
	Severe	Less Severe	Normal Controls
Boys:			
N	10	14	19
Age (in years), M (SD)	2.6 (.81)	2.7 (.57)	2.7 (.38)
SES, M (SD)	52 (13)	53 (13)	55 (11)
Race:			
Caucasian	10	14	17
Black	0	0	2
Problems:			
Present	3	9	8
Absent	7	5	11
Girls:			
N	13	15	19
Age (in years), M (SD)	2.8 (.44)	2.7 (.42)	2.7 (.33)
SES, M (SD)	52 (13)	50 (14)	53 (12)
Race:			
Caucasian	12	12	17
Black	0	3	2
Asian	1	0	0
Problems:			
Present	7	8	9
Absent	6	7	10

by consensual identification. Child behavior was then coded in the following three categories: verbal or physical sharing, helping, comforting and caretaking. (Warning of danger and distracting from distress, although in the coding system, were extremely rare and were not used.) Total number of acts and number of different types of acts were scored. All coding was done from videotapes. Coders were blind to diagnostic data about the children and mothers. Kappas for coding of child behavior ranged from .73 to .98, based on 20 cases.

Experimental data. On the second day of observation, a standard situation was introduced in which the mother was asked to sit down with her child to look at a book of photographs of infants, each expressing a distinct emotion. The mother was instructed to talk about the babies as she might in showing the child a picture book. After completing the book, she was to return to the picture of the crying baby and to express her own sadness and concern. By this simulation, we hoped to tap into how the child responded to mother's sad affect. The child's responding was coded for number of attempts to comfort the mother and number of different types of intervention (verbal sympathy or concern, physical comfort, helping behavior). Intercoder reliabilities were based on 21 cases (kappas were .93 for number and .82 for types of interventions).

Attachment relationship. The attachment relationship was assessed by the Strange Situation (Ainsworth, Blehar, Waters, & Wall, 1978) and on classifications according to the Ainsworth scoring guidelines. When the Cassidy and Marvin (1987/89) classification system for preschool age children became available, the older children were reclassified using this system (see DeMulder & Radke-Yarrow, 1991). Because of sample size, attachment classification for the present analyses was either secure ($n = 51$) or insecure ($n = 39$).

Organization of analyses. The scores on prosocial behavior were the separate sums of all prosocial acts in the naturalistic setting and in the experimental situation. The child's repertoire of caring acts was the number of different kinds of prosocial behavior. The scores of two outliers in the naturalistic setting and three outliers in the experimental situation (five different children, all offspring of depressed mothers) were brought in to equal one greater than the score of the next highest child (Tabachnick and Fidell, 1989). All values of prosocial behavior then ranged between 0 and 3 standard deviations from the mean ($M = 7.94$, SD 6.28 in the naturalistic setting; $M = 1.25$, SD = 1.77 in the experimental situation). In the naturalistic setting, both of the outliers were children of the most severely depressed mothers; their prosocial acts were initially 5 and 9 standard deviations from the mean of prosocial behavior for all children in the study. In the experimental setting, two of the outliers were children of the most severely depressed mothers and one was a child of a less severely depressed mother; their prosocial responding to mother's simulated sadness was initially 4 and 7 standard deviations from the mean of all children.

Pearson correlations were run between frequency and repertoire scores on prosocial behavior. These scores were highly correlated, $r = .69$, $p < .01$, in the naturalistic setting; $r = .81$, $p < .01$, in the experimental situation. Preliminary analyses also revealed similar patterns of findings based on total frequency and repertoire. Therefore, for further analyses, only frequency of prosocial initiations was used.

Frequency of children's prosocial acts was examined in relation to mothers' psychiatric status, gender of child, child's problem status, and attachment relationship. The descriptive data of children's behavior considering each variable separately are presented in the Appendix.

To examine main effects and interactions between the variables (diagnosis, gender, problems, and attachment), $2 \times 2 \times 2 \times 2$ analyses of variance (ANOVAs) were run separately for prosocial behavior in the naturalistic setting and prosocial behavior in the experimental situation. Post-hoc comparisons were Tukey's HSD tests (alpha level = .05). All post-hoc tests were conservatively two-tailed.

Because the sample included a 2-year age span, preliminary analyses were conducted to determine whether there were age differences. Children above the mean age of the sample (M = 33 months) were the "older" group. There were no age differences in the naturalistic setting in frequency of prosocial acts (M = 8.26, SD = 6.77 for younger; M = 8.08, SD = 7.44 for older) or in the experimental situation in frequency of interventions (M = 1.47, SD = 2.40 for younger; M = 1.18, SD = 1.60 for older). In 3×2 ANOVAs, with mother's diagnosis and age of child as the independent variables, there were no significant differences in relation to age in either setting. Age was not considered in further analyses.

RESULTS

Concerned Interventions by Children in Response to Mothers' Simulated Sadness (Experimental Situation)

Mother's simulation of sadness was the single stimulus saliently presented when the child was in close physical proximity to the mother. ANOVAs revealed one significant main effect of mother's diagnosis (depressed vs. well), $F(1, 82) = 6.48$, $p < .01$. Children of depressed mothers intervened more (M = 1.66, SD 2.10) in response to mother's sadness than did children of well mothers (M = .72, SD = 1.03).

There was a significant two-way interaction between attachment and gender, $F(1, 82) = 3.95$, $p < .05$. In post-hoc comparisons, securely attached girls expressed significantly more concern (M = 1.83, SD = 1.97) than securely attached boys (M = .83, SD = 1.30) and more concern than insecurely attached girls (M = .75, SD = 1.2). Insecurely attached boys and girls (M = 1.63, SD = 2.34, for boys; M = .75, SD = 1.25, for girls) did not differ significantly. Securely attached boys (M = .83, SD = 1.30) and insecurely attached boys (M = 1.63, SD = 2.34) did not differ significantly.

Children's interventions were next examined after reclassifying mothers on severity of depression. Surprisingly, there were no main effects. There was a significant two-way interaction between gender and severity, $F(1, 82) = 5.66$, $p = .02$. Post-hoc comparisons revealed the following pattern: Boys intervened with severely depressed mothers significantly more often (M =

2.78, SD = 2.86) than boys with mothers who were well or less severely depressed (*M* = .67, SD = .99). Severity of mother's depression was necessary to bring out concerned responding by boys. Girls' responding to their mother's sadness was not influenced by the mother's diagnosis (*M* = 1.46, SD = 1.94 for severely depressed mothers; *M* = 1.29, SD = 1.70 for others). Boys and girls did not differ in their responding to severely depressed mothers, but girls responded significantly more than did boys to less severely depressed and well mothers.

Children's Prosocial Interventions in the Naturalistic Setting

The mother's simulated sadness presented a focused, high-demand situation for her child. In contrast, naturalistic settings required the child to perceive maternal needs in the midst of competing events and diverse stimuli. Analyses of prosocial responding under these conditions repeated those used with the experimental data.

There was no main effect of mother's diagnosis on frequency of children's prosocial behavior, whether diagnoses were classified as depressed versus well or as severely depressed versus well and less severely depressed (*M* = 8.29, SD = 6.72 for depressed and *M* = 7.47, SD = 5.69 for well; *M* = 9.78, SD = 7.53 for severely depressed and *M* = 7.81, SD = 5.73 for well and less severely depressed combined). There was no main effect of attachment or child problems. There was, however, a main effect of gender, $F(1, 89)$ = 18.11, $p < .000$, with girls showing more prosocial behavior (*M* = 10.49, SD = 6.5) than boys (*M* = 5.16, SD = 4.71).

When comparisons of children's caring behavior involved children of depressed versus well mothers, there were no interactions. However, when severity of illness was the classificatory basis, the picture was very different. There was a significant three-way interaction involving severity of maternal depression, child's problem status, and attachment, $F(1, 89) = 4.01$, $p < .05$ (see Fig. 1).

When children were *without* problematic anxiety and/or disruptive behavior, there were no significant differences in prosocial interventions related to severity of mother's depression or to attachment (Fig. 1, cols. 5–8).

In the *presence* of problems of anxiety and/or disruptive behavior, there were significant differences in children's prosocial behavior relating to severity of maternal depression and security of attachment. The configuration of severe maternal depression, secure attachment, and child problems was associated with the highest frequency in children's prosocial actions (*M* = 16.33, SD = 8.98) (col. 1). In post-hoc comparisons, these children

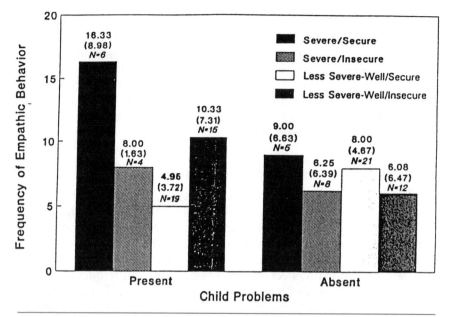

Figure 1. Empathic behavior in the naturalistic setting. Empathic behavior is expresed as mean (standard deviation). Severity of illness represents children of severely depressed mothers versus children of less severely depressed and well mothers combined. There is a significant three-way interaction for severity of illness, child problems, and attachment.

initiated caring behavior significantly more often than (*a*) children with problems, with severely depressed mothers, but with insecure attachment relationships ($M = 8.00$, SD $= 1.63$) (col. 2), (*b*) children with problems with secure attachment relationships but with mothers who were not severely depressed ($M = 4.95$, SD $= 3.72$) (col. 3), and (*c*) children of severely depressed mothers, with secure attachment relationships but no problems ($M = 9.00$, SD $= 6.63$) (col. 5).

When children had problems but their mothers were well or less severely depressed, prosocial responses were more frequent by children with insecure attachment ($M = 10.33$, SD $= 7.31$) than by children with secure attachment ($M = 4.95$, SD $= 3.72$) (cols. 4 and 3). (With Tukey's post-hoc comparisons for three-way interactions, we are limited to pair comparisons in which two independent variables are constant; Keppel, 1982, pp. 302–305.)

The interactions we have seen portray a complex picture that brings into consideration the child's regulatory status (psychiatric assessment of anxiety and disruptive-oppositional behavior), level of stress introduced by severe maternal depression, and attachment classification. Children's high caring in the configuration of severe maternal depression, secure attachment, and presence of affective and regulatory problems prohibits a simple interpretation of the processes involved in young children's prosocial behavior toward their mothers. It also raises questions regarding the nature of processes linking maternal depression and child behavior.

SUMMARY AND DISCUSSION

The study began with the assumptions that maternal depression exposes children to many experiences of maternal emotional distress and neediness and that these cumulative experiences have consequences for children's social and emotional development, specifically, for their coping with the needs and distress of others. The findings indicate that differences in young children's caring behavior are related to mothers' depression in complex ways. Mothers' diagnosis of depression by itself was not a strong or consistent predictor of children's caring behavior. However, as the analyses indicate, prediction depended on a more functional definition or assessment of maternal depression and the presence of other interacting variables, including child characteristics. These variables in concert influenced children's caring behavior.

Severity of depression exposes children to more maternal distress and takes a higher toll on children's well-being (Keller et al., 1986). The findings on children's caring behavior reflect this contextual impact *in interaction* with specific child characteristics. Boys and girls are differently responsive. Girls, overall, exhibited more caring behavior toward their mothers than boys and the level of their caring behavior was little influenced by differences in mothers' psychiatric status. Sadness expressed by mothers brought out girls' caring interventions equally, regardless of maternal diagnosis. Only boys with severely depressed mothers were moved to interventions equal to girls' interventions. The gender difference is of interest regarding the transmission of problems in families with depressed mothers, especially in light of the differences in depression in male and female adults. How girls and boys react differently across development to maternal distress is worthy of further study.

Children's own psychosocial stress or well-being was a second child characteristic that entered into their responding to their mothers' distress. A configuration of severe maternal depression, secure attachment relationship with a severely depressed mother, and psychiatrically assessed child problems of affect regulation and/or impulse control was associated with the highest frequency of children's prosocial acts. These findings raise important questions concerning the underlying processes of prosocial behavior. Is the elevated level of these children's prosocial acts an expression of positive concern for mother? Is this concern for mother qualified by concern for self? What are the long-term consequences of very high levels of caring behavior by young children of severely depressed mothers? The interaction of severity of maternal depression, child problems, and mother-child attachment needs to be viewed in the perspective of the other configurations. When mothers are not depressed or not severely depressed, the dynamics appear to be different: In this situation, the children who have problems and who are insecurely attached perform more prosocial acts. Here, anxious concern for self is a possible motivator.

When we examine children of well or less severely depressed mothers with secure attachment relationships and without problems of affect regulation, their frequencies of caring behavior are neither extremely high nor extremely low (Fig. 1, col. 7). They may conform to the findings in the literature (Eisenberg & Lennon, 1983) of prosocial behavior fostered by positive rearing experiences. What seems clear from our data is that young children's prosocial behavior and empathy are heterogeneous with respect to underlying processes, especially under conditions of risk.

In summarizing and integrating the findings from this study, we have emphasized the signals in our data regarding the different processes that appear to underlie overt acts of caring. The patterns of mother and child variables have provided clues. This study is exploratory and its findings need to be replicated. They are robust, however, in indicating a heterogeneity of conditions defining and determining young children's prosocial and empathic behaviors. They underscore both the limitations of attempting to understand this aspect of children's development solely in terms of the frequency of caring behavior and the inadequacy of single explanatory models for the development of caring behavior.

We have speculated regarding different mechanisms that may account for prosocial and emotionally empathic behavior in young children. There is need to design studies and procedures that will enable us to identify when and how varied processes support or interfere with the development of this behavior in children. Moreover, there is need for follow-up of children who show extremes of caring behavior.

APPENDIX
Caring Behavior in Experimental Situation and Naturalistic Setting by Mother's Diagnosis, Attachment, and Child Problems

| | Mother's Psychiatric Status | | | | | | | |
| | Well | | | Less Severely Depressed | | | Severely Depressed | | |
Child Characteristics	(N)	M	(SD)	(N)	M	SD	(N)	M	(SD)
Experimental situation:									
Total group	(36)	.72	(1.03)	(25)	1.36	(1.80)	(22)	2.00	(2.39)
Secure attachment	(24)	.75	(1.03)	(12)	1.83	(2.08)	(11)	2.09	(2.21)
Insecure attachment	(12)	.67	(1.07)	(13)	.92	(1.44)	(11)	1.91	(2.66)
Problems absent . . .	(20)	.80	(1.11)	(9)	.56	(1.13)	(12)	2.25	(2.73)
Problems present	(16)	.63	(.96)	(16)	1.81	(1.92)	(10)	1.70	(2.00)
Boys	(18)	.50	(.92)	(12)	.92	(1.08)	(9)	2.78	(2.86)
Girls	(18)	.94	(1.10)	(13)	1.77	(2.24)	(13)	1.46	(1.94)
Naturalistic setting:									
Total group	(38)	7.47	(5.69)	(29)	7.10	(5.87)	(23)	9.78	(7.53)
Secure attachment	(26)	7.46	(4.64)	(14)	4.86	(3.70)	(11)	13.00	(8.22)
Insecure attachment	(12)	7.50	(7.74)	(15)	9.20	(6.82)	(12)	6.83	(5.24)
Problems absent . . .	(21)	7.70	(5.05)	(12)	6.67	(6.08)	(13)	7.31	(6.36)
Problems present	(17)	7.24	(6.54)	(17)	7.41	(5.89)	(10)	13.00	(8.01)
Boys	(19)	4.79	(3.58)	(14)	4.86	(5.91)	(10)	6.30	(5.06)
Girls	(19)	10.16	(6.20)	(15)	9.20	(5.17)	(13)	12.46	(8.17)

REFERENCES

Ainsworth, M., Blehar, M., Waters, E., & Wall, S. (1978). *Patterns of attachment: A psychological study of the Strange Situation.* Hillsdale, NJ: Erlbaum.

Billings, A., & Moos, R. (1985). Children of parents with unipolar depression: A controlled 1-year follow-up. *Journal of Abnormal Child Psychology, 14,* 149–166.

Brody, L. R. (1985). Gender differences in emotional development: A review of theories and research. *Journal of Personality, 53,* 102–149.

Cassidy, J., Marvin, R., & MacArthur Working Group on Attachment. (1987/89). *Attachment organization, in three and four year olds: Coding guidelines.* Unpublished scoring manual.

Cicchetti, D., & Schneider-Rosen, K. (1986). An organizational approach to childhood depression. In M. Rutter, C. Izard, & P. Read (Eds.), *Depression in young people: Developmental and clinical perspectives* (pp. 71–134). New York: Guilford.

Davenport, Y. B., Zahn-Waxler, C., Adland, M. L., & Mayfield, A. (1984). Early child-rearing practices in families with a manic-depressive parent. *American Journal of Psychiatry,* **141**, 230–235.

DeMulder, E., & Radke-Yarrow, M. (1991). Attachment with affectively ill and well mothers: Concurrent behavioral correlates. *Development & Psychopathology,* **3**, 227–242.

Dunn, J. (1988). *The beginnings of social understanding.* Oxford: Basil Blackwell.

Eisenberg, N., Fabes, R. Muller, P., Fultz, J., Shell, R., Mathy, R., & Reno, R. (1989). Relation of sympathy and personal distress to prosocial behavior: A multi-method study. *Journal of Personality and Social Psychology,* **57**, 55–66.

Eisenberg, N., & Lennon, R. (1983). Sex differences in empathy and related capacities. *Psychological Bulletin,* **94**, 100–131.

Eisenberg-Berg, N., & Lennon, R. (1980). Altruism and the assessment of empathy in the preschool years. *Child Development,* **51**, 552–557.

Gordon, D., Burge, M., Hammen, C., Adrian, C., Jaenicke, C., & Hiroto, D. (1989). Observations of interactions of depressed women and their children. *American Journal of Psychiatry,* **146**, 50–55.

Harder, D., Kokes, R., Fisher, L., & Strauss, J. (1980). Child competence and psychiatric risk: Relationships of parent diagnostic classifications and parent psychopathology severity to child functioning. *Journal of Nervous and Mental Disease,* **168**, 343–347.

Hay, D. F. (1979). Cooperative interactions and sharing between very young children and their parents. *Developmental Psychology,* **15**, 647–653.

Hoffman, M. L. (1982). Development of prosocial motivation: Empathy and guilt. In N. Eisenberg (Ed.), *The development of prosocial behavior* (pp. 281–313). New York: Academic Press.

Hollingshead, A. B. (1975). *Four-Factor Index of Social Status.* Unpublished manuscript, Yale University, Sociology Department, New Haven, CT.

Hops, H., Biglan, A., Sherman, L., Arthur, J., Friedman, L., & Osteen, V. (1987). Home observations of family interactions of depressed woman. *Journal of Consulting and Clinical Psychology,* **55**, 341–346.

Jaenicke, C., Hammen, C., Zupan, B., Hiroto, D., Gordon, D., Adrian, C., and Burge, D. (1987). Cognitive vulnerability in children at risk for depression. *Journal of Abnormal Child Psychology,* **15**, 559–572.

Keller, M. B., Beardslee, W. R., Dorer, D. J., Lavori, P. W., Samuelson, H., & Klerman, G. R. (1986). Impact of severity and chronicity of parental affective illness on adaptive functioning and psychopathology in children. *Archives of General Psychiatry,* **43**, 930–937.

Keppel, G. (1982). *Design and analysis* (2d ed.). Englewood Cliffs, NJ: Prentice-Hall.

Klimes-Dougan, B., & Kistner, J. (1990). Responses of physically abused preschoolers to distressed peers. *Developmental Psychology,* **26,** 599–602.

Kochanska, G., Radke-Yarrow, M., Kuczynski, L., & Friedman, S. (1987). Normal and affectively ill mothers' beliefs about their children. *American Journal of Orthopsychiatry,* **57,** 345–350.

Main, M., & George, C. (1985). Response of abused and disadvantaged toddlers to distress in playmates: A study in the day care setting. *Developmental Psychology,* **4,** 407–412.

Murphy, L. B. (1937). *Social behavior and child personality.* New York: Columbia University Press.

Radke-Yarrow, M. (1989). Family environments of depressed and well parents and their children: Issues of research methods. In G. R. Patterson (Ed.), *Aggression and depression in family interactions* (pp. 48–67). Hillsdale, NJ: Erlbaum.

Radke-Yarrow, M., Nottelmann, E., Belmont, B., & Welsh, J. (1993). Affective interactions of depressed and nondepressed mothers and their children. *Journal of Abnormal Child Psychology,* **21,** 683–695.

Radke-Yarrow, M., Nottelmann, E., Martinez, P., Fox, M. B., & Belmont, B. (1992). Young children of affectively ill parents: A longitudinal study of psychosocial development. *Journal American Academy of Child and Adolescent Psychiatry,* **31,** 68–77.

Rheingold, H., Hay, D., & West M. (1976). Sharing in the second year of life. *Child Development,* **47,** 1148–1158.

Spitzer, R., & Endicott, J. (1977). *The schedule for affective disorders and schizophrenia: Lifetime version.* New York: New York State Psychiatric Institute, Biometrics Research.

Spitzer, R., Gibbon, M., & Endicott, J. (1973). *Global Assessment Scale.* New York: New York State Department of Mental Hygiene.

Stein, A., Gath, D., Bucker, J., Bond, A., Day, A., and Cooper, P. (1991). The relationship between postnatal depression and mother-child interaction. *British Journal of Psychiatry,* **158,** 46–52.

Tabachnick, B., & Fidell, L. (1989). *Using multivariate statistics.* New York: Harper & Row.

Tronick, E. Z., Ricks, M., & Cohn, S. F. (1982). Maternal and infant affective exchange: Patterns of adaptation. In T. Field & A. Fogel (Eds.), *Emotion and early interaction* (pp. 83–100). Hillsdale, NJ: Erlbaum.

Weissman, M., & Klerman, G. (1977). Sex differences in the epidemiology of depression. *Archives of General Psychiatry,* **34,** 98–111.

Weissman, M., & Paykel, E. (1974). *The depressed woman: A study of social relationships.* Chicago: University of Chicago Press.

Yarrow, M. R., & Waxler, C. Z. (1978). Emergence and functions of prosocial behaviors in young children. In M. S. Smart and R. C. Smart (Eds.), *Infants: Development and relationships* (pp. 77–81) New York: Macmillan.

Zahn-Waxler, C., Kochanska, G., Krupnick, J., & McKnew, D. (1990). Patterns of guilt in children of depressed and well mothers. *Developmental Psychology, 26,* 51–59.

Zahn-Waxler, C., Radke-Yarrow, M., Wagner, E., & Chapman, M. (1992). Development of concern for others. *Developmental Psychology, 28,* 126–136.

Zahn-Waxler, C., Robinson, J., & Emde, R. (1992). The development of empathy in twins. *Developmental Psychology, 28,* 1038–1047.

5

Child Maltreatment, Attachment, and the Self System: Emergence of an Internal State Lexicon in Toddlers at High Social Risk

Marjorie Beeghly
Harvard Medical School, Boston
Children's Hospital, Boston
Dante Cicchetti
University of Rochester

The ability to talk about the internal states (ISs) and feelings of self and other is an age-appropriate development of late toddlerhood hypothesized to reflect toddlers' emergent self-other understanding and to be fundamental to the regulation of social interaction. This study examined the effects of child maltreatment on the emergence of low-socioeconomic status 30-month-old toddlers' IS lexicons. Children's lexicons were derived both from maternal interviews and from observations of children's spontaneous IS utterances in four laboratory contexts. Results from both data sources indicated that mal-

Reprinted with permission from *Development and Psychopathology*, 1994, Vol. 6, 5–30. Copyright © 1994 Cambridge University Press.

We are grateful to the families who participated in this investigation. We also thank the staff of the Harvard Child Maltreatment Project for their diligent efforts, especially Vicki Carlson, Anne Churchill, and Carol Kottmeier. Kathleen Holt provided invaluable statistical assistance, and Doug Barnett assisted in the coding of the Strange Situation protocols reported in this study. In addition, Cliff Calloway, Amanda Hanrahan-Veith, Kathryn Howell, Brad Johns, Thomas Kelly, Marthe Outcault, Jeannine Page, Paula Shea, and James Sucich deserve special recognition for their significant efforts in transcribing and/or coding internal state language. Fred Rogosch and Sheree L. Toth provided helpful feedback on a prior version of this manuscript. Partial support of this research was provided to Dante Cicchetti and Marjorie Beeghly from the John D. and Catherine T. MacArthur Foundation Transition Network on Early Childhood and to Dante Cicchetti from the National Center on Child Abuse and Neglect (90-C01929), the William T. Grant Foundation, the National Institute of Mental Health (RO1-MH37960), the Smith-Richardson Foundation, Inc., the Spencer Foundation, and the Spunk Fund, Inc.

treated toddlers produced significantly fewer IS words, fewer IS word types, and proportionately fewer IS words denoting physiological states and negative affect than nonmaltreated toddlers. In addition, maltreated toddlers were more context bound in IS language use and more restricted in their attributions of internal states to self and other. Gender differences were also observed. Individual differences in children's IS language production were significantly related to general linguistic maturity in both groups but to toddlers' conversational skills only in the comparison group. In addition, a cumulative risk model describing the effects of the child's attachment relationship with the caregiver on early IS language was tested. Toddlers most severely at risk (maltreated/insecure) had the most compromised IS language. Thus, secure attachment may serve as a protective mechanism against self-dysfunction in maltreated toddlers.

The ability to talk about the feelings, emotions, and other internal states (ISs) of self and other is an age-appropriate development of late toddlerhood hypothesized to reflect toddlers' emergent self-other understanding and to be fundamental to the regulation of social interaction (Bretherton, 1991; Cicchetti, Ganiban, & Barnett, 1991; Dunn & Brown, 1991; Harris, 1989; Stern, 1985; see also Johnson-Laird, 1983). The emergence of this ability may be viewed as part of a larger developmental transformation during toddlerhood characterized not only by general linguistic advances (e.g., lexical growth, the ability to talk in sentences [Bates, O'Connell, & Shore, 1987; Bloom, 1991]), but also by specific developments reflecting toddlers' emerging self-other differentiation, including an increase in self-descriptive utterances (Kagan, 1981), shifting personal pronouns (Bates, 1990), a growing empathic concern for others (Zahn-Waxler, Radke-Yarrow, Wagner, & Chapman, 1992), the emergence of the ability to tease and deceive (Dunn & Brown, 1991; Lewis, Stanger, & Sullivan, 1989), the "social" emotions such as guilt and shame (Barrett & Campos, 1987; Kagan & Lamb, 1987; Lewis, Sullivan, Stanger, & Weiss, 1989), and active agency during symbolic play (Beeghly, 1993; Bretherton & Beeghly, 1989; Leslie, 1987; Piaget, 1962; Watson & Fischer, 1977).

During the past decade, a rapidly growing body of research has focused on the extent and significance of young children's ability to talk about the inner states of themselves and others in their social environments (see recent reviews by Bretherton, 1991; Dunn & Brown, 1991; Harris, 1989; Ridgeway, Waters, & Kuczaj, 1985; Smiley & Huttenlocher, 1989; Wellman, 1988). This research has demonstrated that IS words first emerge early in the 2nd year and increase dramatically during the 3rd. Not only are there marked increases in the diversity of toddlers' IS lexicons, but also the range of social agents (other persons, toys, photographs) to whom ISs are imputed proliferates and becomes increasingly decentered, abstract, and decontextualized. Moreover, age-related changes in the content of toddlers' IS utterances also have been observed. By age 2½, for example, words about sensory perceptions, physiological states, and volition are most common in children's IS lexicons, followed by words for the basic emotions such as joy, anger, sadness, fear, and disgust and words denoting moral approval ("good girl"). In contrast, utterances about social and moral obligation ("supposed to," "have to") and cognitive processes (thought, knowledge, memory, etc.) are still relatively rare. Note that the latter category has been shown to increase in frequency after 30 months (Shatz, Wellman, & Silber, 1983; Wellman, 1988).

It is important to clarify that "IS words" in this literature refer primarily to those words that have explicit reference to internal states ("mad," "happy") rather than words that have implicit connotations of emotion, motivation, or intention (Bromley, 1977). Moreover, toddlers' IS words do not yet have their full adult meaning but, rather, appear to be based on concrete, observable aspects of experience or behavior (see Beckwith, 1991; Bloom & Beckwith, 1989; Gopnik & Astington, 1988). Nevertheless, by 2½ years, toddlers appear to use IS words in appropriate contexts and to discuss the stages of nonpresent persons as well as the causes and consequences of ISs for self and other (Bretherton & Beeghly, 1982; Bretherton, Fritz, Zahn-Waxler, & Ridgeway, 1986; Dunn, Bretherton, & Munn, 1987).

Moreover, parental language to toddlers about ISs has been shown to mirror their children's abilities and becomes increasingly other oriented as children grow in linguistic and conceptual maturity (Beeghly, Bretherton, & Mervis, 1986; Dunn et al., 1987). Participating in family discussions about emotions and ISs is thought to be an important way children acquire and refine an IS lexicon, particularly if these discussions involve the child directly (Dunn et al., 1987). Moreover, such interchanges promote the establishment of close relationships by encouraging toddlers to share their experiences and feelings and to negotiate conflicts and misunderstandings. In her longitudinal home observations, for example, Dunn and her colleagues (Dunn et al., 1987; Dunn, Brown, & Beardsall, 1991a) reported that a high proportion of families' conversations involved discussions about feeling and emotions states. Notably, individual differences in the amount of this talk were stable over time and predicted children's perspective taking abilities several years later, even when children's language skills were controlled analytically (see Denham, McKinley, Couchoud, & Holt, 1990, for other correlates of early emotion language).

The purpose of the present study was to examine the impact of low social status and child maltreatment on the emergence of an IS lexicon in 30-month-old toddlers. Because the extant IS literature has focused primarily on low risk samples drawn from middle-socioeconomic status (SES) backgrounds, it was unclear whether or not maltreated and nonmaltreated toddlers from extremely low-SES homes would exhibit similar developmental progressions in their ability to use IS language. Although low SES is associated with mild developmental delays (McLloyd & Wilson, 1991) and with parenting styles hypothesized to interfere with early language learning (Barnes, Gurgreund, Satterly, & Wells, 1983; Snow, 1984), child maltreatment has been documented to place low-SES children at even greater jeopardy for compromised developmental outcomes, particularly for aspects of development relevant to the acquisition of an IS lexicon (e.g., early language and communicative development [e.g., Cicchetti & Beeghly, 1987; Coster & Cicchetti, 1993], affective communication during early social interactions [Gaensbauer & Sands, 1979], affective regulation during visual self-recognition tasks [Schneider-Rosen & Cicchetti, 1991], infant-caregiver attachment formation [Carlson, Cicchetti, Barnett, & Braunwald, 1989; Crittenden & Ainsworth, 1989; Egeland & Sroufe, 1981; Lyons-Ruth, Connell, Zoll, & Stahl, 1987]). In addition, child maltreatment has also been documented to have deleterious effects on the socioemotional and regulatory abilities of older children (e.g., Aber & Cicchetti, 1984; Alessandri, 1991; Cicchetti et al., 1991; Jaffe, Wolfe, & Wilson, 1990; Lynch & Cicchetti, 1991; Starr & Wolfe, 1991; Vondra, Barnett, & Cicchetti, 1989). For these reasons, we expected maltreated toddlers from low-SES homes to show compromised patterns of early IS language production, even when controlling for the effects of poverty.

For example, Coster, Gersten, Beeghly, and Cicchetti (1989) reported significantly delayed language and communicative skills in a sample of low-SES maltreated 2½-year-olds, relative to cognitively and demographically matched controls. The maltreated children's language was markedly impoverished in productivity, complexity, and content. Moreover, children were especially delayed in particular pragmatic skills that serve to initiate and sustain conversation (e.g., questions, descriptive utterances, discourse skills). Similar language deficits have also been reported for older maltreated children (e.g., Blager & Martin, 1976).

We also hypothesized that the quality of children's attachment relationships with the caregiver might serve as a moderating factor in maltreated children's IS language development, because maltreated children are significantly more likely than nonmaltreated children to be insecurely attached. From both a psychodynamic and an attachment perspective

(Bowlby, 1982; Bretherton, 1987; Mahler, Pine, & Bergman, 1975), the quality of a child's early relationships with the caregiver (e.g., attachment security) should have a significant impact on multiple domains of the emerging self system, including children's ability to talk about ISs, via its hypothesized links with children's budding representational development ("internal working models"; Bowlby, 1982; Bretherton, 1987; Crittenden, 1990; Sroufe, 1990).

In support of this, attachment security has been related to individual differences in self-development such as visual self-recognition (Schneider-Rosen & Cicchetti, 1984); executive function and mastery pride (e.g., Matas, Arend, & Sroufe, 1978); pro-social behavior and empathy (e.g., Kestenbaum, Farber, & Sroufe, 1989), featural knowledge of self and mother (Pipp, Easterbrooks, & Harmon, 1992), and greater action complexity for self and mother during symbolic play (Pipp et al., 1992). In older children, attachment also has been related to affective regulation, use of emotion language, emotional awareness, and interpersonal planning skills (Greenberg, Kusche, & Speltz, 1991).

In addition, attachment security has been shown to serve as a protective factor for children's general language abilities, but only for high-risk children (Gersten, Coster, Schneider-Rosen, Carlson, & Cicchetti, 1986; Morisset, Barnard, Greenberg, Booth, & Spieker, 1990). For example, in their longitudinal high-risk sample, Morissett et al. (1990) found that children at highest risk who were classified as secure in infancy had significantly higher developmental quotients at 24 months and more advanced language skills as assessed by the Preschool Language Scale at 36 months than the highest risk insecure children. Similarly, Gersten et al. (1986) found that attachment security had a significant protective effect on low-SES, maltreated, 24-month-old toddlers' language development, even though maltreatment status was unrelated to toddlers' language at this age.

Deficits in maltreated children's IS language profiles, as well as their communicative development more generally, might also be expected in the light of the negative, disorganized affective-linguistic environments reported for maltreating families (Bronfenbrenner, 1979; Prizant & Wetherby, 1990). In striking contrast to low-risk, middle-class families (e.g., Dunn et al., 1987; Mervis, 1984; Snow, 1984), maltreating families are reported to spend less time in conversations and discussions than nonmaltreating families. For instance, Silber (1990) reported that, during a conflict negotiation task, maltreating families were less likely to engage in sustained, task-focused verbal interaction and had children who were less likely to initiate conversation than demographically matched nonmaltreating families.

In addition, maltreating parents, who fall at the extreme end of the continuum of caretaking casualty (Sameroff & Chandler, 1975), are reported to provide their children with chronically insensitive care (Crittenden & Ainsworth, 1989; Trickett, Aber, Carlson, & Cicchetti, 1991) and to have less optimal interactive styles than nonmaltreating caregivers. Though variable across families, these interactive styles have been described as overly controlling, hostile/punitive, neglecting, and/or inconsistent (Belsky & Vondra, 1989; Bousha & Twentyman, 1984; Grusec & Walters, 1991; Lyons-Ruth et al., 1987; Silber, Bermann, Henderson, & Lehmann, 1993; Wasserman, Green, & Allen, 1983).

In the present study, we assessed the productive IS language abilities of maltreated and nonmaltreated children from low-SES homes when children were 2½ years old, a time when IS language is rapidly increasing and significant effects of the social environment on language development have been demonstrated (Coster et al., 1989; Moriset et al., 1990). To maximize validity, child language data were derived from two sources: structured maternal interviews and direct observations of toddlers' IS language during social interaction in four laboratory contexts.

Maternal interviews were included because children's use of certain categories of IS words such as emotion words may occur less frequently in laboratory contexts as compared to other situations (Bretherton et al., 1986; Dunn et al., 1987). In addition, considerable support for the concurrent and predictive validity of maternal interviews for assessing toddlers' early lexical development (e.g., Fenson et al., 1991) and early IS vocabulary (Bretherton & Beeghly, 1982; Bretherton et al., 1986) has recently been generated, at least in low-risk samples. However, less is known about the validity of maternal interviews in extremely low-SES samples or for families at high psychological risk, such as maltreating families.

In view of the more general language delays observed for maltreated children during the 3rd year (Coster et al., 1989), we expected to find significant negative effects of maltreatment of the productivity, diversity, and decontextualization of children's IS lexicons. Decontextualized language was of interest because references to nonpresent persons and events increase in frequency during the 3rd year and reflect more advanced linguistic and conceptual development (Hood & Bloom, 1979; Sachs, 1983). Moreover, in light of the socioaffective comorbidities associated with child maltreatment, including disturbances in the self system (Cicchetti, 1991), we expected to find effects of maltreatment on the semantic content of their IS language as well as on their ability to use IS words for self and other.

In addition to specific effects of maltreatment, we also were interested in whether individual differences in children's IS language in both groups were related to gender differences or to children's general linguistic maturity, as has been reported for low-risk toddlers. Finally, we assessed the possible moderating effects of children's attachment relationship with the caregiver on their IS language profiles, using a cumulative risk approach (Sameroff & Seifer, 1990). We anticipated that children at the highest risk (maltreated, insecure children) would have the most compromised IS language abilities.

METHODS

Subjects

Forty toddlers (17 girls and 23 boys) and their biological mothers participated in the present study (*M* toddler age = 31 months, 22 days; range = 30 months, 0 days, to 33 months, 29 days). Subjects were participants in a larger longitudinal prospective study of the developmental consequences of child maltreatment (Cicchetti & Rizley, 1981; see also Coster et al., 1989, for further description of the current sample). All toddlers were clinically normal and free of any physical impairments or brain injury. All families were from urban, English-speaking, low-income homes, with 93% receiving Aid to Families with Dependent Children (AFDC). Eighty percent of the study mothers were single parents, with no spouse or partner living in the home. Thirty-four (85%) were Caucasian, four (10%) were African American, and two (5%) were Hispanic.

Maltreated group. Fifty percent of the study toddlers (9 girls and 11 boys) had been maltreated while living with one or both of their biological parents. The mothers of these maltreated children were indicated as either the sole or coperpetrator in each case. Maltreatment was documented by a legal record filed with the Department of Social Services (DSS) and verified by a follow-up interview with the family's protective service social worker. All maltreating families were being monitored by public or private social service agencies. At the time this project was conducted (1979–1985), the families recruited in the present study were representative of the statewide population of newly confirmed maltreatment cases reported by the DSS (see Cicchetti & Manly, 1990).

Comparison group. An additional 20 toddlers (8 girls and 12 boys) and their mothers were recruited to serve as demographically matched, non-maltreated controls. Comparison families were recruited by advertisements in welfare offices, neighborhoods, and newspapers. All comparison toddlers and families were verified as having no history of abuse or neglect as documented by legal record and corroborated by home interview. Demographic and maternal characteristics of the maltreated and nonmaltreated groups are presented in Table 1. Groups did not differ significantly on any of the following important demographic variables: (a) household prestige ratings (Nock & Rossi, 1979), a 100-point rating of SES summarizing each household member's ability to command cultural, social, and economic resources; (b) ethnicity; (c) maternal age; (d) marital status; (e) maternal educational level; (f) religion; (g) family income; (h) maternal employment status; and (i) presence or absence of a spouse or partner in the

TABLE 1
Sample Characteristics

	Maltreated (N = 20)	Nonmaltreated (N = 20)
Maternal age		
M	28.33	25.66
SD	5.70	5.15
Maternal ethnicity		
Caucasian	16 (80%)	18 (90%)
African American	3 (15%)	1 (5%)
Other	1 (5%)	1 (5%)
Maternal education level (highest grade completed)		
M	10.10	11.40
SD	2.17	2.04
Partner/spouse living in home	4 (20%)	4 (20%)
Number of children in home		
M	2.50	1.65**
SD	0.89	0.93
Currently receiving Aid to Families with Dependent Children	17 (85%)	20 (100%)
Socioeconomic status (household prestige score)		
M	47.03	47.89
SD	5.64	2.76
Maternal employment status		
Unemployed/homemaker	14 (70%)	15 (75%)
Unemployed/student	2 (10%)	3 (15%)
Employed part-time	4 (20%)	2 (10%)

Note: Maltreated and nonmaltreated groups did not differ significantly on any maternal and demographic variable, with the exception of number of children in the home.
**$p < .01$.

home. Only one significant group difference was observed: Maltreating families were significantly more likely to have a larger number of children living in the home relative to nonmaltreating families.

Types of maltreatment. To identify the types of maltreatment documented for each maltreated toddler and for each toddler's immediate family, a trained graduate-level research associate interviewed the social workers of each family using a modification of Giovannoni and Becerra's (1979) 87-item checklist. This well-validated instrument tallies specific incidents and conditions of maltreatment and identifies the perpetrator for each incident. The social workers' interviews were then reviewed by two Ph.D.-level psychologists who identified the following types of maltreatment in this sample: physical abuse, physical neglect, and emotional mistreatment. No sexual abuse was documented in this sample. Interrater agreement for placement of children and families into maltreatment categories was 100%.

The majority of toddlers and their families were documented with multiple types of maltreatment; therefore, it was not feasible to test the impact of particular maltreatment types on children's IS language. Overall, 55% of the maltreated toddlers and 75% of their families were documented with two or more types of maltreatment: 7 (35%) toddlers had been physically abused, 16 (80%) had experienced physical neglect, and 12 (60%) had been emotionally abused. Somewhat higher rates of maltreatment were documented for the maltreated toddlers' families, suggesting that some study children may have been exposed to a greater variety of maltreatment than documented for them as individuals: 13 (65%) families were filed on for physically abusing their children, 17 (85%) for physically neglecting children, and 12 (60%) for emotional mistreatment.

Procedure

Children and mothers participated in two laboratory sessions spaced 2 weeks apart when children were within approximately 1 month of their 30-month birthdays. The first laboratory session (Visit 1) included three tasks administered in the following order: (a) the Strange Situation (Ainsworth, Blehar, Waters, & Wall, 1978), (b) a semistructured stranger-child play session (30 min), and (c) an Emotions Picture Book session with mother and child (5 min). The second laboratory session (Visit 2) included three contexts administered in the following order: (a) a semistructured mother-child play session (30 min); (b) the Peabody Picture Vocabulary Test–Revised (PPVT-R; Dunn & Dunn, 1981), a measure of receptive single-word vocabulary and an estimate of verbal IQ; and (c) an unstructured mother-child free-play session (20 min). In addition, mothers were interviewed about their children's current ability to produce IS words. All laboratory procedures at Visit 1 and Visit 2 except the PPVT-R and maternal interview were videotaped from behind a one-way mirror. All experimenters, interviewers, and research assistants were unaware of family diagnostic status.

Maternal Interview

Mothers were interviewed about their toddlers' current use of IS words utilizing a comprehensive interview adapted from Bretherton and Beeghly (1982). From a list of 50 target words divided into the 10 semantic categories described below, mothers were asked to identify those words their children could currently produce and to indicate whether they used them for self, other persons, toys, or pictures. Only words for which verbatim examples and contextual information could be given were counted. Maternal interviews were audiotaped for later data reduction. Specific IS words targeted in the interview were derived from prior research detailing toddlers' use of IS words (e.g., Bretherton & Beeghly, 1982) and included those words that explicitly referred to the ISs of themselves and others. Words denoting affective behavior (e.g., kiss, cry) were also included, because young children commonly use these terms to refer to affective states (Bretherton et al., 1986; Smiley & Huttenlocher, 1989).

The IS categories targeted in the present study included the following: sensory perception (sight, hearing, smell, taste, touch, pain, temperature); physiology (hunger, thirst, and states of consciousness such as sleep, fatigue, and arousal); positive affect (love, affection, kindness, happiness, joy, surprise); negative affect (hate, disgust, anger, sadness, fear, distress); affective behavior (words referring to affective behavior used by many language-learning toddlers to denote emotional states: kiss, hug, cry, laugh); moral judgment (good/bad person, moral conformity and nonconformity); obligation (permission, compulsory or imperative behavior); volition (desire, need); ability (task ability, mastery); and cognition (knowledge, thought, memory, insight, uncertainty).

Data reduction. Audiotapes of the maternal IS language interviews were transcribed verbatim and scored to produce the following summary variables:

1. Diversity of IS words. The number of different IS words reported was tallied across categories.

2. Semantic content. The proportion of IS words in each semantic category, relative to total reported IS words, was also calculated.

3. Self-other differentiation. Two summary scores reflecting the range and flexibility with which toddlers use IS words for self and other social agents were derived: (a) the proportion of IS utterances used to describe a single agent only (e.g., self) relative to total IS utterances, and (b) a self–other differentiation score, calculated by summing (for each IS word reported) the number of IS words for which the child used all three categories of social agents: self, other persons, toy/pictures.

Laboratory Observations

Toddlers' spontaneous production of IS utterances was also assessed during four different laboratory contexts, yielding a total of 80 min of videotaped interactive behavior for each child. Play contexts were included because IS language production is reported to occur frequently during pretend play (Beeghly et al., 1986; Dunn et al., 1987). The Emotions Picture Book task was included to elicit talk about emotions and other states directly. These four contexts are described below.

Stranger-child semistructured play. At Visit 1, a 30-min stranger-child semistructured play session was administered in a laboratory playroom furnished with a standard set of age-appropriate toys (e.g., a doll-house, puppets, trucks, story books, blocks, a toy piano) and a bean-bag chair for the adult situated to one side of the room. The play session was divided into three 10-min segments to allow an examination of the child's communicative and self-regulatory behavior during both structured and unstructured conditions. During the first and last 10-min segments, the stranger was asked to sit on the bean-bag chair provided for her and to refrain from initiating social interaction or directing the child's play. However, if the child initiated social interaction, the adult was asked to respond naturally. During the middle 10-min segment, the adult was asked to engage the child in playful interaction.

Emotions Picture Book task. In this task, the mother-child dyad was seated together in a large easy chair with the Emotions Picture Book and instructed to talk about the pictures together. The ensuing interchange was videotaped for 5 min from behind a one-way mirror. The Emotions Picture Book contained a series of photographs of children and adults in a variety of emotion-arousing situations (e.g., happy children at a birthday party; angry children struggling over a toy; a crying child getting an injection at the doctor's office; an adult scolding a child for breaking a potted plant).

Mother-child semistructured play. A 30-min semistructured mother-child play session was administered at Visit 2 that was identical in form and length to the stranger-child play session administered at Visit 1.

Unstructured mother-child free play. A second mother-child play session with a different set of age-appropriate toys was also included at Visit 2. During this 15-min session, mothers were given no specific directions other than "play with your child as you normally would at home."

Data reduction. Trained, reliable coders who were unaware of child diagnostic status transcribed verbatim all spontaneous child utterances containing IS words (see definition, earlier) from videotapes of adult-child interaction made during each of the four laboratory contexts. Along with each child IS utterance, relevant contextual information and any contingent adult utterances were also transcribed. Any questions that arose during transcription were resolved in conference with the first author. Reliability was assessed for 20% of the transcripts (range 88–100%). Each transcribed utterance containing a targeted IS word was further coded for semantic content and attributional focus (i.e., about self, other, toys, or pictures). Semantic content and self–other differentiation were defined and calculated exactly as for the analogous variables derived from the maternal interviews, described earlier. In addition, each observed IS utterance was further scored for decontextualization of use, that is, whether or not the child used the term to refer to nonpresent states (see later).

For analytic purposes, IS language variables were combined across contexts due to low frequencies for some categories of IS words. The following summary IS variables were derived from transcribed utterances in all four laboratory contexts:

1. Frequency and diversity of IS words. The absolute frequency of IS words as well as the number of different IS words were tallied across contexts.

2. Semantic categories. The proportion of IS words classified into each semantic category, relative to total IS words, was also calculated.

3. Self–other differentiation. Two summary scores reflecting children's flexibility in their attributions of ISs to self and other social agents were derived that are analogous to those derived from the maternal interviews: (a) the proportion of IS utterances used to describe self only, relative to total IS utterances; and (b) a total self–other differentiation score, relative to total IS utterances, calculated in the following way. For each different IS word produced, a point was scored for each different social agent that the child was reported to describe with that word (self, other person, toy, picture), resulting in a maximum self–other differentiation score of 4 per word. Word scores were then summed across lexical items and averaged (relative to the total number of different IS words).

4. Decontextualization of use. A summary score reflecting children's ability to use IS words in a decontextualized manner (i.e., in utterances referring to the inner states of nonpresent persons, or past, future, conditional, or hypothetical states, or in queries or negations about the existence of ISs). Each word was awarded 1 point for each instance of decontextualized use observed, resulting in a maximum possible decontextualization score of 6 per word. A score of 0 was also possible if children had not yet begun to discuss nonpresent states. Scores were then summed across words in each category and averaged (relative to the total number of different IS words produced). Decontextualization of IS word use was not included in the maternal interviews.

Table 2 provides brief definitions and verbatim examples of the semantic categories, self/other attribution, and decontextualized use scored in the present study.

General Linguistic Maturity

To determine the relationship of children's IS word production to their general linguistic maturity, indices of children's receptive and productive language ability were also derived, as follows.

Receptive language. Children's single-word receptive vocabulary and general verbal intelligence were estimated using the PPVT-R, a structured, forced-choice pictorial comprehensive test requiring no verbal output from the child. To reduce possible examiner effects on child performance, the PPVT-R was administered by the same familiar experimenter who had greeted the family and conducted the earlier play session. For analytic purposes, raw scores as well as standard scores (population $M = 100$, $SD = 15$) were included in the statistical analyses to safeguard against possible basement effects in this inner-city sample (children were at the youngest test age normed for the PPVT-R).

Expressive language. Two estimates of children's expressive language maturity were also included from data available from Coster et al. (1989). These measures were calculated from complete, reliable transcripts of consecutive, verbatim child utterances produced during the two mother-child play contexts described earlier.

1. Mean length of utterance (MLU; Brown, 1973). MLU in morphemes was calculated according to Brown's specifications as a measure of utterance complexity and an estimate of children's linguistic and syntactic maturity.

TABLE 2
Semantic Categories of Toddlers' Internal State (IS) Words

IS Category	Brief Definition	About Self or Others	Decontextualized Use
Sensory perception	Words explicitly referring to sensory perception: vision, hearing, smell, taste, or touch, including pain and tactile sensation	"Feels soft" "Lookin' at you" "See bottle" "Ouch" "Mommy smell it"	"See Grandma" (referring to future) "Don't watch me" "Hear that?"
Physiological states	Words explicitly referring to states of arousal, fatigue, sleep, hunger, thirst, or illness (feel sick)	"Baby sick" "Too tired"	"Not sleepy, Ma" "I was starving"
Positive affect	Words explicitly referring to positive affect, affection, pleasure, or sympathy (e.g., like, love, be silly, have fun, be funny)	"Love my baby" "Me havin' fun" "I like toys!"	"Having fun, Ma?" "Maggie silly" (referring to past)
Negative affect	Words explicitly referring to negative affect, dislike, displeasure, or disgust	"Yucky" "I hate it" "Mad at you"	"Bobby sad?" (referring to past) "Mommy mad?"
Affective behavior	Words explicitly referring to behavior denoting affective states (e.g., kiss, hug, cry)	"Hug dolly" "Baby kissin' Grover"	"Don't cry"
Moral judgment	Words explicitly referring to moral judgment of persons	"Bad dolly!" "Me good girl" "I being bad"	"Billy bad boy" (referring to past) "I be good" (referring to future)
Obligation	Words explicitly referring to obligation or permission	"You supposed to watch me" "Have to share"	"Don't let him" "Can I go outside?"
Volition	Words explicitly referring to volition and desire	"I want a large burger" "I need that truck"	"No wanna" "Need a tissue Ma?"
Ability	Words explicitly referring to ability and mastery	"That's easy!" "I can jump"	"I can't!" "Too hard, Mom?"
"Cognition"	Words referring to mental states or processes, even if used in routines (e.g., knowledge, thought, memory, uncertainty)	"I know" "I think it's a cat"	"I dunno" "Guess!"

2. Mean length of episode (MLE; Brown, 1980a, 1980b). Children's ability to maintain conversation at the discourse level (conversational relatedness) was estimated using MLE. MLE refers to the average length of children's sustained conversationally relevant episodes produced during playful interaction with an adult. According to Brown, a child's utterance is judged to be conversationally relevant if it is appropriately tied semantically and pragmatically to the adult's conversational act or to the context at hand. MLE was calculated by dividing the total number of a child's conversationally relevant acts that were unbroken by a nonrelevant act by the total number of the child's communicative acts.

Quality of Attachment

To evaluate the quality of the child's attachment to the caregiver, toddlers and mothers were videotaped in the Strange Situation paradigm (Ainsworth et al., 1978) as the first laboratory assessment conducted at Visit 1. The Strange Situation is a well-established, standardized procedure in which the child experiences a series of eight increasingly stressful episodes including being left alone and interacting with a stranger in an unfamiliar setting. The entire procedure lasts about 25 min and is videotaped. Attachment security was of interest in the present study because of its hypothesized role as either a protective factor or an added risk factor in the early language development of maltreated children.

Strange Situation behavior at 30 months was scored by two individuals with extensive experience in coding both infant and preschool attachment and demonstrated reliability in scoring Strange Situation behavior in both high- and low-risk samples. All discrepancies were resolved by repeated viewing of the videotapes by the coders until consensual agreement was reached. Videotapes were classified according to the MacArthur Preschool Attachment Coding System (Cassidy & Marvin, 1992). The following major classifications were analyzed: secure (Type B), insecure–avoidant (Type A), insecure–ambivalent (Type C), insecure controlling–disorganized (Type D), and insecure–other (mixed strategy—e.g., A/C). For analytic purposes, a dichotomous variable (secure/insecure) was used in the present study. Overall agreement for the major classifications was 92%.

RESULTS

The results are presented in four sections. First, group comparisons on indices of children's general expressive and receptive linguistic maturity are presented as a background for interpreting the specific analyses of IS language that follow. Next, group differences in the diversity, semantic content, attributional focus (self–other differentiation), and decontextualization of children's IS word production are reported, as derived from both the maternal interviews and laboratory observations. Third, results of two sets of correlation analyses are presented: (a) relationships between children's IS language production and their general linguistic maturity and (b) the degree of correspondence between mothers' reports of their children's current IS language production competencies and our direct observations. Coefficients are presented for the entire sample as well as for each group separately. In the fourth and final section, results are presented that (a) demonstrate the toxic effects of maltreatment on attachment security at 30 months and (b) compare the IS language profiles of the highest risk children in this sample (maltreated, insecure) to children at moderate or low risk, using a cumulative risk approach.

Unless otherwise specified, effects of maltreatment and child gender on toddlers' IS language were tested with a series of 2 (Group) $\times$ 2 (Gender) multiple analyses of variance (MANOVAs). Gender was included as an independent variable in the model because, although the literature is inconsistent, gender has been associated both with rate of linguistic maturity (e.g., Fenson et al., 1991) and with individual differences in language about feelings and other ISs in early childhood (e.g., Dunn et al., 1987; Fivush, 1989).

General Linguistic Maturity

Receptive language. No significant main effects for maltreatment were observed for children's receptive abilities as estimated by the PPVT-R, using either standard scores or raw scores. Thus, there was no indication that the maltreated children showed greater receptive deficits at 30 months than their nonmaltreated counterparts. The mean standard score for the sample as a whole was 92 (SD = 17, range 62–138). Although this average falls below the population mean of 100, it is, nonetheless, within the normal range for this age group. Children's mean raw score on the PPVT-R was 15 (SD = 11, range = 3–54). There were no significant main effects of gender or gender by maltreatment interactions for PPVT-R scores.

Expressive language. In contrast, maltreated toddlers had significantly poorer scores than nonmaltreated toddlers on both measures of expressive language: linguistic maturity (i.e., MLU) and conversational relatedness (i.e., MLE); Wilks's lambda for overall maltreatment effects = .68, p = .002. The average MLU in the maltreated group was 2.11 (SD = 0.48, range =

1.37–3.06) compared to an average of 2.77 (SD = 0.68, range = 1.43–3.73) in the nonmaltreated group, $F(3, 36)$ = 10.9, p = .002. A noteworthy finding is that the average MLUs in both groups were lower than that typically reported for similarly aged children from the middle SES (see Bates et al., 1987). For instance, Bretherton and Beeghly (1982) reported an average MLU of 2.77 for a sample of 30 28-month-old, middle-class children who were nearly 3 months younger than the present sample. Similarly, maltreated toddlers' average MLE scores were significantly lower than those of their nonmaltreated counterparts (maltreated: M = 2.19, SD = 0.48, range = 1.41–3.44; nonmaltreated: M = 3.23, SD = 1.09, range = 1.74–6.10), $F(3, 36)$ = 13.06, p = .001. Interestingly, MLE was significantly correlated with MLU (r = .56, p = .01) in the comparison group but not in the maltreated group, suggesting possible disorganization among different language domains for maltreated children. There were no significant main effects of gender or maltreatment by gender interactions for MLU or MLE.

IS Word Production: Maternal Reports and Laboratory Observations
Frequency and diversity of IS words. Group means, standard deviations, and ranges for mothers' reports of the number of different IS words produced by their toddlers and for the frequency and diversity of children's IS words spontaneously produced in the laboratory are provided in Table 3.

Similar main effects of maltreatment were observed in both the reported and observed data sets. In the maternal reports, maltreated toddlers produced fewer IS word types than nonmaltreated toddlers, $F(3, 34)$ = 4.18, p = .05. In the laboratory-based data, as hypothesized, maltreated toddlers produced significantly fewer IS words overall, ($F(1, 35)$ = 8.35, p = .007) and fewer different IS words ($F(1, 35)$ = 9.36, p = .004) than nonmaltreated toddlers; Wilks's lambda for maltreatment effects = .77, p = .03. There were no significant gender effects or maltreatment by gender interactions for either the reported or observed data.

Semantic content of IS words. Group means, standard deviations, and ranges for the proportional semantic content variables as derived from maternal report and from direct observations are in Table 4.

Controlling for the size of the IS lexicon, significant group differences in semantic content were found in the laboratory data set; Wilks's lambda for overall maltreatment effects = .60, p = .01, Wilks's lambda for gender effects = .66, p = .04, and Wilks's lambda for maltreatment by sex effects = .63, p = .02. Univariate analyses revealed that maltreated toddlers produced proportionately fewer IS words describing physiological states ($F(3, 35)$ = 5.27, p = .03), negative affect ($F(3, 35)$ = 13.98, p = .0007), and moral

TABLE 3
Frequency and Diversity of Toddlers' Internal State (IS) Words:
Maternal Report and Laboratory Observations

	Maltreated	Nonmaltreated
Maternal report		
Number of different IS words		
M	26.00	32.17*
SD	9.45	8.73
Range	9.00–42.00	12.00–47.00
Laboratory observations		
Number of different IS words		
M	9.95	16.35**
SD	5.48 ˙	6.7
Range	3.00–26.00	7.00–28.00
Total frequency of IS words		
M	41.45	77.65**
SD	31.31	43.90
Range	6.00–122.00	26.00–207.00

*$p < .05$. **$p < .01$.

obligation ($F(3, 35) = 4.80$, $p = .04$) than nonmaltreated toddlers. The main effect for negative affect was qualified by a significant interaction effect with gender such that maltreated girls used negative affect words less often than all other groups, $F(1, 35) = 15.68$, $p = .0004$.

Two significant gender effects were also found: Girls used proportionately fewer words about negative affect ($F(1, 35) = 3.93$, $p = .005$) but more affective behavior words than boys ($F(1, 35) = 4.69$, $p = .04$). There was also a marginally significant trend for girls to use more positive affect words than boys, $F(1, 35) = 3.07$, $p = .09$.

No significant group differences were observed for the maternal report data. Thus, during laboratory observations, maltreated toddlers were significantly less likely to talk about physiological states, negative affect, and moral obligation than their nonmaltreated counterparts but could not be distinguished on other more "task-oriented" categories of IS words (e.g., perception, volition, cognition[1]). In contrast, no significant main effects of maltreatment in the semantic content of children's IS language were found in the maternal report data.

---

[1] Note that toddlers' "cognitive" words at this age were almost exclusively routines (e.g., "I don't know") or used to modulate assertions ("I think it goes there") rather than references to abstract mental states (see also Shatz et al., 1983).

TABLE 4
Semantic Content of Toddlers' Internal State Words

	% IS Words							
	Maltreated				Nonmaltreated			
	M %	(*SD*)	Range	% 1[a]	*M* %	(*SD*)	Range	% 1[a]
Reported								
Perception	28.04	(7.85)	19.00–55.00	100	26.81	(3.99)	16.67–33.33	100
Physiology	16.16	(6.20)	0.00–25.00	95	16.14	(3.37)	12.00–25.00	100
Positive affect	15.92	(5.18)	0.00–23.81	95	17.92	(2.78)	14.29– 21.74	100
Negative affect	11.26	(4.24)	4.76–20.00	100	10.89	(2.92)	4.35–16.22	100
Affective behavior	9.03	(3.87)	3.85–20.00	100	9.94	(4.39)	5.26–25.00	100
Moral judgment	5.89	(3.05)	0.00–11.11	95	4.70	(2.49)	0.00– 9.52	94
Obligation	2.02	(3.11)	0.00–11.11	40	1.62	(1.75)	0.00– 4.35	50
Volition	5.99	(4.19)	0.00–14.29	80	7.00	(1.96)	2.90– 9.09	100
Ability	4.07	(2.37)	0.00– 8.00	80	3.02	(2.19)	0.00– 5.99	72
Cognition	1.03	(1.51)	0.00– 4.00	35	1.68	(1.43)	0.00– 4.00	61
Observed								
Perception	40.34	(23.80)	9.10–90.47	100	31.03	(13.08)	14.29–63.22	100
Physiology	2.05	(2.86)	0.00– 8.82	45	5.95**	(6.89)	0.00–29.03	85**
Positive affect	3.83	(6.41)	0.00–25.00	55	2.32	(2.07)	0.00– 7.69	80†
Negative affect	1.10	(1.99)	0.00– 7.00	35	3.69***	(2.92)	0.00–12.50	63†
Affective behavior	5.92	(8.13)	0.00– 2.69	65	6.69	(7.80)	0.00–35.71	100**
Moral judgment	3.46	(6.36)	0.00–18.52	40	2.09	(3.10)	0.00–12.62	60
Obligation	3.53	(4.73)	0.00–18.18	50	6.82*	(4.92)	0.00–15.38	80*
Volition	27.83	(19.66)	0.00–78.56	95	28.97	(14.29)	8.69–53.85	100
Ability	7.24	(9.19)	0.00–36.36	65	9.64	(8.95)	0.00–34.69	80
Cognition	4.71	(7.33)	0.00–26.08	50	3.26	(5.03)	0.00–21.43	60

[a]Percentage of toddlers reported to use at least one word from a particular category.
†$p < .10$. *$p < .05$. **$p < .01$. ***$p < .001$.

Nonparametric (chi-square) analyses were also performed for the semantic content data. In these analyses, the percentages of toddlers in each group reported to use at least one IS word in each category were compared. Nonparametric analyses were included as an alternative to MANOVA in light of the relatively low frequencies observed for some categories of IS words at 30 months. These percentages are presented in Table 4 for both the maternal report and laboratory data.

Chi-square results largely corroborated the MANOVA results for both the maternal report and the laboratory data: Whereas no significant group differences were observed for the maternal report data, significantly fewer maltreated than nonmaltreated toddlers produced at least one word about physiological states (9 vs. 17, respectively, $\chi^2(1) = 7.03$, $p = .008$), affective behavior (13 vs. 19, respectively, $\chi^2(1) = 8.1$, $p = .004$), and moral obligation (10 vs. 16, respectively, $\chi^2(1) = 3.96$, $p = .05$). Similar albeit nonsignificant trends (ps < .10) were also observed for positive and negative affect.

Distribution of IS word categories. Despite group differences observed for particular categories of IS words, roughly similar distributions in toddlers' relative production of IS word types were observed within each group, as seen in Table 4. Thus, virtually 100% of toddlers produced words for perceptual and volitional states, whereas somewhat fewer produced words about affective and other feeling states and moral judgment; only a minority used words for moral obligation and cognitive processes.

Self–other attributions and decontextualization in IS word use. Group means, standard deviations, and ranges for maternal reports and for laboratory observations of the degree of self–other differentiation in toddlers' use of IS words are presented in Table 5. Toddlers' decontextualization scores derived from laboratory observations are also presented in Table 5. These variables were corrected for the size of toddlers' IS corpora.

Similar findings were observed in both the maternal report and the laboratory data. Mothers in the maltreatment group reported that their toddlers used IS words in a more restricted way, that is, were more likely to use IS words to describe a single rather than multiple social agents, $F(1, 34)$ = 6.59, p = .01. Similarly, maltreated toddlers were less likely to use the same IS word to describe the internal states of a variety of social agents (self, others, pictures), $F(1, 34)$ = 7.41, p = .01, Wilks's lambda for overall maltreatment effects = .81, p = .03. No significant gender or maltreatment by gender effects were observed for these variables.

Similarly, in the laboratory data, maltreated toddlers were more likely than their cognitively-matched controls to use IS words in a restricted manner, that is, to refer only to a single agent ($F(1, 35)$ = 5.28, p = .03), but less likely to use the same IS word to describe the ISs of a variety of social agents (self, others, toys, pictures) ($F(1, 35)$ = 9.10, p = .005) and less likely to decontextualize IS language ($F(1, 35)$ = 9.05, p = .005), Wilks's lambda for overall maltreatment effects = .70, p = .008. As in the maternal report data, no significant overall gender effects or interaction effects were found.

Correlation Analyses

IS language and general linguistic maturity. Correlations relating children's IS language production to their general expressive and receptive language maturity are presented in Table 6. These correlations demonstrate that, for both the maternal report and the laboratory data in both the maltreatment and comparison groups, children's overall IS word productivity was significantly related to the complexity of their expressive language in general, as measured by MLU. In addition, for the laboratory-based data, the

TABLE 5
Self–Other Differentiation and Decontextualization in Use of
Internal State (IS) Words: Maternal Report and Laboratory Observations

	Maltreated	Nonmaltreated
Maternal report		
% IS words used for self or one agent only		
M	41.11	21.43**
SD	21.43	16.25
Range	5.12–85.71	0.00–57.00
Self–other differentiation[a]		
M	0.24	0.45
SD	0.24	0.23
Range	0.00–0.84	0.00–0.83
Laboratory observations		
% IS words used for self only		
M	36.17	21.4*
SD	19.96	16.2
Range	8.00–75.00	0.00–57.0
Self–other differentiation[a]		
M	1.18	1.32**
SD	0.14	0.15
Range	1.00–1.40	1.00–1.62
Decontextualization in use of IS words[a]		
M	0.54	0.76**
SD	0.17	0.25
Range	0.20–0.81	0.38–1.29

Note: Mothers were not interviewed about their toddlers' decontextualized use of IS words.
[a]See text for definitions. Proportional value relative to total IS lexicon.
†$p < .10$. *$p < .05$. **$p < .01$. ***$p < .001$.

children's flexibility in attributing internal states to self and other and their ability to use IS language in decontextualized ways were also significantly correlated with children's expressive language maturity. Moreover, the majority of the laboratory-derived IS variables were also significantly correlated with children's receptive language maturity (PPVT-R scores).

A somewhat contrasting pattern of correlation coefficients was observed for the maternal report data. Although maternal reports of children's IS language were correlated with children's MLU, they were not significantly correlated with children's PPVT-R scores in either group. In addition, a striking group difference emerged for children's reported flexibility in

TABLE 6
Correlations Between Toddlers' General Linguistic Maturity and
Their Production of Internal State (IS) Words (Reported and Observed)

| | General Linguistic Maturity | | | |
| | Expressive | | Receptive | |
	MLU[a]	MLE[b]	PPVT-R[c]	PPVT-R[d]
Maternal report				
Number of different IS words				
Whole sample	.63***	.43**	.23	.25
Maltreated	.55**	−.11	.03	.09
Nonmaltreated	.61**	.56**	.40	.35
Self–other differentiation score[e]				
Whole sample	.53***	.48**	.10	.11
Maltreated	.29	.13	−.08	−.08
Nonmaltreated	.50*	.49*	.23	.22
% IS words used for single agent				
Whole sample	−.40**	−.41**	.04	−.41**
Maltreated	−.20	.06	.33	.30
Nonmaltreated	−.29	−.43+	−.28	−.26
Laboratory observations				
Total frequency of IS words				
Whole sample	.75***	.49**	.42*	.42*
Maltreated	.85***	.04	.48+	.65**
Nonmaltreated	.59**	.45*	.28	.37
Number of different IS words				
Whole sample	.75***	.58***	.41*	.42*
Maltreated	.77***	−.002	.49+	.65**
Nonmaltreated	.63**	.63**	.35	.27
Self–other differentiation[e]				
Whole sample	.80***	.57**	.40*	.40*
Maltreated	.75***	−.02	.47+	.62**
Nonmaltreated	.72**	.58**	.35	.27
Decontextualization score[e]				
Whole sample	.76***	.60***	.34+	.37+
Maltreated	.69***	.01	.47+	.64+
Nonmaltreated	.68***	.55**	.29	.28

[a]MLU = mean length of utterance in morphemes. [b]MLE = mean length of episode. [c]Peabody Picture Vocabulary Test – Revised, standard score. [d]Raw score. [e]Raw score.
†$p < .10$. *$p < .05$. **$p < .01$. ***$p < .001$.

using the same IS words for both self and other: Whereas nonmaltreating mothers' reports of their toddlers' ability to use IS language for self and other agents was significantly correlated with their children's MLU ($r = .50$, $p = .05$), maltreating mothers' reports of the same dimensions were not.

In sum, the laboratory-derived data for both maltreated and non-maltreated toddlers and the maternal report data for the nonmaltreating mothers (but not the maltreating mothers) are largely consistent with prior research in middle-class samples documenting significant relationships between children's IS language production and their general expressive and receptive language maturity.

Validity of maternal reports. To assess the validity of the maternal interviews in this inner-city sample and for maltreating mothers in particular, mothers' reports of their children's IS language were correlated with direct observations of toddlers' IS language produced in the laboratory. These correlation coefficients are presented in Table 7. Again, strikingly different patterns were observed for the maltreated and comparison groups (Table 8). Comparison mothers' reports were significantly correlated with laboratory observations of their toddlers' IS word production, attesting to the validity of structured maternal report measures of lexical development for these extremely low-SES mothers. In contrast, maltreating mothers' reports of their toddlers' IS language were not correlated significantly with laboratory observations, especially toddlers' ability to use IS words for self and other agents. These findings suggest that it is maltreatment and its comorbidities (e.g., family dysfunction, neglect, violence), rather than poverty per se, that may have deleterious effects on the accuracy of maternal reports of their toddlers' developmental skills.

Maltreatment, Attachment, and IS Language Production

The distribution of attachment classifications in the low-SES comparison group was highly similar to that reported in the literature for low-risk samples (Spieker & Booth, 1988): 63% were secure, 16% were insecure–avoidant, 10% were insecure–ambivalent, and 11% were insecure controlling–disorganized or insecure–other. In contrast, a significantly lower rate of security and a higher rate of insecure controlling–disorganized or insecure–other (e.g., mixed strategy) classifications was observed in the maltreated group, $\chi^2(4) = 9.36$, $p = .05$. Only five maltreated toddlers (25%) were classified as secure, 40% were insecure controlling–disorganized or insecure–other, 25% were insecure–avoidant, and 10% were insecure–ambivalent.

To examine the possible moderating role of the quality of the child's attachment to the caregiver in either buffering or compromising their early production of IS language, three a priori groups of toddlers varying in cumulative risk were created: (a) low risk (nonmaltreated/secure toddlers, $n = 12$), (b) moderate risk (maltreated/secure toddlers or nonmaltreated,

TABLE 7

Correlations Between Maternal Reports of Children's Internal State (IS) Words
and Laboratory Observations of Children's IS Words

	Maternal Report	
Laboratory Observations	No. different IS words	Self–other differentiation
Total frequency of IS words		
Whole sample	.45**	.45**
Maltreated	.23	.03
Nonmaltreated	.48*	.55**
Number of different IS words		
Whole sample	.64***	.61***
Maltreated	.40†	.18
Nonmaltreated	.77***	.79***
Self–other differentiation		
Whole sample	.64***	.62***
Maltreated	.38†	.14
Nonmaltreated	.77***	.80***

†$p < .10$. *$p < .05$. **$p < .01$. ***$p < .001$.

insecure toddlers, $n = 12$), and (c) high risk (maltreated/insecure toddlers, $n = 15$).

For the laboratory observations, toddlers in the highest risk group showed more compromised IS language than toddlers in either the moderate- or low-risk groups, as follows: High-risk toddlers produced fewer IS words ($F(2, 33) = 3.44$, $p = .04$) and fewer IS word types ($F(2, 33) = 4.39$, $p = .02$), Wilks's lambda for overall maltreatment effects = .71, $p = .02$. Moreover, the high-risk toddlers were more context bound in their use of IS words ($F(2, 32) = 4.56$, $p = .02$) and less likely to use IS words for both self and other ($F(2, 32) = 6.52$, $p = .02$) relative to the other groups, Wilks's lambda for overall maltreatment effects = .60, $p = .01$. Notably, the low- and moderate-risk groups did not differ significantly. No significant gender or interaction effects were seen.

Similar findings were observed for maternal reports of toddlers' flexibility in their attributions of internal states to self and other, Wilks's lambda for overall risk group effects = .69, $p = .03$. Specifically, toddlers in the highest risk group were reported to use proportionately more IS words to refer to a single agent only ($F(2, 31) = 6.70$, $p = .004$) and to have

TABLE 8

Cumulative Risk: Effects of Attachment Quality on Maltreated and
Nonmaltreated Toddlers' Internal State (IS) Language Production

| Language Variable | Attachment/Maltreatment Risk Group[a] | | | | | |
| | Group 1: Low Risk (N = 12) | | Group 2: Moderate Risk (N = 12) | | Group 3: High Risk (N = 15) | |
	M	*(SD)*	*M*	*(SD)*	*M*	*(SD)*
General linguistic ability						
Mean length of utterance	2.66	(0.70)	2.65	(0.75)	2.08	(0.47)
Mean length of episode	2.83	(0.87)	3.12	(1.19)	2.16	(0.54)[b]
PPVT-R (standard score)	92.33	(9.66)	94.33	(25.28)	91.00	(15.94)
PPVT-R (raw score)	14.11	(5.09)	18.56	(16.50)	14.18	(8.85)
Maternal report						
Number of different IS words	29.92	(8.44)	33.10	(10.83)	25.00	(8.57)
Self–other differentiation[c]	0.37	(0.24)	0.49	(0.22)	0.20	(0.25)[b]
% IS words used for single agent only[c]	27.85	(22.80)	17.46	(12.59)	46.33	(21.38)[d]
Laboratory observation						
Total frequency of IS words	77.58	(50.16)	71.00	(36.73)	37.87	(29.86)[b]
Number of different IS words	14.67	(6.79)	16.42	(7.88)	9.20	(4.33)[b]
% IS words about self only[c]	21.58	(19.14)	28.33	(18.49)	36.69	(18.57)
Self–other differentiation[c]	1.30	(0.17)	1.33	(0.09)	1.14	(0.13)[b]
Decontextualization score[c]	0.82	(0.29)	0.63	(0.21)	0.54	(0.15)[e]

Note: PPVT-R = Peabody Picture Vocabulary Test – Revised.
[a]Group 1 = secure/nonmaltreated, Group 2 = secure/maltreated and insecure/nonmaltreated, Group 3 = insecure/maltreated toddlers. [b]Student Neuman-Keuls ($p < .05$): Groups 1, 2 > 3. [c]Relative to size of total IS corpus. [d]Student Neuman-Keuls ($p < .05$): Groups 1, 2 < 3. [e]Student Neuman-Keuls ($p < .05$): Groups 2, 3 > 1.

significantly lower self-other differentiation scores ($F(2,31) = 5.04$, $p = .01$) than toddlers in the moderate- or low-risk groups.

DISCUSSION

Summary

In this study, the impact of child maltreatment on the emergence of an IS lexicon was examined in a sample of toddlers from extremely low-SES homes (over 90% of the study families were receiving AFDC). The effects of child gender, general linguistic maturity, and the quality of the child's attachment relationship with the caregiver on characteristics of children's IS word production were also assessed.

Our findings are consistent with a growing pool of evidence suggesting that maltreatment has toxic effects on toddlers' early self-development and sociocommunicative abilities over and above the effects attributable to poverty. Evidence from both maternal interviews and direct observations of children's spontaneous language in the laboratory confirmed our expectations that the IS lexicons of maltreated toddlers were significantly delayed, impoverished, and pragmatically restricted, relative to demographically and cognitively matched, nonmaltreated controls. Thus, maltreated toddlers produced fewer IS words and fewer IS word types than their nonmaltreated counterparts, were more restricted in their ability to attribute IS to self and other agents, and were more context bound in their IS language use. These findings are consistent with more general deficits reported for maltreated toddlers' expressive language, which were described for this sample during maternal play contexts by Coster et al. (1989).

Notably, in the present study, group differences in children's IS language could not be explained entirely on the basis of differences in children's general linguistic maturity. Although individual differences in children's IS language were significantly related to their overall level of language maturity in both groups (a finding consistent with those reported for middle-class children), significant group differences in the content, attributional flexibility, and decontextualization of children's IS language were found even when the size of children's IS corpora and children's receptive abilities were controlled. Moreover, when moderating effects of the child's attachment relationship with the caregiver were considered, toddlers at the highest risk (maltreated and insecure) had the worst IS language profiles. Each of these aspects of IS language will be discussed in turn below.

Semantic Content

Distributions in the IS categories used by our low-SES toddlers were roughly similar to those reported for middle-class children in the literature: Perception and volition words were used proportionately most frequently by both maltreated and nonmaltreated children, followed by words about feelings and affective states (Bretherton & Beeghly, 1982). In contrast, words for cognitive processes were rarely observed. Moreover, when cognitive terms were observed, they were used primarily in routines ("dunno") or to modulate assertions ("I think it'll fit") rather than as references to abstract mental states. These latter findings are consistent with prior research documenting the relatively late emergence of mental state terms in middle-class samples (e.g., Bretherton & Beeghly, 1982; Dunn et al., 1987; Wellman, 1988).

Despite general distributional similarities in both the observed and reported data, significant main effects of maltreatment were found for particular IS categories in the laboratory data. Specifically, maltreated toddlers produced significantly fewer words denoting physiological feeling states (fatigue, hunger, thirst, illness, states of consciousness), negative affect (anger, sadness, disgust, fear), and obligation (permission, social or moral obligation). In contrast, no differences were observed for IS words more commonly produced to direct or guide behavior during task-oriented interactions, such as perception and volition.

Several possible explanations may be considered for the content differences observed for maltreated children. At a pragmatic level, maltreated children may have been trying to keep conversations with adults focused on the external and as "impersonal" as possible, an avoidant strategy that effectively minimizes intimate social interaction and, presumably, opportunities for further maltreatment or emotional injury. Characteristically, avoidant interactive styles during free play with mother (Coster et al., 1989) and during stressful conditions (e.g., separations, reunions) have been reported for maltreated toddlers (Carlson et al., 1989; Cicchetti et al., 1991; Crittenden & Ainsworth, 1989).

On a more general level, differences in the amount and content of children's IS language may be explained in part by characteristics of the affective-linguistic environment reported for maltreating families (e.g., Silber, 1990; Wolfe, 1985), which appear to be inconsistent with those hypothesized to facilitate vocabulary growth (see Mervis, 1990, and Snow, 1984, for reviews). This may be particularly true for the acquisition of terms for emotions and feeling states, because these words are thought to be acquired most readily during child-focused family discussions about emotions and negotiations of disputes and conflicting goals (Dunn & Brown, 1991). In contrast, the emotional climate of maltreating families, as reported earlier, has been characterized as highly disorganized, dysregulated, and noncontingent. Moreover, maltreating parents are reported to engage in maladaptive patterns of interactive behavior with their children that effectively preclude prolonged discussions about emotions (e.g., Burgess & Conger, 1978; Howes & Cicchetti, 1993). In such a climate, maltreated children may have learned that it is unacceptable, threatening, or even dangerous to talk about feelings and emotions, particularly negative ones.

A similar tendency to repress or deny negative feelings has been reported for older maltreated children. For example, Crittenden and DiLalla (1988) found that some insecurely attached/maltreated children showed a worrisome degree of "compulsive compliance"; that is, they did not express negative feelings overtly and were passively compliant with their mothers. Similarly, Vondra et al. (1989) found that maltreated school-age children were more likely to idealize their parents by exaggerating positive qualities and denying negative feelings or disturbances in the relationship (see also Lynch & Cicchetti, 1991).

An additional, and not necessarily mutually exclusive, interpretation of the emotional language data is that the use of negative emotion terms, references to the self, and the self's desires has provoked responses in the mother that generate anxiety in the child that necessitate regulation and control. Thus, maltreated children, in an attempt to control their anxiety, may modify their language (and perhaps even their thinking) to preclude the anxiety engendered by certain aspects of language and discourse in general.

Although possibly effective as a coping strategy during toddlerhood, a strategy of denying or repressing negative emotions may lead to a restricted or disorganized emotions lexicon and fewer dyadic exchanges about feeling states. Notably, these exchanges are thought to promote the acquisition of interpersonal regulatory skills and an increasingly differentiated self–other understanding (Bretherton, 1991; Cassidy, 1988). In support of this, Greenberg et al. (1991) observed that the behavior problems of deaf children, who had impoverished communicative skills, could be minimized if they were taught signs for emotions and feelings. Ultimately, these communicative and regulatory problems could contribute to future communicative, cognitive, and socioemotional problems (Cassidy & Kobak, 1988; see also Radke-Yarrow & Sherman, 1990). Although direct links between IS language and regulatory skills of maltreated children have not been established, maltreatment has, in fact, been associated with significant problems in emotion regulation later in childhood (Rieder & Cicchetti, 1989).

Gender Differences

Few significant main effects of gender or interaction effects of gender with maltreatment were observed. Gender was not related to children's overall linguistic maturity, lexical diversity, attributional flexibility, or decontextualization of their IS language. However, two notable exceptions were found that deserve mention, although findings were inconsistent across the two data sets (no significant differences in content were observed via maternal report). First, girls produced more utterances about affective behavior in the laboratory than boys, a finding similar to that reported by

Dunn et al. (1987) and Fivush (1989). It may be that greater talk about emotions by girls reflects a greater interest or propensity for social attunement. In support of this idea, in their studies of early prosocial behavior, Zahn-Waxler et al. (1992) reported that girls showed more concern to distress produced by others than boys and were more likely to "join in" the emotional experiences of others through imitation.

Our second gender finding—that maltreated girls were least likely to produce words about negative affect—stands in striking contrast to these gender findings but is consistent with reports of gender differences in children's coping styles under conditions of extreme or chronic stress. In their review of coping and resilience in high-risk children, for instance, Masten, Best, and Garmezy (1990) reported that an internalizing pattern of response to stressful circumstances (i.e., being disengaged but not disruptive) was more common in girls than in boys. Although such a coping strategy may have short-term adaptiveness, Masten et al. (1990) hypothesized that this response, if persistent or extreme, may be associated with vulnerability to affective or anxiety disorders, particularly during later adolescence.

Self-Other Differentiation

Individual differences in children's ability to use IS words for a variety of social agents, as derived from both laboratory observations and maternal reports, were positively correlated with indices of general language maturity, a developmental association similar to those reported for low-risk, middle-class toddlers (Bretherton & Beeghly, 1982; Dunn et al., 1987). Nevertheless, a significant main effect of maltreatment on children's ability to attribute ISs to self and other was also observed in both laboratory and maternal report data sets, even when controlling for the size of children's IS corpora. Specifically, maltreated toddlers were more restricted than MA-matched controls in their ability to use the same IS word for a variety of social agents, including self, other persons, toys, and photographs. To the extent that this linguistic ability reflects children's differentiating self and other understanding, this finding suggests that maltreated children may be more delayed in this domain than would be expected on the basis of their receptive language abilities.

Moreover, group differences in the correlational patterns of toddlers' linguistic abilities with self–other differentiation scores were also noted: Whereas nonmaltreated toddlers' ability to use IS words for self and other was significantly correlated with all general language indices (MLU, MLE,

PPVT-R), maltreated toddlers' self–other differentiation scores were not significantly related to their discourse abilities (MLE, conversational relatedness). Interestingly, maltreated children's MLE scores were unrelated to their utterance complexity (MLU) and to every IS measure, whether observed or reported. These correlational differences suggest some degree of disorganization at the interface of maltreated children's self and socio-communicative systems (Cicchetti, 1991).

Decontextualization in IS Language

Verbal references to the inner states of nonpresent persons, to past, future, conditional, or hypothetical states, were relatively rare at 30 months and were significantly correlated with indices of toddlers' general linguistic maturity. This finding is consistent with prior research in middle-class samples reporting an age-related increase in linguistic decontextualization (Bretherton, 1991; Hood & Bloom, 1979; Wellman, 1988). Notably, maltreated toddlers were significantly more context bound than nonmaltreated toddlers, controlling for overall IS vocabulary size, suggesting an important association between socioaffective experience and language development (Bronfenbrenner, 1979; Howlin & Rutter, 1987; Prizant & Wetherby, 1990).

Moderating Effects of Attachment

A significantly lower rate of attachment security and higher rate of insecure controlling–disorganized and insecure–other classifications were found for maltreated children at 30 months, relative to demographically matched nonmaltreated children. This finding is consistent with other studies reported for younger toddlers in the burgeoning maltreatment literature on attachment formation (e.g., Cicchetti & Lynch, 1993). In contrast, the distribution of secure and insecure attachment classifications in the nonmaltreated group, despite their SES risk, were consistent with those reported for low-risk samples (see review by Spieker & Booth, 1988). Notably, children who were both maltreated and insecure showed more compromised IS language and conversational relatedness (MLE) that did either a moderate-risk (insecure/nonmaltreated or secure/maltreated) or a low-risk (secure/nonmaltreated) group. Again, results point to the striking effects of cumulative risk on the organization of socioemotional and communicative development in this low-SES sample.

Validity of Maternal Reports

This study also provides at least general support for the validity of the maternal interviews in this low-SES sample, particularly the nonmaltreating mothers, based on two findings. First, similar maltreatment effects were observed for analogous IS variables in both the maternal interview and the laboratory data sets, at least for the major IS language variables (diversity, self–other differentiation). Second, mothers' reports of the diversity of their children's IS words in both the maltreatment and comparison groups were also significantly related to their children's concurrent expressive language maturity (MLU), as derived during laboratory play contexts. Thus, mothers' reports of their children's IS language abilities in this low-SES sample appear to be tapping at least general aspects of their children's language maturity. The accuracy of the maternal interviews were undoubtedly enhanced by three factors: the interviews were highly structured, information about children's *current* abilities was requested, and concrete examples were required for every lexical item (see Bretherton & Beeghly, 1982).

Our findings also suggest, however, that cumulative risk factors (poverty, maltreatment) within a low-SES sample may compromise caregivers' ability to provide accurate information about their children's developmental abilities. Thus, significant autocorrelations between maternal reports and laboratory observations were observed only for mothers in the lower risk comparison group. These findings suggest that maltreating mothers are less accurate reporters of their children's use of IS language.

In sum, our findings suggest that maltreatment has a significant compromising effect on dimensions of children's productive language that reflect their emerging understanding of self and other: IS language. These findings could not be explained entirely on the basis of demographic characteristics relevant to delayed language acquisition (Barnes et al., 1983; McLloyd & Wilson, 1991) or the maltreated children's lower general linguistic maturity. Furthermore, effects of maltreatment on IS language were exacerbated by the "double jeopardy" of a concurrent insecure attachment relationship with the caregiver.

Because IS language is critical to the regulation of social interaction and an early index of self–other understanding, our data bode poorly for later self-development in maltreated children. Due to the hierarchical organization of ontogenesis within and across psychological and biological domains, the early self-dysfunction manifested by maltreated toddlers is likely to eventuate in further disruptions in the development of the self.

To end on a more positive note, not all maltreated toddlers evidenced perturbations in self-development. Securely attached maltreated toddlers did not exhibit the dysfunctions revealed by the insecurely attached maltreated children. Thus, secure attachment may be a protective mechanism (Rutter, 1987) ameliorating the link between maltreatment and self-disturbances. In the future, researchers must continue to elucidate the processes whereby maltreated children develop competent outcomes despite the experience of adversity (Cicchetti & Garmezy, 1993; Cicchetti, Rogosch, Lynch, & Holt, 1993).

REFERENCES

Aber, J. L., & Cichetti. D. (1984). The socioemotional development of maltreated children: An empirical and theoretical analysis. In H. Fitzgerald, B. Lester, & M. W. Yogman (Eds.), *Theory and research in behavioral pediatrics* (Vol. 2, pp. 147–205). New York: Plenum Press.

Ainsworth, M. D. S., Blehar, M., Waters. E., & Wall, S. (1978). *Patterns of attachment.* Hillsdale NJ: Erlbaum.

Alessandri, S. M. (1991) Play and social behavior in maltreated preschoolers. *Development and Psychopathology, 3,* 191–205.

Barnes, S., Gurgreund, M., Satterly, D., & Wells, G. (1983). Characteristics of adult speech which predict children's language development. *Journal of Child Language, 10,* 65–84.

Barrett, K. C., & Campos, J. J. (1987). Perspectives on emotional development II: A functionalist approach to emotions. In J. D. Osofsky (Ed.), *Handbook of infant development* (pp. 555–578). New York: Wiley.

Bates, E. (1990). Language about me and you. Pronominal references and the emerging concept of self. In D. Cicchetti & M. Beeghly (Eds.), *The self in transition* (pp. 165–182). Chicago: University of Chicago Press.

Bates, E., O'Connell, B., & Shore, C. (1987). Language and communication in infancy. In J. Osofsky (Ed.), *Handbook of infant development* (2nd ed.). New York: Wiley.

Beckwith, R. T. (1991). The language of emotion, the emotions, and nominalist bootstrapping. In D. Fry & C. Moore (Eds.), *Children's theories of mind: Mental states and social understanding* (pp. 77–96). Hillsdale, NJ: Erlbaum.

Beeghly, M. (1993). Parent–child play as a window on infant competence. In K. MacDonald (Ed.), *Parent–child play: Descriptions and implications* (pp. 71–112). New York: State University of New York Press.

Beeghly. M., Bretherton, I., & Mervis, C. (1986). Mothers' internal state language to toddlers. *British Journal of Developmental Psychology, 4,* 247–260.

Belsky, J., & Vondra, J. (1989). Lessons from child abuse: The determinants of parenting. In D. Cicchetti & V. Carlson (Eds.), *Child maltreatment: Theory and* research on the causes and consequences of child abuse and neglect (pp. 153–202). New York: Cambridge University Press.

Blager, F., & Martin, H. (1976). Speech and language of abused children. In H. P. Martin (Ed.), *The abused child* (pp. 83–92). Cambridge, MA: Balinger.

Bloom, L. (1991). *Language development: From two to three.* New York: Cambridge University Press.

Bloom, L., & Beckwith, R. (1989). Talking with feeling: Integrating affective and linguistic expression in early language development. *Cognition and Emotion, 3,* 313–342.

Bousha, D., & Twentyman, C. (1984). Mother–child interactional style in abuse, neglect, and control groups: Naturalistic observations in the home. *Journal of Abnormal Psychology, 93,* 106–114.

Bowlby, J. (1982). *Attachment and loss: Vol. 1. Attachment* (2nd ed.). New York: Basic Books.

Bretherton, I. (1987). New perspectives on attachment relations: Security, communication, and internal state working models. In J. D. Osofsky (Ed.), *Handbook of infant development* (pp. 1059–1100). New York: Wiley.

Bretherton, I. (1991). Intentional communication and the development of an understanding of mind. In D. Frye & C. Moore (Eds.), *Children's theories of mind: Mental states and social understanding* (pp. 49–75). Hillsdale, NJ: Erlbaum.

Bretherton, I., & Beeghly, M. (1982). Talking about internal states: The acquisition of an explicit theory of mind. *Developmental Psychology, 18,* 906–921.

Bretherton, I., & Beeghly M. (1989). Pretense: Acting "as if." In J. J. Bridges & N. H. Hazen (Eds.), *Action in social context: Perspectives on early development* (pp. 239–271). New York: Plenum Press.

Bretherton, I., Fritz, J., Zahn-Waxler, C., & Ridgeway, D. (1986). Learning to talk about emotions: A functionalist perspective. *Child Development, 55,* 529–548.

Bretherton, I., McNew, S., & Beeghly-Smith, M. (1981). Early person knowledge as expressed in gestural communication: When do infants acquire a "theory of mind"? In M.E. Lamb & L. R. Sherrod (Eds.), *Infant social cognition* (pp. 333–373). Hillsdale, NJ: Erlbaum.

Bromley, D. B. (1977). Natural language and the development of self. In C. B. Keasey (Ed.), *Nebraska Symposium on Motivation* (pp. 117–167). Lincoln: University of Nebraska Press.

Bronfenbrenner, U. (1979). *The ecology of human development.* Cambridge, MA: Harvard University Press.

Brown, R. (1973). *A first language: The early stages.* Cambridge, MA: Harvard University Press.

Brown, R. (1980a). *Coding child utterances for conversational relevance.* Unpublished coding manual, Harvard University, Cambridge, MA.

Brown, R. (1980b). The maintenance of conversation. In D. R. Olson (Ed.), *The social foundations of language and thought.* New York: Norton.

Burgess, R., & Conger, R. (1978). Family interaction in abusive, neglectful, and normal families. *Child Development, 49,* 1163–1173.

Carlson, V., Cicchetti, D., Barnett, D., & Braunwald, K. (1989). Disorganized/disoriented attachment relationships in maltreated infants. *Developmental Psychology, 25,* 525–531.

Cassidy, J. (1988). Child–mother attachment and the self at age six. *Child Development, 57,* 331–337.

Cassidy, J., & Kobak, R. R. (1988). Avoidance and its relationship to other defensive processes. In J. Belsky & T. Nezworski (Eds.), *Clinical implications of attachment* (pp. 300–323). Hillsdale, NJ: Erlbaum.

Cassidy, J., & Marvin, R., with the MacArthur Working Group on Attachment Beyond Infancy. (1992). *Attachment organization in preschool children: Procedure and coding manual.* Unpublished manuscript, University of Virginia, Charlottesville.

Cicchetti, D. (1984). The emergence of developmental psychopathology. *Child Development, 55,* 1–7.

Cicchetti, D. (1991). Fractures in the crystal: Developmental psychopathology and the emergence of self. *Developmental Review, 11,* 271–287.

Cicchetti, D., & Beeghly, M. (1987). Symbolic development in maltreated youngsters: An organizational perspective. *New Directions in Child Development, 36,* 47–68.

Cicchetti, D., & Carlson, V. (Eds.). (1989). *Child maltreatment: Theory and research on the causes and consequences of child abuse and neglect.* New York: Cambridge University Press.

Cicchetti, D., Carson, V., Braunwald, K., & Aber, J. L. (1987). The Harvard child maltreatment project: A context for research on the sequelae of child maltreatment. In R. Gelles & J. Lancaster (Eds.), *Research in child abuse: Biosocial perspectives* (pp. 277–298). Chicago: Aldine Press.

Cicchetti, D., Ganiban, J., & Barnett, D. (1991). Contributions from the study of high risk populations to understanding the development of emotion regulation. In J. Garber & K. Dodge (Eds.), *The development of emotion regulation and dysregulation* (pp. 15–49). New York: Cambridge University Press.

Cicchetti, D., & Garmezy, N. (Eds.). (1993). Milestones in the development of resilience [Special issue]. *Development and Psychopathology, 5*(4), 497–502.

Cicchetti, D., Lynch, M. (1993). Toward an ecological/transactional model of community violence and child maltreatment: Consequences for children's development. *Psychiatry, 56,* 96–118.

Cicchetti, D., & Manly, J. T. (1990). A personal perspective on conducting research with maltreating families: Problems and solutions. In G. Brady & I. Sigel (Eds.), *Methods of family research: Vol. 2. Families at risk* (pp. 87–133). Hillsdale, NJ: Erlbaum.

Cicchetti, D., & Rizley, R. (1981). Developmental perspectives on the etiology, intergenerational transmission, and sequelae of child maltreatment. In R. Rizley & D. Cicchetti (Eds.), *Developmental perspectives on child maltreatment* (Vol. II, pp. 31–57). San Francisco: Jossey-Bass.

Cicchetti, D., Rogasch, F. A., Lynch, M., & Holt, K. D. (1993). Resilence in maltreated children: Processes leading to adaptive outcome. *Development and Psychopathology, 5* (4), 629–647.

Coster, W., & Cicchetti, D. (1993). Research on the communicative development of maltreated children: Clinical implications. *Topics in Language Disorders, 13*, 25–38.

Coster, W., Gersten, M. S., Beeghly, M., & Cicchetti, D. (1989). Communicative functioning in maltreated toddlers. *Developmental Psychology, 25*, 1020–1029.

Crittenden, P. M. (1988). Relationships at risk. In J. Belsky & T. Nezworski (Eds.), *Clinical implications of attachment* (pp. 136–174). Hillsdale, NJ: Erlbaum.

Crittenden, P. M. (1990). Internal representational models of attachment relationships. *Infant Mental Health Journal, 11*, 259–277.

Crittenden, P. M. & Ainsworth, M. (1989). Attachment and child abuse. In D. Cicchetti & V. Carlson (Eds.), *Child maltreatment: Theory and research on the causes and consequences of child abuse and neglect* (pp. 432–463). New York: Cambridge University Press.

Crittenden, P. M, & DiLalla, D. L. (1988). Compulsive compliance: The development of an inhibitory coping strategy in infancy. *Journal of Abnormal Child Psychology, 16*, 585–599.

Denham, S., McKinley, M., Couchoud, E., & Holt. R. (1990). Emotional and behavioral predictors of peer status in young preschoolers. *Child Development, 61*, 1145–1152.

Dunn, J., Bretherton. I., & Munn, P. (1987). Conversations about feeling states between mothers and their young children. *Developmental Psychology, 21*, 132–139.

Dunn, J., & Brown. J., (1991). Relationships, talk about feelings, and the development of affect regulation in early childhood. In J. Garber & K. A. Dodge (Eds.). *The development of emotion regulation and dysregulation* (pp. 89–108). New York: Cambridge University Press.

Dunn, J., Brown. J., & Beardsall, L. (1991a). Family talk about feeling states and children's later understanding of others' emotions. *Developmental Psychology, 27*, 448–455.

Dunn, J., Brown, J., Slomkowski, C., Tesla, C., & Youngblade, L. (1991b). Young children's standing of other peoples' feelings and beliefs: Individual differences and their antecedents. *Child Development, 62*, 1352–1366.

Dunn, L. M., & Dunn, L. (1981). *The Peabody Picture Vocabulary Test—Revised.* Circle Pines, MN: American Guidance Service.

Egeland, B., & Sroufe, L. A. (1981). Developmental sequelae of maltreatment in infancy. *New Directions for Child Development, 11*, 77–92.

Emde, R., Johnson, W., & Esterbrooks, M. A. (1987). The do's and don'ts of early moral development: Psychoanalytic tradition and current research. In J. Kagan & S. Lamb (Eds.), *The emergence of morality in young children* (pp. 245–276). Chicago: University of Chicago Press.

Fenson, L., Dale, P. S., Resnick, J. S., Thal, D., Bates, E., Hartung, J. P., Pethick, S., & Reilly, J. S. (1991). *Technical manual for the MacArthur Communicative Development Inventories.* San Diego: San Diego State University.

Fivush, R. (1989). Exploring sex differences in the emotional content of mother-child conversations about the past. *Sex Roles, 20*, 675–691.

Gaensbauer, T. J., & Sands, S. K. (1979). Distorted affective communications in abused/neglected infants and their potential impact on caretakers. *Journal of the American Academy of Child Psychiatry, 18*, 236–250.

Gersten, M., Coster, W., Schneider-Rosen, K., Carlson, V., & Cicchetti, D. (1986). The socio-emotional bases of communicative functioning: Quality of attachment, language development, and early maltreatment. In M. E. Lamb, A. L. Brown, & B. Rogoff (Eds.), *Advances in developmental psychology* (Vol. 4, pp. 105–151). Hillsdale, NJ: Erlbaum.

Giovannoni, J., & Becerra, R. M. (1979). *Defining child abuse.* New York: The Free Press.

Gopnik, A., & Astington, J. (1988). Children's understanding of representational change and its relation to the understanding of false-belief and the appearance-reality distinction. *Child Development, 59*, 26–37.

Greenberg, M. T., Kusche, C. A., & Speltz, M. (1991). Emotional regulation, self-control, and psychopathology: The role of relationships in early childhood. In D. Cicchetti & S. Toth (Eds.), *Rochester Symposium on Developmental Psychopathology: Vol. 2. Internalizing and externalizing expressions of dysfunction* (pp. 21–55). Hillsdale, NJ: Erlbaum.

Grusec, J. E., & Walters, G. E. (1991). Psychological abuse and childrearing belief systems. In R. H. Starr & D. A. Wolfe (Eds.), *The effects of child abuse and neglect: Issues and research* (pp. 186–202). New York: Guilford Press.

Harris, P. L. (1989). *Children and emotion: The development of psychological understanding.* New York: Basil Blackwell.

Hood, L., & Bloom, L. (1979). What, when, and how about why: A longitudinal study of early expressions in causality. *Monographs of the Society for Research in Child Development, 44* (2, Serial No. 181).

Howlin, P., & Rutter, M. (1987). The consequences of language delay for other aspects of development. In W. Yule & M. Rutter (Eds.), *Language development and language disorders* (pp. 271–294). Philadelphia: Lippincott.

Jaffe, P. G., Wolfe, D. A., & Wilson, S. K. (1990). *Children of battered women: Vol. 21. Developmental clinical psychology and psychiatry.* Newbury Park, CA: Sage.

Johnson-Laird, P. N. (1983). *Mental models: Towards a cognitive science of language, inference, and consciousness.* Cambridge, MA: Harvard University Press.

Kagan, J. (1981). *The second year: The emergence of self awareness.* Cambridge, MA: Harvard University Press.

Kagan, J., & Lamb, S. (1987). *The emergence of morality in young children.* Chicago: University of Chicago Press.

Kestenbaum, R., Farber, E. A., & Sroufe, L. A. (1989). Individual differences in empathy among preschoolers: Relation to attachment history. In N. Eisenberg (Ed.), *Empathy and related emotional responses* (pp. 51–56). San Francisco: Jossey-Bass.

Leslie, A. M. (1987). Pretense and representation: The origins of "theory of mind." *Psychological Review, 94,* 412–426.

Lewis, M., Stanger, C., & Sullivan, M. W. (1989). Deception in three year olds. *Developmental Psychology, 25,* 439–443.

Lewis, M., Sullivan, M. W., Stanger, C., & Weiss, M. (1989). Self-development and self-conscious emotions. *Child Development, 59,* 146–156.

Lynch, M., & Cicchetti, D. (1991). Patterns of relatedness in maltreated and non-maltreated children: Connections among multiple representation models. *Development and Psychopathology, 3,* 207–226.

Lyons-Ruth, K., Connell, D. B., Zoll, D., & Stahl, J. (1987). Infants at social risk: Relations among infant maltreatment, maternal behavior, and infant attachment behavior. *Developmental Psychology, 23,* 223–232.

Mahler, M., Pine, F., & Bergman, A. (1975). *The psychological birth of the infant.* New York: Basic Books.

Main, M., Kaplan, N., & Cassidy, J. (1985). Security in infancy, childhood, and adulthood: A move to the level of representation. In I. Bretherton & E. Waters (Eds.), Growing points of attachment theory and research (pp. 66–104). *Monographs of the Society for Research in Child Development, 50*(1–2, Serial No. 209).

Main, M., & Solomon, J. (1990). Procedures for identifying infants as disorganized/disoriented during the Ainsworth Strange Situation. In M. Greenberg, D. Cicchetti, & E. M. Cummings (Eds.), *Attachment in the preschool years: Theory, research, and intervention* (pp. 121–160). Chicago: University of Chicago Press.

Masten, A. S., Best, K. M., & Garmezy, N. (1990). Resilience and development: Contributions from the study of children who overcome adversity. *Development and Psychopathology, 2,* 425–444.

Matas, L., Arend, R., & Sroufe, L. A. (1978). Contiuity of adaptation in the second year: The relationship between quality of attachment and later competent functioning. *Child Development, 49,* 547–555.

McLloyd, V. C., & Wilson, L. (1991). The strain of living poor: Parenting, social support, and child mental health. In A. C. Huston (Ed.), *Children in poverty: Child development and public policy* (pp. 105-135). New York: Cambridge University Press.

Mervis, C. B. (1984). Early lexical development: The contributions of mother and child. In C. Sophian (Ed.), *Origins of cognitive skills* (pp. 339-370). Hillsdale, NJ: Erlbaum.

Morrisset, C., Barnard, K. E., Greenberg, M. T., Booth, C. L., & Spieker, S. J. (1990). Environmental influences on early language development: The context of social risk. *Development and Psychopathology, 2,* 127-149.

Nock, S., & Rossi, P. (1979). Household types and social standing. *Social Forces, 57,* 1325-1345.

Oates, R. K., Peacock, A., & Forrest, D. (1984). The development of abused children. *Developmental Medicine and Child Neurology, 26,* 649-656.

Piaget, J. (1962). *Play, dreams, and imitation in childhood.* New York: Norton.

Pipp, S., Easterbrooks, M. A., & Harmon, R. (1992). The relation between attachment and knowledge of self and mother in one- to three-year-old infants. *Child Development, 63,* 738-750.

Prizant, B. M., & Wetherby, A. M. (1990). Toward an integrated view of early language and communication development and socioemotional development. *Topics in Language Disorders, 10,* 1-16.

Radke-Yarrow, M., & Sherman, T. (1990). Hard growing: Children who survive. In J. Rolf, A. S. Masten, D. Cicchetti, K. H. Nuechterlein, & S. Weintraub (Eds.), *Risk and protective factors in the development of psychopathology* (pp. 97-119). New York: Cambridge University Press.

Ridgeway, D., Waters, E., & Kuczaj, S. (1985). Acquisition of emotion-descriptive language: Receptive and productive vocabulary norms for ages 18 months to 6 years. *Developmental Psychology, 21,* 901-908.

Rieder, C., & Cicchetti, D. (1989). Organizational perspective on cognitive control functioning and cognitive-affective balances in maltreated children. *Developmental Psychology, 25,* 382-393.

Rutter, M. (1987). Psychosocial resilience and protective mechanisms. *American Journal of Orthopsychiatry, 57,* 316-331.

Sachs, J. (1983). Talking about the there and then: The emergence of displaced reference in parent–child discourse. In K. E. Nelson (Ed.), *Child language* (Vol. 4, pp. 1-28). New York: Gardner Press.

Sameroff, A., & Chandler, M. (1975). Reproductive risk and the continuum of caretaking casualty. In F. Horowitz (Ed.), *Review of child development research* (Vol. 4, pp. 187-244). Chicago: University of Chicago Press.

Sameroff, A. J., & Seifer, R. (1990). Early contributors to developmental risk. In J. Rolf, A. S. Masten, D. Cicchetti, K. H. Nuechterlein, & S. Weintraub (Eds.), *Risk and protective factors in the development of psychopathology* (pp. 52-66). New York: Cambridge University Press.

Schneider-Rosen, K., & Cicchetti, D. (1984). The relationship between affect and cognition in maltreated infants: Quality of attachment and the development of visual self-recognition. *Child Development, 55,* 648–658.

Schneider-Rosen, K., & Cicchetti, D. (1991). Early self-knowledge and emotional development: Visual self-recognition and affective reactions to mirror self-images in maltreated and nonmaltreated toddlers. *Developmental Psychology, 27,* 471–478.

Shatz, M., Wellman, H. M., & Silber, S. (1983). The acquisition of mental verbs: A systematic investigation of the first reference to mental state. *Cognition, 14,* 301–321.

Silber, S. (1990). Conflict negotiation in child abusing and nonabusing families. *Journal of Family Psychology, 3,* 368–384.

Silber, S., Bermann, E., Henderson, M., & Lehman, A. (1993). Patterns of influence and response in abusing and nonabusing families. *Journal of Family Violence, 8,* 27–38.

Smiley, P., & Huttenlocher, J. (1989). Young children's acquisition of emotion concepts. In C. Saarni & P. L. Harris (Eds.), *Children's understanding of emotions* (pp. 27–49). New York: Cambridge University Press.

Snow, C. E. (1984). Parent–child interaction and the development of communicative ability. In R. L. Schiefelbusch & J. Pickar (Eds.), *The acquisition of communicative competence.* Baltimore, MD: University Park Press.

Spieker, S. J., & Booth, C. L. (1988). Maternal antecedents of attachment quality. In J. Belsky & T. Nezworski (Eds.), *Clinical implications of attachment.* Hillsdale, NJ: Erlbaum.

Sroufe, L. A. (1990). An organizational perspective on the self. In D. Cicchetti & M. Beeghly (Eds.), *The self in transition: Infancy to childhood* (pp. 281–308). Chicago: University of Chicago Press.

Starr, R., & Wolfe, D. (Eds.). (1991). *The effects of child abuse and neglect: Issues and research.* New York: Guilford Press.

Stern, D. N. (1985). *The interpersonal world of the infant.* New York: Basic Books.

Trickett, P., Aber, J. L., Carlson, V., & Cicchetti, D. (1991). Child rearing characteristics and child development in two samples of physically abusive families. *Developmental Psychology, 27,* 148–158.

Tronick, E. (1989). Emotions and emotions communication in infants. *American Psychologist, 44,* 112–119.

Vondra, J., Barnett, D., & Cicchetti, D. (1989). Perceived and actual competence among maltreated and comparison school children. *Development and Psychopathology, 1,* 237–255.

Wasserman, G., Green, A., & Allen, R. (1983). Going beyond abuse: Maladaptive patterns of interaction in abusing mother–infant pairs. *Journal of the American Academy of Child Psychiatry, 22,* 245–252.

Watson, M., & Fischer, K. (1977). A developmental sequence of agent use in late infancy. *Child Development, 48*, 828–836.

Wellman, H. M. (1988). First steps in the child's theorizing about the mind. In J. W. Astington, P. L. Harris, & D. R. Olson (Eds.), *Developing theories of mind* (p. 64–92). New York: Cambridge University Press.

Wolfe, D. A. (1985). Child abusive parents: An empirical review and analysis. *Psychological Bulletin, 97*, 462–482.

Zahn-Waxler, C., Radke-Yarrow, M., Wagner, E., & Chapman, M. (1992). Development of concern for others. *Developmental Psychology, 28*, 126–136.

Part II

BIOLOGICAL/GENETIC ISSUES

The three papers in Part II reflect growing interest and concern with the identification of biological correlates of psychiatric disorder in children and adolescents and their mechanisms of action. In Chapter 6, "Genetic Mechanisms in Childhood Psychiatric Disorders," Lombroso, Pauls, and Leckman provide a timely update of recent advances in the genetics of child psychiatric and developmental disorder. The methods and procedures of classical genetic investigation including twin, family, and adoption studies, segregation analysis, and linkage inquiries are described and critically reviewed, as are the intercellular processes governing the production of protein from genomic DNA. The status of current understanding of the genetics of autism, affective disorder, specific reading disorders, attention-deficit hyperactivity disorder, and Tourette's syndrome—all conditions investigated by these techniques—is summarized. Although the evidence for a genetic contribution is strong, no specific mutations have yet been identified for any of these illnesses.

Studies directed toward the clarification of the molecular etiologies of developmental disorders, particularly those in which cytogenetic abnormalities point directly to the chromosomal region of interest, have progressed further. Advances in DNA recombinant technology have led to the identification of specific mutations affecting different aspects of DNA to RNA processing in Fragile X syndrome, Prader-Willi syndrome, and Waardenberg syndrome. Although it has been hoped that similar methodologies can be successfully applied to the study of psychiatric and behavioral disorder, the task of demonstrating single mutations for more complex neurobehavior disorders is fraught with difficulty. The authors' discussion of the limitations of underlying genetic assumptions, as well as the importance of considering both genetic and environmental contributions to the variable expression of psychiatric illness within a developmental context, provides a useful framework for evaluating ongoing research in this rapidly expanding area of inquiry.

The second paper (Chapter 7) in Part II, by Dorn, Mazzocco, and Hagerman, illustrates an approach to the further specification of the range of phenotypic variation in a condition for which the specific genetic abnormality has been identified. The recent discovery of the fragile X mental-retardation (FMR-1) gene and the subsequent identification of an abnormal

167

expansion of cytosine-guanine-guanine (CGG) nucleotide repeats in both affected and unaffected Fragile X persons have led to a growing awareness that carriers of the FMR-X gene may exhibit a broad spectrum of involvement. In males, the full syndrome usually includes a characteristic physical appearance, mental retardation, and behavioral disorders including attention-deficit hyperactivity disorder, impulsivity, anxiety, compulsive behaviors, perseveration, angry outbursts, and sometimes self-injurious behavior.

Dorn and coworkers have developed an innovative strategy to explore the possibility that carrier males might well manifest a more subtle form of the full syndrome. Retrospective data concerning fragile X carrier adult males and nonfragile X control males were collected via the family informant method. Each informant was the parent or relative of a child referred to a regional developmental assessment clinic serving fragile X families nationwide. Pedigree or DNA analyses were employed to determine the carrier status of each informant's father. Twenty-four daughters of fragile X fathers and 32 daughters of control fathers were interviewed by an examiner, using standardized instruments, who was blind to the father's carrier status. The finding that fragile X males exhibited a higher incidence of psychopathology involving symptoms of ADHD, alcohol abuse and dependence, and obsessive-compulsive symptoms, is consistent with the hypothesis that some carrier males may indeed be mildly affected carriers. Additional research to clarify relationships between behavioral and cognitive status, as well as between these clinical features and the number of CGG repeats within the FMR-gene are clearly needed. The possibility that psychopathology may also be an indicator of carrier status within a family in which the gene is suspect, demands that careful consideration be given to the determination of carrier status of at-risk, but cognitively able, males during childhood.

In the final paper in Part II, McKenna, Gordon, and Rapoport discuss the relevance of recent advances in neurobiological research to the understanding of childhood-onset schizophrenia as well as the adult forms of the disorder. Although variability in the onset of schizophrenia has long been recognized, little by way of systematic research has been directed toward those rarely occurring individuals whose psychotic symptoms have become manifest before puberty. The seminal work of Kolvin provided the basis for the modern DSM separation between autism and childhood-onset schizophrenia. Nevertheless, questions about the specificity of diagnostic criteria, differentiation from pervasive developmental disorder particularly as it may present in children with normal intelligence, as well as continuity with adult forms of the disorder are still incompletely resolved. Recent advances in genetics, neuroimaging, and pharmacology have contributed to a growing consensus that later-onset schizophrenia is a heterogeneous neurodevelopmental disorder in which genetics as well as environmental factors affecting prenatal development are of etiological significance. Compared with adult-onset schizophrenics, samples of schizophrenic children may be more homogeneous, and certainly less affected by chronic neuroleptic treatment, substance abuse, or the consequences of institutionalization. The application of newly developed methods of biological investigation may well contribute to further clarification of salient environmental insults or neurodevelopmental abnormalities.

The present paper constitutes both a status report and a programmatic outline. Two questions inform the discussion of research in the areas of genetics, physiology, neuropsychology, functional imaging, neurochemistry, and pharmacology: (1) whether a "novel" neurobiological mechanism will be found for childhood-onset schizophrenia; and (2) whether biological studies will validate subgrouping by prodrome, phenomenology, comorbidity, or prognosis. Although the account of the history of schizophrenia in childhood is incomplete, the work of Lauretta Bender being conspicuous for its absence, the provisional roadmap for the future that this review provides is of value to investigators and to consumers of research alike.

6

Genetic Mechanisms in Childhood Psychiatric Disorders

Paul J. Lombroso, David L. Pauls, and James F. Leckman
Yale University, New Haven, Connecticut

Objective: *This review summarizes research findings on the genetics of several childhood psychiatric disorders.* **Method:** *One hundred fifty papers were reviewed from the past several decades and were selected because they have suggested that genetic factors may play a role in the etiology of certain childhood disorders. This review is not meant to be exhaustive but rather has emphasized those disorders for which a genetic etiology has been proposed by different research groups.* **Results:** *The more classical approaches to genetic research are reviewed and critiqued. The status of research for a number of childhood disorders is summarized. The molecular basis for several developmental disorders is presented and the prospects for arriving at a similar molecular understanding for other childhood psychiatric illnesses are discussed.* **Conclusions:** *Genetic factors play a determining role for certain developmental disorders. However, the molecular basis for other psychiatric disorders has yet to be elucidated and there are complicating factors that bear on genetic research of complex behavioral disorders.*

Major advances have been made over the past two decades in elucidating some of the underlying genetic and molecular mechanisms involved in a number of medical and neurological disorders including Huntington's disease, amyotrophic lateral sclerosis, Duchenne and Becker muscular

Reprinted with permission from the *Journal of the American Academy of Child and Adolescent Psychiatry*, 1994, Vol. 33(7), 921–938. Copyright © 1994 by the American Academy of Child and Adolescent Psychiatry.

From the Child Study Center, Yale University, New Haven, CT.

This work was supported in part by NIH and ADAMHA grants MH00856, MH44843, MH49351, MH00508, NS16648, HD03008, RR00125, and RR06022.

dystrophies, cystic fibrosis, and a variety of blood dyscrasias. For many of these disorders, evidence for a genetic involvement came from initial twin and family studies that pointed to the etiological importance of major genes. For others, evidence for a genetic etiology was based on cytogenetic abnormalities. The enormous progress in molecular biological and recombinant DNA techniques has led to the isolation and characterization of genes with mutations responsible for these syndromes.

Although genetic factors have been implicated in a number of mental, behavioral, and developmental disorders of childhood onset, the majority of human disease genes isolated and characterized to date have not been implicated in the pathogenesis of childhood psychiatric disorders. This article will first review some of the methodological approaches that have been used to investigate the genetics of childhood psychiatric disorders. Table 1 summarizes the evidence for a number of psychiatric illnesses for which a genetic contribution has been demonstrated (reviewed by Lombroso et al., 1990; Pauls, 1990; Rutter et al., 1990a,b). The majority of these disorders have been studied using more traditional approaches which first establish the importance of genetic factors through twin, family, and adoption studies. If family data are available, segregation analysis can then be performed to determine the best genetic model to explain the aggregation data. If transmission patterns are consistent with relatively simple inheritance, linkage studies and physical mapping can then be done to determine the chromosomal location of the gene of interest. Although a large body of data exists that supports the contention that specific genetic etiologies will be found for childhood psychiatric disorders, no specific mutations have yet been identified for any of these illnesses. Listed in Table 1, however, are three developmental disorders for which specific molecular etiologies have been discovered. These conditions can be used as models for illnesses with known genetic mutations that lead to childhood developmental disorders. For two of these disorders, the traditional approaches were not necessary because cytogenetic abnormalities directly pointed to the chromosomal region of interest. In the last section, the formidable difficulties involved in demonstrating single mutations for some of the more complex neurobehavioral disorders are reviewed and the importance of environmental factors is stressed.

TWIN STUDIES

Twin studies are a powerful research strategy used to assess the contribution of genetic factors in the etiology of childhood psychiatric disorders;

TABLE 1
Current Status of Research on the Genetic Basis for Several Childhood Psychiatric Disorders

Diagnosis	Twin/Adoption Studies Indicate Heritability	Segregation Analyses Support Major Gene Involvement	Linkage Studies Under Way	Chromosomal Region Identified	Specific Mutation Identified
Autism	Yes	Yes	Yes	No	No
Dyslexia	Yes	Yes	Yes	Reported, not replicated	No
ADHD	Yes	Yes	No	No[a]	No[a]
Conduct disorder	Yes	No	No	No	No
Tourette's syndrome	Yes	Yes	Yes	No	No
OCD[b]	Yes	Yes	Yes	No	No
Affective disorders[b]	Yes	Yes	Yes	Reported, not replicated	No
Schizophrenia[b]	Yes	Yes	Yes	Reported, not replicated	No
Fragile X syndrome	—[c]	Yes	Yes	Yes	Yes
Prader-Willi syndrome	—[c]	—[c]	—[c]	Yes	Yes
Waardenburg syndrome	—	—	—	Yes	Yes

Note: ADHD = attention-deficit hyperactivity disorder; OCD = obsessive-compulsive disorder.

[a] A disorder caused by mutation in the thyroid receptor-β gene has been associated with ADHD and is probably responsible for only a very small fraction of ADHD probands (see text).

[b] In adults only.

[c] Genetic basis initially established by cytogenetic observations.

this methodology has been recently reviewed (LaBuda et al., 1993). This approach was developed in response to the debate over whether genetic or environmental factors were the determinants in behavioral disorders. The theoretical basis for twin studies is relatively straightforward. Monozygotic (MZ) twins arise from the same fertilized egg and share identical genes. Dizygotic (DZ) twins arise from two separately fertilized eggs, and, similar to nontwin siblings, share on average 50% of their genes. The importance of genetic factors can thus be assessed by comparing the degree to which MZ and DZ twin pairs and their siblings have similar phenotypes. MZ co-twins should both have a genetic illness at a higher frequency than DZ twins. For MZ twins, the concordance rate will approach 100% for a condition that is minimally influenced by the environment (including fully penetrant single-gene disorders). For DZ twins the maximum concordance is 50%. This is the case for a fully penetrant autosomal dominant gene. However, if a condition is caused by a fully penetrant autosomal recessive gene, the expected concordance rate for DZ twins is 25%.

Twin studies have also been useful for studying disorders that do not follow classical Mendelian transmission patterns. For such complex disorders, in which more than one gene may play an etiological role, the concordance rate found among MZ twins should likewise be higher than the rate obtained for DZ twins. This higher concordance rate has been taken as evidence for a genetic contribution in various childhood disorders.

The results from twin studies have indicated that many illnesses thought to be influenced by genetic factors rarely have a concordance rate of 100%. This has been interpreted as evidence that environmental factors play a significant role in determining which children with a specific genetic vulnerability for a disorder will actually express it. The study of MZ twins who are discordant for an illness may identify environmental factors, such as perinatal stresses or socioeconomic factors, that significantly impinge on the developing child (Pauls, 1985). These kinds of investigations may also clarify what factors are at work among those children with a genetic vulnerability who do not develop mental illness.

A common critique of twin studies relates to the assumption that twins raised in the same family share the same environment. It is possible that MZ and DZ twins have very different responses to, or are affected differently by, a common environment. This issue has been investigated by Cohen et al. (1975), who found no significant differences for the parameters measured. It remains possible, however, that additional as yet unidentified environmental factors will have different effects on children with identical genes. For example, during intrauterine development, MZ twins frequently have different growth rates (with one twin pair significantly smaller) or suffer congenital malformations differentially, even though their development occurred in an environment that appears identical. The assumption that a shared environment has the same effect on twins needs to be reexamined. But as has been pointed out (Rowe, 1983), not only must environmental differences be demonstrated but, in addition, it is necessary to show that these differences are etiologically important in influencing the expression of a particular disorder.

FAMILY AND ADOPTION STUDIES

Family aggregation studies have also been used to study the genetic factors involved in psychiatric disturbances. The overall paradigm for these investigations is based on the premise that if an illness has a genetic component, then the frequency of that illness will be higher among the biological relatives of identified probands when compared to the prevalence in the general population. This design has been used for years in the behavioral disorder field, and much of the data have been used to support the hypothesis of a genetic involvement in different syndromes.

A major critique of such studies is that it is not possible to control for environmental factors that may play an etiological role. The fact that a particular disorder is found with a higher frequency among relatives suggests that some factor, either genetic or environmental, is important. The resemblance among family members is as likely to be due to a common environment, such as cultural or socioeconomic factors, as it is to a genetic input. Family aggregation studies by themselves are not powerful enough to discriminate between these two variables; however, it should be added that if the transmission pattern is consistent with Mendelian inheritance, it is unlikely that the illness is environmentally caused.

In an effort to address the problems inherent in this approach, adoption or cross-fostering studies were developed. This methodology attempts to look more closely at the role played by environmental factors. Adoption studies rely on the premise that when a disorder has a genetic basis, the frequency of a disorder among members of the biological family will be higher than the frequency of that disorder among members of the adoptive relatives. Conversely, when environmental factors are etiologically more significant than the genetic ones, the frequency for an illness among relatives of the adoptive parents may be higher than among the relatives of the biological parents.

Few adoption studies have been conducted for childhood psychiatric disorders. Adoption studies are difficult to do and their use in the study of childhood disorders reflects this. One major problem has been the difficulty of obtaining reliable information about both biological parents of adoptees, including diagnostic data from the biological parents' childhood. This is due partly to privacy issues involved at the time of placement, but also it reflects the fact that the biological father is often unavailable for examination. In addition, the timing of the adoption may have significant effects on the behavior of interest. For example, environmental influences will be significantly greater for a child who spends the first 3 years of life with his or her biological parents compared to the infant who is adopted at 3 days of age. Moreover, the environmental effects of 9 months in utero will always be present, and this is a critical period that affects the early development of the CNS. Finally, attempts are often made by adoption agencies to select families similar to the biological parents. This practice, termed selective placement, will add to the difficulty in interpreting the findings, as the assumption of a different environment is once again open to question. These difficulties with adoption studies have combined to make them less attractive to current investigators in the field of childhood psychiatric disorders.

SEGREGATION ANALYSIS

Family aggregation studies provide the appropriate data to test specific genetic hypotheses based on specific segregation patterns. Segregation is defined as the separation of alleles during meiosis. When the genetic model being tested is a simple Mendelian model, the expected ratios of genotypes are easily calculated and can quickly be compared to the observed ratios among the siblings of the affected probands. The expected ratios are conditioned on the most likely genotype of the parent given the specific genetic hypothesis. For simple traits, those that follow a Mendelian pattern, these analyses are sufficient. However, for complex traits that do not show a simple Mendelian pattern, additional parameters need to be added into the model and one relies more heavily on tests of genetic hypotheses under more general models rather than simple estimation of segregation ratios. This analysis allows estimation of the parameters of a specific model using nuclear family data and is known as segregation analysis.

Segregation analyses can give maximum likelihood estimates of the ascertainment probability and other parameters of the genetic model being used (Elandt-Johnson, 1970; Elston and Stewart, 1971; Morton et al., 1971). Statistical techniques can then be used to compare different hypotheses about the relationships of genotypes to phenotypes. The main drawback of most such analyses is that it must be assumed that the disorder being studied in all families is homogeneous and that the families represent a random sample from a homogeneous distribution of environments. For most common diseases, both of those assumptions are questionable.

Pedigree analysis using large multigenerational pedigrees is conceptually similar to segregation analysis of nuclear family data, but is generally considered more powerful because each pedigree contains more relationships. Specific hypotheses currently testable by pedigree analysis methods include single-locus inheritance, polygenic inheritance, and multilocus inheritance, among others (Cannings et al., 1978; Elston and Yelverton, 1975; Elston and Namboodiri, 1977; Lange and Elston, 1975; Lange et al., 1976). Parameters in the single-locus and multilocus models include the allele frequencies, the penetrances of all genotypes, and the transmission probabilities. A potential difficulty is that analyses of large pedigrees may be biased in favor of one specific hypothesis if only "interesting" pedigrees are analyzed. By establishing rules for the sequential sampling of pedigrees, it is possible to correct for such biases while avoiding unnecessary study of uninformative families (Cannings and Thompson, 1977).

LINKAGE STUDIES

In the absence of a known biological defect, linkage analysis studies are the most powerful method available to demonstrate that a genetic etiology exists for a given disorder. This approach assumes a fairly simple genetic etiology and should only be used after more classical methodologies, such as twin or adoption studies, have suggested that genetic factors are at work. Linkage analysis allows the determination of the relative position between different genetic loci and can identify the chromosomal location of a gene of interest. In this approach, known genetic loci, termed markers, are used and the analyses are designed to examine whether these markers are located near a particular gene.

Our 46 chromosomes (22 autosomal pairs and the X and Y chromosome) are made up of a linear arrangement of approximately 3×10^9 nucleotides, which encode for the approximately 100,000 genes which are expressed at some time in our bodies. During meiosis within fertilized gametes, chromosome pairs line up next to each other and exchange pieces of DNA during a process termed homologous recombination. This process ensures that genetic mixing occurs between maternal and paternal chromosomes.

The frequency of recombination can be used to determine the relative distance between genes on a chromosome. Two genes that are located on separate chromosomes will be passed independently from one another. In contrast, genes that lie close to each other on a chromosome will tend to be passed together, as the probability of a recombination event between them will be less than if they were on separate chromosomes or at either ends of the same chromosome.

Before more modern and sophisticated techniques, linkage analysis was done purely on the basis of a distinctive phenotype. For example, it was noted that certain forms of color blindness seemed to occur in individuals who also have a particular bleeding disorder, and when one was passed from a parent to a child, the other was transmitted as well. This is an example of close linkage between two genes each of which causes a recognizable disorder. It was later determined that the gene for one type of hemophilia is, in fact, closely linked to genes involved in color vision.

The next advance in linkage analysis came when it was recognized that investigators could use the inherent variability of certain serum proteins as markers. This variability, termed polymorphism, stems from the fact that a single protein from two individuals can contain slight changes in amino acid sequence which may have no effect on the protein's enzymatic or functional activity but which allow the proteins to be distinguished. In this way, many different blood types have been found in the population, and some have met the criteria for being useful markers in linkage studies: they were highly polymorphic or distinguishable and could be followed unambiguously as the gene that encoded for them was passed from one generation to the next. If a particular protein variant was noted to be frequently transmitted from parent to child in association with a particular syndrome, then that disorder was determined to be closely linked to the gene encoding for the serum protein. And if the chromosomal location of the serum marker was known from previous investigation, then one could confidently assert that the chromosomal location for the disorder of interest was near the gene that encoded the serum protein.

Unfortunately, there were not a sufficient number of polymorphic proteins available for linkage studies. To make further advances, a new methodology needed to be developed. This was accomplished when it was realized that DNA fragments themselves could be used as markers in linkage analyses (Botstein et al., 1980). Most DNA fragments obtained from any two individuals will differ slightly in their nucleotide sequence, the result of mutations that have occurred in the population. The vast majority of these mutations are silent, that is, they occur in regions of DNA that either do not encode for protein or, if they do occur in a coding sequence, do not change the activity of the protein. Even though these slight nucleotide variations are silent in a functional sense, molecular techniques have advanced to the point where it is relatively easy to detect these nucleotide variations between any two individuals. Thus, if one could identify the maternal or paternal contribution to these DNA markers, one could then conduct linkage studies. Over the past decade, a large group of highly polymorphic DNA fragments have been isolated and found to be evenly spaced throughout the human genome (NIH/CEPH Collaborative Mapping Group, 1992). If one looks at a sufficient number of such markers, one will eventually be found that is closely linked to a given genetic disorder. Establishing linkage between a specific disorder and a DNA marker is the first step in establishing the chromosomal localization for the disorder and, hopefully, is followed by the actual cloning and characterization of the gene of interest. It needs to be stated that, at the present time, linkage studies are only useful for those genes that have a major effect on the phenotype of interest. Currently, linkage studies cannot help to identify genes of small effect.

AUTISM

Twenty-five years ago, Rutter (1968) reviewed the twin literature on autism and concluded that because of ascertainment and design problems, the data could not be interpreted as supporting a genetic hypothesis. In 1976, Hanson and Gottesman again reviewed the literature and also concluded that the cause was unlikely to be genetic. We have come full circle since then, primarily because of better design and implementation of twin and family studies (Piven and Folstein, 1992).

Folstein and Rutter (1977) were the first to address these issues by obtaining a more complete and unbiased sample of same-sex twin pairs. Their study included 21 twins who had been located in a systematic search of schools, hospitals, and national registries. These 21 twin pairs consisted of 11 MZ and 10 DZ pairs. Four of the MZ twins and none of the DZ twins were concordant for autism. A recent and carefully designed twin study (Steffenburg et al., 1989) showed even higher concordance rates among MZ twins. This study also included 21 twin pairs (11 MZ and 10 DZ and one set of MZ triplets), and the concordance rate among MZ twins was 90% while none occurred among the DZ twins.

Folstein and Rutter (1977) proposed that autism might be the more severe expression of an underlying cognitive disability. They hypothesized that several factors would contribute to produce the more severe illness in affected probands, while siblings not exposed to these factors with the same genetic vulnerability would express only milder cognitive difficulties. When these investigators reexamined their twin pairs and looked for milder cognitive disabilities, they found that the concordance rate among

MZ twins increased from 35% to 80% while the concordance rate among DZ twins increased from 0% to 10%, a highly significant finding.

If this hypothesis is true, then one should find a higher incidence of both autism and milder cognitive disorders among the siblings of autistic children. A family study was conducted by August and coworkers (1981) to further test this hypothesis. Seventy-one siblings of 41 autistic probands were included in the study. A control group consisted of 38 siblings of 15 individuals with Down syndrome. Comparisons were made with impaired children to control for the possibility that having an impaired child was detrimental to the cognitive development of his or her siblings.

The results indicated that both milder cognitive difficulties and autism were increased among the siblings of probands when compared to the siblings of control children with Down syndrome. Approximately 15% of the siblings of autistic probands had cognitive difficulties, while only 2.5% of the siblings of Down probands had cognitive difficulties. In addition, the rate for autism itself was approximately 3% compared to 0% among the siblings of the Down probands. The incidence for autism among siblings was similar to that originally reported by Rutter (1968), who pointed out that even though this was a low recurrence rate, it represented greater than a 50-fold increase to the prevalence of autism in the general population. It should be noted that not all studies have supported the hypothesis proposed by Folstein and Rutter (1977). Another study (Freeman et al., 1989) presented data indicating that the first-degree relatives of autistic probands do not have a higher rate of cognitive disabilities when compared to the general population.

In a small percentage of cases, autism has been associated with several single-gene disorders including tuberous sclerosis, untreated phenylketonuria, and neurofibromatosis (reviewed in Folstein and Rutter, 1988). A small proportion of children diagnosed as autistic are later found to have fragile X syndrome (August, 1983; Brown et al., 1982). In addition, congenital injuries and a number of intrauterine infections such as rubella and cytomegalovirus have been associated with the disorder. It remains unclear what the relationship is between these various etiologies and the pathophysiology of autism, or whether these are related, in turn, to idiopathic autism. It is likely that a number of different molecular mechanisms will be discovered, mutation in any one of which will result in the phenotype of autism.

AFFECTIVE DISORDERS

It is not uncommon for considerably more work to be published on the genetic basis of adult psychiatric disorders than among similar disorders found in childhood. This is true with the major affective disorders; relatively little has been reported regarding the inheritance of this group of disorders among children. Several groups have examined the children of depressed parents who are thought to be at higher risk for developing affective disorders and have compared these rates to those found among normal controls. These rates have been consistently elevated (Hammen et al., 1990; Kashani et al., 1985; Orvaschel et al., 1988; Weissman et al., 1984, 1987). However, less work has been conducted that examines families ascertained through childhood probands.

One of the earliest works to suggest that prepubertal children do indeed suffer from major depressive disorder (MDD) and that their family members have a higher incidence of MDD was a study conducted by Puig-Antich and his collaborators (1989). They examined first- and second-degree relatives of children with major depression and compared the rates within family members to rates among relatives of two control groups—a group with psychiatric disorders other than affective disorders and a group with no psychiatric diagnoses. All family members ascertained were interviewed by structured interviews and the mother of the proband was usually directly interviewed. The rates for psychiatric disorders in general (0.27) were significantly higher among the relatives of the depressed children than among the relatives of the normal control group (0.06). In addition, the rate for MDD among the first-degree relatives was 0.53 for the probands but 0.28 for the relatives of the normal control group. MDD rates were not significantly elevated among the relatives of the psychiatric control group when compared to the normal control group; however, their rates for other psychiatric disorders were significantly elevated.

Strober and collaborators (1988) conducted a similar study to examine the rates of affective disorder among the relatives of an older group of adolescents. They compared the families of 50 probands who had the diagnosis of bipolar affective disorder to the families of 30 adolescents with schizophrenia. Relatives were interviewed with structured schedules in face-to-face meetings. The incidence of bipolar affective disorder was significantly elevated (15%) among the relatives of probands when compared to the incidence of bipolar disorder among the controls (0%). When the recurrence rate for all affective disorders was obtained, these were also found to be elevated among the bipolar probands (30%) when compared to the schizophrenics (4%). It is interesting to note that among the early symptoms observed in prepubertal onset probands were hyperactivity and/or conduct difficulties, and the association of affective disorders with attention deficit disorder has also been found by other groups (Biederman et al., 1991a,b; Puig-Antich et al., 1989).

SPECIFIC READING DISORDERS

Specific reading disability (RD) has been written about for almost 100 years since its initial description by Morgan (1896) and Kerr (1897). It is a relatively common learning disability with a prevalence of 10% among school-age children and with a male-female ratio of approximately 4:1. It is characterized by an inability to read despite adequate intelligence, schooling, and socioeconomic opportunity.

Over the years, it has become clear that the term RD has been used to describe a broad range of children with difficulties in reading. This has made comparisons between studies difficult and attempts have been made over the past 20 years to identify more homogeneous subgroups of RD. The Colorado Family Reading Study (Decker and DeFries, 1980; DeFries and Decker, 1981) has identified at least four subgroups among the large number of probands it has been following. More than 90% of their children had either (1) a spatial/reasoning deficit; (2) a coding/speed deficit; (3) a specific reading deficit only; or (4) a mixed or global deficit. Studies such as theirs emphasize the need for a careful assessment of RD probands to identify and include in genetic studies only those children with similar disabilities.

The aggregation of RD within families has been recognized since the turn of the century (Fisher, 1905; Stephenson, 1907; Thomas, 1905). Hallgren in 1950 published one of the largest family studies of RD which confirmed both the higher incidence of RD among first-degree relatives (41%) as well as the higher male-female occurrence rate (4:1). This study also proposed that the data were consistent with an autosomal dominant mode of transmission with a sex modifier that protected women from expressing the disorder. A more recent study by Pennington et al. (1991) investigated four independently ascertained samples (204 families with 1,698 individuals) and obtained results which were consistent with a major locus transmission in three of the samples and with a polygenic transmission in the fourth.

Twin studies support the hypothesis that RD is a genetic disorder. A review of the literature in 1967 (Zerbin-Rudin, 1967) found that 100% of MZ twins were concordant for RD compared to only 35% for DZ twin pairs. More recent twin studies (Balkwin, 1973; DeFries et al., 1987; Stevenson et al., 1987) are generally in agreement with these earlier findings, although with lower concordance rates ranging from 30% to 80% for MZ twins.

Linkage analyses have also been conducted with RD families (Smith et al., 1990) and have been recently reviewed (Pennington, 1990). Because of the heterogeneous nature of dyslexia, attempts have been made to find large, multigenerational families in which RD is found among many family members. This strategy will maximize the chances of studying the effects of a single gene, although it makes the assumption that all cases of RD in a single family will be caused by the same gene.

The first linkage study of RD (Smith et al., 1983) reported a linkage to a region on the short arm of chromosome 15. However, more recent attempts by the same group to extend these findings (Kimberling et al., 1985) and of a second group (Bisgaard et al., 1987) to confirm the earlier results have been unsuccessful.

ATTENTION-DEFICIT HYPERACTIVITY DISORDER

Attention-deficit hyperactivity disorder (ADHD) is one of the most commonly diagnosed disorders of childhood, with prevalence estimates as high as 10% among the pediatric age group (Rutter, 1983). The disorder appears to be heterogeneous, with a variety of known etiologies such as head trauma (Rutter, 1981), intrauterine exposure to toxins (Shaywitz et al., 1983), and infections (Shaywitz and Shaywitz, 1982). However, in the majority of cases, no etiology has been determined.

The evidence that some forms of ADHD have a genetic component come from a number of family aggregation, adoption, and twin studies over the past 30 years (reviewed in Pauls, 1990). However, these results must be reviewed with some caution because of methodological problems including the heterogeneous population of probands in various studies and the frequency with which the diagnosis has been made in the past.

A number of investigators have looked at the incidence of ADHD among first-degree family members of affected children. An early study by Morrison and Stewart (1971) reported a significant increase in the parents (20%) of ADHD probands compared to a matched control group (5%). When other relatives were included in the analysis, the frequency of hyperactivity was even higher. This study relied on the retroactive collection of data from the family members and, thus, must be interpreted with caution. A family study by Cantwell (1972) found a similar increase in hyperactivity among the relatives of hyperactive probands when compared to control families.

More recent family studies by Biederman and his collaborators have also demonstrated a higher incidence of ADHD among first-degree relatives of affected probands. Earlier works presented the results of systematic family studies in which all family members of ADHD probands and a control group of unaffected children used standardized forms (Biederman et al., 1986, 1987a). ADHD was diagnosed more than five times more frequently among the relatives of affected children than among the controls. The rates for a number of other diagnoses were also found to be significantly increased among relatives including conduct disorder, oppositional disorder, and major affective disorders. The presence of other disorders among the first-degree relatives (Biederman et al., 1991a,b) points to a considerable degree of comorbidity in the population studied and makes the interpretation of the findings problematic. However, a later study (Biederman et al., 1987b) of those families found to have a higher incidence of conduct and oppositional disorder demonstrated that these difficulties were confined to families in which the proband also had a conduct disorder. A more recent publication has provided further evidence for a genetic etiology in ADHD (Biederman et al., 1992), while other studies have attempted to compare the familial rate in the families of affected boys (Biederman et al., 1990) and girls (Faraone et al., 1991).

Adoption paradigms have been used to study children with ADHD, although these studies contain a number of methodological difficulties intrinsic to separation studies that were discussed earlier. Morrison and Stewart (1973) reported on the adoptive parents of hyperactive children and found a lower incidence of hyperactivity among these parents than among a control group which consisted of biological parents who were raising their own ADHD children. The study relied on self-report data and was unable to compare rates for the biological parents of the probands, for whom no information was available. A second adoption study (Cantwell, 1975) reported essentially the same results, with a much higher incidence of hyperactivity found among the biological families raising a hyperactive child than among the adoptive relatives. These studies must be interpreted with caution because of selective placement by adoption agencies, that is, adoptive families must be interviewed before they are allowed to adopt and are not allowed to do so if there exists a high level of psychopathology.

Several early twin studies (Scarr, 1966; Vandenberg, 1962; Willerman, 1973) provided some data suggesting that within this population genetic factors were important. A more recent twin study by Goodman and Stevenson (1989a,b) used parent and teacher questionnaires to assess the level of ADHD among MZ and DZ twin pairs. Their findings suggested that there was a group of twins with pervasive hyperactivity (present both at home and at school) in which an important component of the hyperactivity could be explained by genetic factors. More recent twin studies have replicated these earlier findings (Stevenson, 1992).

In a recent study by Hauser and coworkers (1993), subjects with generalized resistance to thyroid hormone were studied for the presence or absence of ADHD. This hormonal disorder is caused by mutations in the thyroid receptor-β gene and is characterized by reduced responsiveness of peripheral and pituitary tissues to the actions of thyroid hormone. The study included 49 affected and 55 unaffected family members of whom 52 were adults and 52 were children (<18 years of age). Among the adults, 50% of the affected patients had had ADHD as children, compared with 7% of the unaffected subjects (p < .001). Among the children, 70% of the affected children were given the diagnosis of ADHD, compared with 20% of the unaffected children (*p* < .001). In this study sample, ADHD is strongly associated with a specific mutation giving rise to generalized resistance to thyroid hormone.

It is unlikely that a substantial number of patients with ADHD will now be found to have generalized resistance to thyroid hormone, which is a rare disorder. However, future studies should build on the findings from this study and investigate whether additional mutations in thyroid-related proteins, as well as other hormones, are linked to specific subgroups of children with ADHD. These investigations may provide new insights and clarity to the underlying mechanisms at work in this heterogeneous population of patients.

TOURETTE'S SYNDROME

Tourette's syndrome (TS) is a chronic disorder that first appears in childhood and is characterized by motor and phonic tics that wax and wane over the course of an individual's lifetime. In addition, TS patients often report the experience of obsessions and compulsions in conjunction with their tic symptomatology.

Gilles de la Tourette described the disorder more than 100 years ago and was the first to suggest that the illness aggregated in certain families. Neurobiological, neuroimaging, and pharmacotherapeutic studies have pointed to the basal ganglia and regions of the frontal cortex in the pathophysiological process of TS, with the central monoaminergic pathways often being implicated.

A number of twin and family aggregation studies as well as linkage analyses have been undertaken to elucidate the underlying molecular mechanisms operative in TS. The data support the hypothesis that TS, chronic tic (CT) disorder, and obsessive-compulsive disorder (OCD) are passed vertically across generations as a single autosomal dominant gene (Eapen et al., 1993; Pauls and Leckman, 1986; Pauls et al., 1991; Van de Wetering, 1993).

Price et al. (1985) published a report that compared the concordance rate for MZ (0.53) and DZ (0.08) twins. The data for this study had been obtained by telephone interviews. A follow-up study (Walkup et al., 1987), which used direct interviews of all probands, found that the concordance rate among MS twins increased to 1.0 when both TS and CT were included; this finding points to the need for careful, face-to-face interviews to avoid underestimation of the true incidence of a disorder.

Twin studies have also been conducted to investigate the contribution of environmental factors in individuals with a genetic vulnerability for TS. Leckman and coworkers (1990) and, more recently, Hyde and coworkers (1992) have looked for nongenetic factors that mediate the expression of TS during the perinatal period. Both groups studied MS twin pairs and found a significant correlation between prenatal complications, such as severe maternal nausea and/or vomiting during the first trimester, and the severity of current tic symptomatology.

In addition to the twin work, a number of family aggregation studies have been published. Two earlier studies appeared in the 1970s (Eldridge et al., 1977; Shapiro et al., 1978) and demonstrated a higher incidence of TS in the families of identified probands. Shortly thereafter, these findings were extended by Kidd et al. (1980), who investigated whether other forms of tic disorder beside TS tended to aggregate in TS families. This study demonstrated that chronic tics were found at a significantly higher frequency than could be explained by chance alone. Over the next decade, five separate groups (Baron et al., 1981; Comings et al., 1984; Devor, 1984; Kidd and Pauls, 1982; Price et al., 1987) published additional family aggregation results and found a higher incidence of TS and CT in the families of TS probands.

These studies also attempted to answer whether one gene or several genes were involved and to determine the specific mode of transmission. The data from these studies suggested single-gene transmission. However, there was less agreement on the specific inheritance mode: three of the groups (Baron et al., 1981; Comings et al., 1984; Price et al., 1987) presented data suggesting autosomal dominant transmission with sex-specific penetrances, while the remaining two groups were unable to rule out an additive model.

The association of TS with OCD was mentioned earlier. The data in support of this association have been extensive over the years. A number of uncontrolled clinical studies have suggested this connection (Cummings and Frankel, 1985; Fernando, 1967; Jagger et al., 1982; Kelman, 1965; Montgomery et al., 1982; Morphew and Sim, 1969; Nee et al., 1980, 1982; Stefl, 1984; Yaryura-Tobias et al., 1981). More recent controlled family studies have been conducted and support the earlier results (Frankel et al., 1986; Green and Pitman, 1986; Robertson et al., 1988; Walkup et al., 1987). At the present time, it is generally accepted that TS is associated with a higher incidence of certain forms of OCD in the first-degree relatives of TS probands.

Pauls and coworkers (Pauls and Leckman, 1986; Pauls et al., 1991) conducted a family study in which they suggested that OCD without a tic disorder occurred more frequently in the female family members of identified TS probands. If that were true, then the previous finding that TS/CT occurs in males at a 4:1 ratio over females would need to be modified. While it is true that males are more likely to get TS/CT, vulnerable females are at a greater risk of developing OCD. To test the hypothesis that OCD cosegregates with tic disorders, Pauls and Leckman (1986) conducted segregation analyses to test specific transmission models. Their data supported an autosomal dominant hypothesis regardless of whether they included only relatives with TS, relatives with TS or CT, or relatives with TS, CT, and OCD. These segregation analyses have been replicated by a number of additional studies (Eapen et al., 1993; Pauls et al., 1990, 1991; Van de Wetering, 1993).

TS is one of the few childhood psychiatric disorders in which extensive linkage analyses have been conducted. However, despite an international effort by several laboratories, no DNA marker has yet been found linked to TS with at least 50% of the genome already excluded.

SPECIFIC MUTATIONS IN
THREE DEVELOPMENTAL DISORDERS

The more classical strategies are necessary when there are no other clues to the chromosomal location of a gene of interest. There are a number of disorders, however, in which a cytogenetic abnormality is present in one or more chromosomes and, thus, points directly to the genomic region where further studies are needed. Klinefelter's syndrome (47, XXY karyotype), Turner's syndrome (X monosomy), XYY syndrome, and Down syndrome are examples of developmental disorders in which a chromosomal abnormality and an associated abnormal protein product presumably lead directly to the clinical phenotypes, although the mechanisms for these abnormalities are not yet understood.

In fragile X syndrome, more information is available regarding the molecular basis for the disorder. This syndrome is the most common inherited form of mental retardation and is second only to Down syndrome as a known cause for genetically determined mental retardation. The clinical symptoms can vary widely from case to case, but usually involve moderate to severe mental retardation, macro-orchidism, and a distinctive facies. The syndrome gets its name from the fact that many affected individuals have an unstable site on the long arm of the X chromosome that apparently breaks apart and can thus be detected cytogenetically. When lymphocyte cultures from these individuals are grown in the absence of the vitamin folate, an apparent gap occurs within this region on the X chromosome (Sutherland, 1977). The cytogenetic abnormality was noted to be associated with a specific phenotype in affected males, which was strong evidence for an X-linked genetic abnormality. Subsequent linkage studies showed that the fragile chromosomal region was indeed the locus of the disorder. Understanding this disorder and the ability to accurately diagnose it has progressed from the initial characterization of the fragile X site 20 years ago (Lubs, 1969) to the recent cloning of the gene responsible for this disorder (Verkerk et al., 1991).

The isolation and characterization of the fragile X, mental retardation gene (*FMR-1*) has permitted clinicians to finally understand some of the more baffling aspects of the genetics of this syndrome. One of the peculiarities of fragile X syndrome was the fact that certain individuals carried the fragile site, but did not express the full clinical picture. In addition, it appeared that what was passed from one generation to the next was an increasingly severe form of the disorder. Thus, for example, an asymptomatic grandparent would pass a genetic vulnerability to a mother, who might show some symptoms (e.g., mild mental retardation) but who would more commonly show varying degrees of learning difficulties and vulnerabilities toward certain emotional problems. In the next generation, however, the developmental disabilities become more severe, and a proband would appear to the clinician with the complete symptomatic picture of fragile X syndrome. This progression of severity from one generation to the next is termed "anticipation" by geneticists and, in fragile X syndrome, has come to be known as the "Sherman paradox." The characterization of the *FMR-1* gene has resulted in a more complete understanding of the mechanisms involved in these interesting familial patterns. To understand these mechanisms, it is helpful to review the "basic dogma" of genetics (reviewed in Leckman, 1990).

The flow of genetic information within any cell is from DNA to RNA to the eventual production of proteins. This sequence typically involves a number of highly regulated steps, and interruption of any of these steps can disrupt the production of functional protein (Fig. 1). The first step, termed transcription, involves the synthesis of a gene's RNA message. Adjacent to and upstream from the gene is a region called the promoter, which regulates the transcription of the gene. The promoter also indicates where on the

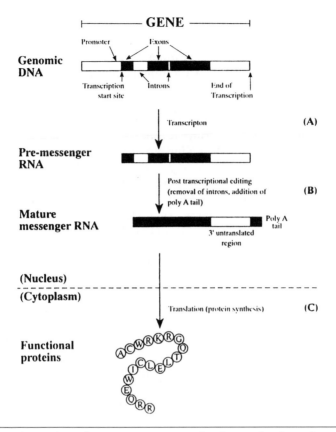

Figure 1. A number of steps are necessary for the production of protein from genomic DNA. Disruption of any of these highly regulated steps can lead to the production of either a dysfunctional protein or no protein. Three different developmental disorders are described in which mutations have been identified which disrupt each of these steps. *A:* In fragile X syndrome, a mutation within the *FMR-1* gene is thought to directly disrupt the transcription of *FMR-1* message. *B:* In Prader-Willi syndrome (PWS), a mutation within the coding region of a small nuclear ribonucleoprotein leads to the production of nonfunctional protein that is unable to properly edit other, still unidentified RNA messages. The mutation in PWS leads to a disruption of posttranscriptional editing because one of the proteins involved in that machinery is mutated. *C:* In Waardenburg syndrome, a mutation has been found in the coding region of the *PAX-3* gene, and nonfunctional *PAX-3* protein is produced. The *PAX-3* gene product is a transcription factor that regulates the transcription of other proteins presumed, though not yet demonstrated, to be involved in the development of the CNS. This type of mutation within the coding region of genes, seen in both PWS and Waardenburg syndromes, leads to the disruption of other steps in the DNA to RNA processing.

DNA molecule transcription will be initiated. The DNA molecule then acts as a template for the formation of a complementary, RNA copy, called pre-RNA. The second step involves the proper processing of preRNA into mature message, and the eventual transport of mature message from the nucleus to the cytoplasm where it will be translated into protein.

In the case of fragile X syndrome, it appears that it is the initial transcription step that is disrupted in the majority of fragile X patients. The resulting lower level of transcription leads to lower levels of *FMR-1* message (Pieretti et al., 1991). The exact mechanism by which transcription is disrupted remains unclear, but two hypotheses have been proposed. The first involves the unusual finding of many copies of a particular repeat of three bases, cytosine-guanine-guanine (CGG) (Fu et al., 1991). This triplet of nucleotides is normally repeated among healthy individuals from 6 to 54 times, but in fragile X individuals the number of repeated triplets increases to between 200 and more than 1,000 CGG repeats (Fu et al., 1991). Relatives, who are carriers for the mutant gene but show milder clinical symptoms, have an intermediate number of CGG repeats. It has been suggested that the unusually long repeat found in the *FMR-1* primary transcript is inherently unstable and disrupts the ongoing transcription process, so that lower levels of *FMR-1* mRNA are produced. A second mechanism that has been proposed is that the long triplet repeat affects the ability of the promoter region itself to regulate transcription. This has been suggested because of the identification of a second unstable region in fragile X patients, one that lies in the promoter region and that has been found to be abnormally modified in a process termed methylation (Vincent et al., 1991). In addition, the instability within the promoter region is thought to contribute to the chromosomal breakage that led to the syndrome's name (Oberle et al., 1991).

FMR-1 mRNA message has been detected preferentially within regions of the human brain and testes (Hinds et al., 1993), and abnormally low amounts of message were detected in fragile X patients (Pieretti et al., 1991). It is thought, although not proven, that the low level of message leads to a low level of *FMR-1* protein and to the symptoms of the disorder. Relatives who are carriers of the fragile X gene, with an intermediate number of repeats, presumably have less disruption of transcription and some functional *FMR-1* protein. It is not yet known whether the intermediate amount of message and protein is responsible for the milder cognitive deficits found in some fragile X relatives. In fact, the actual function of the *FMR-1* protein remains unknown and its role both in adult tissue and during development is being actively studied in a number of laboratories. These studies will help to clarify the role of the *FMR-1* in the pathogenesis of the full fragile X syndrome as well as the milder cognitive disabilities seen in some relatives.

Theoretically, a similar clinical phenotype should be found by disrupting other key steps in the pathway from DNA to functional *FMR-1* protein. Indeed, individuals have been described with the identical symptoms of fragile X syndrome who lack the cytological findings on their X chromosome. Some of these individuals have now had their *FMR-1* gene characterized and appear to have the normal number of CGG repeats. Instead, a second type of mutation has been found that lies within the portion of the message that encodes for the protein. This mutation within the coding region itself leads directly to the production of dysfunctional *FMR-1* protein, leading to the fragile X phenotype but the absence of cytogenetic findings. One would predict that such individuals would be among the most severely affected fragile X patients because of the complete absence of functional protein, while patients with the triplet repeat form can have varying levels of functional protein as a consequence of the variable amount of transcriptional disruption. In addition, families with a mutation within the coding region should not show anticipation from one generation to the next. A report of such a mutation in the protein coding region has been recently described (DeBoulle et al., 1993).

It should be pointed out that similar triplet repeats have been described for several other disorders, including myotonic dystrophy, spinobulbar muscular atrophy and, most recently, for Huntington's disease and spinocerebellar ataxia. It is intriguing that for five neuropsychiatric disorders, the elongation of a trinucleotide repeat sequence has been discovered, suggesting that this mutational mechanism may prove important as the etiology for a number of human genetic diseases (reviewed in Ross et al., 1993).

The molecular basis for two other developmental disorders has recently been elucidated. Children with Prader-Willi syndrome (PWS) are characterized by a number of developmental delays, including mental, psychomotor, and growth retardation. In addition, they show a characteristic facies, small hands and feet, and a lesion of the hypothalamus which results in hypogonadism and hyperphagia with obesity (Prader et al., 1956). Using classical cytogenetic techniques, PWS was found to be associated with a small deletion of the long arm of chromosome 15 (Ledbetter et al., 1981). Attention then focused on the identification of genes localized to this region that might serve as candidate genes. Recently, a gene was mapped to the region that is deleted in PWS (Ozcelik et al., 1992), and the protein encoded for by the gene was produced in an inactivated form in a mouse model for PWS (Cattanach et al., 1992).

The mutation involved in PWS disrupts the second step in the DNA to protein axis. As is shown in Figure 1, after a gene is transcribed from DNA into its primary RNA transcript, the transcript must be further processed before mature message (mRNA) can be faithfully translated into protein. The steps involved in this processing include the excision of noncoding regions (termed introns) and the religation of coding regions (termed exons) in a precise and orderly manner to generate mature messenger RNA. This series of steps from preRNA to mature mRNA is termed "splicing," and it involves the cooperative actions of a number of small proteins within the nucleus called small nuclear ribonucleoprotein particles (SNRPs). One of the consequences of this biological processing is that a single gene can contain the genetic code for several proteins. This occurs through the splicing together of different combinations of exons into related messages, each of which has been adapted to the specialized environment of particular cell types. It has been suggested that one mechanism for the tissue-specific expression of certain proteins results from the tissue-specific expression of various SNRPs. In this way, proteins found within neurons of the brain are present there because of the actions of neuron-specific splicing proteins.

A small nuclear protein involved in splicing was recently discovered (McAllister et al., 1989) and found to be predominantly expressed within neurons of the brain (Schmauss et al., 1992). It is precisely this protein that is mutated in PWS. The now inactive SNRP can no longer splice together alternative mRNAs within neurons of the CNS. It should be pointed out that the message(s) that are no longer properly processed are not themselves mutated in PWS. In fact, these protein(s) have not yet been identified, although it is presumed that their absence leads to the clinical symptoms seen in PWS. One can speculate that individuals with a similar symptomatic profile will be identified whose splicing proteins are found to be intact, but in whom specific mutations have occurred within the coding regions of these target proteins.

In Waardenburg syndrome, affected individuals are characterized by deafness, a typical facies, and various pigmentation abnormalities. The mutation that causes this syndrome was recently identified (Baldwin et al., 1992; Morell et al., 1992; Tassabehji et al., 1992). As was mentioned above, approximately one third of the genes expressed in our bodies are specifically localized within the CNS. Some of these proteins are expressed only within the adult brain and are expressed during particular developmental time periods. In considering genes that may affect the development of the brain, particular attention has been given to a family of proteins termed homeobox proteins. These proteins, also termed master control genes, are found in many different species of animals and have been shown to be important in regulating critical steps in the development and differentiation of various tissues throughout the body (reviewed in Leckman, 1991).

They act, in part, by controlling the expression of additional genes and their protein products in a precise and orderly fashion during development.

Recently, a homeobox protein called *PAX-3* was found to be mutated in Waardenburg syndrome. Several families have now been studied and six different single nucleotide mutations have been found which alter or abolish a highly conserved sequence within the protein coding region (Baldwin et al., 1992; Morell et al., 1992; Tassabehji et al., 1993). It is assumed, although not yet demonstrated, that these mutations result in a decrease, or loss, of the ability of *PAX-3* to control the expression of other genes important in the development of the CNS (reviewed in Gruss and Walther, 1992). Given the fact that more than 30,000 genes are specifically transcribed in the CNS and require accurate regulation and processing, it is not unreasonable to propose that other developmental disorders will be caused by mutations in transcription and splicing factors.

COMPLICATING FACTORS

A major transformation has occurred in the field of human genetics over the past 20 years. This has been due primarily to the discovery of highly polymorphic DNA markers which has allowed researchers to map the human genome (NIH/CEPH Collaborative Mapping Group, 1992) and has facilitated the cloning of several genes responsible for human illnesses. Huntington's disease and cystic fibrosis are examples of the successful application of these techniques, and it was thought that similar methodologies could be applied to the study of psychiatric and behavioral disorders (Merikangas et al., 1989; Pardes et al., 1989). On the other hand, the initial reports of linkage for bipolar disorder (Egeland et al., 1987) and schizophrenia (Sherrington et al., 1988) have not been replicated (Detera-Wadleigh et al., 1987; Kelsoe et al., 1989; Kennedy et al., 1988).

There are a number of reasons why these initial studies may have been unsuccessful. Risch (1990) and Pauls (1993) discuss several issues that arise in studying complex psychiatric illnesses. First, the application of traditional linkage methodologies assumes that a single gene contributes significantly to the expression of the disease being studied. Although the inability to accurately specify the correct genetic model may not be a fatal flaw (Clerget-Darpoux et al., 1986), the effect of misspecification may be significant enough to mask linkage. Second, most studies of psychiatric illness done to date have assumed genetic homogeneity of the illness under investigation. This is probably not the case, given the high prevalence for most neuropsychiatric illness in the general population. This means that there may be several different mutations at separate loci that can each "cause" a disorder. Alternatively, the disorder may be the result of the impact of several genes acting in concert but each having a small effect in isolation. Although efforts are under way to develop strategies to address these possibilities, either possibility will confound traditional linkage analysis.

A third critical issue is the use of the correct phenotypic definition. To date, all studies have assumed that a particular phenotypic spectrum represents a unitary genetic disorder being transmitted within these families. This assumption may be incorrect. For example, in all of the linkage studies of affective disorder, bipolar disorder has been considered as part of a spectrum of illnesses that included unipolar MDD. While it is true that the rate of MDD is elevated among families of bipolar probands, it has not yet been determined that all MDD in families of bipolar patients represents a variant expression of the same genetic factors that predispose to bipolar disorder. Linkage studies that have made this assumption would include cases with variant MDD as positive diagnoses when in fact they were not. Too many such false-positives would doom linkage studies.

Linkage studies have often relied on large multigenerational families for their analyses. This has been the case because of the increased statistical power possible in single, large families, as well as the assumption that a given disorder is genetically homogeneous within a single family. However, a number of limitations stemming from the use of large multigenerational pedigrees have been described and should be kept in mind (Greenberg, 1992). Large pedigrees do not guarantee homogeneity; in fct, the more branches that are included from a family, the more likely it is that a separate susceptibility gene for the disorder will appear through an individual marrying into the family. Results from large families may also be sensitive to changes in the phenotypes of critical individuals in the family (Hodge and Greenberg, 1992; Kennedy et al., 1988). In addition, not only are large families hard to find, but they are less useful for other kinds of studies. For these reasons, some investigators are turning to the analysis of large samples of smaller families. Such samples allow the examination of hypotheses about the transmission of possible subtypes of disorders and the application of a wider range of analytic methodologies (Falk and Rubenstein, 1987; Haseman and Elston, 1972; Weeks and Lange, 1992).

GENES AND ENVIRONMENT

Although a large body of evidence has accumulated to suggest that genetic factors play an important role in the etiology of major psychiatric illness, it is also clear that environmental factors play a critical part. Perhaps the strongest evidence favoring a role for environmental factors is the fact that among MZ twins, there is never a 100% concordance rate for any psychiatric disorder that has been systematically studied in twin paradigms. Basic scientists who for years have studied the growth and development of the brain, no longer debate whether environmental or genetic factors are of paramount importance. It is now accepted that both factors contribute to the development of the organism, and the emphasis in current research is on just how the two sets of factors interact during critical periods of growth and maturation (reviewed in Rubenstein et al., 1990).

It will be useful for future research to permit the examination of both genetic and environmental contributions to the variable expression of psychiatric illness. Although in most studies of psychiatric illnesses it has been possible to demonstrate that genes contribute to their etiology, it is clear that genetic factors are not both necessary and sufficient for the expression of any behavioral disorder. It is possible that the genetic mechanism for a specific illness will only be identified when the impact of nongenetic factors on the expression of the illness has been adequately described. It may also be the case that only with the careful documentation of environmental factors will it be possible to determine the phenotype that is inherited. Environmental factors may mask the true phenotype and make it impossible to understand the impact on genetic factors for the "core phenotype."

Finally, in studies that examine the impact of the environment, it will be important that the research takes place in a developmental context. Studies in developmental psychology have shown that early life experiences have a significant impact on later mental health. The work of Bowlby (1969, 1988) has clearly demonstrated that the quality of an infant's attachment to its mother has a strong predictive power for later childhood as well as adult behavior. What is less well understood is how the genetic endowment of both parent and child may influence this attachment. Not all children respond in the same way to specific events. Different genotypes or temperamental predispositions may mediate response to different caregiving environments and may even elicit differences in caregiving. Documentation of the influence of both genetic and nongenetic factors on behavior requires prospective longitudinal studies of children at genetic risk.

CONCLUSIONS

The evidence that genetic factors are important in the etiology of many childhood psychiatric disorders is clearly suggested by this review of the literature. Two general approaches have been used to establish a role for specific genetic factors. The more traditional approach attempts to first demonstrate the importance of genetic factors through twin, adoption, or family studies. If successful, then segregation analyses can be performed on the data to determine whether the vulnerability for a particular disorder can be explained by a specific genetic model. Linkage analysis is then undertaken to establish the general chromosomal region of interest. Finally, a finer map can be constructed and the gene of interest eventually cloned and characterized.

The second approach takes genes that have already been isolated and asks whether they can be considered as candidates for specific syndromes. This approach short cuts several steps in the more traditional approach by making the assumption that mutations in certain proteins lead to illness and looks for the illnesses associated with the already cloned genes. When a particular chromosomal abnormality is detected for a disorder, candidate genes, known from previous mapping studies to be located near the region of interest, can be further tested for linkage with a particular disorder. This approach has limited applicability as it can be useful for only those disorders in which identified chromosomal abnormalities are recognized. When a disorder is not associated with any chromosomal abnormality, candidate genes can still be used in linkage studies. In this case, the candidate genes are selected on the basis of a particularly interesting aspect of the gene. Thus, several of the dopamine receptors have been used as candidate genes in linkage studies based on the dopamine hypothesis, although none of them have yet been demonstrated to be associated with any human disease.

The advances in DNA recombinant technology have permitted the isolation and characterization of genes specifically involved in human medical illnesses and will clearly continue at an ever-increasing pace. Until recently, no mutation had been discovered for any of the childhood psychiatric disorders. With the recent publication of the molecular basis for several developmental syndromes, the current climate is changing and we are encouraged to think that the next decade will bring us closer to our ultimate goal of understanding and eventually treating these disabling disorders.

REFERENCES

August GJ (1983), A genetic marker associated with infantile autism. *Am J Psychiatry* 140:813

August GJ, Stewart MA, Tsai L (1981), The incidence of cognitive disabilities in the siblings of autistic children. *Br J Psychiatry* 138:416–422

Baldwin C, Hoth C, Amos J, da Silva E, Milunsky A (1992), An exonic mutation in the HuP2 paired domain gene causes Waardenburg's syndrome. *Nature* 355:637–638

Balkwin H (1973), Reading disability in twins. *Dev Med Child Neurol* 15:184–187

Baron M, Shapiro E, Shapiro A, Ranier JD (1981), Genetic analysis of Tourette syndrome suggesting a major gene effect. *Am J Hum Genet* 33:767–775

Biederman J, Faraone SV, Keenan K, Knee D, Twuang MT (1990), Family-genetic and psychosocial risk factors in *DSM-III* attention deficit disorder. *J Am Acad Child Adolesc Psychiatry* 29:526–533

Biederman J, Faraone SV, Keenan K, Steingard R, Tsuang MT (1991a), Familial association between attention deficit disorder and anxiety disorders. *Am J Psychiatry* 148:251–256

Biederman J, Faraone SV, Keenan K, Tsuang MT (1991b), Evidence of familial association between attention deficit disorder and major affective disorders. *Arch Gen Psychiatry* 48:633–642

Biederman J, Faraone SV, Keenan K et al. (1992), Further evidence for family-genetic risk factors in attention deficit hyperactivity disorder. *Arch Gen Psychiatry* 49:728–738

Biederman J, Munir K, Knee D et al. (1986), A family study of patients with attention deficit disorder and normal controls. *J Psychiatr Res* 20:263–274

Biederman J, Munir K, Knee D et al. (1987a), High rate of affective disorders in probands with attention deficit disorder and in their relatives: a controlled family study. *Am J Psychiatry* 144:330–333

Biederman J, Munir K, Knee D et al. (1987b), Conduct and oppositional disorder in clinically referred children with attention deficit disorder: a controlled family study. *J Am Acad Child Adolesc Psychiatry* 26:724–727

Bisgaard ML, Eiberg H, Moller N, Niebahr E, Mohr J (1987), Dyslexia and chromosome 15 heteromorphism: negative lod score in a Danish study. *Clin Genet* 32:118–119

Botstein D, White R, Skolnick M, Davis R (1980), Construction of a genetic linkage map in man using restriction fragment length polymorphisms. *Am J Hum Genet* 32:312–331

Bowlby J (1969), *Attachment and Loss.* New York: Basic

Bowlby J (1988), *A Secure Base.* New York: Basic

Brown W, Jenkins E, Friedman E et al. (1982), Association of fragile X syndrome with autism. *Lancet* 1:100

Cannings C, Thompson EA (1977), Ascertainment in the sequential sampling of pedigrees. *Clin Genet* 12:208–212

Cannings C, Thompson EA, Skolnick MH (1978), Probability functions on complex pedigrees. *Advances in Applied Probability* 10:26–61

Cantwell D (1972), Psychiatric illness in the families of hyperactive children. *Arch Gen Psychiatry* 27:414–417

Cantwell D (1975), Genetic studies on hyperactive children. Psychiatric illness in biologic and adoptive parents. In: *Genetic Research in Psychiatry*, Fieve R, Rosenthal D, Brill H, eds. Baltimore: Johns Hopkins Press, pp 275–280

Cattanach BM, Barr JA, Evans EP et al. (1992), A candidate mouse model for Prader-Willi syndrome which shows an absence of Snrpn expression. *Nature Genetics* 2:270–274

Clerget-Darpoux F, Bonaiti-Pellie C, Hochez J (1986), Effects of misspecifying genetic parameters in the lod score analysis. *Biometrics* 42:393–399

Cohen D, Dibble E, Grawe J, Pollin W (1975), Reliably separating identical from fraternal twins. *Arch Gen Psychiatry* 32:1371–1378

Comings DE, Comings BG, Devor EJ, Cloninger CR (1984), Detection of a major gene for Gilles de la Tourette syndrome. *Am J Hum Genet* 36:586–600

Cummings JL, Frankel M (1985), Gilles de la Tourette syndrome and the neurological basis of obsessions and compulsions. *Biol Psychiatry* 20:1117–1126

DeBoulle K, Verkerk AJ, Reyniers E et al. (1993), A point mutation in the *FMR-1* gene associated with fragile X mental retardation. *Nature Genetics* 3:31–35

Decker SN, DeFries JC (1980), Cognitive abilities in families with reading disabled children. *Journal of Learning Disabilities* 13:53–58

DeFries JC, Decker SN (1981), Genetic aspects of reading disability: the Colorado Family Reading Study. In: *Neuropsychological and Neuropsycholinguistic Aspects of Reading Disability*, Aaron PG, Malatesha M, eds. New York: Academic Press

DeFries JC, Fulker DW, LaBuda MC (1987), Evidence for a genetic etiology in reading disability of twins. *Nature* 329:537–539

Detera-Wadleigh S, Berrettini W, Goldin L, Boorman D, Anderson S, Gershon E (1987), Close linkage of c-Harvey-ras-1 and the insulin gene to affective disorder is ruled out in three North American pedigrees. *Nature* 325:806–808

Devor EJ (1984), Complex segregation analysis of Gilles de la Tourette syndrome: further evidence for a major locus mode of transmission. *Am J Hum Genet* 36:704–709

Eapen N, Pauls D, Robertson M (1993), Evidence for autosomal dominant transmission in Gilles de la Tourette syndrome—United Kingdom Cohort Study. *Br J Psychiatry* in press

Egeland J, Gerlhard D, Pauls D et al. (1987), Bipolar affective disorder linked to DNA markers on chromosome 11. *Nature* 325:783–787

Elandt-Johnson RC (1970), Segregation analysis for complex modes of inheritance. *Am J Hum Genet* 22:129–140

Eldridge R, Sweet R, Lake CR, Ziegler M, Shapiro A (1977), Gilles de la Tourette's syndrome: clinical, genetic, psychologic, and biochemical aspects in 21 selected families. *Neurology* 27:115–124

Elston RC, Namboodiri KK (1977), Family studies of schizophrenia. In: Proceedings of the 41st Session of the International Statistics Institute

Elston RC, Stewart J (1971), A general model for the genetic analysis of pedigree data. *Hum Hered* 21:523–542

Elston RC, Yelverton KC (1975), General models for segregation analysis. *Am J Hum Genet* 27:31–45

Falk CT, Rubenstein P (1987), Haplotype relative risks: an easy reliable way to construct a proper control sample for risk calculations. *Ann Hum Genet* 51:227–233

Faraone SV, Biederman J, Keenan K, Tsuang MT (1991), A family-genetic study of girls with *DSM-III* attention deficit disorder. *Am J Psychiatry* 148:112–117

Fernando SM (1967), Gilles de la Tourette's syndrome. *Br J Psychiatry* 113:607–617

Fisher JH (1905), A case of congenital word-blindness (inability to learn to read). *Ophthalmic Review* 24:315–318

Folstein S, Rutter M (1977), Infantile autism: a genetic study of 21 twin pairs. *J Child Psychol Psychiatry* 18:297–321

Folstein S, Rutter M (1988), Autism: familial aggregation and genetic implications. *J Autism Dev Disord* 18:3–30

Frankel M, Cummings JL, Robertson MM, Trimble M, Hill M, Benson F (1986), Obsessions and compulsions in the Gilles de la Tourette syndrome. *Neurology* 36:379–382

Freeman BJ, Ritvo ER, Mason-Brothers A et al. (1989), Psychometric assessment of first-degree relatives of 62 autistic probands in Utah. *Am J Psychiatry* 146:361–364

Fu Y, Kuhl D, Pizzuti A et al. (1991), Variations of the CGG repeat at the fragile site results in genetic instability: resolution of the Sherman paradox. *Cell* 67:1047–1058

Goodman R, Stevenson J (1989a), A twin study of hyperactivity. I. An examination of hyperactivity scores and categories derived from Rutter teacher and parent questionnaires. *J Child Psychol Psychiatry* 30:671–689

Goodman R, Stevenson J (1989b), A twin study of hyperactivity. II. The aetiological role of genes, family relationships and perinatal adversity. *J Child Psychol Psychiatry* 30:691–709

Green RC, Pitman RK (1986), Tourette syndrome and obsessive compulsive disorder. In: *Obsessive Compulsive Disorders: Theory and Management*, Jenike M, Baer L, Minicheillo W, eds. Littleton, MA: PSG

Greenberg DA (1992), There is more than one way to collect data for linkage analysis. *Arch Gen Psychiatry* 49:745–750

Gruss P, Walther C (1992), Pax in development. *Cell* 69:719–722

Hallgren B (1950), Specific dyslexia. *Acta Psychiatr Neurol Scand* 65(suppl):1–287

Hammen C, Burge D, Burney E, Adrian C (1990), Longitudinal study of diagnoses in children of women with unipolar and bipolar affective disorder. *Arch Gen Psychiatry* 47:1112–1117

Hanson D, Gottesman I (1976), The genetics, if any, of infantile autism and childhood schizophrenia. *J Autism Child Schizophr* 6:209–234

Haseman JK, Elston RC (1972), The investigation of linkage between a quantitative trait and a marker locus. *Behav Genet* 2:3–19

Hauser P, Zametkin A, Martinez P et al. (1993), Attention-deficit-hyperactivity disorder in people with generalized resistance to thyroid hormone. *N Engl J Med* 328:997–1001

Hinds HL, Ashley CT, Sutcliffe JS et al. (1993), Tissue specific expression of *FMR-1* provides evidence for a functional role in fragile X syndrome. *Nature Genetics* 3:36–43

Hodge SE, Greenberg DA (1992), Sensitivity of lod scores to changes in diagnostic status. *Am J Hum Genet* 50:1053–1066

Hyde T, Aaronson B, Randolph C, Rickler K, Weinberger D (1992), Relationship of birth weight to the phenotypic expression of Gilles de la Tourette's syndrome in monozygotic twins. *Neurology* 42:652–658

Jagger J, Prusoff BA, Cohen DJ, Kidd K, Carbonari C, John K (1982), The epidemiology of Tourette's syndrome: a pilot study. *Schizophr Bull* 8:267–278

Kashani JH, Burk JP, Horwitz B, Reid J (1985), Differential effect of subtype of parental major affective disorder on children. *Psychiatry Res* 15:195–204

Kelman DH (1965), Gilles de la Tourette's disease in children: a review of the literature. *J Child Psychol Psychiatry* 6:219–226

Kelsoe J, Ginns E, Egeland J et al. (1989), Re-evaluation of the linkage relationship between chromosome 11p loci and the gene for bipolar affective disorder in the Old Order Amish. *Nature* 342:238–243

Kennedy J, Giuffra L, Moises H et al. (1988), Evidence against linkage of schizophrenia to markers on chromosome 5 in a northern Swedish pedigree. *Nature* 336:167–169

Kerr J (1897), School hygiene, in its mental, moral and physical aspects. Howard medical prize essay. *Journal of the Royal Statistical Society* 60:613–680

Kidd KK, Pauls DL (1982), Genetic hypotheses for Tourette syndrome. In: *Gilles de la Tourette Syndrome*, Friedhoff AJ, Chase TN, eds. New York: Raven Press

Kidd KK, Prusoff BA, Cohen DJ (1980), The familial pattern of Tourette syndrome. *Arch Gen Psychiatry* 37:1336–1339

Kimberling W, Fain P, Ing P, Smith S, Pennington B (1985), Genetic linkage studies of reading disability with chromosome 15 markers (abstract). Presented at the 15th annual meeting of Behavior Genetics Association, Pennsylvania State University

LaBuda MC, Gottesman II, Pauls DL (1993), Usefulness of twin studies for exploring the etiology of childhood and adolescent psychiatric disorders. *Am J Med Genet* 48:47–59

Lange K, Elston RC (1975), Extensions to pedigree analysis. I: Likelihood calculations for simple and complex pedigrees. *Hum Hered* 25:95–105

Lange K, Westlake J, Spence MA (1976), Extensions to pedigree analysis. II: Recurrence risk calculations under the polygenic threshold model. *Hum Hered* 26:337–348

Leckman JF (1990), Genes and developmental neurobiology. In: *Child and Adolescent Psychiatry: A Comprehensive Textbook*, Lewis M, ed. Baltimore: William and Wilkins, pp 3–11

Leckman JF (1991), Genes and the genesis of the CNS: hints from the homeobox. *Journal of Child and Adolescent Psychopharmacology* 1:207–211

Leckman JF, Dolnansky ES, Hardin MT et al. (1990), Perinatal factors in the expression of Tourette's syndrome: an exploratory study. *J Am Acad Child Adolesc Psychiatry* 29:220–226

Ledbetter D, Riccardi V, Airhart S, Strobel R, Keenan B, Crawford J (1981), Deletion of chromosome 15 as a cause of the Prader-Willi syndrome. *N Engl J Med* 304:325–329

Lombroso PJ, Pauls DL, Leckman JF (1990), Genetic factors in the etiology of childhood psychiatric disorders. In: *Brain and Behavior in Child Psychiatry*, Rothenberger A, ed. New York, Berlin: Springer-Verlag, pp 106–122

Lubs HA (1969), A marker X chromosome. *Am J Hum Genet* 21:231–244

McAllister G, Roby-Shemkovitz A, Amara S, Lerner M (1989), A comparison of the rat U snRNP-associated protein N: description of a potential Sm epitope. *EMBO J* 8:1177–1181

Merikangas K, Spence A, Kupfer D (1989), Linkage studies of bipolar disorder: methodologic and analytic issues. *Arch Gen Psychiatry* 46:1137–1141

Montgomery MA, Clayton PJ, Friedhoff AJ (1982), Psychiatric illness in Tourette syndrome patients and first-degree relatives. In: *Gilles de la Tourette Syndrome*, Friedhoff AJ, Chase TN, eds. New York: Raven Press.

Morell R, Friedman T, Moeljopawiro S, Hartono S, Asher J (1992), A frameshift mutation in the HuP2 paired domain of the probable human homolog of murine Pax-3 is responsible for Waardenburg syndrome type 1 in an Indonesian family. *Human Molecular Genetics* 1:243–247

Morgan W (1896), A case of congenital word-blindness. *Br Med J* 2:1543–1544

Morphew JA, Sim M (1969), Gilles de la Tourette's syndrome: a clinical and psychopathological study. *Br J Med Psychol* 42:293–301

Morrison J, Stewart M (1971), A family study of hyperactive child syndrome. *Biol Psychiatry* 3:189–195

Morrison J, Stewart M (1973), The psychiatric status of the legal families of adopted hyperactive children. *Arch Gen Psychiatry* 28:888–891

Morton NE, Yee S, Lew R (1971), Complex segregation analysis. *Am J Hum Genet* 23:602–611

Nee LE, Caine ED, Polinsky RJ, Eldridge R, Ebert M (1980), Gilles de la Tourette syndrome: clinical and family study of 50 cases. *Ann Neurol* 7:41–49

Nee LE, Polinsky RJ, Ebert MH (1982), Tourette syndrome: clinical and family studies. In: *Gilles de la Tourette Syndrome*, Friedhoff AJ, Chase TN, eds. New York: Raven Press, pp 291–295

NIH/CEPH Collaborative Mapping Group (1992), A comprehensive genetic linkage map of the human genome. *Science* 258:67–86

Oberle I, Rousseau F, Heitz D et al. (1991), Instability of a 550-base pair DNA segment and abnormal methylation in fragile X syndrome. *Science* 252:1097–1101

Orvaschel H, Walsh-Allis G, Ye W (1988), Psychopathology in children of parents with recurrent depression. *J Abnorm Child Psychol* 16:17–28

Ozcelik T, Leff S, Robinson W et al. (1992), Small nuclear ribonucleoprotein polypeptide N (SNRPN) an expressed gene in the Prader-Willi syndrome critical region. *Nature Genetics* 2:265–269

Pardes H, Kaufman C, Pincus H, West A (1989), Genetics and psychiatry: past discoveries, current dilemmas, and future directions. *Am J Psychiatry* 146:435–443

Pauls DL (1985), Strategies for the genetic study of child psychiatric disorders. In: *Psychiatry*, vol 2, Michels R, Cavenar J, Brodie H et al., eds. Philadelphia: Lippincott, chapter 10, pp 1–10

Pauls DL (1990), Genetic influences on child psychiatric conditions. In: *Child and Adolescent Psychiatry: A Comprehensive Textbook*, Lewis M, ed. Baltimore: Williams & Wilkins, pp 351–363

Pauls DL (1993), Behavioural disorders: lessons in linkage. *Nature Genetics* 3:4–5

Pauls DL, Leckman JF (1986), The inheritance of Gilles de la Tourette's syndrome and associated behaviors. *N Engl J Med* 315:993–997

Pauls DL, Pakstis A, Kurlan R et al. (1990), Segregation and linkage analyses of Gilles de la Tourette's syndrome and related disorders. *J Am Acad Child Adolesc Psychiatry* 29:195–203

Pauls DL, Raymond C, Leckman JF, Stevenson J (1991), A family study of Tourette's syndrome. *Am J Hum Genet* 48:154–163

Pennington BF (1990), The genetics of dyslexia. *J Child Psychol Psychiatry* 31:193–201

Pennington BF, Gilger JW, Pauls D, Smith SA, Smith SD, DeFries JC (1991), Evidence for major gene transmission of developmental dyslexia. *JAMA* 266:1527–1534

Pieretti M, Zhang F, Fu Y et al. (1991), Absence of expression of the *FMR-1* gene in fragile X syndrome. *Cell* 66:817–822

Piven J, Folstein S (1992), The genetics of autism. In: *Innovations in Autism*, Bauman M, Kemper T, eds. Baltimore: Johns Hopkins University Press

Prader A, Labhart A, Willi H (1956), Ein syndrom von adiposita, kleinwuchs, kryptorchidismus und oligophrenie nach myotonie-artigem zustand in neuge-borenalter Schweiz. *Med Wochenschr* 81:1260–1261

Price RA, Kidd KK, Cohen DJ, Pauls DL, Leckman JF (1985), A twin study of Tourette's syndrome. *Arch Gen Psychiatry* 42:815–820

Price RA, Pauls DL, Kruger SD, Caine ED (1987), Family data support a dominant major gene for Tourette syndrome. *Psychiatry Res* 24:251–261

Puig-Antich J, Goetz D, Davies M et al. (1989), A controlled family history study of prepubertal major depressive disorder. *Arch Gen Psychiatry* 46:406–418

Risch N (1990), Genetic linkage and complex diseases, with special reference to psychiatric disorders. *Genet Epidemiol* 7:3–16

Robertson MM, Trimble MR, Lees AJ (1988), The psychopathology of Gilles de la Tourette: a phenomenological analysis. *Br J Psychiatry* 152:383–390

Ross CA, McInnis MG, Margolis RL, Li S (1993), Genes with triplet repeats: candidate mediators of neuropsychiatric disorders. *Trends in Neuroscience* 16:254–260

Rowe D (1983), Biometrical genetic models of self-reported delinquent behavior: a twin study. *Behav Genet* 13:473–489

Rubenstein JL, Lotspeich L, Ciaranello RD (1990), The neurobiology of developmental disorders. In: *Advances in Clinical Child Psychology*, Lahey BB, Kazdin AE, eds. New York: Plenum Publishing Corp, pp 1–52

Rutter M (1968), Concepts of autism: a review of research. *J Child Psychol Psychiatry* 9:1–25

Rutter M (1981), Psychological sequelae of brain damage in children. *Am J Psychiatry* 138:1533–1544

Rutter M (1983), Behavioral studies: questions and findings on the concept of a distinctive syndrome. In: *Developmental Neuropsychiatry*, Rutter M, ed. New York: Guilford Press

Rutter M, Bolton P, Harrington R, Le Couteur A, Macdonald H, Simonoff E (1990a), Genetic factors in child psychiatric disorders. I. A review of research strategies. *J Child Psychol Psychiatry* 31:3–37

Rutter M, Macdonald H, Le Couteur A, Harrington R, Bolton P, Bailey A (1990b), Genetic factors in child psychiatric disorders. II. Empirical findings. *J Child Psychol Psychiatry* 31:39–83

Scarr S (1966), Genetic factors in activity motivation. *Child Dev* 37:663–673

Schmauss C, Brines M, Lerner M (1992), The gene encoding the small nuclear ribonucleoprotein-associated protein N is expressed at high levels in neurons. *J Biol Chem* 267:8521–8529

Shapiro AK, Shapiro ES, Bruun RD, Sweet RD (1978), *Gilles de la Tourette Syndrome*. New York: Raven Press

Shaywitz S, Cohen D, Shaywitz B (1983), Pharmacotherapy of attention deficit disorder. In: *Pediatric Update*, Swaiman K, ed. New York: Elsevier

Shaywitz S, Shaywitz B (1982), Biologic influences in attention deficit disorders. In: *Developmental-Behavioral Pediatrics*, Levine M, Carey W, Crocker A, Gross R, eds. Philadelphia: WB Saunders

Sherrington R, Brynjolfsson J, Petursson H et al. (1988), Localization of a susceptibility locus for schizophrenia on chromosome 5. *Nature* 336:164–167

Smith SD, Kimberling WJ, Pennington BF, Lubs H (1983), Specific reading disability: identification of an inherited form through linkage analysis. *Science* 219:1345–1347

Smith SD, Pennington BF, Kimberling WJ, Ing PS (1990), Familial dyslexia: use of genetic linkage data to define subtypes. *J Am Acad Child Adolesc Psychiatry* 29:204–213

Steffenburg S, Gillberg C, Hellgren L et al. (1989), A twin study of autism in Denmark, Finland, Iceland, Norway and Sweden. *J Child Psychol Psychiatry* 30:405–416

Stefl ME (1984), Mental health needs associated with Tourette syndrome. *Am J Public Health* 74:1310–1313

Stephenson S (1907), Six cases of congenital word-blindness affecting three generations of one family. *Ophthalmoscope* 5:482–484

Stevenson J (1992), Evidence for a genetic etiology in hyperactivity in children. *Behav Genet* 22:337–344

Stevenson J, Graham P, Fredman G, McLoughlin V (1987), A twin study of genetic influences on reading and spelling ability and disability. *J Child Psychol Psychiatry* 28:229–247

Strober M, Morrell W, Burroughs J, Lampert C, Danforth H, Freeman R (1988), A family study of bipolar I disorder in adolescence: early onset of symptoms linked to increased familial loading and lithium resistance. *J Affect Disord* 15:255–268

Sutherland G (1977), Fragile sites on human chromosomes, demonstration of their dependence on the type of tissue culture medium. *Science* 197:245–255

Tassabehji M, Read AP, Newton VE et al. (1992), Waardenburg syndrome patients have mutations in the human homologue of the Pax-3 paired box gene. *Nature* 355:635–636

Tassabehji M, Read AP, Newton VE et al. (1993), Mutations in the PAX3 gene causing Waardenburg syndrome type 1 and type 2. *Nature Genetics* 3:26–30

Thomas CJ (1905), Congenital "word blindness" and its treatment. *Ophthalmoscope* 3:380–385

Van de Wetering BJ (1993), A genetic study of the Gilles de la Tourette syndrome in the Netherlands. Dissertation, Erasmus University, Rotterdam, The Netherlands

Vandenberg S (1962), The hereditary abilities study: hereditary components in a psychological test battery. *Am J Hum Genet* 14:220–237

Verkerk AJ, Pieretti M, Sutcliffe J, Fu Y, Kuhl DP, Warren ST (1991), Identification of a gene (FMR-1) containing a CGG repeat coincident with a breakpoint cluster region exhibiting length variation in fragile X syndrome. *Cell* 65:905–914

Vincent A, Heitz D, Petit C, Dretz C, Oberle I, Mandel JL (1991), Abnormal pattern detected in fragile X patients by pulsed-field gel electrophoresis. *Nature* 349:624–626

Walkup JT, Leckman JF, Price RA, Cohen D (1987), Non-genetic factors associated with the expression of Tourette syndrome. In: Proceedings of the 34th annual meeting of the American Academy of Child and Adolescent Psychiatry

Weeks DE, Lange K (1992), A multilocus extension of the affected-pedigree-member method of linkage analysis. *Am J Hum Genet* 50:859–868

Weissman MM, Gammon D, John K et al. (1987), Children of depressed parents. *Arch Gen Psychiatry* 44:847–853

Weissman MM, Prusoff BA, Gammon GD, Merikangas K, Leckman J, Kidd K (1984), Psychopathology in the children (ages 6–18) of depressed and normal parents. *J Am Acad Child Psychiatry* 23:78–84

Willerman L (1973), Activity level and hyperactivity in twins. *Child Dev* 44:288–293

Yaryura-Tobias JA, Neziroglu F, Howard S, Fuller B (1981), Clinical aspects of Gilles de la Tourette syndrome. *Orthomolecular Psychiatry* 10:263–268

Zerbin-Rudin E (1967), Congenital word-blindness. *Bulletin of the Orton Society* 17:47–54

7

Behavioral and Psychiatric Disorders in Adult Male Carriers of Fragile X

Margaret B. Dorn, Michele M. M. Mazzocco, and Randi J. Hagerman
*The Children's Hospital,
Denver University of Colorado Health Sciences Center*

Objective: *In the present study we examined the incidence of psychiatric and behavioral problems among male carriers of the fragile X gene.* **Method:** *Retrospective data on carrier males were gathered using the family informant method. Each of 56 fragile X carrier women was interviewed about her father by an examiner blind to the father's carrier status. The interviewer administered measures of (1) behaviors related to DSM-III-R Axis I disorders, (2) adult attention-deficit hyperactivity disorder (ADHD) behaviors, (3) parental bonding skills, and (4) abusive behaviors. The endorsements from 24 women with fragile X fathers were compared with endorsements from 32 women with nonfragile X fathers.* **Results:** *The results show a higher incidence of psychopathology among the fragile X males (relative to nonfragile X fathers) for behaviors related to adult ADHD, parental bonding, abuse; and particularly for alcohol abuse/dependence and obsessive-compulsive disorder behaviors.* **Conclusions:** *These findings support the hypotheses that some "nonpenetrant" males may*

Reprinted with permission from the *Journal of the American Academy of Child and Adolescent Psychiatry*, 1994, Vol. 33(2), 256–264. Copyright © 1994 by the American Academy of Child and Adolescent Psychiatry.

This research was supported by USPHS Grant 5 T32 MH15442; partial support was provided by grant MH45916 United States National Institute of Mental Health, a grant from the Joslins Department Store, and grant RR-69 from the General Clinical Research Program, National Center for Health Research. The authors thank the study participants; W. Ted Brown, M.D., Ph.D., Faye Levinson, M.S.; William Seltzer, Ph.D.; Annette Taylor, Ph.D.; William E. Sobesky, Ph.D.; and Dennis Luckey, Ph. D.; and Barrett Jeffers, M.S., both of the Kempe Research Center at the Children's Hospital of Denver.

*indeed be mildly affected carriers and that there is a broad spectrum
of involvement among carrier males.*

Fragile X syndrome, the leading cause of hereditary mental retardation, was first identified by Lubs in 1969. The name fragile X was adopted for this genetic syndrome when cytogenetic technology made it possible to see the microscopic break or fragile site at the Xq27.3 location on the X chromosome. The recent discovery of the fragile X mental retardation (FMR-1) gene (Verkerk et al., 1991) led to the identification of an abnormal expansion of cytosine-guanine-guanine (CGG) nucleotide repeats (Fu et al., 1991; Yu et al., 1991) in both affected and unaffected fragile X persons. It is believed that the degree of expansion in those affected inhibits protein synthesis and thus leads to the full syndrome. However, the exact relationship between the number of CGG repeats and the cognitive, psychiatric, and physical phenotype is not yet known, particularly among less affected persons.

Although the phenotype for those most severely affected has been described (Hagerman, 1991), more recently attention has been drawn to the entire spectrum of involvement associated with this gene. This spectrum includes unaffected carriers, mildly affected carriers with learning disabilities (LD) (Mazzocco et al., 1992; Miezejeski et al., 1986) and/or emotional problems (e.g., Reiss et al., 1988), and those with the full syndrome who are severely affected with mental retardation and psychopathology. The prevalence of the full fragile X syndrome is 1/1000 individuals (Optiz, 1986), but the prevalence rate (which includes affected, unaffected and mildly affected carriers of the fragile X gene) is estimated to be 1/625 (Sherman, 1992).

Although both males and females can inherit the abnormal FMR-1 gene, the incidence of mental retardation (MR) is greater among males with the fragile X gene than it is among females with the gene. It is not surprising, therefore, that a significant portion of fragile X-related research has been focused on affected males. Researchers have identified that males affected by fragile X usually have, in addition to MR, behavioral disorders including: attention-deficit hyperactivity disorder (ADHD), impulsivity, anxiety, compulsive behaviors, perseveration, angry outbursts, and sometimes self-injurious behaviors. In addition, these males have a characteristic physical phenotype that includes a long face and prominent ears (Hagerman, 1991).

In contrast, male and female carriers of the gene who have fewer than 200 CGG repeats in the FMR-1 gene have been considered unaffected by the gene. Nonmentally retarded carrier males have been regarded as completely unaffected cognitively, emotionally, and physically (Laird 1987; Laird et al., 1991). Female carriers similarly have been regarded as unaffected, until recently. Evidence from recent studies of normal IQ women carriers of fragile X suggests that variability exists for cognitive (Grigsby, 1990; Mazzocco et al., 1992) and social-emotional (Hagerman and Sobesky, 1989; Reiss et al., 1988) features. However, the variability of affectedness appears primarily among women with cytogenetic fragility $\geqslant 2\%$ and not among carriers with $<2\%$ cytogenetic fragility (Freund et al., 1992; Mazzocco et al., 1992). Whereas these studies show a continuum of involvement among female carriers, only a few case reports are available on the variability of involvement among male carriers (Hagerman, 1991; Loesch et al, 1987). Emerging molecular genetic data (Brown, 1993, personal communication; Yu et al., 1991) and anecdotal clinical data (e.g., Loesch et al., 1987) led us to question whether these supposedly asymptomatic male carriers are truly "unaffected."

The present study is the first to systematically investigate the incidence of behavioral and psychiatric disorders among males who are carriers of the fragile X gene. We predicted that a greater percentage of carrier males (relative to control males) would exhibit behavioral and psychiatric symptoms. We specifically hypothesized that carrier males would manifest a more subtle form of the severe symptomology documented for the full syndrome, as described above. Therefore, the behaviors we examined were abusive and antisocial behaviors, alcohol abuse and dependence, attentional and impulsivity difficulties, and obsessive-compulsive disorder (OCD) behaviors.

METHOD

Retrospective data concerning fragile X carrier adult males and non-fragile X controls males were collected via the family informant method (Andreasen et al., 1977; Mannuza et al., 1985). This method was chosen for two reasons. First, it is often difficult to interview carrier males directly because they are most often identified when their affected grandchild is diagnosed with fragile X syndrome. By this time, the carrier grandfather may be deceased or is likely to be elderly and thus not available, capable, or willing to participate in a direct interview study. Second, a family informant's report may be at least as accurate, if not more accurate, than a proband's report when the behaviors in question include observable psychiatric symptomology and pathological behaviors (Andreasen et al., 1977; Stabenau, 1990; Zimmerman et al., 1988). One difficulty reported for this method is the incidence of underreporting (Andresaen et al., 1986). Thus the family informant method can be considered a conservative estimate of behavior in the proband.

Subjects

Family informants were recruited from a regional developmental assessment clinic at a hospital that serves fragile X families nationwide. Each informant was a parent or relative of a child referred to the clinic for a fragile X assessment or a nonfragile X family member control subject. The majority of parents who accompanied their child to the clinic were mothers. Therefore, we included only women as informants in this study because of availability: there were not enough men available as informants to statistically examine gender differences. None of the women interviewed was herself referred for clinical assessment, therefore eliminating one possible source of ascertainment bias.

Sixty-eight informant daughters were interviewed individually by the same female examiner (M.B.D.) who was blind to the carrier status of the informant and of her parents. The interview questions pertained to the informant's father's behavior during her first 18 years of life. Each of 62 informants was from a fragile X family. The remaining six informants were from nonfragile X families, and were included in the study to ensure that the interviewer was blind to the informant's DNA status. However, to maintain a conservative control group of informants from fragile X families only, the data from these six women were not included in our analyses.

For 26 informants, the father was the carrier of the fragile X gene. For the remaining 36 informants, the mother was the carrier. In the majority of cases, maternal versus paternal inheritance was determined via pedigree analysis; specifically by identifying a diagnosed and affected individual with fragile X from the paternal or maternal side of the family. If the study informant had an affected brother, then maternal inheritance was implicated. For the few families for which maternal or paternal inheritance was not implicated by pedigree, DNA analyses were performed to determine carrier status of the parents. The former group of 26 informants constituted the "daughters of fragile X fathers" group, whereas the latter group of 36 women served as the control group.

Among the 62 informants from fragile X families were six pairs of sisters from whom we were able to obtain estimates of informant data validity. Data from only one randomly selected sister from each pair were included in the overall analyses to ensure independent ratings of fathers within each group. Therefore, our final sample consisted of 24 daughters of fragile X fathers and 32 daughters of control fathers. These two subgroups of informant daughters were similar in age and fragile X status (Table 1). Among the former group, we know that all of the informant daughters were obligate carriers of the abnormal FMR-1 gene; among the latter group, among the 31 (of 32) for whom fragile X status is known, 21 (68%) are known carriers (Table 1).

Instruments

Carrier and control fathers' behaviors (as reported by their daughters) were assessed using four instruments: the Family Informant Schedule Criteria, an adult ADHD checklist, an abuse questionnaire, and the Parental Bonding Instrument.

The first and probably the single most important measure used was the Family Informant Schedule Criteria (FISC) (Mannuzza et al., 1985; revised 1990). The FISC is a well-known structured interview designed to parallel 14 *DSM-III-R* Axis I diagnostic categories plus one Axis II disorder category (antisocial personality disorder). It is a revision of the Family History Research Diagnostic Criteria (FH-RDC)(Andreasen et al., 1977). Informant data from the FH-RDC measure of parental *DSM-III* diagnoses have been shown to correlate with probands' self-reports of psychopathology as obtained on the Schedule for Affective Disorders and Schizophrenia (SADS) (Andreasen et al., 1981). Thus the FH-RDC, on which the FISC is based, has gained research support as a valid family informant measure (Zimmerman et al., 1988).

The FISC variables of primary interest in this study were these categories: panic disorder, social phobia, general anxiety disorder, major depression, dysthymia, obsessive compulsive disorder, alcohol dependence and abuse, and adult antisocial personality disorder. Each informant was

TABLE 1
Characteristics of Informants

$N = 56$	With Fra (X) Fathers, $n = 24$		With Control Fathers, $n = 32$	
Mean (SD)				
Full-scale IQ	$n = 11$	99.1 (10.8)	$n = 28$	102.9 (13.4)
Age	$n = 24$	37.5 (8.3)	$n = 32$	33.3 (7.8)
% (no.) of informants who test positive for Fra X	$n = 24$	100% (24)	$n = 31$[a]	68% (21)

[a] Fragile X carrier status unknown for one informant.

asked to respond "yes" or "no" to each of the 16 probe items. If a "yes" response was given to any probe item, the interviewer administered an additional 20 or more in-depth questions to determine whether the father's behavior met the full criteria for the disorder in question. The additional items allowed the examiner to assign a diagnostic score of "2" (yes, possible) or "3" (yes, probable) to each of the 15 *DSM-III-R* categories; a score of "1" was assigned to "no" responses. (See Mannuzza et al., 1985, revised 1990, for a detailed description of the FISC). The FISC dependent variables examined in this study included one score per each of the 15 categories, as described above, and one overall score that reflected whether the father in question was likely to have had one or more *DSM-III-R* psychiatric disorders.

The Adult Attention-Deficit Hyperactivity Disorder (A-ADHD) checklist is an adaptation of a self-report measure of the frequency of 18 symptoms of adult ADHD (Barkley, 1990). These 18 symptoms relate specifically to hot-temperedness, hyperactivity, attention deficits, impulsivity, and impatience. For each of the 18 items, daughters indicated the degree of presence of each symptom with a four-point rating scale ranging from "0" (not at all) to "3" (very much). The primary dependent measure obtained was the total score (ranging from 0 to 54) across these 18 items and individual scores for hot-tempered, impatient, and impulsive behaviors—characteristics easily observed by daughters and associated with affected fragile X males. Thus, one overall and three individual scores were obtained from and examined with this measure.

The Parental Bonding Instrument (PBI)(Parker et al., 1979) is a family informant retrospective interview that has gained research support as a valid indicator of parent/child relationships (Parker, 1983). It includes 25 items that correspond to two factor-analytically derived dimensions: (1) care (a measure of warmth and acceptance) and (2) control (a measure of coldness and rejection). Each item was scored on a four-point scale ranging from "very much *unlike* my father" to "very much *like* my father." The PBI was adapted for use as a retrospective, family informant interview. The two variables obtained from this measure included total scores across items pertaining to "care" and items pertaining to "control."

The Abuse Questionnaire was developed by Dorn and Sobesky in 1992 (unpublished questionnaire) to serve as an additional indicator of psychopathology. This structured interview was designed to measure the incidence of physical, verbal, and/or sexual abuse, none of which are examined with the previously described instruments. The Abuse Questionnaire includes three items pertaining to each of these types of abuse, as reported relative to father's abusiveness to: (1) informant, (2) father's spouse, and (3) informant's siblings. Informants rated the nine items described above on a two-point scale corresponding to "no, abuse did not occur" or "yes, abuse occurred." In addition to these nine items, an overall score ("yes" or "no") indicated the presence of *any type* of abusive behavior between the father and other family member(s). Thus, 10 dependent variables were obtained from the Abuse Questionnaire.

RESULTS

Preliminary analyses revealed no significant age differences across the two groups of informants. For the two groups of informants for whom FSIQ scores were available (11 of the 24 informant daughters of fragile X fathers and 28 of the 32 informant daughters of control fathers), there were no significant FSIQ differences. Age and FSIQ were thus not included in the subsequent analyses. Of primary interest was whether fragile X fathers differed from control fathers on any measure of behavioral or psychiatric disorder. For each continuous variable, t tests were performed to address this question. For each categorical variable, two-tailed Fisher's Exact tests were performed. We report all differences significant at the $<.05$ level.

FISC

Sixteen scores (i.e., one overall score and one score for each of 15 diagnostic categories) were obtained from the FISC. For each of following six categories (panic disorder with agoraphobia, agoraphobia, bipolar disorder, cyclothymia, substance abuse, and schizophrenia), only one or no endorsements were assigned from our 56 informants. Thus, no analyses were carried out for these six categories. Fisher's Exact procedures were carried out for the remaining scores. The results indicate the distribution of endorsements corresponding to scores of "1," "2," or "3," differed across the two groups of fathers. Significant differences in the distribution were seen for the overall FISC score, OCD behaviors, and alcohol abuse/dependence, $p < .01$. Sixty-three percent of fragile X fathers received an overall FISC score of "3" (indicating that, "yes, a diagnosis is probable"), compared with 25% of control fathers. Similarly, 25% of fragile X fathers received a score of "3" for OCD-related behaviors, whereas no control father received this endorsement. Finally, 46% of fragile X fathers received a score of "3" for alcohol abuse/dependence whereas this score was received by 13% of control fathers (Table 2).

TABLE 2
Rates of Psychiatric Disorder as Reported by Informant Daughters
of Fragile X and Control Fathers

	Fra (X) Fathers $n = 24$		Control Fathers $n = 32$		Fisher's Exact p
Family Information Schedule Criteria % with score = 3 (probable):					
Overall	63%	(15)	25%	(8)	.005
Axis I related behaviors					
Panic	13%	(3)	3%	(1)	.300
Social phobia	8%	(2)	0%		.179
Obsesive-compulsive disorder	25%	(6)	0%		.004
Alcohol abuse	46%	(11)	13%	(4)	.007
Dysthymia	33%	(8)	16%	(5)	.200
V-Code behaviors					
Adult Antisocial	13%	(3)	3%	(1)	.072
Abuse: Scored yes/no % Yes responses					
Any type of abuse	46%	(11)	28%	(9)	.260
Verbal abuse of informant	38%	(9)	16%	(5)	.117
Physical abuse of informant	17%	(4)	13%	(4)	.713
Verbal abuse of spouse	42%	(10)	22%	(7)	.146
Physical abuse of spouse	29%	(7)	9%	(3)	.080

No significant differences were seen for the seven remaining FISC scores. However, among many measures for which differences did not reach statistical significance, the differences seen were in the direction predicted. For panic disorder, social phobia, dysthymia, and Axis II adult antisocial behaviors, scores of "3" were assigned at least twice as frequently for fragile X fathers as for control fathers (Table 2.) There were no differences seen for simple phobia, major depression, or substance abuse.

Abusive Behaviors

Ten scores can be obtained from the Abuse Questionnaire. Abusive behavior was predicted to be endorsed for fragile X fathers, but we did not expect the informants to endorse sexual abuse items because of the highly personal nature of the items. As predicted, only one endorsement for sexual abuse occurred from among our 56 informants. For this reason, the three questions pertaining to sexual abuse were not analyzed. This left seven scores remaining: one overall score and six specific scores pertaining to physical or verbal abuse, as described earlier. Each score reflected a "yes" or "no" response. For each of these seven measures, a two-tailed Fisher's Exact test was performed to examine whether the number of fathers receiving endorsements for abusive behaviors differed as a function of group status (fragile X versus nonfragile X control). Statistical significance was not reached for any of the measures. However, for all seven measures, "yes" responses occurred more frequently among fragile X fathers than for control fathers. Differences approached significance on two measures: when compared to control fathers, fragile X fathers were more than three times as likely to be endorsed as having been physically abusive to their spouse ($p = .059$) and were more than twice as likely to be endorsed as having been verbally abusive to the informant ($p = .08$; Table 2). All remaining differences were also in the direction predicted.

Adult ADHD

A t test was employed to examine overall scores on the A-ADHD measure. The results indicate that fragile X fathers had higher scores, indicating more attention-deficit hyperactivity disorder behaviors, $t = 2.16, p < .05$ (Table 3). The A-ADHD scale measures the likelihood of adult ADHD, with higher scores indicating a greater likelihood. It is worth noting that the group mean for fragile X fathers (16.8), although higher than the group mean for control fathers (10.5), does not approach the maximum possible score of 54. This suggests that the fragile X fathers, while receiving higher scores than control fathers, were not endorsed as having all ADHD related behaviors.

The ADHD behaviors of particular interest in this study were impatience, hot-temperedness, and/or impulsivity. A Fisher's Exact test revealed no group differences on scores for impatience, $p = .53$. Fisher's Exact tests also revealed that group differences in impulsivity and hot-temperedness approached but did not reach significance. Fifty percent (12/24) of fragile X fathers were endorsed as being impulsive compared with 31% (10/32) of control fathers. Although the frequency of overall hot-temperedness ratings did not differ across groups, the highest intensity endorsements (i.e., scores of "3") were assigned to 33% (8/24) of the fragile X fathers and to 16% (5/32) of the control fathers. Therefore, our findings suggest that fragile X

TABLE 3

Group Means and Standard Deviations on Parental Bonding Instrument (PBI)
and Adult-Attention-Deficit Hyperactivity Disorder (A-ADHD)
Scores Assigned to Fathers by Informants

	Fra (X) Carrier Fathers $n = 24$		Control Fathers $n = 32$		
	$\overline{X}$	SD	$\overline{X}$	SD	p
PBI					
Care score	17.7	10.2	22.7	8.2	.046
Control score	12.0	7.9	11.2	5.9	
A-ADHD					
Total score	16.8	13.0	10.5	8.7	.035

carrier fathers, relative to controls, may have a higher incidence of some
adult ADHD behaviors but do not demonstrate remarkable differences.

Parental Bonding Instrument (PBI)

Two *t* tests were employed to examine whether parental behaviors related to warmth/affection or to coldness/rejection differed between our two
groups of fathers. The results indicate that fragile X fathers were less caring
($\overline{X}$ score = 17.65) than were control fathers ($\overline{X}$ score = 22.7), $p < .05$. There
was no difference between the two groups on coldness/rejection scores,
$p = .6$.

Validity of Informant Data

Although not a component of the study design, the validity of informants' reports was addressed through the six instances for which two informants reported on one father. There were two sets of daughters each
reporting on one fragile X father, and four sets of daughters each reporting
on one control father. (Data from only one of each sister pair were included
in the primary analyses, as aforementioned.) For each set, we calculated the
percentage of responses in agreement in proportion to the total number of
responses given. Specifically, we examined endorsements for the 17 items
pertaining to behaviors that were not directed toward the informant (such
as parental bonding behaviors). We defined "agreement" for Likert scale

items as those within one point of each other; agreement on the adult ADHD overall scores were defined as those within one standard error; and yes/no items were in agreement if exactly the same. However, among the 87 responses in agreement (from the 102 responses received across the six fathers each of whom had two informants), only three responses were *not* identical; the remaining 84 responses were identical. The average percentage of agreement within each sister pair was 85% (rates of agreement between individual pairs of sisters were 59, 82, 82, 88, 100, and 100%).

DISCUSSION

The primary hypothesis addressed in this study was that the incidence of behavioral and psychiatric disorders would be higher among fragile X fathers relative to control fathers. Our findings support this hypothesis for many of the behaviors examined. The incidence rates between the two groups of fathers include statistically significant differences for the *DSM-III-R* overall FISC score and OCD behavior score. Moreover, additional differences in alcohol abuse/dependence, adult ADHD, and parental caring scores were significant at least at the $p < .05$ level. The differences seen among scores for which significance was only approached were in the direction predicted. For seven of these differences, the frequency with which a behavior was endorsed by an informant was at least twice as great among fragile X fathers as it was for control fathers.

The most dramatic differences seen were for Axis I OCD behaviors and alcohol abuse/dependence. For OCD behaviors, 21% of fragile X fathers versus 0% of the control fathers were reported to have had repetitive, compulsive behaviors that significantly interfered with social activities or relationships with others. However, the daughters' reports could not support the *DSM-III-R* OCD criteria that these obsessive behaviors were performed in conjunction with a fear. Therefore, our data support that OCD *behaviors* occur with greater frequency in fragile X fathers relative to controls; but these data cannot support the formal diagnosis of OCD.

In contrast, the data for alcohol abuse/dependence do fulfill the *DSM-III-R* diagnostic criteria. Forty-six percent of fragile fathers versus 13% of X control fathers were endorsed with behaviors that met the DSM-III-R criteria for alcohol abuse or dependence. The incidence among fragile X fathers far exceeds the observed prevalence of 5% as reported for the male general population (Helzer and Pryzbeck, 1988; Plomin, 1991) and even exceeds the prevalence rate of 25% reported for first-degree relatives of known alcoholics (Mednick et al., 1987).

In addition to OCD behaviors and alcohol abuse/dependency, some additional behavior disorders and Axis I and II psychiatric disorders occurred with greater frequency among fragile X fathers relative to control fathers. As predicted, there were no group differences on measures of agoraphobia, panic disorder with agoraphobia, bipolar disorder, cyclothymia, and schizophrenia. Yet relative to control fathers, twice as many fragile X fathers were reported to have dysthymia and verbally abusive behaviors; three times as many fragile X fathers were reported to have been physically abusive to their spouse; and four times as many fragile X fathers were reported to have panic disorder and antisocial personality disorder (APD) behaviors. Although the *adult* criteria for the formal Axis II diagnosis of APD was endorsed by informants, the informants were unable to report on the presence of *adolescent* conduct disorder behaviors in their fathers. Therefore, we are limited to reporting the notable frequency of adult APD *behaviors* in fragile X fathers versus controls, in the absence of information necessary to meet the full *DSM-III-R* APD criteria.

The incidence of APD behaviors among the control fathers was identical to the rate of APD reported in the *DSM-III-R* for the general population (3%), whereas the 13% incidence rate of APD behaviors among the fragile X fathers approaches the 15% rate of APD reported in the *DSM-III-R* for first-degree relatives of a diagnosed APD father. The fragile X fathers in our sample are all carriers of the abnormal FMR-1 gene, but none of these fathers are first-degree relatives of each other.

In addition to the significant differences described above, tendencies for behavior and/or psychiatric difficulties were seen for adult ADHD and parental caring behaviors. The higher adult ADHD scores among fathers who are fragile X carriers are slight and at most suggest the possibility of these characteristics as components of the carrier male phenotype.

Interpretation of the Family Informant Data

Our findings clearly indicate that a higher percentage of fragile X fathers have a tendency for behavioral and psychiatric disorders relative to control fathers. Interpretation of these data warrants the consideration of potential confounds, including the use of the family informant method, the nature of our informant sample, and the comorbidity of the behaviors examined in this study. If we are to argue that the abnormal FMR-1 gene is related to behaviors reported for fathers, we need to first consider the role each of the above potential confounds may have on the reported behaviors. As described earlier, the family informant method has gained support, particularly for studies concerning psychopathology in a parental proband (Andreasen et al., 1977; Stabenau, 1990). This method of data collection is particularly sensitive to observable behaviors, including OCD, abusive, and adult antisocial behaviors; alcohol abuse/dependence; and other observable behaviors examined in this study. A discussion of each of the two remaining potential confounds is presented below.

The subjects included in this study were primarily fragile X carrier women, a group for which cognitive and emotional deficits have been reported (e.g., Freund et al., 1992; Grigsby et al., 1990; Mazzocco et al., 1992; Miezejeski et al., 1986; Reiss et al., 1988). If this group is *less* reliable as informants than is a nonfragile X group, one might question the quality of reports received in this study. Such an argument is countered by two important features of our informant group. First, if fragile X carrier status affects reliability of reporting, then the quality of reporting should be comparably affected across groups because the majority of all informants were fragile X carriers. Thus any group differences reported would then be in addition to the potential effect of informant carrier status. Second, the informant daughters who participated in this study were representative of women with normal FSIQ scores, not of affected women.

The remaining question concerns to what extent we may attribute our findings to the fathers' genetic status (fragile X versus control). One possibility is that the high frequency of occurrence for each of the behavior problems reported in this study results from the abnormal FMR-1 gene. However, heritability rates for any behavior rarely exceed 50% (Plomin, 1990). An alternative explanation gains support from the extensive literature on the comorbidity of alcoholism and Axis I psychiatric disorders as well as personality disorders. For instance, APD is reported to be the most prevalent personality disorder associated with alcoholism (Hesselbrock et al., 1984; Nace, 1984; Stabenau, 1984) but also has been linked to genetic factors independent of family history of alcohol abuse (Cloninger and Reich, 1983). Alcoholism appears to heighten one's risk for generalized anxiety disorder, social phobia (Ross et al., 1988); panic disorder (Helzer and Pryzbeck, 1988), and OCD (Nace and Isbell, 1991). These increased risks for dual diagnoses appear to have genetic components, especially for males.

The prevalence of dual diagnoses of these disorders suggests that comorbidity, independent of the FMR-1 gene, may in part explain the high incidence rates of these disorders as seen in the fragile X carrier males. Therefore, the behaviors reported with greater frequency for fragile X fathers may be related to each other, rather than related only to the abnormal FMR-1 gene itself. Nevertheless, our preliminary findings show that these behavioral and psychiatric disorders occur for a higher percentage of fragile X fathers relative to control fathers. Moreover, these incidence rates exceed those reported for the general population and approach or exceed those known for first-degree relatives of persons diagnosed with a psychiatric disorder, including alcohol abuse and APD.

To this point we have focused on the portion of fragile X fathers for whom psychiatric disorders were reported. It is important to question the differentiating factors that lead to an affected versus unaffected phenotype. One explanation as to why only a portion of the fragile X fathers is reported to have behavioral and psychiatric disorders pertains to the potential effect of the number of CGG repeats in carrier males (as determined by polymerase chain reaction). An examination of this relationship may additionally address which phenotypic characteristics may be primary (versus secondary) effects of the gene; as well as whether the number of CGG repeats predicts the likelihood that a fragile X carrier male will have psychiatric or behavioral difficulties.

The primary focus of this study was to examine the potential effect of a gene (the abnormal FMR-1 gene) on psychopathology. Although we cannot argue a clear cause-effect relationship owing to the potential confounds described above, we can argue that we found a greater incidence of several behavioral and psychiatric disorders among males who carry the abnormal FMR-1 gene relative to control males. Carrier males do not have the expanded number of CGG repeats (i.e., more than 200) that is associated with the full fragile X syndrome and MR. Nevertheless, we have found a subpopulation of carrier males with behavioral and psychiatric disorders. We hypothesize that these carrier males have a higher number of CGG repeats within the abnormal FMR-1 gene than do those carrier males without behavioral and psychiatric disorders or perhaps have some variation in methylation or gene function. However, other environmental influences or gene interactions could be responsible for the disorders reported in this study. In addition, the small amplification status (<200 CGG repeats) could predispose a person to other genetic and environmental factors that may lead to the disorders described here.

The implications to be drawn from these findings pertain to identification of carriers as well as to treatment issues. Identification of family members who may be at risk for carrying the FMR-1 mutation (as well as of members who are at risk for being affected by the gene) typically has been directed toward males with significant cognitive deficits. Our findings suggest that psychopathology also can be an indicator of carrier status within a family in whom the gene is suspect. As our findings do not allow us to examine the relation between psychopathology and cognitive functioning (as cognitive performance was not examined), they lead us to question whether psychopathology occurs regardless of an person's level of cognitive abilities. Directing this question toward "unaffected" male carriers would contribute toward our understanding of this relationship or toward whether the behavioral and cognitive components of the fragile X phenotype involve two separate (or at least not directly causal) modalities.

Regardless of the level of cognitive functioning among our group of fragile X fathers, the evidence for a higher incidence of psychopathology speaks to the importance of identifying carrier males in childhood and to consider their *potential* risk for psychopathology. Clinical attention is particularly appropriate given the success reported for childhood intervention of attention and conduct difficulties (e.g., Barkley 1990; Greenfield 1988; Hesselbrock 1986). The incidence of precursors to adult psychopathology among carrier boys deserves research attention to clarify this issue. Although the underlying mechanisms that lead to our findings are in need of additional investigation, our preliminary report supports the hypotheses that *some* carrier males may indeed be mildly affected carriers and that there is a broad spectrum of involvement among fragile X carrier males.

REFERENCES

Andreasen NC, Enticed J, Spitzer RI, Winokur G (1977), The family history method using diagnostic criteria. *Arch Gen Psychiatry* 34:1229–1235

Andreasen NC, Grove WM, Shapiro RW, Keller, MB, Hirschfeld RMA, McDonald-Scott P (1981), Reliability of Lifetime diagnosis: a multi-center collaborative perspective. *Arch Gen Psychiatry* 38:400–405

Andreasen NC, Rice J, Enticed J, Reich T, Coryell W (1986), The family history approach to diagnosis: how useful is it? *Arch Gen Psychiatry* 43:421–429

Barkley RA (1990), *Attention Deficit and Hyperactivity Disorder: Diagnosis and Treatment. A Handbook for Diagnosis and Treatment.* New York: The Guilford Press

Cloninger CR, Reich T (1983), Genetic heterogeneity in alcoholism and sociopathy. In: *Genetics of Neurological and Psychiatric Disorders*, eds, Kety SS, Rowland LP, Sidman RL, Matthysee SW. New York: Raven Press, pp 145–166

Freund LS, Reiss AL, Hagerman RJ, Vinogradov S (1992), Chromosome fragility and psychopathology in obligate female carriers of the fragile X chromosome. *Arch Gen Psychiatry* 49:54–60

Fu YH, Kuhl DPA, Pizzuti A, et al (1991), Variation of the CGG repeat at the fragile X site results in genetic instability: resolution of the Sherman Paradox. *Cell* 67:1047–1058

Greenfield B, Hechtman L, Weiss G (1988), Two subgroups of hyperactives as adults: co-relations of outcome. *Can J Psychiatry* 33:505–508

Grigsby JP, Kemper MB, Hagerman RJ, Myers CS (1990), Neuropsychological dysfunction among affected heterozygous fragile X females. *Am J Med Genet* 35:28–35

Hagerman RJ (1991), Physical and behavioral phenotype. In: *Fragile X Syndrome, Diagnosis, and Research*, eds, Hagerman RJ, Silverman AC. Baltimore, MD: Johns Hopkins University Press

Hagerman RJ, Sobesky WE (1989), Psychopathology in fragile X syndrome. *Am J Orthopsychiatry* 59:142–152

Helzer JE, Pryzbeck TR (1988), The co-occurrence of alcoholism with other psychiatric disorders in the general population and its impact on treatment. *J Stud Alcohol* 49:219–224

Hesselbrock MN (1986), Childhood behavior problems and adult antisocial personality disorder in alcoholism. In: *Psychopathology and Additive Disorders*, ed. Meyer RE. New York: Guilford Press

Hesselbrock MN, Hesselbrock VM, Babor TF, Stabenau JR, Meyer RE, Weidenman M (1984), Antisocial behavior, psychopathology, and problem drinking in the natural history of alcoholism. In: *Longitudinal Research in Alcoholism*, eds, Goodwin DW, van-Dusen KT, Mednick SA. Boston: Kluwer-Nijhoff Publishing, pp 197–214

Laird CD (1987), Proposed mechanism of inheritance and expression of the human fragile-X syndrome of mental retardation. *Genetics* 117:587–599

Laird CD, Lamb MM, Sved J, Thorne J (1991), Modeling the inheritance and expression of fragile X syndrome, with emphasis on the X-inactivation imprinting model. In: *Fragile X Syndrome: Diagnosis, Treatment and Research*, eds, Hagerman RJ, Silverman AC. Baltimore, MD: Johns Hopkins University Press

Loesch DZ, Hay DA, Sutherland GRR, Halliday J, Judge C, Webb GC (1987), Phenotypic variation in male transmitted fragile X: genetic inferences. *Am J Med Genet* 27:401–417

Lubs HA (1969), A marker X chromosome. *Am J Hum Genet* 21:231–244

Mannuzza S, Fyer AJ, Enticed J, Klein DF (1985; rev 1990), *The Family Informant Schedule and Criteria (FISC).* New York: New York State Psychiatric Clinic

Mazzocco MMM, Pennington BF, Cronister-Silverman A, Hagerman RJ (1992), Specific frontal lobe deficits among women with the fragile X gene. *J Am Acad Child Adolesc Psychiatry* 32:1141–1148

Mednick SA, Moffit TE, Stack, S (1987), The causes of crime: new biological approaches. In: *Biological Risk Factors for Psychosocial Disorders*, eds, Rutter M, Casaer P. New York: Cambridge University Press, p 109

Miezejeski CM, Jenkins EC, Hill AL, Wisiewski K, French JH, Brown, TW (1986), A profile of cognitive deficit in females from fragile X families. *Neuropsychologia* 24:405–409

Nace EP, Isbell PG (1991), Alcohol. In: *Clinical Textbook of Addictive Disorder*, eds, Frances RJ, Miller SI. New York: Guilford Press

Nace EP (1984), Epidemiology of alcoholism and prospects for treatment. *Annu Rev Med* 35:293–309

Opitz JM (1986), On the gates of hell and a most unusual gene. Editorial Comment. *Am J Med Genet* 23:1–10

Parker G, Tupling H, Brown LB (1979), A parental bonding instrument. *Br J Med Psychol* 52:1–10

Parker G (1983), *Parental Overprotection. A Risk Factor in Psychological Development.* New York: Grune & Stratton

Plomin R (1991), Genetic risk and psychosocial disorders: links between the normal and the abnormal. In: *Biological Risk Factors for Psychosocial Disorders*, eds, Rutter, M, Casaer P. New York: Cambridge University Press, pp 101–138

Plomin R (1990), The role of inheritance in behavior. *Science* 248:183–188

Reiss AL, Hagerman RJ, Vinogradov S, Abrams M, King RJ (1988), Psychiatric disability in female carriers of the fragile X chromosome. *Arch Gen Psychiatry* 45:25–30

Ross HE, Glaser FB, Germanson T (1988), The prevalence of psychiatric disorders in patients with alcohol and other drug problems. *Arch Gen Psychiatry* 45:1023–1031

Sherman SL (1992), *Epidemiology and Screening.* Presented at the National Fragile X Foundation Third International Conference, Snowmass, CO, June 16–20, 1992

Stabenau JR (1990), Additive independent factors that predict risk for alcoholism. *J Stud Alcohol* 51:164–173

Stabenau JR (1984), Implications of family history of alcoholism, antisocial personality, and sex differences in alcohol dependence. *Am J Psychiatry* 141:1178–1182

Verkerk AJMH, Pieretti M, Sutcliffe JS et al. (1991), Identification of a gene (FMR-1) containing a CGG repeat coincident with a breakpoint cluster region exhibiting length variation in fragile X syndrome. *Cell* 65:905–914

Yu S, Pritchard M, Kramer E et al. (1991), Fragile X genotype characterized by an unstable region of DNA. *Science* 252:1179–1181

Zimmerman M, Coryell W, Pfohl B, Stangl D (1988), The reliability of the family history method for psychiatric diagnoses. *Arch Gen Psychiatry* 45:320–322

8

Childhood-Onset Schizophrenia: Timely Neurobiological Research

Kathleen McKenna, Charles T. Gordon, and Judith L. Rapoport

Child Psychiatry Branch, National Institute of Mental Health, Bethesda, Maryland

Objective: *To review timely research on childhood-onset schizophrenia in view of advances in biological research on, and neurodevelopmental theories of, the later-onset disorder.* **Method:** *Research issues are outlined including further clarification of ICD- and DSM-defined childhood schizophrenia, and differentiation from autism "spectrum" and other subtle, chronic developmental disorders. Key neurobiological advances are reviewed for which child studies are relevant and feasible.* **Conclusion:** *It is anticipated that narrowly defined childhood-onset schizophrenics will constitute a predominately male population. A high rate of family illness or chromosomal and/or brain developmental abnormalities, which will be instructive regarding the pathophysiology of later-onset schizophrenia, is expected.*

Schizophrenia has been described in children as young as 5 years of age (Cantor et al., 1982; Green et al., 1984), but little systematic research has focused on this rare disorder. The treated prevalence of schizophrenia in children younger than 15 years of age is an estimated 0.14/1000, almost 50 times less than for children with onset between 15 and 54 years of age (Beitchman, 1985; Volkmar et al., 1988). The term "childhood-onset schizophrenia" (COS) is defined as approximately prepubertal onset of psychotic

---

Reprinted with permission from the *Journal of the American Academy of Child and Adolescent Psychiatry*, 1994, Vol. 33(6), 771–781. Copyright © 1994 by the American Academy of Child and Adolescent Psychiatry.

Accepted July 26, 1993.

symptoms before age 12 years. Until recently it was applied to children with not only schizophrenia, but also what now would be considered dissociative and affective disorders, autism, "organic brain syndromes," neurological disorders, and even mental retardation (Prior and Werry, 1986). Over the past 20 years, however, differentiation of various severely disabling childhood disorders has progressed so that it is now generally accepted that autism and childhood-onset schizophrenia are separate disorders on the basis of phenomenology, genetics, and biological correlates, and degenerative neurological disorders have also been distinguished from COS. However, *DSM-III-R* and *DSM-IV* (American Psychiatric Association, in preparation) defined schizophrenia are still used to include a range of childhood conditions having psychotic symptoms that need to be differentiated (Gordon et al., in press).

Variability in age at onset of schizophrenia has been noted since the earliest descriptions of the illness in adults (Bleuler, 1911; De Sanctis 1908; Kraepelin, 1919), but the significance of this variability is not known, nor is it known if some childhood-onset schizophrenia is continuous with later-onset illness. Schizophrenia in adults is considered a heterogeneous disorder in which genetic and environmental factors affecting prenatal brain development play etiological roles and there is growing consensus that schizophrenia is a neurodevelopmental disorder (Feinberg, 1982; Murray et al., 1992a; Weinberger, 1987). Recent advances in genetics, neuroimaging, and pharmacology offer new approaches to the nature of the developmental insult. Each of these advances has implications for childhood-onset illness.

Earlier-onset illness may, for example, reflect a more salient early brain "lesion," premature endocrine influence on brain development, greater familial genetic "loading" or instructive genetic abnormalities, increased environmental insult (e.g., viral infection), fewer protective factors, or greater psychosocial stress. Increased familiarity has been observed in the earliest-onset cases of a variety of other diseases of multifactorial origin (Childs and Scriver, 1986), and in one study, male schizophrenics with onset before age 17 had an increased familial risk for schizophrenia compared with a later-onset group (Pulver et al., 1990), but this finding remains controversial, as the age of onset in schizophrenia is probably influenced by other genetic factors not closely related to disease liability (Kendler and Maclean, 1990).

Compared with adult-onset schizophrenics, these children might represent a more homogeneous patient group, and one less confounded by neuroleptic treatment, substance abuse, and chronic illness, and/or institutionalization. Study of early-onset schizophrenia, cases that "ought not to occur," may give unique insight into later-onset disease by revealing more salient environmental insults or neurobiological abnormalities. This review outlines the development of the current concept of childhood schizophrenia and addresses the most appropriate diagnostic and neurobiological questions in view of advances in neurobiological research on later-onset schizophrenia.

PHENOMENOLOGY AND DIAGNOSIS

Development of Current Concept

In 1908, De Sanctis described a group of young children with normal and abnormal premorbid development who either abruptly or insidiously exhibited catatonia, stereotypies, negativism, mannerisms, outbursts of anger, echolalia, and emotional blunting (De Sanctis, 1908). Some children experienced intellectual deterioration. De Sanctis (1908) considered a range of factors to be etiological including heredity, paternal alcoholism, infections or toxic diseases, "psychic trauma," and developmental factors. These heterogeneous conditions, which would now include autism, childhood-onset schizophrenia, and postencephalitic and deteriorating neurological disorders, were termed "dementia praecocissima" (Boyle, 1990).

The need for differentiating between organic dementia and early-onset schizophrenia was addressed by Heller, who defined a specific early-onset dementia that he termed "dementia infantalis," later to be known as Heller's syndrome (Heller, 1930). Kraepelin (1919) noted that in 3.5% of adult patients, signs of "psychic weakness" such as "mental disability" or "hebephrenia" had existed in childhood, suggesting that children developing schizophrenia early may appear retarded. Most of Kraepelin's patients, who had normal development until age 4 followed by personality change and stereotypies, would today be diagnosed as atypical pervasive developmental disorder.

Potter elaborated on the developmentally specific manifestations of schizophrenia (Potter, 1933), and emphasis on developmental stage at onset of illness remains a focal concern and source of confusion (Despert, 1938; Group for the Advancement of Psychiatry, 1966; Lutz, 1937). Potter distinguished these children from those who were mentally retarded and astutely pointed out in each case that the sensorium was clear, thus differentiating them from children with organic dementias.

Internationally, other subgroupings of psychotic children have been proposed, similar to *DSM-III-R* mood disorders. Various psychotic disorders also have been described which must be differentiated from normal perceptual experiences. These include "confusion or oneiroid syndromes" or "delusion syndromes" with no *DSM* counterpart that may represent childhood dissociative states (Leonhard, 1991; Stutte, 1969). Other more subtle subtypes of COS (Remschmidt, 1988) such as "later onset," "prepubertal schizophrenia" which have similarities to adult schizophrenia need further documentation. Leonhard (1991) described "early onset catatonia" as a specific childhood syndrome characterized by motor abnormalities, negativism, and speech abnormalities including mutism; however, the overlap between this syndrome and autism is unclear.

Differentiation from Autism

Kanner initially conceptualized his severely disturbed subgroup of children as having a form of schizophrenia but later described them as having a separate syndrome, "infantile autism" (Kanner, 1943). The important distinction between schizophrenia and autism was established by Kolvin (Kolvin et al., 1971a,b) and later by Rutter (1972), who found marked differences in symptom pattern, family history, perinatal events, and neurological deficits (Kolvin et al., 1971a,b).

Kolvin's study of 33 patients with a schizophrenic psychosis before they were 15 years old began the modern systematic approach to this group. Onset was most often after age 11, when the children were just entering puberty, but there were 13 children in whom the disorder began between age 7 and 11 years.

Preexisting abnormalities of personality or behavior and insidious onset were typical. Symptoms were similar to those in adults with thought blocking, delusions (typically of persecution), and hallucinations (typically auditory). Mannerisms and grimacing were common. One in 10 parents were schizophrenic, a percentage similar to that seen in adult patients.

The major difference between child and adult cases was the preponderance of male patients. Premorbid uneven development such as mild, transient speech delay was common. One third of the children showed some "soft" evidence of organic cerebral dysfunction, and delayed motor-milestones had intriguing resemblance to the nonpsychotic antecedents of later-onset psychosis (Murray et al., 1992a; Offord, 1974; Walker and Lewire, 1990).

Controversy over continuity between autism and schizophrenia is still sparked by occasional case reports documenting early autism with the emergence of schizophrenia in adolescence and young adulthood (Fish, 1977; Petty et al., 1984), but studies of larger samples of autistic children aged 15 years and older, found a 0.67% rate of schizophrenia, which is no higher than that expected in the general population (Volkmar and Cohen, 1991), arguing for the existing separation of the disorders.

More subtle research questions concerning the relationship between childhood schizophrenia and "spectrum" of pervasive developmental disorder (PDD) remain today; however, in one study 40% of prepubertal schizophrenics had prior autistic symptoms (Watkins et al., 1988) although this was not seen consistently (Russell et al., 1989), and differentiation at any age in the presence of normal intelligence from atypical PDD (not otherwise specified) may be arbitrary (Volkmar et al., 1988). Thus premorbid characteristics such as language difficulties, motor abnormalities, and social impairments should be correlated with biological measures.

Other childhood-onset psychiatric and developmental disorders are less likely to be mislabeled as *DSM-III-R/DSM-IV* schizophrenia. Social impairments, oddities of verbal and nonverbal communication, and peculiar fantasies are characteristic of children with Asperger's syndrome and schizotypal personality disorder (Kay and Kolvin, 1987; Rumsey et al., 1986; Szatmari et al., 1989). Major depression in childhood may be accompanied by hallucinations and delusions (Chambers et al., 1982) but these are more easily recognized. However, early bipolar disorders may be misdiagnosed (Kydd and Werry, 1982; Werry et al., 1991). Dissociative disorders may be initially misdiagnosed as psychotic disorders (McKenna, unpublished).

Differentiation from Neurological Disorder

The distinction between childhood-onset schizophrenia and degenerative neurological disorders is well established. "Organicity" was emphasized by Heller after finding cerebral deterioration in children believed to be schizophrenic (Heller, 1930); however, "Heller's syndrome" was discarded in 1969 as too heterogeneous. The lipoidoses, tuberous sclerosis, infantile spasms, subacute sclerosing panencephalitis, congenital syphilis, and metachromatic leukodystrophy all can cause childhood psychosis (Corbett et al., 1977; Davison and Bagley, 1969; Hyde et al., 1992; Malamud, 1959; Slater and Glithero, 1963). In early stages of neurological illness, incoherence, loosening of associations, inappropriate affect, and deterioration of functioning may mimic schizophrenia (Caplan et al., 1987). However, the presence of dementia as well as the severity and pervasiveness of the psychotic symptoms should suggest brain pathology even before the appearance of focal neurological signs (Corbett et al., 1977).

In contrast to the relatively clear status of degenerative neurological disorder, is the categorization of patients with *indirect* evidence of more subtle developmental difficulties, called here "multidimensionally impaired" ("MDI") (Gordon et al., in press; McKenna et al., 1994). Children with normal intelligence accompanied by multiple cognitive and language impairments who might meet *DSM-III-R* and *DSM-IV* criteria for schizophrenia are numerically most important and least characterized. Mood lability and social ineptness are present but social withdrawal is not. Most children also meet criteria for attention-deficit hyperactivity disorder. Such children may report fleeting hallucinations particularly under stress and may exhibit odd thinking, especially if a language disorder is present.

The question of whether this group represents an early stage of schizophrenia or bipolar disorder, "sub-clinical" seizure disorder, or dissociative disorder remains to be untangled (Mallenhaum and Russell, 1987; Lowenstein, 1991). These "MDI" children do not, however, resemble the pattern of the more subtle withdrawn or "unexpressive" prodrome described retrospectively for adult-onset schizophrenia (Klein and Klein, 1969; Offord, 1974; Walker and Lewire, 1990), nor do they meet criteria for schizotypal or borderline personality disorder.

Although this group may be a "miscellaneous category" for subjects not fitting any disorder, they may prove interesting in terms of magnetic resonance imaging (MRI) evidence for early brain injury or chromosomal abnormalities (McKenna, unpublished).

DSM-III-R, DSM-IV, and Childhood Schizophrenia

The *DSM* diagnostic system has fostered the most systematic studies of childhood schizophrenia to date which have essentially supported and extended Kolvin's (1971) work. *DSM-III-R* defined schizophrenic children can be reliably rated as having had hallucinations (in 83%) and delusions (in 54%) (Green et al., 1984, 1992). The presence of such symptoms does not vary with age, but their expression is predictably colored by developmental level (Russell et al., 1989). The positive symptom (type I)/negative symptom (type II) distinction postulated for schizophrenia (Andreasen and Olsen, 1982; Crowe, 1985) will probably not be useful for schizophrenic children, as most seem to have both symptoms (Green et al., 1992; Russell et al., 1989; Werry et al., 1991).

The application of *DSM-III-R* (or *DSM-IV*) criteria in the evaluation of disturbed children still needs improvement; e.g., standardized instruments must be adapted to developmental level. In the absence of delusions, a diagnosis of schizophrenia may be given because of overall "thought disordered" presentation not appropriate to developmental level (Russell et al., 1989). Children with serious social impairments may report a "voice" telling them "Don't go near those big kids," which is difficult to distinguish from an anxious thought.

The identification of thought disorder in the presence of developmental language disorders can be a major problem. The deemphasis on thought disorder in *DSM-IV* and focus on disorganized speech (frequent derailment or incoherence) rather than "loose association" of *DSM-III-R* does not solve this problem. Communication (i.e., language) disorder is common in psychiatrically disturbed children (Cantwell et al., 1979).

Because of the competing operational definitions of schizophrenia, with no clarity at this time as to which are most valid particularly for a pediatric sample, an "operationalized polydiagnostic approach" (e.g., Farmer et al., 1991) is needed. Diagnostic groupings will depend on the question being asked. For example, the concept of schizophrenia "spectrum" disorders will be important for family studies. Neurobiological abnormalities (e.g., brain imaging measures) may relate to dimensional rather than dichotomous measures. For this reason, symptoms of schizophrenia, "atypical" PDD, "organic brain syndromes," and motor and cognitive impairments should be measured in both dimensional (e.g., *DSM-IV*, ICD-10) and dichotomous fashion for examination in relation to neurobiological measures discussed below.

NEUROBIOLOGY

Advances in the neurobiological correlates of schizophrenia should stimulate studies of child populations to address questions of etiology, continuity between child and adult disorders, treatment, etc. The following sections summarize those questions most timely for psychotic children. Two questions that run through these sections are whether a "novel" neurobiological mechanism will be found for COS that might shed light on the later-onset disorder such as chromosomal abnormalities or brain lesions that may provide "premature" forms of later-onset disorder. A second question is whether subgrouping by prodrome, phenomenology, comorbidity, or prognosis will be validated by biological studies.

Prepubertal Status

An overarching concept for COS research will be the neurobiological basis for the early onset of psychosis. Prepubertal status must be systematically determined using endocrine and physical measures so that neurobiological measures are examined in relation to puberty and to chronological age. For example, evidence of premature pubertal processes would be of particular importance for theories of pubertal biological trigger mechanism in schizophrenia. For this reason, Tanner staging, serum, follicle-stimulating hormones, luteinizing hormones, growth curves, and other data to pinpoint adrenarche must be obtained in early onset cases.

Genetics

Children with early-onset schizophrenia may come from families with greater prevalence of the disorder and therefore family pedigrees for psychiatric disorders must be completed. However, individual case studies of chromosomal abnormalities have been important for later linkage studies in several genetically based pediatric diseases (Orkin, 1986), and early cases should also have chromosomal analysis. The clinical history of pre- and perinatal events, minor physical anomalies, and dermatoglyphics will also be important in patient evaluation, particularly for males (Murray et al., 1992a). Moreover, self-selected research subjects, who often come from better-functioning (less genetically impaired) families, may be more likely to have had prenatal insult and/or chromosomal mutations.

Physiology: Eye-Tracking and Autonomic Responsivity

Smooth pursuit eye-tracking impairment in adult schizophrenics and their first-degree relatives appears to be trait related (i.e., a measure of susceptibility not presence of disorder), occurring in 50% to 85% of patients, compared to 8% of normals (Holzman, 1987, 1989; Holzman et al., 1974; Iacono and Koening, 1983; Siever et al., 1990). Eye-tracking abnormalities have been reported in adolescents at risk for schizophrenia (offspring of a schizophrenic parent) and study of children as young as 4 years old is feasible (Kowler and Martins, 1982; Pavlidus, 1980). The developmental sequence for smooth pursuit tracking abilities, as demonstrated on infrared oculography, parallels neurointegrative, especially frontal lobe, development. Fixation reaches an adult pattern by age 7, although saccadic latency for visually guided saccades develops up to age 14. Smooth pursuit gain (eye velocity relative to target velocity) is also comparable to that seen in adults by age 14 (Ross et al., 1993).

Studies of eye-tracking patterns in children with schizophrenia represent one way to assess continuity between childhood and later-onset schizophrenia. Although some eye movement abnormalities are diagnostically nonspecific, smooth pursuit abnormalities, particularly anticipatory saccades during smooth pursuit eye movements, are believed specific for vulnerability to schizophrenia. Specificity for childhood-onset schizophrenia would support the distinction from other severe childhood disorders discussed in previous sections.

The study of autonomic physiology has been of interest with adult schizophrenics who show unusually high resting arousal rates, slow adaptation, and attenuated autonomic reactivity to significant stimuli and situations (Zahn, 1988). Preliminary data indicate that childhood-onset schizophrenics show a similar pattern to that of adult schizophrenics, and a dissimilar pattern from that seen with other severely impaired obsessive-compulsive, hyperactive, and conduct-disordered groups (Gordon et al., in press).

Neuropsychology

Deficits of controlled, attentional processing have been reported in schizophrenic children (Asarnow and Sherman, 1984; Erwin et al., 1986) and could underlie illogical thinking and loose associations. Schizophrenic children are impaired in their ability to process visual information (Asarnow and Sherman, 1984; Erwin et al., 1986), regulate attention, and discriminate target stimuli (Asarnow et al., 1986); the inattention generally precedes psychosis. Auditory processing impairments might also account for some behavioral manifestations of childhood schizophrenia (Sherman and Asarnow, 1985).

Frontal lobe dysfunction, implicated in schizophrenic adults (Cohen et al., 1987; Goldberg and Weinberger, 1988; Weinberger et al., 1986) but not systematically assessed in schizophrenic children, is of interest in relation to ongoing frontal myelination during childhood and adolescence, and addresses continuity with adult schizophrenia. Pediatric instruments to assess frontal lobe functioning in children are now available (Welsh and Pennington, 1988), and neuropsychological and physiological measures may be studied in relation to various biological markers of frontal lobe function (such as smooth pursuit eye movements), as well as to neuroanatomic and functional brain imaging. In a recent position emission tomography (PET) study of 11 unmedicated childhood-onset schizophrenics attention deficits on the Continuous Performance Test may have accounted for striking right posterior parietal hypometabolism seen with PET (Gordon et al., in press).

Neuroanatomic and Functional Imaging

Brain development has become a central focus of schizophrenia research (Murray et al., 1992a; Weinberger, 1987). Normal excess production of neurons, synapses, and dendritic spines early in development and synaptic pruning and programmed cell death occur throughout childhood and adolescence paralleling age-related changes in cerebral glucose metabolism. Increases in cerebral glucose metabolism are seen until age 3 or 4 and are maintained until age 9, followed by a decline to adult levels by late adolescence, a time concurrent with usual onset of psychosis (Chugani et al., 1987; Feinberg et al., 1990).

The proliferation and migration of neurons, followed by neuronal cell death, provides a complex sequence for hypothetical environmental, developmental, and genetic models of childhood-onset schizophrenia. Particularly relevant may be the specialized temporary junctions that allow the cell to keep in contact with guiding fibers, and nerve cells adhesion molecules that assist in the process during migration as possible processes that might be aberrant (Feinberg, 1982; Murray et al., 1992b; Weinberger, 1987). The report of a transmissible growth-promoting agent in the CSF of drug-free schizophrenics suggests studies that might support an hypothesis of abnormal reinnervation after injury in patients with schizophrenia particularly in limbic projection sites (Steven, 1992).

Hypothetically, early injury, infection, or abnormality of development in the brain can cause anomalous sprouting and synaptic reorganization in projection sites, the extent of which depends on the nature and site of the initial injury or dystrophy and on genetic and hormonal factors regulating tissue growth and repair (Stevens, 1992). Gonadal and adrenal hormones, for example, are known to be potent neurotrophic substances (Gorski, 1985) and may be implicated in mediating the pubertal onset of psychotic symptoms. Neuroimaging (MRI) comparisons of pre- and postpubertal onset cases can address these postulated relationships.

Such neurodevelopmental models have obvious relevance for childhood schizophrenia (Weinberger, 1987). If continuous with the adult disorder, childhood-onset schizophrenia is due to the same fixed "lesion," in interaction with a combination of genetic or nongenetic factors such as early viral CNS infection, autoimmune mechanisms, or pregnancy/birth complication that would lead to biological maldevelopment. Psychotic symptoms might then be expressed earlier if the developmental processes outlined above occurred earlier (Feinberg, 1982; Murray et al., 1992b; Stevens, 1992; Turner et al., 1986), whereas premorbid symptoms such as language deficit, poor motor skills, or social withdrawal would be similar to those noted in many adult-onset cases (Feinberg, 1982).

MRI has revolutionized the study of normal and pathological human brain development. New quantification techniques enable measurement of relative gray and white matter and, by inference, myelination, as well as cortical and subcortical volumes. Therefore more specific neuroanatomical hypotheses can be tested. Adult schizophrenics have been reported to show enlarged cerebral ventricles (Andreason et al., 1990; Kelsoe et al., 1988; Suddath et al., 1989), reduced medial temporal lobe hippocampal amygdala volume (Barta et al., 1990; Dauphinais et al., 1990; Suddath et al., 1989), and smaller superior temporal gyral volume (Barta et al., 1990). Abnormalities in limbic structures and in the corpus callosum (which develops embryologically in association with limbic structures) (Nasrallah et al., 1986; Stratta et al., 1989; Suddath et al., 1990; Swayze et al., 1990) all suggest a neurodevelopmental basis. In adult schizophrenics, brain imaging abnormalities are more marked in men (Castle and Murray, 1991) and those patients with poor childhood adjustment (Murray et al., 1992b), suggesting that MRI studies in COS will target a population with identifiable quantitative differences.

Neuroanatomical imaging studies have reported a variety of brain abnormalities in several severe childhood psychiatric disorders such as autism (Bauman and Kemper, 1985; Courchesne et al., 1988; Gaffney et al., 1987; Murakami et al., 1989; Ritvo et al., 1986). Within a sample of children with various psychiatric disturbances, a subgroup with "schizophrenia" had enlarged left ventricular horns (Hendren et al., 1991).

As noted, schizophrenia-like symptoms occur in a variety of pediatric brain disorders (Corbett et al., 1977; Hyde et al., 1992; Rutter, 1977; Slater and Glithero, 1963; Wilcox and Nasrallah, 1987), but childhood-onset schizophrenics (like their adult counterparts) will usually not exhibit diagnosable neuropathology (Hendren et al., 1991). Because of the hypothesized greater likelihood of developmental brain lesions and abnormality in COS, virtually all these brain areas should be examined to see how quantitative abnormalities evolve, and how these relate to puberty and to symptom development, an approach made feasible by MRI (Holland et al., 1986).

Functional imaging such as PET, single photon emission computerized tomography, and potentially, spectral and dynamic MRI, will complement MRI and neuropathological investigations. A limited use of PET in children with low-dose radiation and modified technique has gained approval for some pediatric studies (Gordon et al., in press), although functional MRI technology will soon obviate this issue.

Although PET studies in autistic adults have failed to show localized abnormalities (Herold et al., 1988; Rumsey et al., 1985), the correlational patterns of glucose utilization among various brain areas showed abnormalities consistent with mesolimbic dysfunction (Horwitz et al., 1988) which is hypothesized to occur in schizophrenia (Weinberger, 1987).

A single cerebral blood flow study in schizophrenic adolescents (Chabral et al., 1986) has, similar to PET studies in adult schizophrenics, demonstrated diminished activity of the dorsolateral prefrontal cortex (Berman et al., 1986; Goldberg and Weinberger, 1988; Weinberger et al., 1986; Weinberger et al., 1988). An ongoing PET study in childhood-onset schizophrenia at the National Institute of Mental Health to date has not shown this pattern (Gordon et al., in press).

Neurochemistry

There are no neurochemical studies of *DSM-III-R*-diagnosed schizophrenic children. In adult patients, lower CSF and higher plasma levels of homovanillic acid (HVA) are associated with positive symptoms, and there is a fall in plasma HVA with improvement in psychosis ratings (Bowers et al., 1984; Picker et al., 1986) consistent with decreased frontal cortical dopamine release and/or metabolism coupled with increased subcortical activity (Pickar et al., 1986, 1990). The latter was not observed in a single unpublished study of haloperidol treatment of COS (Spencer, K., personal communication).

CSF studies in pediatric psychiatric patients (Kruesi et al., 1988, 1990), carried out with the cooperation of children as young as 6 years without undue distress or untoward effects, may be important for the study of childhood psychoses.

Lower baseline levels of CSF HVA have been associated with cortical atrophy in adult schizophrenia (Van Kammen et al., 1986) and should be examined in relation to the "secondary" psychoses in childhood. Serotonin challenge studies in which the release of hormones under the control of the 5-HT system (cortisol, prolactin, and growth hormone) are studied after stimulation with 5-HT agonist or antagonists have been inconsistent in adult schizophrenics. However, because hyperserotonemia is well established in a subgroup of 25% to 35% of autistic children (Hanley et al., 1977) as well as in retarded populations (Stahl, 1977) and may be present in a subgroup of adult schizophrenics (Bieich et al., 1988), the subject deserves re-examination in childhood-onset schizophrenia in relation to measures of "autistic spectrum" pathology.

A "high 5-HT" subgroup of childhood-onset schizophrenics, if identified, might represent an autism-related subgroup with an earlier onset and atypical childhood history, continuous with negative symptom-type later-onset schizophrenia.

DRUG TREATMENT

The first controlled study of the efficacy of treatment with neuroleptics in schizophrenic children is only now in progress. Earlier single-blind, double-blind, and placebo-controlled neuroleptic trials in schizophrenic adolescents have shown modest superiority of neuroleptics (Pool et al., 1976; Realmuto et al., 1984). In an ongoing study (Spencer, 1991) 19 schizophrenic children, aged 5 to 11 years, have demonstrated consistent improvement with haloperidol, using doses from 0.5 to 3.5 mg/day (average 0.02 to 0.12 mg/kg per day).

It is unlikely, however, that neuroleptic response will define a diagnostic entity, because antipsychotic drugs are effective for several pediatric neuropsychiatric conditions including infantile autism (Faretra et al., 1970; LeVann, 1969; Pool et al., 1976; Realmuto et al., 1984), pervasive developmental disorder (Joshi et al., 1988), motor stereotypies in mental retardation (Joshi et al., 1988), and Tourette's syndrome (Feinberg and Carroll, 1979; Bruun, 1984) usually at doses less than that used in adult schizophrenics. Very low doses of haloperidol are also beneficial for attention-deficit hyperactivity disorder (Werry, 1988). Thus the efficacy of dopamine-blocking agents will be difficult to interpret because of the very broad usefulness of these agents in child psychiatry.

Pharmacokinetic studies of haloperidol and other neuroleptics in prepubertal psychotic children can address possible pharmacokinetic differential response to neuroleptics between adults and children (Morselli et al., 1982, 1983).

Clozapine, a dibenzodiazepine, is an "atypical" anti-psychotic compound possessing antipsychotic properties with limited extrapyramidal side effects (Baldessarini and Frankenburg, 1991; Kane et al., 1988). Although there is a risk of agranulocytosis with clozapine that varies from 0.47 to 134 cases/1000 (phenothiazine rates vary from 0.004 to 7/1000) (Lieberman et al., 1989), careful monitoring allows safe use. Recent open studies of schizophrenic adolescents considered unresponsive to or intolerant of typical neuroleptics found 75% of the subjects improved and tolerated the medication well with improvement in both positive and negative symptoms (Birmaher et al., 1992; Remschmidt, 1991; Siefen and Remschmidt, 1986). A controlled study of clozapine in the treatment of childhood-onset schizophrenia is under way at the National Institute of Mental Health with preliminary encouraging results. If abnormalities in the serotonin system are associated with negative symptoms, clozapine may be particularly helpful with these symptoms in children with negative symptoms given its 5-HT- 2 receptor blockade (Bieich et al., 1988). The newer generation of atypical antipsychotics such as risperidone will avoid the hematological problems of clozapine and may find a place in the treatment of childhood disorders owing to their combined serotonergic and dopaminergic effects.

SUMMARY AND FUTURE DIRECTIONS

The study of childhood-onset schizophrenia is only beginning but clinical and biological observations already provide testable hypotheses. Equally important, the treatment of patients with early-onset schizophrenia and other severely impaired children has been unsatisfactory and the understanding of this severely disturbed population of children remains critical.

The diagnosis of schizophrenia is currently being applied too broadly (Gordon et al., in press). Other childhood disorders may exhibit psychotic symptoms but lack the personality deterioration, thought disorder, avolition, disorganization, and extreme social withdrawal that is usual in schizophrenic children (at least as we understand them). These children also do not resemble the more subtle nonpsychotic prodrome described for later-onset schizophrenia (Walker and Lewire, 1990).

The task of validating a childhood version of a probably heterogenous and poorly understood adult disease may seem overwhelming. However, the combined phenomenological and neurobiological approach that we have outlined can address several issues simultaneously.

Relevant psychiatric contrast groups, particularly the "multidimensionally impaired," or "multiple complex developmental disorder" (Tobin et al., 1993) child, atypical PDD, and attention-deficit hyperactivity disorder groups should be studied in addition to normal controls. By using several interlocking diagnostic paradigms, and taking into account measures of other behaviors (including thought disorder, autistic behaviors, language skills, and attention disorders), using dimensional and dichotomous approaches to diagnosis, a clinical data base can be related to the neurobiological measures or pharmacological response.

A narrowly defined group of schizophrenic children is expected to show continuity on biological measures with later-onset disorder and/or to provide instructive phenocopies. It is likely that many children currently diagnosed as "psychotic" will not be continuous with later-onset schizophrenia, although drug treatment studies are likely to classify a broad array of childhood symptoms as responsive. These studies will help meet the needs of a severely ill population and complement the broader field of research.

REFERENCES

Andreasen NC, Olsen S (1982), Negative vs. positive schizophrenia. *Arch Gen Psychiatry* 39:789–794

Andreason N, Erhhardt JC, Swazye VW, et al. (1990), Magnetic resonance imaging of the brain in schizophrenia. *Arch Gen Psychiatry* 47:35–44

Asarnow RF, Sherman T (1984), Studies of visual information processing in schizophrenic children. *Child Dev* 55:249–261

Asarnow RF, Sherman T, Strandburg R (1986), The search for the psychobiological substrate of childhood onset schizophrenia. *JAACAP* 25:601–604

Baldessarini RJ, Frankenburg FR (1991), Clozapine: a novel antipsychotic agent. *N Engl J Med* 324:746–754

Barta PE, Pearlson GD, Powers RE, Richards SS, Tune LE (1990), Auditory hallucinations and smaller superior temporal gyral volume in schizophrenia. *Am J Psychiatry* 147:1457–1462

Bauman M, Kemper TL (1985), Histoanatomic observations of the brain in early infantile autism. *Neurology* 35:866–874

Beitchman JH (1985), Childhood schizophrenia: a review and comparison with adult-onset schizophrenia. *Psychiatr Clin North Am* 8:793–814

Berman KF, Zec FC, Weinberger DR (1986), Physiological dysfunction of dorsolateral prefrontal cortex in schizophrenia II. Role of medication, attention, and mental effort. *Arch Gen Psychiatry* 43:126–143

Bieich A, Brown SL, Kahn R, Van Praag HM (1988), The role of serotonin in schizophrenia. *Schizophr Bull* 14:297–315

Birmaher B, Baker B, Kapur S, Quintana H, Ganguli R (1992), Clozapine for the treatment of adolescents with schizophrenia. *JAACAP* 31:160–164

Bleuler E (1911), *Dementia Praecox or the Group of Schizophrenias.* Translated by J. Zinkin. New York: International Universities, 1950

Bowers MB, Swigar M, Jatlow PI, Goicoechea N (1984), Plasma catecholamine metabolites and early response to haloperidol. *J Clin Psychiatry* 45:248–251

Boyle M (1990), Is schizophrenia what it was? A reanalysis of Kraepelin's and Bleuler's population. *J Hist Behav Sci* 26:323–333

Bruun RD (1984), Gilles de la Tourette's syndrome. An overview of clinical experience. *J Am Acad Child Psychiatry* 23:126–133

Cantor S, Evans J, Pearce J, Pezzot-Pearce T (1982), Childhood schizophrenia: present but not accounted for. *Am J Psychiatry* 139:758–762

Cantwell D, Baker L, Mattison R (1979), The prevalence of psychiatric disorder in children with speech and language disorder: an epidemiologic study. *JAACAP* 18:450–461

Caplan R, Tonguay P, Szekely A (1987), SSPE presenting as childhood psychosis. *JAACAP* 26:440–443

Castle D, Murray R (1991), The neurodevelopmental basis of sex differences in schizophrenia. *Psychol Med* 21:565–575

Chabral H, Guell A, Bes A, Moron P (1986), Cerebral blood flow in schizophrenic adolescents. *Am J Psychiatry* 143:130

Chambers WJ, Puig-Antich J, Tabrizi MA, Davis M (1982), Psychotic symptoms in prepubertal major depressive disorder. *Arch Gen Psychiatry* 39:921–927

Childs B, Scriver C (1986), Age at onset and causes of disease. *Perspect Biol Med* 29:437–460

Chugani H, Phelps M, Mazziotta J (1987), Positron emission tomography study of human brain functional development. *Ann Neurol* 22:487–497

Cohen RM, Semple WE, Gross M, et al. (1987), Dysfunction in a prefrontal substrate of sustained attention in schizophrenia. *Life Sci* 40:2031–2039

Corbett J, Harris R, Taylor E, Trimble M (1977), Progressive disintegrative psychosis of childhood. *J Child Psychol Psychiat* 18:211–219

Courchesne E, Yeung-Courchesne R, Press GA (1988), Hypoplasia of cerebellar vermal lobules VI and VII in autism. *N Engl J Med* 318:1349–1354

Crowe TJ (1985). The two-syndrome concept: origins and current status. *Schizophrenia Bull* 11:471–485

Dauphinais D, DeLisi LE, Crow TJ, et al. (1990), Reduction in temporal lobe size in siblings with schizophrenia: a magnetic resonance imaging study. *Psychiatry Res* 35:137–147

Davison K, Bagley C (1969), Schizophrenia-like psychoses associated with organic disorders of central nervous system. In: *Current Problems in Neuropsychiatry*, Herrington RN, ed

De Sanctis S (1908), Dementia praecocissima catatonica. *Folio Neurobiol* 2:9–12

Despert L (1938), Schizophrenia in children. *Psychiatr Q* 12:366–371

Erwin RJ, Edwards R, Tanguay PE, Buchwald J, Letai D (1986), Abnormal P300 responses in schizophrenic children. *JAACAP* 25:615–622

Faretra G, Dooher L, Dowling J (1970), Comparison of haloperidol and fluphenazine in disturbed children. *Am J Psychiatry* 126:1670–1673

Farmer A, McGuffin P, Harvey I, Williams M (1991), Schizophrenia: How far can we go in defining the phenotype? In: *The New Genetics of Mental Illness*, McGuffin P, Murray R, eds. Oxford: Butterworth-Heinmon

Feinberg I (1982), Schizophrenia: caused by a fault in programmed synaptic elimination during adolescence? *J Psychiatr Res* 17:319–334

Feinberg I, Thode H, Chugani H, March JD (1990), Gamma distribution model describes the maturational curves for delta wave amplitude. Cortical metabolic rate and synaptic density. *J Theor Biol* 142:149–161

Feinberg M, Carroll J (1979), Effects of dopamine agonists and antagonists in Tourette's disease. *Arch Gen Psychiatry* 36:979–985

Fish B (1977), Neurobiological antecedents of schizophrenia in children: evidence for an inherited, congenital neurointegrative defect. *Arch Gen Psychiatry* 34:1297–1313

Gaffney GR, Tsai LY, Kuperman S, Minchin S (1987), Cerebellar structure in autism. *J Autism Dev Disord* 141:1330–1332

Goldberg TE, Weinberger DR (1988), Probing prefrontal function in schizophrenia with neuropsychological paradigms. *Schizophr Bull* 14:179–183

Gordon CT, Casanova M, Zametkin A, Zahn T, Hong W, Rapoport JL (in press), Childhood onset schizophrenia: neurobiological characterization and pharmacologic response: NIMH studies in progress. *Schizophr Bull*

Gorski RA (1985), Gonadal hormones as putative neurotrophic substances. In: *Synaptic Plasticity*, Cotman C, ed. New York: Guilford Press

Green W, Padron-Gayol M, Hardesty A, Bassiri M (1992), Schizophrenia with childhood onset: a phenomenological study of 38 cases. *JAACAP* 31:968–976

Green WH, Campbell M, Hardesty AS et al. (1984), A comparison of schizophrenic and autistic children. *JAACAP* 23:399–409

Group for the Advancement of Psychiatry (1966), Psychopathological disorders in children: theoretic considerations and a proposed classification

Hanley HG, Stahl SM, Freedman DX (1977), Hyperserotonemia and amine metabolites in autistic and retarded children. *Arch Gen Psychiatry* 34:521–523

Heller T (1930), About dementia infantilis. *Zeitschrift Kinderfarsch* 37:661–669

Hendren R, Hodde-Vargas J, Vargas L, Orrison WW, Del L (1991), Magnetic resonance imaging of severely disturbed children—a preliminary study. *JAACAP* 30:466–470

Herold S, Frackowiak RSJ, Lecouter AP, Rutter M, Howlin P (1988), Cerebral blood flow and metabolism of oxygen and glucose in young autistic adults. *Psychol Med* 18:823–831

Holland BA, Haas DK, Norman D, Brant-Zawadzki M, Newton TH (1986), MRI of normal brain maturation. *Am J Neurol Radiol* Mar/April 201–208

Holzman PS (1987), Recent studies of psychophysiology in schizophrenia. *Schizophr Bull* 13:49–75

Holzman PS (1989) The use of eye movement dysfunction in exploring the genetic transmission of schizophrenia. *Eur Arch Psychiatry Neurol Sci* 239:43–48

Holzman PS, Proctor LR, Levy DL, Yasillo NJ, Meltzer MY, Hurt SW (1974), Eye tracking dysfunction in schizophrenic patients and their relatives. *Arch Gen Psychiatry* 31:143–151

Horwitz B, Rumsey JM, Grady CL, Rapoport JL (1988), The cerebral metabolic landscape in autism: Intercorrelations of regional glucose utilization. *Arch Neurol* 45:749–755

Hyde T, Ziegler J, Weinberger D (1992), Psychiatric disturbances in metachromatic leukodystrophy: insights into the neurobiology of psychosis. *Arch Neurol* 49:401–406

Iacono WG, Koening WGR (1983), Features that distinguish the smooth-pursuit eye-tracking performance of schizophrenic, affective-disorder, and normal individuals. *J Abnorm Psychol* 92:29–41

Joshi PT, Capozzoli JA, Coyle JT (1988), Low-dose neuroleptic therapy for children with childhood-onset pervasive developmental disorder. *Am J Psychiatry* 145:335–338

Kane J, Honigfeld G, Singer J, Meltzer H (1988), Clozapine for the treatment—resistant schizophrenic. *Arch Gen Psychiatry* 45:789–796

Kanner L (1943), Autistic disturbances of affective contact. *Nervous Child* 2:217–250

Kay P, Kolvin I (1987), Childhood psychoses and their borderlands. *Br Med Bull* 43:570–586

Kelsoe JR, Cadet JL, Pickar D, Weinberger DR (1988), Quantitative neuroanatomy in schizophrenia. *Arch Gen Psychiatry* 45:533–541

Kendler KS, Maclean CJ (1990), Estimating familial effects on age at onset and liability to schizophrenia. 1. Results of a large sample family study. *Genet Epidemiol* 7:409–417

Klein DF, Klein RG (1969), Premorbid asocial adjustment and prognosis. *J Psychiatr Res* 7:35–53

Kolvin I, Ounsted C, Humphrey M, McNay A (1971a), The phenomenology of childhood psychosis. *Br J Psychiatry* 118:385–395

Kolvin I, Ounsted C, Roth M (1971b), Cerebral dysfunction and childhood psychoses. *Br J Psychiatry* 118:407–414

Kowler E, Martins AJ (1982), Eye movements of preschool children. *Science* 215:997–999

Kraepelin E, *Dementia Praecox and Paraphrenia.* Translated by R. Barclay, ed. Edinburgh: S. Livingstone, 1919

Kruesi MJP, Rapoport JL, Hamburger S et al. (1990), Cerebrospinal fluid monoamine metabolites, aggression and impulsivity in disruptive behavior disorders of children and adolescents. *Arch Gen Psychiatry* 47:419–426

Kruesi MJP, Swedo SE, Coffey ML, Hamburger SD, Leonard H, Rapoport JL (1988), Objective and subjective side effects of research lumbar punctures in children and adolescents. *Psychiatry Res* 25:59–63

Kydd RR, Werry JS (1992), Schizophrenia in children under 16 years. *J Autism Dev Disord* 12:343–357

Leonhard K. *Classification of Endogenous Psychoses.* New York: Irvington, 1991

LeVann LJ (1969), Haloperidol in the treatment of behavioral disorders in children and adolescents. *Can Psychiatric Assoc J* 14:217–220

Lieberman JA, Kane JM, Johns CA (1989), Clozapine: guidelines for clinical management. *J Clin Psychiatry* 50:329–338

Lowenstein R (1991), An office mental status examination for complex chronic dissociation symptoms and multiple personality disorder. *Psychiatr Clin North Am* 14:567–604

Lutz (1937), Uber Schizophrenia im Kindersalter. *Schweiz Arch Neurol Neurocher Psychiatr* 39:335–372

Malamud N (1959), Heller's disease and childhood schizophrenia. *Am J Psychiatry* 116:215–218

Mallenhaum R, Russell AT (1987), Multiple personality disorder in an 11 year old boy and his mother. *J Am Acad Child Adoles Psychiatry* 26:436–439

McKenna K, Gordon CT, Lenane M, Kaysen D, Rapoport JL (1994), Looking for childhood-onset schizophrenia: the first 71 cases screened. *J Am Acad Child Adolesc Psychiatry* 33:636–644

Morselli PL, Bianchetti G, Dugas M (1982), Haloperidol plasma level monitoring in neuropsychiatric patients. *Ther Drug Monit* 4:51–58

Morselli PL, Bianchetti G, Dugas M (1983), Therapeutic drug monitoring of psychotropic drugs in children. *Pediatr Pharmacol* 3:149–156

Murakami JW, Courchesne E, Press GA, Yeung-Courchesne R, Hesselink JR (1989), Reduced cerebellar hemisphere size and its relationship to vermal hypoplasia in autism. *Arch Neurol* 46:689–694

Murray R, Jones P, O'Callaghan E, Takei W, Sham P (1992a), Genes, virus and neurodevelopmental schizophrenia. *J Psychiatr Res* 26:225–236

Murray R, O'Callaghan E, Castle D, Lewis S (1992b), A neurodevelopmental approach to the classification of schizophrenia. *Schizophr Bull* 18:319–332

Nasrallah HA, Andreasen NC, Coffman JA, Olson SC, Dunn VD, Ehrhardt JC (1986), A controlled magnetic resonance imaging study of corpus callosum thickness in schizophrenia. *Biol Psychiatry* 21:274–282

Offord D (1974), School performance of adult schizophrenics their siblings and age mates. *Br J Psychiatry* 125:12–19

Orkin S (1986), Reverse genetics and human disease. *Cell* 47:845–850

Pavlidus GT (1980), Eye movements in reading and beyond. *Nurs Mirror* 150:22–26

Petty LK, Ornitz EM, Michelman JD, Zimmerman EG (1984), Autistic children who become schizophrenic. *Arch Gen Psychiatry* 41:129–135

Pickar D, Breier A, Hsaio JK (1990), Cerebrospinal fluid and plasma monoamine metabolites and their relation to psychosis. *Arch Gen Psychiatry* 47:641–648

Pickar D, Labarca R, Doran AR, Wolkowitz OM, Roy A, Breier A, Linnoila M (1986), Longitudinal measurement of plasma homovanillic acid levels in schizophrenic patients: Correlation with psychosis and response to neuroleptic treatment. *Arch Gen Psychiatry* 43:669–676

Pool D, Bloom W, Mielke D, Roniger JJ, Gallant DM (1976), A controlled evaluation of loxitane in seventy-five adolescent schizophrenic patients. *Curr Ther Res* 19:99–104

Potter HW (1933), Schizophrenia in children. *Am J Psychiatry* 12:1253–1270

Prior W, Werry JS (1986), Autism, schizophrenia and allied disorders. In: *Psychopathological Disorders of Childhood*, Quay H, Werry JS, eds. pp 156–210

Pulver A, Brown CH, Wolyniec P et al. (1990), Schizophrenia: age at onset, gender and familial risk. *Acta Psychiatr Scand* 82:344–351

Realmuto GM, Erickson WD, Yellin AM, Hopwood JH, Greenberg LM (1984), Clinical comparison of thiothixene and thioridazine in schizophrenic adolescents. *Am J Psychiatry* 141:440–442

Remschmidt H (1988), Schziophrene Psychosen in Kindersalter. In: *Psychiatrie der Genewart, Band 7, Kinder-und Jugenpsychiatrie*, Kisker KP, Lauter H, Meyer JE, Muller C, Stromgren E, eds

Remschmidt H. *Die behandlung schizophrener psychosen in der adoleszenz mit clozapin*. Vortrag auf dem Workshop Leponex-Pharmakologie und Klinik eines atypischen Neuroleptikums, Nurnberg: 1991

Ritvo ER, Freeman BJ, Scheibel AB et al. (1986), Lower purkinje cell counts in the cerebella of our autistic subjects: initial findings of the UCLA-NSAC autopsy research report. *Am J Psychiatry* 143:862–866

Ross RC, Radant A, Hommer D (1993), A developmental study of smooth pursuit eye movements in normal children from 7 to 15 years of age. *J Am Acad Child Adolesc Psychiatry* 32:783–791

Rumsey J, Andreason N, Rapoport JL (1986), Thought, language, communication, and affective flattening in autistic adults. *Arch Gen Psychiatry* 43:771–777

Rumsey J, Duara R, Grady C et al. (1985), Brain metabolism in autism: Resting cerebral glucose utilization as measured with positron emission tomography. *Arch Gen Psychiatry* 42:448–457

Russell AT, Bott L, Sammons C (1989), The phenomenology of schizophrenia occurring in childhood. *JAACAP* 28:399–407

Rutter M (1972), Childhood schizophrenia reconsidered. *J Autism Child Schiz* 2:315–337

Rutter M (1977), Brain damage syndromes in childhood: concepts and findings. *J Child Psychol Psychiat* 18:1–21

Sherman T, Asarnow RF (1985), The cognitive disabilities of the schizophrenic child. In: *Children with Emotional Disorders and Developmental Disabilities*. Sigman M, ed. Orlando, FL: Grune and Stratton

Siefen G, Remschmidt H (1986), Behandlungsegebnisse mit clozapin bei schizophrenen Jugendlichen. *Z Kinder Jugenpsychiatr* 14:245-257

Siever LJ, Keefe R, Bernstein DP et al. (1990), Eye tracking impairment in clinically identified patients with schizotypal personality disorder. *Am J Psychiatry* 147:740-745

Slater E, Glithero E (1963), The schizophrenia like psychoses of epilepsy. *Br J Psychiatry* 109:95-150

Spencer K (1991), Haloperidol in schizophrenic children. Poster presented at Annual Meeting of the American Academy of Child and Adolescent Psychiatry (abstract). San Francisco, CA, October 1991

Stahl S (1977), The human platelet: a diagnostic and research tool for the study of biogenic amines in psychiatric and neurologic disorders. *Arch Gen Psychiatry* 34:509-516

Stevens J (1992), Abnormal reinnervation as a bsis for schizophrenia: a hypothesis. *Arch Gen Psychiatry* 49:238-243

Stratta P, Rossi A, Gallucci M, Amicarelli I, Passariello R, Casacchia M (1989), Hemispheric asymmetries and schizophrenia: a preliminary magnetic resonance imaging study. *Biol Psychiatry* 25:275-284

Stutte H (1969), Psychosen des Kindersalters. In: *Neurologie-Psychologie-Psychiatrie.* Opritz H, Schmid F, eds. New York: Springer

Suddath RL, Casanova MF, Goldberg TE, Daniel DG, Kelsoe JR, Weinberger DR (1989), Temporal lobe pathology in schizophrenia: a quantitative magnetic resonance imaging study. *Am J Psychiatry* 146:464-472

Suddath RL, Christison GW, Torrey EF, Casanova MF, Weinberger DR (1990), Anatomical abnormalities in the brains of monozygotic twins discordant for schizophrenia. *N Engl J Med* 332:789-794

Swayze VW, Andreasen NC, Ehrhardt JC, Yuh WTC, Alliger RJ, Cohen GA (1990), Developmental abnormalities of the corpus callosum in schizophrenia. *Arch Neurol* 47:805-808

Szatmari P, Bremner R, Nagy J (1989), Asperger's syndrome: a review of clinical features. *Can J Psychiatry* 34:554-560

Towbin K, Dykens E, Pearson G, Cohen D (1993), Conceptualizing "borderline syndrome of childhood" and "childhood schizophrenia" as a developmental disorder. *J Am Acad Child Adolesc Psychiatry* 32:775-782

Turner S, Toone B, Brett-Jones J (1986), Computerized tomographic scan changes in early schizophrenia. Preliminary findings. *Psychol Med* 16:219-225

Van Kammen DP, Van Kammen WB, Mann LS, Seppala T, Linnoila M (1986), Dopamine metabolism in the cerebrospinal fluid of drug-free schizophrenic patients with and without cortical atrophy. *Arch Gen Psychiatry* 43:978-983

Volkmar F, Cohen D, Hoshino V, Rende R, Paul R (1988), Phenomenology and classification of the childhood psychoses. *Psycholog Med* 18:191-201

Volkmar FR, Cohen DJ (1991), Comorbid association of autism and schizophrenia. *Am J Psychiatry* 148:1705–1707

Walker E, Lewire R (1990), Prediction of adult-onset schizophrenia from childhood movies of the patients. *Am J Psychiatry* 147:1052–1056

Watkins J, Asarnow R, Tanguay P (1988), Symptom development in childhood onset schizophrenia. *J Child Psychol Psychiat* 29:865–878

Weinberger DR (1987), Implications of normal brain development for the pathogenesis of schizophrenia. *Arch Gen Psychiatry* 44:660–669

Weinberger DR, Berman KF, Illowsky BP (1988), Physiological dysfunction of dorsolateral prefrontal cortex in schizophrenia: a new cohort and evidence for a monoaminergic mechanism. *Arch Gen Psychiatry* 45:609–615

Weinberger DR, Berman KF, Zec RF (1986), Physiologic dysfunction of dorsolateral prefrontal cortex in schizophrenia: regional cerebral blood flow evidence. *Arch Gen Psychiatry* 43:114–124

Welsh M, Pennington B (1988), Assessing frontal lobe functioning in children: views from developmental psychology. *Dev Neuropsychology* 4:199–230

Werry J, McClellan J, Chard L (1991), Childhood and adolescent schizophrenia. Bipolar and schizoaffective disorder: A clinical outcome study. *JAACAP* 30:457–465

Werry JS (1988), Drugs, learning and cognitive functioning in children—an update. *J Child Psychol Psychiatry* 29:129–141

Wilcox JA, Nasrallah HA (1987), Perinatal distress and prognosis of psychotic illness. *Neuropsychology* 17:173–175

Zahn TP (1988), Studies of autonomic psychophysiology and attention in schizophrenia. *Schizophr Bull* 14:205–208

Part III

CLINICAL ISSUES

Whitehurst and Fischel begin the first paper (Chapter 9) of Part III, on clinical issues, with a brief vignette illustrative of a familiar parental concern. A parent of a two-year-old seeks evaluation for her child because she has become aware that, while other similarly aged children have large vocabularies and are beginning to combine words into sentences, her child is saying only a few single words. Are this parent's concerns an overreaction to normal developmental variation in the rate at which language develops in young children? Or does this child actually have a disorder? And if so, how should it be treated?

A systematic review of recent research on early language development provides the basis for the development of a carefully documented conceptual framework to guide clinicians in their resolution of these questions. The diagnosis of developmental language delay requires distinctions between specific and secondary delay at the broadest level, between expressive and receptive-expressive delay at the next level, and between problems of syntax, semantics, phonology, and pragmatics at the third level. Assessment instruments useful in making these distinctions are described and criteria for norm-based diagnoses are provided. Biologic correlates of specific language delay include gender, genetic factors, perinatal complications, motoric difficulties, and otitis media. While specific language delay is, in part, a function of biologic conditions, social-interactional factors including family size, socioeconomic status, and patterns of misbehavior and discipline appear to be additional risk factors. Family verbal interactions, while most probably not a root cause of specific language delay, can, however, play a role in the maintenance of delayed language.

Whether or not specific language delay is a disorder requiring treatment is a question of considerable practical as well as theoretical importance. The evidence summarized in this review suggests that children under the age of five with specific expressive language delay have relatively low risk of later language or reading impairments, with or without treatment. In contrast, children with secondary language delay and children with specific receptive-expressive delays that persist to the age of four are at risk of later problems. Very high rates of spontaneous resolution make research into the effectiveness of early intervention strategies difficult, and, in fact, studies of this issue are few in number. Nevertheless, interventions for categories of delay with high remission rates may be justifiable if the purchaser of the intervention understands that the goal of treatment is the improvement of current levels of functioning and the reduction of stress within the family. If the goal of treatment is the reduction of long-term risks of impairment, provision of treatment to children with secondary language delays and those with specific receptive-expressive delays that include difficulties with comprehension is indicated. The thinking behind these recommendations, summarized in a carefully constructed decision tree, is eminently sensible, and provides the reader with a framework within which to interpret and integrate results of developmental evaluations for concerned parents.

The magnitude of the problem of suicidality in children and adolescents is clearly established. During recent years a burgeoning of reports clearly documents the growing concern of both professionals and the general public. The frequency of occurrence of suicidal ideation and suicidal attempts among children undergoing psychiatric treatment is sufficiently high to ensure that many clinicians will be called upon to evaluate children who are suicidal. However, as Jacobsen, Rabinowitz, Popper, Solomon, Sokol, and Pfeffer point out in Chapter 10, literature on the assessment of suicidal children, primarily focused on the identification of risk factors, has provided little by way of practical guidance to clinicians about how to talk to children and their parents about suicidal thoughts and actions. These authors fill this gap by sharing their observations based on multiple semi-structured interviews directed toward identifying and characterizing previous and current suicidal ideation. Although the interviews were conducted during the course of an investigation of suicidality in children admitted to a child psychiatry inpatient unit, the distillation of experience is directly relevant to clinical encounters in a variety of different settings.

Interviewing children about suicidal ideation and behavior necessitates that the clinician attend to multiple elements of the interview simultaneously. Interviews may be further complicated by stressful thoughts and feelings that arise in both clinician and patient in reaction to exploring the child's suicidal ideation and behavior. Clinical vignettes effectively illustrate difficulties commonly faced in assessing suicidal intent within a developmental context as well as characteristics of play associated with suicidal states. The importance of interactions between current emotional state and recollection of previous suicidal episodes, the effects of parents' attitudes and the impact of risk factors on cognition and behavior during the interview are thoughtfully explored. Suicidal thoughts and behavior may occur in children of different developmental levels who present with different constellations of risk factors. The examples of specific questions designed to facilitate the process of eliciting detailed descriptions of events and the emotions and cognitions associated with them serve to guide the clinician through this demanding and complex task. Although the authors stress the unique features of evaluating suicidality in children, the underlying principle that accurate assessment is dependent upon unambiguous descriptions of thoughts, feelings, and behavior elicited in a developmentally appropriate context is clearly generalizable across clinical situations.

The analysis of trajectories to delineate developmental patterns is of particular value in identifying the correlates of both continuities and discontinuities in the development of psychopathology. In Chapter 11, Graber, Brooks-Gunn, Paikoff, and Warren utilize this technique to examine the longitudinal course of eating behavior and attitudes in a community-based sample of 116 white upper-middle-class girls followed from young adolescence through young adulthood. The sample was studied initially when they were in the 7th, 8th, or 9th grade (Time 1), again two years later in the 9th, 10th, and 11th grades (Time 2), and finally when they were between the ages of 21 and 23 years of age (Time 3). Time 1 and Time 2 scores obtained on the EAT-26, a measure utilizing a 6-point Likert-type scale to assess dieting behaviors, bulimic behaviors, self-control of eating, and perceived social pressure, provided the basis for establishing four risk trajectories. Girls (60.3%) were considered to be at low risk for having or developing a serious eating problem. Their scores at both Time 1 and Time 2 were below a pre-established cutoff. Girls (14.7%) with chronic eating problems had scores above the cutoff at both times. The early-transient-risk group was composed of girls (12.1%) who had scores above the cutoff at Time 1 and below the cutoff at Time 2, while girls (12.9%) in the late-transient-risk group displayed the reverse pattern. The following correlates of eating problems were examined: attitudes toward eating, physical development, personality, psychopathology, and family relationships.

Results indicated that girls on the chronic-risk trajectory were distinguishable from those in the other three groups for the entire course of the study. They entered puberty earlier, had higher rates of body fat, poorer body image, and were more likely to exhibit comorbid symptoms of depression. Although generalizability of the results to girls from other ethnic and socioeconomic backgrounds is limited, as the authors point out, the identification of risk groups constitutes a first step in the development of prevention and intervention programs to offset the health and mental health risks of disturbed eating behavior. The rates and timing of the onset of eating problems found in the present study justify the development of primary prevention programs for all girls in early adolescence. In addition, secondary prevention should be targeted to "at-risk" adolescents such as early-maturing girls with higher percentages of body fat. Moreover, the identification of trajectories and their correlates are of value to clinicians in evaluating the significance of disturbances in eating behavior in individual patients.

The prevalence of narcolepsy, a neurologic disorder with core symptoms of sleepiness, cataplexy, hypnagogic hallucinations, and sleep paralysis is estimated as between 4–10 per 10,000 individuals in the United States. Although the diagnosis is not commonly made until adulthood, symptoms in most cases are first noted during adolescence or perhaps even earlier. As Dahl, Holttum, and Trubnick (Chapter 12) point out in their review of 16 consecutive cases of polysomnographically proven narcolepsy with onset by 13 years of age, the symptoms of this disorder can easily mimic psychiatric disorders in children and adolescents. Whereas excessive sleepiness was noted in all cases, only one of the 16 patients in this series presented with the classic tetrad of symptoms. Behavioral and emotional disturbances were prominent features of the clinical picture in 12 cases, and 4 patients had been diagnosed with psychiatric disorders including conversion disorder and psychotic depression, before laboratory examination confirmed the presence of narcolepsy. Clinical vignettes vividly illustrate these common diagnostic dilemmas. This detailed and thoughtful summary of clinical observations serves to heighten awareness of the features of narcolepsy as it presents in children and adolescents, and underscores the importance of considering narcolepsy with excessive sleepiness.

The final paper in Part III provides a unique perspective on a problem of considerable clinical as well as social concern. In "Urban Poverty and the Family Context of Delinquency: A New Look at Structure and Process in a Classic Study" (Chapter 13), Sampson and Laub reanalyze data from the Gluecks' historic investigation of 500 delinquents and 500 nondelinquents, born between 1934 and 1935 and raised in the low-income neighborhoods of central Boston. While the Gluecks sought to determine what factors differentiated boys raised in similar poor neighborhoods who became serious and persistent delinquents from boys raised in the same neighborhoods who did not become delinquent or significantly antisocial, Sampson and Laub have utilized the Gluecks' meticulously detailed data base to address the question: by what process does family poverty lead to delinquency within structurally disadvantaged urban environments? Contending that sociological explanations of delinquency tend to focus on the structural consequences of poverty and ignore the role of mediating family processes and behavioral predispositions, while developmental models in psychology tend to emphasize family processes and early antisocial behavior to the neglect of structural context and social disadvantage, the authors propose a model linking structure and process. Specifically they suggest that family poverty inhibits family processes of informal social control, which in turn increases the likelihood of juvenile delinquency.

The data base is clearly described, as are the steps in the analysis. Results show that erratic, threatening, and harsh discipline, inadequate supervision of young children, and impaired parent-child attachment—measures in this model of a construct designated as informal social control—mediate the effects of poverty and other structural factors on the emergence of delinquent behaviors. The mediating processes of informal social control continue to explain a large share of variance in adolescent delinquency, even when the possible confounding effects of difficult children and unstable parents are controlled. The authors raise the possibility that association between childhood and adolescent delinquency may be less of an indication of a latent antisocial trait than a developmental process whereby delinquent children systematically undermine effective strategies of family social control, in turn increasing the odds of later delinquency.

This report underscores the value and importance of data sets deriving from well designed and carefully conducted studies that can be brought to bear on new questions using statistical techniques not available to the original investigators. The findings deriving from this reanalysis of the Gluecks' data, when considered together with those of more recent investigations, add weight to the authors' conclusions that the fundamental causes of delinquency are consistent across time and rooted not in race but in generic family processes—such as supervision, attachment, and discipline—that are systematically influenced by family poverty and structural disadvantage.

9

Practitioner Review: Early Developmental Language Delay: What, If Anything, Should the Clinician Do About It?

Grover J. Whitehurst and Janet E. Fischel

State University of New York, Stony Brook

Early developmental language delay is characterized by slow development of language in preschoolers. The condition is frequent among two- and three-year-olds, causes concern among parents, and generates differences of opinion as to significance among informed professionals. Poorer long-term outcomes are much more likely if language delay persists until the later preschool years, and if the delay is not specific to language and/or includes problems in understanding. Specific language delay in the preschool period is better characterized as a risk factor than a disorder; most children with specific language delay recover to the normal range by five years of age.

INTRODUCTION

Does he hear? Does he understand what is said to him? If the answer to these questions are "yes", the child will talk when what he wishes to communicate cannot be transmitted adequately by means of gestures and pantomime. The parents must avoid pressuring the child to talk . . . (Knobloch & Pasamanick, 1974, p. 290).

Reprinted with permission from the *Journal of Child Psychology and Psychiatry*, 1994, Vol. 35, 613–648. Copyright © 1994 by the Association for Child Psychology and Psychiatry.

Portions of the research reported herein were supported by grants to authors Whitehurst and Fischel by the National Institute of Child Health and Human Development (HD19245), and to author Fischel by the National Institute of Mental Health (MH41603). Preparation of this manuscript was aided by a grant to the senior author from the Pew Charitable Trusts, and a grant to authors Whitehurst and Fischel by the U.S. Administration on Children and Families (90CD095701).

Talking is normal, and not talking is not. While this may seem obvious, too often a child with delayed speech is treated as if speech will begin when the child is ready. Few physicians, confronted by a boy who is old enough to walk but who is isn't would comfort the mother by saying "Well he'll walk when he is ready". . . . Speech and language . . . should occur within a certain range of time, and should not be dismissed as if the child will simply begin talking when ready. (Blager, 1981, pp. 81–82).

A parent brings her two-year-old to a clinician. She has noticed that other two-year-olds have large vocabularies and are putting words together into sentences, while her child says only a few words. She fears something is wrong with her child or perhaps with her. Is she over-reacting to normal developmental variation in the rate at which language develops in young children? Or, does her child actually have a disorder that should be treated?

Professional opinion is divided on the significance of early developmental language delay. Some take the position that most delay that is specific to language is self-correcting and that parents should be reassured that nothing is wrong. Others are of the opinion that specific language delay is a symptom of one or more underlying pathologies, and warrants professional intervention. Twenty years ago, one could hold a version of one or the other of these antithetical views without fear of empirical contradiction. Today, there is a growing body of research on early developmental language delay that is relevant to clinical practice. Our purpose is to review existing research with the goal of helping clinicians ask the right questions of their clients and make informed decisions about the need for further evaluation and treatment. Our concern is with children under five years of age, with particular emphasis on children whose language delays are manifest by two years of age.

CATEGORIES OF DEVELOPMENTAL LANGUAGE DELAY

In many cases delays in language development are secondary to conditions such as mental retardation or hearing loss. In other cases, the causal relations between developmental language delay and associated problems are unclear. Examples include conduct problems, hyperactivity and attention deficits. In still other cases, language impairments occur in isolation from other known developmental problems. Progress in clinical decision making regarding developmental language delay requires that this heterogeneity be recognized and incorporated into diagnostic distinctions.

Specific versus Secondary Delay

The most useful diagnostic distinction is between developmental language delay that is secondary to other conditions (mental retardation, pervasive developmental disorder or autism, physical handicap, hearing loss, brain damage and environmental deprivation), what we will call *secondary language delay*, and developmental language delay that occurs when a child's nonlinguistic cognitive skills and physical abilities are developing normally, what we will call *specific language delay*. For example, a child with severely delayed language and low intelligence would receive a diagnosis of mental retardation with secondary language delay and a child with delayed language and normal intelligence would be diagnosed as having specific language delay.

Many children with specific language delay also have problems outside the cognitive/linguistic arena, particularly in the areas of conduct or activity/attention. We find it useful to designate these children as having *specific language delay with comorbidity*. In both the diagnoses of secondary language delay and specific language delay with comorbidity, the child has a significant problem in addition to language delay. However, instances of normal language development in the face of low IQ are rare, generally the result of known genetic abnormalities, specific to certain modalities of language, and unlikely to result in normal scores on formal language tests (Cromer, 1988; Bellugi, Marks, Bihrle & Sabo, 1988), while cases of completely normal language development in children with problems of conduct or attention are not only frequent but typical. Thus low levels of cognitive development (IQ) appear to impose a limit on the rate of language development in nearly all children, while conduct and attention problems are merely associated with language delay in some children. The diagnostic distinctions between secondary language delay and specific language delay, with or without comorbidity, have clear implications for prognosis and treatment, as we shall subsequently detail.

Expressive Delay versus Receptive-Expressive Delay

For children with specific language delay, with or without comorbidity, it is important to distinguish between problems of expression, what we will call *specific expressive language delay*, and problems of expression and reception, what we will call *specific receptive-expressive language delay*. Problems of expression represent failures to produce language at age-appropriate levels. Problems of reception represent failures to respond to the language of others at age appropriate levels. The most prevalent form of specific language delay is specific expressive delay (Bishop & Edmundson, 1987; Fischel, Whitehurst, Caulfield & DeBaryshe, 1989; Whitehurst, Fischel, Arnold & Lonigan, 1992; Stark & Tallal, 1981). Specific receptive-expressive language delay is also prevalent, but occurs less frequently than specific expressive delay (Bishop & Edmundson, 1987; Paul, 1991; Stark & Tallal, 1981). Children who have receptive delays but not expressive delays are sufficiently rare that we have not afforded them a separate diagnostic label. For example, Bishop and Edmundson (1987) identified no child with problems exclusive to comprehension in their sample of 88 four-year-olds who had been seen by pediatricians or speech-language pathologists because of concern about language development. In our own clinical work with two- and three-year-olds with developmental language delays, we have encountered only one child out of more than 200 who appeared to have normal expressive skills and delayed receptive skills. Significant numbers of children with exclusively receptive problems have been identified in some studies (e.g. Catts, 1993). This usually appears to result from using tests of expressive ability that are known to have inflated norms compared to the tests of receptive ability, and from defining children as having an exclusively receptive delay when their receptive scores fall slightly to one side while their expressive scores fall slightly to the other side of an arbitrary score boundary.

Components of Language

The clinician working with delayed language in the youngest children may find it sufficient to make gross distinctions between problems of expression and problems of reception-expression, with or without corresponding delays in nonlinguistic areas of cognition. However, the accuracy of prognosis for even the youngest child can sometimes be improved by making finer distinctions. These finer distinctions become necessary as children become older and the language of even linguistically delayed children becomes complex. Four categories of language development need to be addressed: phonology, syntax, semantics and pragmatics.

Phonology. Children with phonological problems most frequently have difficulties with articulation, which are generally specific to consonants rather than vowels. Frequent errors include omission (e.g. "ee" instead of "keep"), substitution ("berry" instead of "very"), and cluster reduction ("mell" instead of "smell"). The most problematic consonants are the liquids (/r/, /l/) and the stridents (e.g. /f/, /v/, /s/) (Stoel-Gammon, 1991). While referral to a speech and language professional is necessary for detailed phonological assessment, severe phonological impairment can be detected by anyone who works with children on a regular basis. It is manifest by such a high frequency of consonant omissions, reductions and substitutions that only parents may be able to understand most of the child's utterances. The clinician working with the youngest children with developmental language delay should keep in mind that articulation skills are motor routines that need to be practiced to be performed correctly. Children may show rapid spurts in the development of vocabulary that outpace their phonological abilities, which will catch up in due course.

There is substantial evidence that language impairments during the preschool period that are exclusive to expressive phonology are associated with very low risks of later language or reading problems. For instance, Bishop and Edmundson (1987) found that 78% of a sample of four-year-olds with exclusively phonological delays had no measurable impairments in any areas of speech or language by age of 5½. The subgroup of four-year-olds with exclusively phonological deficits "did particularly well in reading and spelling at 8½ years" (Bishop & Adams, 1990, p. 1040). Even among those children who still had exclusively phonological problems at age 5½ there was no heightened risk of later reading problems. Likewise, Catts (1993), found that correlations between articulation ability in kindergarten and reading ability in first and second grade were low and nonsignificant for a sample of children with speech-language impairments.

On the other hand, phonological problems that are reflected in poor awareness of phonological features during the late preschool period, rather than problems in articulation, seem to predict later reading problems in word recognition (e.g., Catts, 1993; Magnusson & Naucler, 1990). Awareness of phonological features would be reflected in the child's ability to complete rhymes or to identify phonemes (e.g. "Say the word 'sit' without the /s/."). The relation between phonological awareness and early reading occurs in normally developing children as well as those with language delays (e.g. Bradley & Bryant, 1985).

Semantics. Problems of semantics are reflected in a slow rate of acquisition of vocabulary and the meanings associated with words. At its simplest level, the child simply does not understand and/or produce words that are typically part of the repertoire of age mates. Fischel *et al.* (1989) found that children with specific expressive language delay who had fewer than eight words in their expressive vocabularies at 27 months of age were much less likely to demonstrate spontaneous improvement over the next year than children who had from eight to 20 words. A normal vocabulary for a child of this age includes hundreds of words (Fenson, *et al.*, 1993; Rescorla, 1989).

Syntax. Problems of syntax (or grammar) are first evident in restricted utterance length. Multi-word sentences are common in normally developing children by 24 months of age, but are rare in children with specific language delay (Fischel *et al.*, 1989; Rescorla, 1989). Problems in syntax later in development are likely to be reflected in measures of the diversity of a child's grammatical forms as well as utterance length (Scarborough & Dobrich, 1990). For instance, the child with specific language delay may use fewer restrictive clauses (e.g. I want to see the TV show *that I saw at Grandma's house last week*) than his or her normally developing counterpart. Bishop and Adams (1990) found that measures of syntax in general and mean length of utterance in particular, were the best linguistic predictors of reading attainment at age 8½ for children who had been diagnosed as language impaired at age four. Likewise, Magnusson and Naucler (1990) found that low scores on a measure of syntactic production predicted poor spelling ability at the end of first grade for both language impaired and normally developing children.

Pragmatics. Communication or pragmatics involves the ability to construct and interpret messages such that intended meaning is transmitted from one person to another (Lloyd & Beveridge, 1981). Among sophisticated users of a language, this often involves taking aspects of the social, physical and linguistic context into account in formulating or comprehending messages (Whitehurst & Sonnenschein, 1985). For instance, one might alternately describe a particular object as "that thing", "the square", or "the red square" depending on whether it sat alone, next to a triangle, or next to a blue square. Among younger children, communication or pragmatic abilities often hinge on whether the child can make his or her needs known. With very low levels of expressive language, this often depends on gesture. Thal, Tobias and Morrison (1991) found that the existence of good gestural skills discriminated language delayed two-year-olds who caught up over a one-year follow-up from those who remained delayed. Paul and Shiffer (1991) found that two-year-olds with specific receptive-expressive or specific expressive language delay initiated fewer commenting or joint attention interactions with their mothers than normal controls. In the later preschool years, problems of pragmatics become more subtle and related to the understanding or production of extended narrative (Paul, Laszio, McFarland & Midford, 1993). For instance, the child may be less able than age mates to describe what he or she did yesterday, or to describe events in a coherent sequence, tying utterances together by use of devices such as pronouns which refer back to items that have already been mentioned. Bishop and Edmundson (1987) found that the single best linguistic predictor of language development over the course of a year and a half in a group of four-year-olds with delayed language was the ability to tell back a simple story to pictures.

Age as a Critical Dimension

Developmental language delay (specific and secondary) occurs in a progressively smaller proportion of children across the preschool years. For example, from 9 to 17% of two-year-olds (varying with SES) meet a criteria for expressive delay of fewer than 30 words and no word combinations at 24 months of age (Rescorla, 1989). By 36 months of age, estimates of prevalence of specific and secondary delay drop to from 3 to 8% (Silva, 1980; Stevenson & Richman, 1976). Silva's (1980) longitudinal study indicates that the prevalence of secondary and specific forms of developmental language delay drops by another 60% between the ages of three and five. This would indicate a prevalence of 1–3% at age five. Relations between age and prevalence are depicted in Fig. 1.

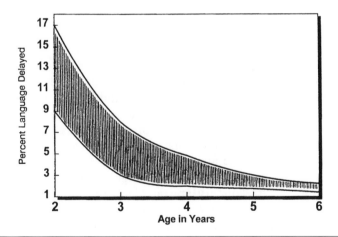

Figure 1. Percentage of children with all forms of developmental language delay over the preschool period. The range at each age is the difference between low and high estimates from various studies of prevalence reported in the text. The percentage of children with specific expressive delay or specific receptive–expressive delay is lower than the range represented in this figure.

ASSESSMENT INSTRUMENTS AND STRATEGIES

We have suggested that the diagnosis of developmental language delay requires distinctions between specific and secondary delay at the broadest level, between expressive and receptive-expressive delay at the next level, and between problems of syntax, meaning, phonology and pragmatics at the third level. Table 1 lists and comments on some assessment instruments that have proven useful in making these diagnostic distinctions.

Differential Diagnosis

The essence of specific language delay as a diagnostic category is the gap between the development of language and nonlinguistic cognitive skills. For instance, a child with a nonverbal performance IQ of 100 and developmental language quotient of 65 would be said to have specific language delay precisely because of the gap between performance on the nonverbal versus verbal tests. The distinctions between specific receptive-expressive delay, and specific expressive delay also have to do with differential levels of performance across domains. For instance, a child with a nonverbal performance IQ of 100, a receptive language quotient of 95, and an expressive language quotient of 65 would be said to have a specific expressive language delay because of the minimal gap between nonverbal performance and receptive performance, on the one hand, and the large gap between nonverbal performance and expressive performance on the other.

A critical nosological issue concerns the importance of the gaps in performance between the nonlinguistic, verbal receptive, and verbal expressive domains, and how they are to be measured and defined. We believe that confusions and ambiguities in the literature on developmental language delay, of which there are many, flow disproportionately from failures to attend to these gaps in performance across domains. There are three major problems in the existing literature.

Secondary versus specific delay. The first problem is a failure to distinguish between children with secondary language delay and children with specific language delay. Several of the classic epidemiological studies of developmental language delay (Fundudis, Kolvin & Garside, 1979; Klackenberg, 1980; Stevenson & Richman, 1976; Silva, Williams & McGee, 1987) have either not separated specific from secondary delay at initial assessment, or have ignored this diagnostic distinction in drawing conclusions. However, other studies have shown that nonverbal IQ is one of the strongest predictors of developmental progress in preschoolers with language delays (Aram, Ekeleman & Nation, 1984; Bishop & Edmundson, 1987). For in-

TABLE 1
Some Instruments for Assessment of Developmental Language Delay in Preschoolers

Test	Purpose	Ages	Comment
Leiter International Performance Scale (Leiter, 1976)	Nonverbal IQ	2–18	Can be administered without verbal instructions; IQs vary in meaning with age
Reynell Developmental Language Scales (2nd revision) (Reynell, 1985)	Language Development	1–7	Separate scales for expressive language and verbal comprehension; children enjoy test materials; British & U.S. norms
Stanford–Binet Intelligence Scale: 4th ed. (Thorndike, Hagen & Sattler, 1986)	IQ & non-verbal IQ	2–adult	Pattern analysis, bead memory, and copying subtests can be used to derive nonverbal IQ; U.S. norms
Templin–Darley Tests of Articulation (2nd ed.) (Templin & Darley, 1968)	Articulation	3–8	Child must fill in blanks in sentences read by examiner and/or label pictures; shorter screening test can be given quickly
The Language Development Survey (Rescorla, 1989)	Expressive vocabulary	2	Parent completed checklist; good validity and easily administered; only appropriate for 24-month-olds
Expressive One-Word Picture Vocabulary Test—revised (Gardner, 1990)	Expressive vocabulary	2–12	Child must label line drawings; sensitive to deficits and advances in expressive skill among younger children
Peabody Picture Vocabulary Test—revised (PPVT—R) (Dunn & Dunn, 1983)	Receptive vocabulary	2.5–18	Child selects picture that represents word used by examiner; British, Spanish, & U.S. versions
MacArthur Communicative Development Inventory Fenson *et al.*, 1993)	Expressive & receptive vocab	8–30 months	Parent-completed inventory of receptive and expressive language; U.S. norms
The Bus Story: A Test of Continuous Speech (Renfrew, 1969; Cowley & Glasgow, 1993)	Pragmatic/ semantics/ MLU	3–8	Child retells a story to a sequential set of pictures; British & U.S. versions
Index of Productive Syntax (Scarborough, 1990)	Grammatical complexity	< 6	Examiner scores occurrence of 56 types of syntactic forms in 100 spontaneous utterances of the child; no norms

stance, Bishop and Edmundson (1987) found that only 11% of a sample of language delayed four-year-olds with Leiter nonverbal IQ scores more than 2 SDs below the mean had positive outcomes at a year later, while 44% of a sample with normal Leiters were functioning well a year later. Likewise, Richman, Stevenson and Graham (1982) found that poor educational outcomes in eight-year-olds with a history of delayed language at age three were limited to children who were retarded in other aspects of development at age three. If the goal is prognostic accuracy, then it is absolutely essential to discriminate specific from secondary language delay.

Degrees of separation. Another approach that is problematic fails to consider the size of the gap between expressive, receptive and nonverbal cognitive skills, opting for categorical rather than quantitative distinctions. Consider the research of Silva *et al.* (1987), who conducted a longitudinal follow-up of children who had been diagnosed with developmental language delay at age three. Children were categorized as having receptive delay, expressive delay, or receptive-expressive delay, based on whether their scores fell 2 SDs or more below the mean on the verbal expression scale, or the verbal comprehension scale, or both the verbal and comprehension scales of the *Reynell Developmental Language Scales* (Reynell, 1969). The investigators then examined differential developmental outcomes for each diagnostic group at the ages of seven, nine and 11. The problem is that no distinctions were made based on the size of the difference between expressive and receptive performance in individual children. Thus a child scoring 2.1 SDs below the mean on expression and 1.9 SDs below the mean on comprehension was categorized as having specific expressive delay, rather than receptive-expressive delay, and was placed in the same category as a child with a size-able gap between expression and reception. Supporting the probability of this type of misclassification, Silva, in an earlier report of this sample, indicated that "in the group with delayed expressive language only there was . . . considerable variation in verbal comprehension ability" (1980, p. 773). We believe that to the degree that the distinctions between specific receptive-expressive delay, specific expressive delay, and secondary language delay are to be useful, they need to be based on appreciable differences in levels of performance across the three domains in question.

What is abnormal? A final problematic approach identifies children as having developmental language delay who are within the normal range of development. For example, Stevenson and Richman (1976) used a 6-month gap between language age and cognitive age at 30 months of age as criteria for language delay. Similarly, Rescorla (1989) defined expressive delay as the child being at least six months behind age norms at 24 months of age. However, this amount of delay represents at its lower bound less than 1 SD from the mean of the population at 30 months, and only slightly more than 1 SD at 24 months. We question the utility of defining a child as delayed whose language ability is low normal or borderline normal.

Recommendations for norm-based diagnoses. Measurement and definitional approaches to developmental language delay will produce confusing data and poor prognostic accuracy if distinctions are blurred between secondary and specific language delay and between problems of expression versus problems of expression and reception. We recommend that in clinical settings the diagnosis of specific receptive-expressive delay be limited to children whose most depressed language quotient (receptive or expressive) is at least 2 SDs below the mean for their age, whose least depressed language quotient (receptive or expressive) is at least 1.5 SDs below the mean, and whose nonverbal intelligence quotient is no more than 1 SD below the mean. The diagnosis of specific expressive delay would require that both performance IQ and receptive language quotient be no more than 1 SD below the mean, while the expressive language quotient would be at least 2 SDs below the mean. These definitions restrict the diagnosis of specific language delay to children who are severely delayed in the domain(s) of language in which they are considered to be impaired, and who are within the normal range in the area of nonverbal cognition.

The issue of the size of the gap between language development and cognitive development or between receptive language and expressive language that is criterial for diagnosis allows only arbitrary solutions, but these solutions are not without consequence. We believe that researchers who are interested in developmental language delay from a theoretical or process orientation might do well to establish lenient criteria, and then use the degree of delay as a process or predictor variable. However, practitioners who are interested in developmental language delay as a clinical disorder ought to use severe criteria for diagnosis in order to limit attention to children whose condition may justify professional time and attention.

Norm-based diagnoses, such as those we have suggested, are preferable to arbitrary, fixed definitions, e.g. no more than 30 words and no word combinations at 24 months of age (Rescorla, 1989). One reason is that a definition that specifies a fixed level of performance at a particular age cannot fit children of other ages. There is no reason to expect that all children with developmental language delay will present to a clinician within a few weeks of their second birthday.

It may seem paradoxical that norm-based definitions could result in changing frequencies of impairment over age, as in Fig. 1. If one defines impairment as being, for example, more than 2 SDs below the mean of the population, should not about 2% of children be impaired at each age? Not necessarily, because the standardization samples typically consist of relatively small numbers of children at any given age and thus underrepresent rare events. With IQ, for instance, the actual distribution derived from testing large numbers of children is known to have a distinct hump at the lower end that includes approximately 6% more cases than would be expected from the normal curve derived from the standardization sample (Dingman & Tarjan, 1960). The same phenomenon is likely for language delay.

CORRELATES OF SPECIFIC LANGUAGE DELAY

The aim of this section is to describe how children with specific language delay and their families differ from children with normal language development and their families. Finding a difference between a diagnostic group and a normal comparison group does not mean, of course, that the difference is causal in the development of the condition that is the basis of the diagnosis. For example, schizophrenics as a group dress less well than the normal population, but no one would conclude that poor clothing causes schizophrenia. At the same time, a search for causes needs to begin with a search for differences: causes must lie somewhere within the set of characteristics that differentiate the clinical group from the rest of the population.

Gender

Male children appear to suffer from most maladies at greater rates than female children. This gender imbalance is extreme with respect to specific language delay. Of the roughly 100 2- and 3-year-olds who have received a diagnosis of specific expressive delay in our research and clinical activities, 84% have been male. Silva (1989) reported a gender imbalance for all types of language delays in three-year-olds of 67% for males. Paul (1991) found that 76% of her sample of expressively and receptively delayed two-year-olds were male, while 82% of Bishop and Edmundson's (1987) sample of language impaired four-year-olds were male. These data indicate clearly and consistently that all types of specific language impairments occur at disproportionate rates among male preschoolers.

Genetic Factors

The etiology and course of various psychological problems are affected by genetic factors. Genetic influences have been documented by means of twin and adoption studies in disorders such as schizophrenia (e.g. Wender, Rosenthal, Kety, Schulsinger & Welner, 1974) and antisocial behavior (e.g. Mednick, Schulsinger, Higgins & Bell, 1974). Language and other cognitive skills show strong genetic loadings in normal populations of preschoolers (Plomin, De Fries & Fulker, 1988). Language delay may be similarly influenced by inherited factors (Ludlow & Cooper, 1983).

The classic behavioral methodology for detecting the heritability of psychological traits is the study of differences between same-sex identical and fraternal twins. The only twin data that are relevant to the genetics of specific language delay are from Bishop (1991), who identified 61 twin pairs ranging from 7 years of age to adults in which at least one member had a current or past specific language impairment. Specific language impairment was defined as having a current nonverbal IQ score of 85 or over, and either a current score below the 5th centile on at least one test of language functioning, or a history of speech therapy or special education for language impairment. Among monozygotic twins with either current or past specific language impairment, 67% of the co-twins also had current or past specific language impairment. Among dizygotic twins, the percentage of affected co-twins was only about half that (32%). While these data suggest a significant genetic component of specific language impairment, it is important to keep in mind that the subjects were school-aged children and adults, not children with transient developmental delays during the preschool period. As we have previously indicated, age is an important dimension in language delay. Individuals who experience language delays in the school years differ in many observable ways from those whose delay resolves during the preschool years: the underlying genetics may be quite different.

Family studies are presently the most relevant source of information about inherited genetic influences on preschoolers with specific language delay. Family studies examine the amount of familial aggregation of disorders, within and across generations. Finding significant family aggregation cannot in and of itself conclusively establish a genetic role in the etiology of a disorder because families share environments as well as genes. However, particular patterns of family aggregation may be better predicted by genetic than environment models, and the absence of familial aggregation may rule out inherited genetic effects.

Bishop and Edmundson (1986) reported family history data from the parents of 56 language-impaired four-year-olds: 46% had blood relatives with a history of language impairment, stuttering or reading disorder. In a control group of normally developing children from similar socioeconomic backgrounds, the percentage with affected relatives was only 15%. Similarly, Tallal, Ross and Curtiss (1989) collected family history data on 76 children with language disorders and without cognitive deficits and 54 matched control children. They found that the mothers of children with language impairments were far more likely than mothers of controls to report that family members had a history of language problems, were held back in school, and had poor writing ability. Consistent with these findings, Paul (1991) reported that a family history of language, speech or learning problems was 3 to 4 times more frequent in two-year-olds with specific language delay than in a normally developing control group.

In opposition to the previous findings of family aggregation, Whitehurst *et al.* (1991) found no differences in family history of speech, language and school problems in 62 two-year-olds with specific expressive delay, versus 55 normally developing children. Further, family history was not predictive of later language development. What explains these seemingly conflicting results? The clearest difference between the studies is that Whitehurst *et al.* limited their sample to children with specific expressive delay, whereas all the other studies included children with receptive-expressive delays and some included children with secondary language delays. Our tentative conclusion is that inherited genetic factors are not involved for the vast majority of two-year-olds with a specific expressive delay, but are likely to be involved for children with specific receptive-expressive delay and children with secondary language delay. Clearly more data and more sophisticated behavior genetic models are needed in this area.

Laterality

Brain laterality as indicated by handedness has often been viewed as related to language development perhaps because of the connection between handedness, cerebral dominance, and Broca's area of the brain: Left-handers experience about 70% left hemisphere localization compared to 85% for right-handers (Springer & Deutsch, 1989). Whitehurst *et al.* (1992) compared handedness (as reported by mothers) in 93 two-year-olds with specific expressive delay and 91 normal controls. The proportion of left-handers was virtually the same in both groups (delayed = .33, normal = .31). Bishop and Edmundson (1987) studied language impaired and normally developing preschoolers on a peg moving task and found no differences between the groups in relative performance with the two hands. Bishop (1990) found that neither hand preference nor relative hand skills differed between normal controls and eight-year-olds who had been language impaired as preschoolers. These data suggest that laterality is not relevant to specific language delay.

Prenatal and Perinatal History

Obstetric complications are known to affect later language development (Cohen, Parmelee, Sigman & Beckwith, 1988). However, the evidence does not support such a relation for specific language delay. In our sample of 91 normal children and 93 two-year-olds with specific expressive delay there were no differences that approached significance on birth weight, rates of prematurity, or obstetric complications (Whitehurst *et al.* 1992). Likewise, Paul (1991) found that neither pre- nor perinatal problems distinguished two-year-olds with specific language delay from normally developing controls. In contrast, Bishop and Edmundson (1986) found a marginally higher frequency of perinatal/neurological risk factors in four-year-olds with language impairments compared to normally developing controls, but this sample differed from the other samples in focusing on older preschoolers with presumably less transient problems.

Motor Deficiencies

Children might be slow to talk because of neurological conditions that make it difficult for them to control the organs of speech or because of neurological immaturity that causes general motor delay. We examined this issue by asking mothers of two-year-olds with specific expressive delay and mothers of normally developing controls whether their child ever experienced any problems in chewing, or ever choked on their food, or ever drooled (Whitehurst *et al.* 1992). Rates of problems in chewing were very low, about 1%, and did not differ in the two populations. However, drooling occurred in significantly more (32%) of the expressively delayed children than the normal sample (21%). Likewise, 23% of the expressively delayed children were reported to choke on their food at least occasionally, versus 9% of the normal children. These data offer support for the hypothesis that oro-motor problems are connected with early specific expressive delay in some children.

Motor problems in young children with specific language delay do not extend to gross clumsiness. Paul (1991) reported no difference between her delayed and normally developing two-year-olds on the motor subscale of the *Vineland Adaptive Behavior Scales* (Sparrow, Bella & Ciccetti, 1984). However, fine motor actions may be another matter. Bishop and Edmundson (1987) asked four-year-olds with specific language delay, secondary language delay, and no language delay to complete a task involving moving pegs from one row to another on a pegboard. Children with language delays (specific or secondary) were slower than the normal controls at completing this task. In a follow-up of the language delayed children through 5½ years of age, improvement of language status was found to correlate highly with improvements in motor skill as measured by the peg-moving task. Follow-up of this sample at 8½ years of age showed that children with persisting language difficulties continued to be slower than normal controls at completing the peg moving test (Bishop, 1990). These findings could reflect either an underlying general neurological immaturity, e.g. slow processing speed, or something more specific to motoric functions.

Otitis Media

Otitis media, inflammation and/or fluid in the middle ear, is a common disease of infancy and early childhood. Approximately 50% of all children experience at least one episode of otitis media during the first year of life, and by three years of age, approximately two thirds of all children experience at least one episode (Howie, 1980). Otitis media is often associated with conductive hearing loss of a transient nature, and may lead to chronic auditory impairment (Bess, 1983).

Several studies have found a relation between an early history of otitis media and later problems in language development. For instance, Teele, Klein and Rosner (1980) followed a cohort of 205 children from birth to three years of age. The presence of otitis media was periodically assessed by otoscopic examination. Tests of speech and language were administered when the children were three years old. Children who had spent prolonged periods of time with otitis media had significantly lower language scores. The correlation between the cumulative duration of otitis media and language scores was strongest for children from the highest SES levels. The amount of time spent with otitis media in the first 6–12 months of life was most strongly associated with poorer language scores.

A relation between otitis media and language scores in a normally developing sample does not necessarily indicate that otitis media is a causative factor in severe language delay. In fact, several studies have found no difference in the overall frequency of otitis media in normally developing versus language delayed preschoolers (Bishop & Edmundson, 1986; Lonigan, Fischel, Whitehurst, Arnold & Valdez-Menchaca, 1992; Paul, 1991). However, one of those studies (Lonigan *et al.*, 1992) found a significant relation between otitis media between 12 and 18 months of age and expressive language improvement between two and three years of age for two-year-olds with specific expressive delay. The relation was the opposite of what one might predict in that expressively delayed children with an early history of otitis media were likely to show more rapid progress in the development of expressive language than expressively delayed children without a history of otitis media.

These findings suggest that specific expressive delay in some two-year-olds is caused by otitis media (perhaps in interaction with or additive to other vulnerabilities) during a critical period for the development of expressive language. When the otitis resolves, language improvement follows. Other children are likely to experience specific expressive delay for reasons that are more central and long lasting. Otitis media does not seem to be a factor in the language progress of children whose language delays persist until four years of age, except perhaps in children who also experience perinatal problems (Bishop & Edmundson, 1986).

Family Size and Birth Order

Data on family size at it relates to developmental language disorders are sketchy. Epidemiological studies by Fundudis *et al.* (1979) and Richman and Stevenson (1977) found that language delay occurred significantly more often among children from large families, but these differences were confounded with socioeconomic status. Whitehurst *et al.* (1992) also found large families over-represented in two-year-olds with specific expressive delay, compared with normally developing controls, but selection biases may have favored small families in the normal control group. Whitehurst *et al.* (1993), in a study of families of 345 four-year-olds with secondary language delay due to conditions associated with poverty, found a significant correlation between number of siblings and language scores, even after controlling for maternal vocabulary and IQ. It seems likely that the relative deprivation of verbal interaction with adults that occurs for children in large families with closely spaced children (Zajonc, 1976) may add to the vulnerabilities that lead children to pass the diagnostic threshold for language delay.

Socioeconomic Status

Rescorla (1989) reported a highly significant inverse relation between socioeconomic status and expressive vocabulary size, and between socioeconomic status and the frequency of expressive delay among two-year-olds seen in pediatric settings. Frequency of delay ranged from 9% in private practice to 17% in a primary-care medical clinic serving inner-city families on public assistance. Unfortunately, Rescorla did not measure receptive language or cognitive ability in her sample. The relations she found between SES and vocabulary size and SES and expressive delay may be due in large part to secondary language delays resulting from non-optimal environments for children reared in poverty. For example, Whitehurst *et al.* (1993) found that the mean language quotient for a sample of normally developing three-year-olds from low-income families attending regular daycare centers in a suburban county in New York was 83, and that over 15% of the sample had expressive language quotients of less than 77. Clearly the conditions that are associated with low levels of family income cause general delays in cognitive development and linguistic development. Whether they also heighten the risk of specific language delays is unknown.

Verbal Interactions in the Family

Related to the possible effects of family size and SES on language development, some studies have suggested that the linguistic environment of language impaired children is qualitatively or quantitatively different from that of normally developing children (Buium, Rynders & Turnure, 1974; Marshall, Hegrenes & Goldstein, 1973; Petersen & Sherrod, 1982; Wulbert, Inglis, Kriegsmann & Mills, 1975). In contrast, other studies have suggested that parental speech to language impaired children is highly similar to that directed to normally developing children (Conti-Ramsden & Friel-Patti, 1983; Cunningham, Siegel, van der Spuy, Clark & Bow, 1985). As with so much other research related to language impairments, research on verbal interactions suffers because various categories of language impairments are aggregated. It is not only possible, but likely, that verbal interactions are substantially different for children with receptive-expressive delays versus those with expressive delays, or articulation difficulties.

Whitehurst *et al.* (1988) focused exclusively on two-year-olds with specific expressive delay and compared their linguistics interactions in the home with two normally developing groups: same aged mates with equivalent receptive skills, and younger children with equivalent expressive skills. We found that expressively delayed children experienced a verbal environment very much like that of normally developing 17-month-olds, and unlike that of 28-month-old normally developing children. These results and similar findings by Paul and Elwood (1991) suggest that the child's delay comes first and causes parents to speak differently, not, vice versa. Nevertheless, parents might play a role in maintaining language delay by providing a less challenging verbal environment than they might if their child's expressive abilities were at age level.

Behavior and Discipline in the Family

The association between language problems and behavioral disorders of childhood has been documented extensively (e.g. Baker & Cantwell, 1982a, b; Beitchman, Nair, Clegg, Ferguson & Patel, 1986; Cantwell & Baker 1980; Jenkins, Bax & Hart, 1980; Paul & James, 1990; Richman & Stevenson, 1977). For example, in a group of 705 randomly sampled three-year-olds, Richman and Stevenson (1977) reported a base-rate prevalence of behavior problems of 14% as assessed by parental responses on a behavior screening interview. Of those children in the sample who exhibited language delay, 58% had concurrent behavior problems. Similarly, Jenkins *et al.* (1980) found an association between low language scores and behavior problems in a sample of 418 preschool children. In this study, behavior problem ratings were obtained from a physician's evaluation of parental responses on a structured behavior interview. Beitchman *et al.* (1986) compared the rates of behavioral and emotional problems in a group of 142 children with diagnosed speech and language disorders and in a normally developing control group. The estimated frequency of psychiatric disorder was 48.7% for the speech and language impaired children, while that for the control group was 12.0%.

While the correlation of language and behavior problems has been documented extensively, research on this relation suffers from the problem encountered again and again in research on the language impaired: the failure to differentiate significantly diverse speech and language syndromes. When studies have differentiated types of language disorder, interesting results have emerged. For example, Baker and Cantwell (1982b) categorized children as exhibiting a pure speech disorder, a combined speech and language disorder, or a pure language disorder. The prevalence of diagnosed psychiatric disorder was much higher for the pure language impaired group (95%) than for the pure speech impaired group (29%), with the combined speech and language impaired group falling in between (45%). The distribution of developmental disorders, such as enuresis and mental retardation, followed the same pattern.

Focusing exclusively on two-year-olds with specific expressive delay, Caulfield, Fischel, DeBaryshe and Whitehurst (1989) examined parent-child interaction and behavior problems using behavioral observations. The delayed group engaged in higher rates of negative behaviors including crying, screaming, hitting, and throwing toys. The delayed group also engaged in a higher frequency of nonverbal communication. Mothers of normal control children engaged in higher rates of nontask oriented conversation and mothers of the expressively delayed children were more likely to use physical discipline.

Caulfield (1989) followed up on the finding of elevated rates of behavior problems in children with specific expressive delay by investigating a frustration model of the relations between language delay and behavior problems. The frustration model holds that a child with inadequate verbal skills for a given situation will exhibit negative behaviors out of frustration. A group of two-year-olds with specific expressive delay and a normally developing group were observed in laboratory tasks that varied in communicative demands. Expressively delayed and normal children had very low rates of misbehavior in a non-verbal pointing task (which was communicatively easy for both groups), while both sets of children had elevated rates of misbehavior in a reading task (which was communicatively impossible for all). However, in the naming task (which was difficult for expressively delayed children and easy for the normal group), the expressively delayed group showed much higher rates of misbehavior such as tantrums and whining. These results support the frustration model of problem behavior in language impaired children by demonstrating that situations that are communicatively difficult generate misbehavior.

Whether the frustration model of the relation between language disorders and misbehavior that applies to expressive deficits is generalizable to other categories of language impairment needs further research. There is some evidence in the literature that problems with verbal comprehension are particularly likely to lead to noncompliance (Kaler & Kopp, 1990), which would suggest that children with secondary language delay or specific receptive-expressive delay might be more at risk of behavior problems than children with exclusively expressive delays. Mawhood, Rutter and Howlin (described in Rutter & Mawhood, 1991) found that school-aged children with profound deficits in language comprehension were at substantial risk of life-long problems in social adjustment. Whether initial problem behaviors in children with language delays flow from deficits in comprehension or from the frustration of being unable to communicate, bidirectional interactions between parent and child are likely to ensue. Parents with weaker discipline skills may be more likely to reward negative forms of child behavior, which may escalate over time and interfere with other areas of development, including language growth. In support of this model, Laplante, Zelazo and Kearsley (1991) trained parents of preschoolers in behavior management of oppositional behavior and found as misbehavior decreased, vocabulary and verbal interaction increased compared to a non-intervention control group.

Summary

The findings reviewed above suggest that specific language delay is, in part, a function of biological conditions. Specifically, males are much more likely to experience specific language delay than are females. Oro-motor problems occur more frequently in two-year-olds with specific expressive delay than in children with normally developing language, and a fine-motor slowness is characteristic of older preschoolers with delayed language. Inherited genetic factors appear to play a special role in many cases of secondary language delay and specific receptive–expressive delay, but appear not to be involved in early specific expressive delay. Otitis media during the 12–18 month time period may be a significant contributor to rapidly resolved specific expressive delay in two-year-olds.

Our survey of research on social-interactional factors identified family size, family socioeconomic status, and patterns of misbehavior and discipline as risk factors for developmental language delay. Family verbal interactions are likely to be important contributors to secondary language delay, particularly in large and/or low SES families, but do not seem to be a root cause of specific language delay. They can, however, play a role in the maintenance of delayed language.

SIGNIFICANCE OF SPECIFIC LANGUAGE DELAY

The question of whether specific language delay is a disorder is of considerable practical importance. For example, one suburban county in New York State (Suffolk), with a population of 1.2 million, spent $118 million in 1992 on preschool educational services for children with special needs (*Newsday*, 1993), with the majority of those served being children with speech and language impairments. If only half of those funds was spent on preschoolers with specific language delay and every county in the United States provided similar levels of service, the result would be an annual expenditure of roughly $12.5 billion, which by way of comparison is more than the annual budget of the government of Ireland.

Disregarding questions of economics, specific language delay generates considerable concern by parents and attention by professionals. Is the concern and attention justified? The fundamental question to answer before a developmental delay is categorized as a disorder is whether it is associated with significant distress for the child or with impairment in important areas of current or future functioning.

Is Specific Language Delay a Disorder?

Evidence in support of treating language delay as a disorder derives from studies demonstrating that it is associated with a variety of undesirable developmental sequelae. More specifically, children with delayed onset of language have more frequent academic problems (e.g. Aram & Nation, 1980; Fundudis *et al.*, 1980; Klackenberg, 1980; Richman *et al.*, 1982; Silva *et al.*, 1987), more behavioral and psychiatric problems (e.g. Baker & Cantwell, 1982a, b; Beitchman *et al.*, 1986), and an elevated frequency of later problems in speech and language (e.g. Aram & Nation, 1980; Aram, Ekelman & Nation, 1984; Klackenberg, 1980).

While these associations are clear, each of the cited studies involved children with secondary as well as specific language delay. It is one thing to indicate that there are undesirable sequelae associated with below average intellectual development and associated language delay. It is quite another thing to link these sequelae to language delay per se. Longitudinal outcome studies that do not make distinctions between specific and secondary language delay, and do not further divide specific language delay into expressive versus receptive-expressive variants, obscure prognostic accuracy and an understanding of underlying processes.

More recent studies of specific language delay have incorporated the diagnostic distinctions we have previously advocated. The picture that emerges from these studies is remarkably consistent:

> Specific language delay in the preschool period is better characterized as a risk factor than a disorder: while some children with specific language delay go on to have learning or language impairments in the school years, the vast majority of children with specific language delay recover to the normal range by five years of age. Children whose language skills are in the normal range by age 5 have low risk of later language or reading disorders. However, they may continue to be weaker in language and reading than in other areas of their development.

Since these conclusions are likely to be controversial, we will review the research on which they are based with some care.

Three roughly contemporary longitudinal investigations in the United States have followed large samples of children who were first diagnosed with specific language delay between 24 and 36 months of age. The New York study (Fischel *et al.*, 1989; Whitehurst *et al.*, 1991, 1992) and the Pennsylvania study (Rescorla & Schwartz, 1990; Rescorla, 1993) only included children with specific expressive delay. The New York study used a more severe criterion for defining expressive delay (≥2.33 SDs below the mean of the standardization sample) than the Pennsylvania study (≥1.1 SDs below the mean). The Oregon study (Paul, 1991; Paul *et al.*, 1993) used criteria for severity of expressive delay equivalent to those used in the Pennsylvania sample, but differed from both the New York and Pennsylvania studies by including children with specific receptive–expressive delay and not differentiating them from children with specific expressive delay. A fourth large-scale longitudinal study, the English study (Bishop & Adams, 1990; Bishop & Edmundson, 1986, 1987), followed a sample of four-year-olds who had been referred for professional help because of concern that their language development was impaired for no obvious reason. Though the overall English sample included children with secondary as well as specific language delay, these and other subtypes were differentiated. Because our focus is on children with preschool language delays, we will not examine several other investigations that have identified children with language impairments at around six years of age and followed them through the early school years (e.g. Catts, 1993; Magnusson & Naucler, 1990).

Phonology. Pholological problems were prevalent at intake among the two-year-olds in all three studies and were resolved with age. In the Oregon sample, the phonological structure of the vocalizations and words of two-year-olds with specific language delay was less complex than that of children with more advanced language (Paul & Jennings, 1992). In the New York sample, progress in expressive vocabulary size over a five-month period was predictable from the proportion of consonants to vowels in the vocalizations of two-year-olds with specific expressive delay: children with few consonants showed slower progress (Whitehurst, Smith, Fischel, Arnold & Lonigan, 1991). Follow-up of children in the New York sample indicated that 35% were below the normal range on articulation at 3½ years of age and 22% were below normal at 5½ years of age (with a mean articulation quotient for the entire sample of 95). This accords well with the results from the Oregon study (Paul *et al.*, 1993), where the children had a mean articulation quotient of 96 at five years of age.

The dominance of vocabulary problems over phonological problems in the early diagnosis of specific language delay may be more a function of adult perception than actual prevalence: Adults are accustomed to frequent errors of articulation in the speech of normally developing two-year-olds and may be unlikely to notice that such errors are more frequent in children with delayed expressive language. Relatedly, there are no standardized tests of phonological skills for two-year-olds. Even if such tests existed, they would be difficult to apply to children with expressive language delays because they are typically very reluctant to use even their limited expressive repertoire. Thus even though limited vocabulary is the striking feature of two-year-olds with specific language delay, it appears that phonological delays are also present from the earliest points that specific developmental language disorder can be diagnosed. Articulation continues to be a problem over the preschool years for some children who are late talkers at two years of age, but the proportion of children experiencing this problem diminishes by five years of age to only slightly more than would be expected in a normal population. As we have already described, children in the age range of 4–5 years whose language impairment is exclusive to articulation do not appear to be at risk of later reading problems (Bishop & Adams, 1990).

Semantics. The three studies of younger children found that the dominant symptom of language delay between two and three years of age was small vocabulary size. The prevalence of this problem decreased dramatically over time. For instance, in the New York sample, 88% of the children were within the normal range (no more than 1 SD below the mean) for expressive vocabulary by 3½ years of age and 96% were within the normal range for vocabulary size by 5½ years of age (Whitehurst *et al.*, 1992). The Pennsylvania sample to have resolved its vocabulary problems even more rapidly (by three years of age), perhaps because they were less severely afflicted at intake than the New York sample (Rescorla, 1993).

Only children in the Pennsylvania sample were followed up on semantic abilities into school. Summarizing these data, Rescorla (1993) says, "follow-up data at ages six through eight suggest that most [specific expressive delayed] children perform normally on standardized language measures and would probably not stand out as language impaired."

If we restrict our attention to standardized tests, we conclude that children who are diagnosed with specific expressive delay at two years of age no longer have semantic deficiencies by five years of age and remain in the normal range through to at least eight years of age.

Syntax. Syntax is not a meaningful dimension of expressive language for children at the stage of single word speech. However, as children with specific expressive delay acquire the ability to produce multi-word utterances, they demonstrate syntactic deficiencies that mirror those that we have described for vocabulary and phonology. In the Pennsylvania sample (Rescorla, 1993), 67–79% of children were below normal on syntax at three years of age (depending on the measure), 56% were below normal at four years of age, and 16% were below normal at five years of age (which is precisely the percentage that should be more than 1 SD below the mean in the general population assuming that performance is distributed as a normal curve). Later follow-up of these children showed that syntactic skills were in the normal range at eight years of age. In the Oregon study, average performance at five years of age was in the normal range for grammatical understanding and grammatical complexity, and the previously language delayed group did not differ from the normal comparison group on those dimensions.

Pragmatics. In a study with only 10 subjects, Thal *et al.* (1991) found that gestural communication was deficient in two-year-olds with specific receptive–expressive delay, but not in children with specific expressive delay. Children with pragmatic deficiencies, who were also the children with receptive delays, did not catch up in expressive language over a one-year follow-up, while children with specific expressive delay, who were also the children who could communicate normally through gesture, did catch up. The perfect correlation between receptive delay and pragmatic delay in this small sample suggests tentatively that both problems are being driven by a common underlying mechanism that is not shared with children who have only expressive delays.

Of children in the New York sample, 26% were more than 1 SD below the mean on the verbal expression subscale of the *Illinois Test of Psycholinguistic Abilities* (Kirk, McCarthy & Kirt, 1968) at three years of age. This test measures the child's ability to produce descriptions of simple objects. However the prevalence of this problem dropped to 16% at 3½ years of age and 7% at 5½ years of age, at which point the mean language quotient for the sample was 105. In the Pennsylvania sample, children scored close to age level on the expressive scale of the *Reynell Developmental Language Scales, Revised* (Reynell, 1977) by three years of age, and above age level at four and five years of age. The *Reynell* expressive scale includes measurement of the child's ability to describe pictorial scenes, which is similar to the test of verbal expression that was employed in the New York study.

At 4 and 5 years of age the Oregon children were behind a normal comparison group on a measure of narrative skills. The Oregon study also found below normal communication skills at five years of age on a parent report instrument (Paul *et al.*, 1993). Recall that children with specific receptive–expressive delay were not differentiated from children with specific expressive delay in the Oregon sample. Thus we do not know whether the communicative and narrative deficiencies at five years of age were limited to children who were delayed in reception at two years of age, or whether later communication problems were also experienced by children with specific expressive delay at age two. A further problem in interpreting the Oregon data is that communication abilities at five years of age were obtained from a parent interview instrument. Parent perceptions of their child's current abilities may well be influenced by knowledge of the child's early language delay. Consistent with this interpretation, children who were language delayed at age two in the Oregon study performed at below normal levels at age five in all domains that were derived from parent report, but were in the normal range on all objective tests (Paul *et al.*, 1993).

Bishop and Edmundson (1987) found that 30% of their sample of four-year-olds with specific and secondary language delay were more than 1.89 SDs below the mean on the Bus Story Test (Renfrew, 1969), a measure of the child's ability to tell back a simple story to pictures. However, by age 5½ the percentage of impaired children had dropped to roughly what would be expected in a normal population.

Reading. The data reviewed above indicate that children with specific expressive delay at two years of age are in the normal range on language abilities by five years of age. Is this catch-up real and lasting, or is it illusory? We have already reviewed data showing that language skills remain in the normal range through to eight years of age (Rescorla, 1993), but perhaps an underlying pathology is still present and expresses itself in other areas of development. A likely candidate for later problems is reading, which presumably draws on some of the same underlying abilities that might lead to language delay during the preschool years.

Scarborough and Dobrich (1990) argued that catch-up in five-year-olds with specific language delay is an illusion due to development occurring in alternating spurts and plateaus. If normally developing children are in a long plateau at five years of age, language delayed children may catch up, only to see their normally developing peers spurt ahead again at some future point. In support of their plateau/sleeper effects model, Scarborough and Dobrich presented follow-up data through to seven years of age for four children who did not use word combinations at 2½ years of age. Though these children caught up to normally developing age mates on most measures of language by five years of age, three of the four were delayed in reading skills at seven years of age compared to a control group of 12 normally developing children who were selected without regard to linguistic abilities and without matching to the delayed sample in any systematic way.

The Scarborough and Dobrich (1990) study has several weaknesses that prevent the data from providing more than suggestive support of their plateau/sleeper effects model. Among the limitations are the arbitrary rather than normative criteria for diagnosis of developmental language delay at age 2½, the very small sample size, a definition of abnormal sequelae of early language delay on the basis of an ad hoc normal comparison group instead of psychometrically valid norms, and the fact that the selection procedure for the language delayed children included the presence of reading problems in family members. Nevertheless, Scarborough and Dobrich's hypothesis of sleeper effects in the area of literacy for children who have previously been language delayed requires thorough evaluation. It is this possibility that is often central to the concerns of parents of young children who are late talkers. Further, many studies on language delayed preschoolers have supported a link to later problems in reading (e.g. Aram *et al.*, 1984; Aram & Nation, 1980; Fundudis *et al.*, 1980; Richman *et al.*, 1982; Silva *et al.*, 1987). Recall, however, that these studies either failed to distinguish specific from secondary language delay or found reading problems only in children who had previously had secondary language impairment (Richman *et al.*, 1982).

Two more recent investigations provide evidence against the Scarborough and Dobrich (1990) hypothesis that children with specific language delay catch up in language by five years of age, only to fall behind in reading a year or two later. In the English study, Bishop and Adams (1990) examined the literacy skills of 83 8½-year-olds whose language development had been delayed at four years of age. Language skills of the same children were examined at age 5½ (Bishop & Edmundson, 1987). Consistent with the catch-up phenomena described previously (Paul, *et al.*, 1993; Rescorla, 1993; Scarborough & Dobrich, 1990; Whitehurst *et al.*, 1992), 44% of the four-year-olds with specific language delay had no measurable language impairment by 5½ years of age. Reading outcomes at age 8½ were examined for this catch-up group, and two non catch-up groups, discriminated by whether their members had specific or secondary language delay at age four.

Bishop and Adams (1990) identified children with reading problems at age 8½ based on gaps between nonverbal IQ and reading scores, a controversial method (Stanovich, 1993). We recoded their data and identified children with reading problems based only on their reading performance being more than 1 SD below the mean. Using this criterion, the group that caught up in language by age 5½ had only 3% of its members with problems in reading accuracy at 8½ years of age, and only 7% with problems in reading comprehension. Among the group that experienced specific language delay at age four and who did not catch up by age 5½, 35% were impaired in reading accuracy and 46% were impaired in reading comprehension at 8½ years of age. The group that experienced the highest risk of reading problems at 8½ years of age consisted of the children who had secondary language delay at age four; these children did not catch up in language at age 5½; further, 63% had problems in reading accuracy and 81% had problems in reading comprehension at age 8½. Interestingly, children who were delayed in reading at 8½ years of age continued to be impaired on expressive and receptive language as well. Thus there was no sleeper effect: Children who were reading impaired at 8½ years of age were language impaired at age four, language impaired at age 5½, and language impaired at age 8½.

The second source of data on the catch up/sleeper effect hypothesis is the first wave of long-term follow-up data from the New York study. We obtained standardized test scores in reading and mathematics from the school records of 22 seven-year-olds who had been diagnosed as having severe specific expressive delay at two years of age. Figure 2 presents these data as a box-whisker plot. Notice that the median performance for the group is above average in both reading and mathematics, and that the overall distribution of scores for reading conforms almost exactly to what would be expected from the normal curve. Thus a history of specific expressive delay did not lead to heightened risk of reading difficulties, defined with respect to norms for the general population of seven-year-olds. Notice, however, that performance in mathematics was significantly higher than performance in reading. We believe this is an important result.

A tentative interpretation of the preliminary data in Fig. 2, when coupled with the low-normal range performance on language tests through to age 8 in the Pennsylvania and Oregon studies, is that some appreciable proportion of children who are diagnosed with specific expressive delay at two years of age have a chronic weakness in one or more of the mechanisms that underlie the acquisition of language and reading. This weakness rarely leads to problems during the school years of sufficient severity to be labeled as abnormal or disordered. However, it is associated with risk of under achievement in language and reading, compared to the child's trajectory in other areas of development.

The Underlying Nature of Specific Language Delay

There is no shortage of theories that seek to identify *the* underlying cognitive deficit that leads to specific developmental language impairment. In a review of the topic, Bishop (1992) lists six general approaches, many of which include several competing models. Of these, Bishop favors the view that children with specific language delays and impairments suffer from limitations in the speed and capacity of their information processing system. In many ways, this is an attractive hypothesis. For example, it can account for the differences between math and reading scores depicted in

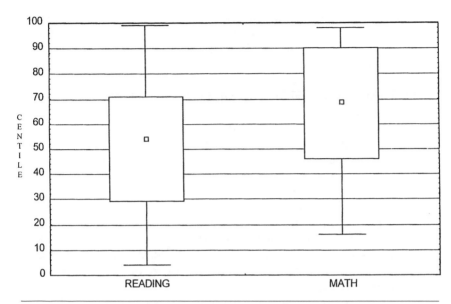

Figure 2. Performance of 22 seven-year-olds on standardized tests of reading and mathematics. These children had severe specific expressive delay at age two. Scores were converted to a standard score scale (Mean = 100, SD = 15). The small rectangle in each box is the median. Each box represents the first 25% of the subjects above and below the median. The whiskers represent the full range of scores of the sample. The difference between reading and mathematics scores is significant (t = 2.40, df = 21, p = .026).

Fig. 2 and the catch-up pattern that is characteristic of so many children with specific language delays.

Consider the mathematics/reading disparity: Reading involves the sub-task of decoding, i.e. translating letters into words, words into sentences, and so forth. Decoding is a massively parallel process that requires simultaneous recognition of letters and other units of written language in real time (Seidenberg & McClelland, 1989). Children who are relatively slow at rapid, simultaneous processing of information will presumably have more difficulty in the early stages of reading. Their reading problems might be expected to diminish over the elementary school years as the decoding process becomes more practiced and routinized (Gough, 1991). In contrast, mathematics in the early school years consists primarily of simple arithmetic computations that are less dependent on rapid processing of multiple inputs. Of course, simple arithmetic requires decoding, as does reading, but arithmetic symbols are smaller in number, much more regular, and far less dependent on context for interpretation than letters. A printed arithmetic problem sits there for contemplation. Similar contemplation of a letter disrupts the fast moving assembly process that is necessary for reading. Thus one would expect children with slow processing speed to have more difficulty in learning to read than in learning to compute.

With regard to language delays, making sense of information that arrives through the auditory channel is similar to reading in that it requires simultaneous processing of multiple inputs at rapid rates (Tallal, 1976). Also similar to the process for reading, the stress on processing mechanisms should diminish over time and the child's delay should resolve as the child gradually integrates smaller sound units (e.g. phonemes) into larger perceptual units (e.g. syllables and words). Thus children whose underlying difficulty is processing speed should be delayed as they encounter a new language acquisition task (e.g. vocabulary recognition), but should catch up as more of the processing chores become chunked and routinized. This is, of course, exactly the pattern we have described for most children with specific language delay.

Though the speed of processing hypothesis is parsimonious and is consistent with some of the salient characteristics of children with specific language delay, it fails to account for the large gap between receptive and expressive skill in children who have specific expressive delay. One would imagine that a deficiency in the speed and capacity of a child's information processing system of sufficient magnitude to cause over a year's lag in the development of expressive language at 30 months of age would also affect the comprehension of language. Yet two-year-olds with specific expressive delay test in the normal range on receptive vocabulary and are consistently described by parents as able to follow complex verbal instructions, e.g. "If you will go upstairs and get my keys off the dresser we will go to MacDonald's." Why would deficiencies in general processing speed or auditory processing speed have such a differential impact on language output?

Bishop and Edmundson (1987) offer an explanation for the preponderance of expressive problems in children with specific language impairments by suggesting that receptive language is less vulnerable than expressive language to underlying impairment. But why is receptive language less vulnerable? On another tack, Bishop (1992, p. 11) defends the processing speed hypothesis by suggesting that most children with specific language impairment also "have deficits in phonology, vocabulary and grammar even when these abilities are tested receptively without requiring speech production." But that is not true by definition for children with specific expressive delay, who are the majority among younger children with specific language delay.

The processing speed hypothesis is attractive in its parsimony, its ability to account for catch-up effects in language delayed children, and its ability to account for superior mathematics versus reading performance in second grade for children who had specific expressive delay at age two. However, this hypothesis encounters difficulties with the phenomena of early specific expressive delay. Not only does the processing speed hypothesis run up against the marked asymmetry in expression versus reception, it also fails to account for the lack of aggregation of language and reading problems in the families of these children, the heightened probability of oro-motor but not general motor problems in a significant portion of this population, and the role of otitis media in early resolving cases.

Here is not the place to attempt to resolve issues concerning the causes of developmental language delays, but it is worth noting some of the possibilities and attendant complexities. One possibility is that all forms of specific language delay might be integratable within a *unitary* model that has not yet been articulated, e.g. a revised speed of processing model that specifies why efferent pathways should be remarkably more vulnerable than afferent pathways (see Fig. 3). Such a resolution would be in keeping with much modern theorizing that sees specific language impairment as nothing more than the lower end of the normal curve of language development (Bishop, 1992; Dale & Cole, 1991; Leonard, 1988; Rutter, 1984).

A second possibility is that *specific* language delay is heterogeneous in etiology and outcome, with each symptom due to a different *specific* cause (see Fig. 3). Bishop and Edmundson (1987) reject this possibility on the basis of their demonstration of what they call a *hierarchy of vulnerability*. This term encompasses two claims for which there is considerable empirical support: (1) that components of language can be ordered hierarchically in terms of the likelihood that they will be affected in a case of language delay, i.e. expressive phonology > expressive syntax + morphology > expressive semantics > receptive language, and (2) that children who change symptoms over time will move up rather than down the hierarchy of vulnerability, e.g. moving from expressive phonological and syntactic problems at age four to exclusively phonological problems at age 5½ and not vice versa. Their point is that one would not expect to find these reliable patterns among symptoms if each symptom were due to a specific cause. However, while the data underlying the hierarchy of vulnerability support the role of some unitary deficiency in children with language delays of varying degrees of severity, they do not rule out the operation of specific factors

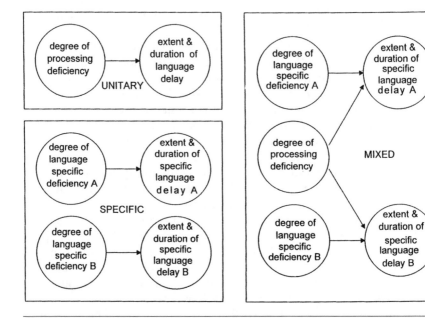

Figure 3. Three models of developmental language delay. In the unitary model, all forms of language delay are caused by the same underlying deficiency, which varies in degree. In the specific model, different symptoms of language delay (e.g. specific expressive delay vs. specific receptive–expressive delay) are caused by different underlying deficiencies. In the mixed model, children with language delay share a common deficiency, which interacts with specific weaknesses to generate specific symptoms.

as well. It is also worth noting that the frequency and patterning of language delays vary so greatly with age that data taken from one age group, e.g. four-year-olds, may have little relevance to other age groups, e.g. children whose expressive delay has resolved prior to age four.

A final possibility for future theories of the etiology of specific language delay is a *mixed* model that posits both a common weakness in children with specific language delays (e.g. slow processing speed), and additional heterogeneous factors that generate different outcomes (e.g. otitis media during a critical period for children with early resolving specific expressive delay) (see Fig. 3). In such a model the common weakness could vary in intensity and lead directly to clinical levels of delay in the extreme (e.g. mental retardation and secondary language delay in children with very slow processing speed). At milder levels, the common weakness could be a vulnerability, a predisposing factor, which when combined with one or more other influences, could generate a substantial level of delay in a specific modality (e.g. specific expressive delay). In the absence of these other factors (e.g. oro-motor weakness), or with enough time to develop compensating strategies (e.g. increased oro-motor maturity), levels of delay could fall within the normal range (e.g. low-normal reading scores contrasted with high-normal mathematics scores in previously language delayed seven-year-olds). We do not believe that current data allow a clear choice between unitary and mixed models of etiology for developmental language delays. However, we prefer the heuristic consequences of the mixed model in that it seeks to identify both how children with language delays are similar, and how they are different.

WHAT, IF ANYTHING, SHOULD THE CLINICIAN DO ABOUT SPECIFIC LANGUAGE DELAY

One recommendation that follows unambiguously from the previous review is that cases of developmental language delay need to be carefully assessed and followed. Accurate assessment affords important information about likely sequelae during the school years. In particular, poor outcomes vary directly with two factors: the generality of delay, and age at which impairments persist. Figure 4 displays these relations. The categories on the impairment axis in the figure are cumulative for most children, e.g. a child with problems in expressive semantics is also likely to have the problems that are listed prior to semantics on the axis, vocab + syntax and phonology. While the figure does not assign particular values of risk to age impairment, it does allow relative predictions. Thus a five-year-old with impaired nonverbal IQ (and by implication impairments in all of the language categories as well) would have the highest risk of poor outcomes in school, while a two-year-old with an exclusively phonological impairment would have the lowest risk.

Figure 4 and the research described previously inform but do not compel decisions concerning treatment of children with developmental language delay. All treatment decisions exist within a complex cost–benefit matrix. Among the factors that must be considered are the direct costs of treatment to parents or taxpayers, indirect costs to participants or society that might take forms such as the redirection of parental time and attention away from other children in the family, the potentially deleterious effects of labeling the child, the costs (both direct and indirect, immediate and deferred) of nontreatment, and the efficacy of available treatments. As with

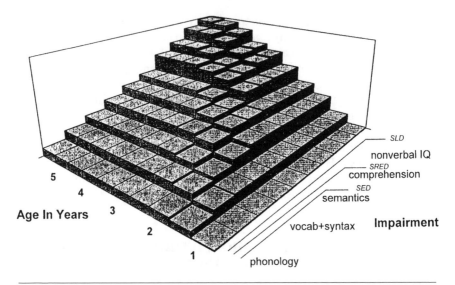

Figure 4. A risk surface for predicting poor outcomes in school from preschool developmental language delay. Long-term risks rise with age and degree of impairment. Forms of impairment are listed by specific language form (e.g. phonology) and are grouped into specific expressive delay (SED), specific receptive–expressive delay (SRED) and secondary language delay (SLD).

the risk surface depicted in Fig. 4, only relative weights can be derived. For example, nearly everyone would agree that an inexpensive, demonstrably effective treatment for five-year-olds with specific receptive-expressive delay would be more justifiable than an expensive treatment of unproven effectiveness for two-year-olds with specific expressive delay.

Going beyond ranking of treatment in terms of relative costs and benefits to decisions about where to draw the line on treatment of individual cases is highly subjective. Informed professionals can and do differ. For example, Paul *et al.* (1993, p. 3) describe the Oregon children who had specific language delay at age two as scoring "at the low end of the *normal range* [emphasis added] in most expressive language skills, as well as reading readiness" at age five. They then conclude that "the need for preventive intervention at the preschool or kindergarten level . . . is indicated, in order to increase their chances for success in school." In contrast, Whitehurst *et al.* (1991, p. 68), commenting on similar findings from children in the New York study, conclude that "most two-year-olds with [specific expressive delay] . . . will eventually achieve normal levels of expressive development without special help." Paul *et al.* (1993) see performance in the low normal range as warranting intervention, while Whitehurst *et al.* (1991) do not. One cannot say that we are right and Paul is wrong, or vice versa, only that the cost-benefit matrix is different for the two positions.

Comparison of Treatments

If a parent or professional is inclined to consider developmental language delays worthy of treatment, how should treatment be delivered and to whom? One typical treatment for specific language delay involves placement in a therapeutic school environment that combines milieu therapy (Cole, Dale & Mills, 1990: Haynes & Naidoo, 1991; Warren & Kaiser, 1988) with occasional one-on-one speech therapy. Another typical treatment involves weekly in-office treatment by a private speech clinician. A third form of treatment, also milieu based, occurs in the home, using the parent as the agent of change (Whitehurst *et al.*, 1991; Zelazo, Kearsley & Ungerer, 1984). We know of no systematic comparative study of such treatments, and no well-designed studies of any of these therapies that have used measures of school success as outcomes. Note that there are many studies showing that specific speech and language teaching procedures can lead to the child's acquisition of particular language forms (see reviews by Leonard, 1981, and Warren and Kaiser, 1988). An important question, however, is whether such specific instruction has any measurable long-term benefit for the child.

Few early interventions for handicapping conditions have been the subject of outcome research (Fischel, 1985), so there is nothing remarkable about the absence of data on the effectiveness of preschool-based treatment of developmental language delays. However, there are reasons to be cautious about the long-term efficacy of speech and language therapy. Aram and Nation (1980) found no relation between involvement in preschool intervention for speech and language problems and the occurrence of problems for children during their school years. Bishop and Edmundson (1987) found that language outcomes for a group of preschool language impaired children could be predicted from the severity of the child's initial impairment, but not from the amount of therapy the child had received. Cantwell (1987) reported similar findings. We found no correlation between progress in expressive language for two-year-olds with specific expressive delay and involvement in typical community-based speech therapy (Whitehurst *et al.*, 1991). Long-term follow-up of children in our home-based treatment for two-year-olds with specific expressive delay was not encouraging: While the intervention and the control group differed in both clinical and statistical terms at the end of the five-month treatment period, there were no longer any significant differences between the groups by 3½ years of age, primarily because by that age nearly all of children in the control group had resolved the problems in expressive language that had been the target of their intervention.

As a practical matter, it is very difficult to demonstrate long-term effects for preschool interventions for specific language delays given the very high rates of spontaneous resolution for all forms of language delays that we have previously documented as occurring throughout the preschool period. We believe that interventions for those categories of delay and ages of child with high remission rates (see Fig. 4) may be justifiable if (1) they improve the child's current level of functioning and reduce anxieties and stress within the child's family, and (2) the purchaser of the intervention (parent or public) understands that it is these short-term outcomes they are buying.

If the definition of expected benefits shifts from short-term relief to the reduction of long-term risks of impairment, then we would restrict treatment of children under four years of age to those with secondary language delays (e.g. mentally retarded children or children suffering from severe environmental deprivation). We would restrict treatment of four- and five-year-olds to those with secondary language delays and those with specific receptive–expressive delays that include difficulties with comprehension. We would not treat children with exclusively phonological problems until age five or six, unless those problems were interfering substantially with social development. Our treatment of choice for most forms of language delay, specific or secondary, would be a milieu therapy (Warren & Kaiser, 1986; Whitehurst *et al.*, 1991; Zelazo *et al.*, 1984), home or preschool based, that takes advantage of full day teaching opportunities in the child's natural environment. Therapy for language delayed children with oppositional behavior or hyperactivity-attention deficit problems should include a strong behavior management component (e.g. Webster-Stratton, 1984). We see no evidence that children with secondary language delay need or benefit from milieu therapies any more or less than children with specific language delay (Cole, *et al.*, 1990).

In general, all children, even those with superior language skills, can benefit from an environment that affords frequent opportunities for responsive verbal interaction with an adult over content that is appropriately challenging to the child (e.g. Whitehurst *et al.*, 1988). However, public policy generally restricts expenditures for early interventions to children who are thought to need such help to achieve normal levels of functioning in school and later life. Children under the age of five with specific expressive lan-

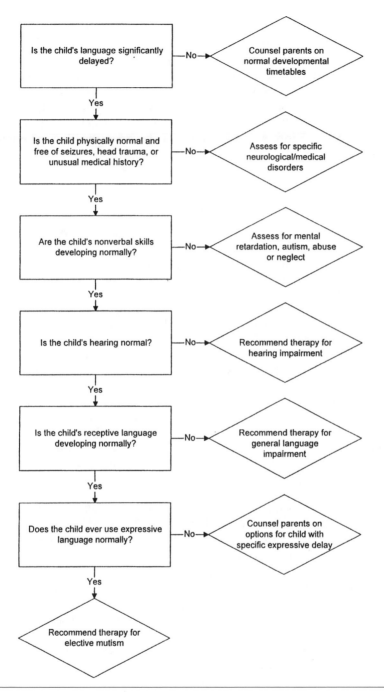

Figure 5. A decision tree for evaluating developmental delay from the perspective of reducing long term risks.

guage delay have relatively low risk of later language or reading impairments, with or without treatment. In contrast, children with secondary language delay and children with specific receptive–expressive delay that persists to age four are at risk of later problems. We believe that demonstrably effective early interventions for these children are badly needed and justify public support. A decision tree based on the reduction of long-term risks of language and reading disorders is presented in Fig. 5.

REFERENCES

Aram, D. M., Ekelman, B. L. & Nation, J. E. (1984). Preschoolers with language disorders: 10 years later. *Journal of Speech and Hearing Research*, **27**, 232–244.

Aram, D. M. & Nation, J. E. (1980). Preschool language disorders and subsequent language and academic difficulties. *Journal of Communication Disorders*, **13**, 159–170.

Baker, L. & Cantwell, D. P. (1982a). Developmental, social and behavioral characteristics of speech and language disordered children. *Child Psychiatry and Human Development*, **12**, 195–206.

Baker, L. & Cantwell, D. P. (1982b). Psychiatric disorders in children with different types of communication disorders. *Journal of Communication Disorders*, **15**, 113–126.

Beitchman, J. H., Nair, R., Clegg, M., Ferguson, B. & Patel, P. G. (1986). Prevalence of psychiatric disorders in children with speech and language disorders. *Journal of the American Academy of Child Psychiatry*, **25**, 528–535.

Bellugi, U., Marks, S., Bihrle, A. & Sabo, H. (1988). Dissociation between language and cognitive functions in Williams syndrome. In D. V. M. Bishop & K. Mogford (Eds), *Language development in exceptional circumstances* (pp. 177–189). Edinburgh: Churchill Livingstone.

Bess, F. H. (1983). Hearing loss associated with middle ear effusion. Workshop on effects of otitis media on the child. *Pediatrics*, **71**, 639–652.

Bishop, D. V. M. (1990). Handedness, clumsiness and developmental language disorders. *Neuropsychologia*, **28**, 681–690.

Bishop, D. V. M. (1991). The biological basis of specific language impairment. In P. Fletcher (Ed.), *Specific speech and language disorders in children*. London: Whurr.

Bishop, D. V. M. (1992). The underlying nature of specific language impairment. *Journal of Child Psychology and Psychiatry*, **33**, 3–66.

Bishop, D. V. M. & Adams, C. (1990). A prospective study of the relationship between specific language impairment, phonological disorders and reading retardation. *Journal of Child Psychology and Psychiatry*, **31**, 1027–1050.

Bishop, D. V. M. & Edmundson, A. (1986). Is otitis media a major cause of specific developmental language disorders? *British Journal of Disorders of Communication*, **21**, 321–338.

Bishop, D. V. M. & Edmundson, A. (1987). Language-impaired 4-year-olds: distinguishing transient from persistent impairment. *Journal of Speech and Hearing Disorders*, **52**, 156–173.

Blager, F. B. (1981). Speech and language evaluation. In W. K. Frankenburg, S. M. Thornton & M. E. Cohrs (Eds), *Pediatric developmental diagnosis* (pp. 79–93). New York: Thieme-Stratton.

Bradley, L. & Bryant, P. E. (1985). *Rhyme and reason in reading and spelling.* Ann Arbor: University of Michigan Press.

Buium, N., Rynders, J. & Turnure, J. (1974). Early maternal linguistic environment of normal and Down's syndrome language-learning children. *American Journal of Mental Deficiency*, **79**, 52–58.

Cantwell, D. (1987, November). *Children with communication disorders—a group at psychiatric risk.* Presented at Psychiatry Grand Rounds, State University of New York, Stony Brook NY.

Cantwell, D. P. & Baker, L. (1980). Psychiatric and behavioral characteristics of children with communication disorders. *Journal of Pediatric Psychology*, **5**, 161–178.

Catts, H. W. (1993). The relationship between speech-language impairments and reading disabilities. *Journal of Speech and Hearing Research*, **36**, 948–958.

Caulfield, M. B. (1989). Communication difficulty: a model of the relation of language delay and behavior problems. *Society for Research in Child Development Abstracts*, **7**, 212.

Caulfield, M. B., Fischel, J. E., DeBaryshe, B. D. & Whitehurst, G. J. (1989). Behavioral correlates of developmental expressive language disorder. *Journal of Abnormal Child Psychology*, **17**, 187–201.

Cohen, S. E., Parmelee, A. H., Sigman, M. & Beckwith, L. (1988). Antecedents of school problems in children born preterm. *Journal of Pediatric Psychology*, **13**, 493–508.

Cole, K. N., Dale, P. S. & Mills, P. (1990). Defining language delay in young children by cognitive referencing: are we saying more than we know? *Applied Psycholinguistics*, **11**, 291–302.

Conti-Ramsen, C. & Friel-Patti, S. (1983). Mothers' discourse adjustments to language-impaired and nonlanguage-impaired children. *Journal of Speech and Hearing Disorders*, **48**, 360–367.

Cowley, J. & Glasgow, C. (1993). *The Renfrew bus story—U.S. edition.* Wilmington, D.E.: authors.

Cromer, R. (1988). The cognitive hypothesis revisited. In F. Kessel (Ed.), *The development of language and language researchers.* Hillsdale, N. J.: LEA.

Cunningham, C. E., Siegel, L. S., van der Spuy, H. I. J., Clark, M. L. & Bow, S. J. (1985). The behavioral and linguistic interactions of specifically language-delayed and normal boys with their mothers. *Child Development*, **56**, 1389–1403.

Dale, P. S. & Cole, K. N. (1991). What's normal? SLI in an individual differences perspective. *Language, speech, and hearing services in schools*, **22**, 80–83.

Dingman, H. F. & Tarjan, G. (1960). Mental retardation and the normal distribution curve. *American Journal of Mental Deficiency*, **64**, 991–994.

Dunn, L. M. & Dunn, L. M. (1983). *Peabody picture vocabulary test—revised (PPVT—R)*. Circle Pines, MN: American Guidance Service.

Fenson, L., Dale, P. S., Reznick, J. S., Thal, D., Bates, E., Hartung, J., Pethick, S. & Reilly, J. S. (1993). *Researcher's Guide and Technical Manual for the MacArthur Communicative Development Inventories*. San Diego, CA: Singular Press.

Fischel, J. E. (1985). Infant intervention: an examination of methods and efficacy. In G. J. Whitehurst (Ed.), *Annals of child development, Vol. 2* (pp. 161–194). Greenwich, CT: JAI Press.

Fischel, J. E., Whitehurst, G. J., Caulfield, M. B. & DeBaryshe, B. D. (1989). Language growth in children with expressive language delay. *Pediatrics*, **82**, 218–227.

Fundudis, T., Kolvin, I. & Garside, R. F. (1979). *Speech retarded children: their psychological development*. London: Academic Press.

Fundudis, T., Kolvin, I. & Garside, R. F. (1980). A follow-up of speech retarded children. In L. A. Hersov, M. Berger, & A. R. Nichol (Eds), *Language and language disorders in childhood*. New York: Pergamon Press.

Gardner, M. F. (1990). *Expressive one-word picture vocabulary test—revised*. Novato, CA: Academic Therapy Publications.

Gough, P. B. (1991). The complexity of reading. In R. R. Hoffman & D. S. Palermo (Eds), *Cognition and the symbolic processes* (pp. 141–149). Hillsdale, NJ: LEA.

Haynes, C. & Naidoo, S. (1991). *Children with specific speech and language impairment*. London: MacKeith Press.

Howie, V. M. (1980). Developmental sequelae of chronic otitis media: a review. *Developmental and Behavioral Pediatrics*, **1**, 34–38.

Jenkins, S., Bax, M. & Hart, H. (1980). Behaviour problems in pre-school children. *Journal of Child Psychology and Psychiatry*, **21**, 5–17.

Kaler, S. R. & Kopp, C. B. (1990). Compliance and comprehension in very young toddlers. *Child Development*, **61**, 1997–2003.

Kirk, S. A., McCarthy, J. J. & Kirk, W. D. (1968). *Illinois test of psycholinguistic abilities*. Urbana, IL: University of Illinois Press.

Klackenberg, G. (1980). What happens to children with retarded speech at 3? Longitudinal study of a sample of normal infants up to 20 years of age. *Acta Paediatrica Scandinavia*, **69**, 681–685.

Knobloch, H. & Pasamanick, B. (1974). *Gesell and Amatruda's Developmental Diagnosis* (3rd Ed.). New York: Harper & Row.

Leonard, L. B. (1981). Facilitating linguistic skills in children with specific language impairment. *Applied Psycholinguistics*, **2**, 89–118.

Leonard, L. B. (1988). Is specific language impairment a useful construct? In S. Rosenberg (Ed.), *Advances in applied psycholinguistics* (pp. 1–39). Cambridge, England: Cambridge University Press.

Lloyd, P. & Beveridge, M. (1981). *Information and meaning in child communication.* London: Academic Press.

Lonigan, C. J., Fischel, J. E., Whitehurst, G. J., Arnold, D. S. & Valdez-Menchaca, M. C. (1992). The role of otitis media in the development of expressive language delay. *Developmental Psychology*, **28**, 430–440.

Ludlow, C. L. & Cooper, J. A. (Eds) (1983). *Genetic aspects of speech and language disorders.* New York: Academic Press.

Magnusson, E. & Naucler, K. (1990). Reading and spelling in language-disordered children—linguistic and metalinguistic prerequisites: report on a longitudinal study. *Clinical Linguistics & Phonetics*, **4**, 49–61.

Marshall, N., Hegrenes, J. & Goldstein, S. (1973). Verbal interactions: mothers and their retarded children versus mothers and their nonretarded children. *American Journal of Mental Deficiency*, **77**, 415–419.

Mednick, S. A., Schulsinger, F., Higgins, J. & Bell, B. (1974). *Genetics, environment and psychopathology.* Amsterdam: North Holland/Elsevier.

Newsday (1993). Suffolk's sane way to trim handicapped pre-K bills. April 19, author.

Paul, R. (1991). Profiles of toddlers with slow expressive language development. *Topics in Language Disorders*, **11**, 1–13.

Paul, R. & Elwood, T. J. (1991). Maternal linguistic input to toddlers with slow expressive language development. *Journal of Speech and Hearing Research*, **34**, 982–988.

Paul, R. & James, D. (1990). Language delay and parental perceptions. *Journal of the American Academy of Child and Adolescent Psychiatry*, **29**, 669–670.

Paul, R. & Jennings, P. (1992). Phonological behavior in toddlers with slow expressive language development. *Journal of Speech and Hearing Research*, **35**, 99–107.

Paul, R., Laszio, C. M., McFarland, L. S. & Midford, N. (1993). Language outcomes in late-talkers: kindergarten. *Society for Research in Child Development Abstracts*, **9**, 534.

Paul, R. & Shiffer, M. (1991). Expression of communicative intentions in normal and 'late talking' young children. *Applied Psycholinguistics*, **12**, 419–431.

Petersen, G. A. & Sherrod, K. B. (1982). Relationship of maternal language to language development and language delay of children. *American Journal of Mental Deficiency*, **86**, 391–398.

Plomin, R., DeFries, J. C. & Fulker, D. W. (1988). *Nature and nurture during infancy and early childhood.* New York: Cambridge.

Renfrew, C. E. (1969). *The bus story: a test of continuous speech.* Oxford, U.K.: Author.

Rescorla, L. (1989). The language development survey: a screening tool for delayed language in toddlers. *Journal of Speech and Hearing Disorders,* **54**, 587–599.

Rescorla, L. (1993). Outcome of toddlers with specific expressive delay (SELD) at ages 3, 4, 5, 6, 7, & 8. *Society for Research in Child Development Abstracts,* **9**, 566.

Rescorla, L. & Schwartz, E. (1990). Outcome of specific language delay (SELD). *Applied Psycholinguistics,* **11**, 393–408.

Reynell, J. K. (1969). *Reynell developmental language scales. Experimental Edition.* Windsor, England: NFER-Nelson.

Reynell, J. K. (1977). *Reynell developmental language scales (revised).* Windsor, England: NFER-Nelson.

Reynell, J. K. (1985). *Reynell developmental language scales (second revision).* Windsor, England: NFER-Nelson.

Richman, N. & Stevenson, J. (1977). Language delay in 3-year-olds. *Acta Pediatricia Belgium,* **30**, 213–219.

Richman, N., Stevenson, J. & Graham, P. (1982). *Preschool to school: A behavioural study.* London: Academic Press.

Rutter, M. (1984). Issues and prospects in developmental neuropsychiatry. In M. Rutter (Ed.), *Developmental neuropsychiatry.* Edinburgh: Churchill Livingstone.

Rutter, M. & Mawhood, L. (1991). The long-term psychosocial sequelae of specific developmental disorders of speech and language. In M. Rutter & P. Casaer (Eds), *Biological risk factors for psychosocial disorders* (pp. 233–259). Cambridge: Cambridge University Press.

Scarborough, H. (1990). Index of Productive Syntax. *Applied Psycholinguistics,* **11**, 1–22.

Scarborough, H. S. & Dobrich, W. (1990). Development of children with early language delay. *Journal of Speech and Hearing Disorders,* **33**, 70–83.

Seidenberg, M. S. & McClelland, J. E. (1989). A distributed, developmental model of word recognition and naming. *Psychological Review,* **96**, 523–568.

Silva, P. A. (1980). The prevalence, stability and significance of developmental language delay in preschool children. *Developmental Medicine and Child Neurology,* **22**, 768–777.

Silva, P. A., Williams, S. & McGee, R. (1987). A longitudinal study of children with developmental language delay at age three: later intelligence, reading and behavior problems. *Developmental Medicine and Child Neurology,* **259**, 630–640.

Sparrow, S., Bella, D. & Ciccetti, D. (1984). *Vineland Adaptive Behavior Scales.* Minneapolis, MN: American Guidance Service.

Springer, S. P. & Deutsch, G. (1989). *Left brain, right brain.* New York: W. H. Freeman.

Stanovich, K. (1993). A model for studies of reading disability. *Developmental Review*, **13**, 225–245.

Stark, R. E. & Tallal, P. (1981). Selection of children with specific language deficits. *Journal of Speech and Hearing Disorders*, **46**, 14–122.

Stevenson, J. & Richman, N. (1976). The prevalence of language delay in a population of three-year-old children and its association with general retardation. *Developmental Medicine and Child Neurology*, **18**, 431–441. Stoel-Gammon, C. (1991). Normal and disordered phonology in two-year-olds. *Topics in Language Disorders*, **11**, 21–32.

Tallal, P. (1976). Rapid auditory processing in normal and disordered language development. *Journal of Speech and Hearing Research*, **19**, 561–571.

Tallal, P., Ross, R. & Curtiss, S. (1989). Familial aggregation in specific language impairment. *Journal of Speech and Hearing Disorders*, **54**, 167–173.

Teele, D. W., Klein, J. O. & Rosner, B. A. (1980). Epidemiology of otitis media in children. *Annals of Otology, Rhinology and Laryngology*, **89**, 5–6.

Templin, M. & Darley, F. (1968). *Templin–Darley tests of articulation* (2nd Edn.). Iowa City, IA: University of Iowa Bureau of Educational Research and Service.

Thal, D., Tobias, S. & Morrison, D. (1991). Language and gesture in late talkers: a 1-year follow-up. *Journal of Speech and Hearing Research*, **34**, 604–612.

Thorndike, R. L., Hagen, E. P. & Sattler, J. M. (1986). *Stanford–Binet intelligence scale: fourth edition.* Chicago: Riverside Publishing Company.

Warren, S. F. & Kaiser, A. P. (1986). Incidental language teaching: a critical review. *Journal of Speech and Hearing Disorders*, **51**, 291–299.

Warren, S. F. & Kaiser, A. P. (1988). Research in early language intervention. In S. L. Odom & M. B. Karnes (Eds), *Early intervention for infants and children with handicaps: an empirical base* (pp. 89–108). Baltimore: Paul H. Brookes.

Webster-Stratton, C. (1984). Randomized trial of two parent-training programs for families with conduct disordered children. *Journal of Consulting and Clinical Psychology*, **52**, 666–678.

Wender, P. H., Rosenthal, D., Kety, S. S., Schulsinger, F. & Welner, J. (1974). Cross-fostering: a research strategy for clarifying the role of genetic and experiential factors in the etiology of schizophrenia. *Archives of General Psychiatry*, **30**, 318–325.

Whitehurst, G. J., Arnold, D. S., Epstein, J. N., Angell, A. L., Smith, M. & Fischel, J. E. (1993). A picture book intervention in daycare and home for children from low-income families. *Society for Research in Child Development Abstracts*, **9**, 219.

Whitehurst, G. J., Arnold, D. S., Smith, M., Fischel, J. E., Lonigan, C. J. & Valdez-Menchaca, M. C. (1991). Family history in developmental expressive language delay. *Journal of Speech and Hearing Research*, **34**, 150–157.

Whitehurst, G. J., Epstein, Angell, A., Payne, A., Crone, D. & Fischel, J. E. (1993). *An emergent literacy curriculum for Head Start: first year outcomes.* Showcase presentation, Second National Head Start Research Conference, Washington, D.C.

Whitehurst, G. J., Falco, F. L., Lonigan, C., Fischel, J. E., Valdez-Menchaca, M. C., Debaryshe, B. D. & Caulfield, M. (1988). Accelerating language development through picture-book reading. *Developmental Psychology*, **24**, 552–558.

Whitehurst, G. J., Fischel, J. E., Arnold, D. S., & Lonigan, C. J. (1992). Evaluating outcomes with children with expressive language delay. In S. F. Warren & J. Reichle (Eds), *Causes and effects in communication and language intervention, Vol. 1* (pp. 277–313). Baltimore: MD: Brookes Publishing.

Whitehurst, G. J., Fischel, J. E., Lonigan, C. J., Valdez-Menchaca, M. V., Arnold, D. S. & Smith, M. (1991). Treatment of early expressive language delay: if, when and how. *Topics in Language Disorders*, **11**, 55–68.

Whitehurst, G. J., Fischel, J. E., Lonigan, C. J., Valdez-Menchaca, M. C., DeBaryshe, B. D. & Caulfield, M. B. (1988). Verbal interaction in families of normal and expressive language delayed children. *Developmental Psychology*, **24**, 690–699.

Whitehurst, G. J., Smith, M., Fischel, J. E., Arnold, D. S. & Lonigan, C. J. (1991). The continuity of babble and speech in children with expressive language delay. *Journal of Speech and Hearing Research*, **34**, 1121–1129.

Whitehurst, G. J. & Sonnenschein, S. (1985). The development of communication: a functional analysis. *Annals of child development*, **2**, 1–48.

Wulbert, M., Inglis, S., Kriegsmann, E. & Mills (B.). Language delay and associated mother-child interaction. *Developmental Psychology*, **11**, 61–70.

Zajonc, R. B. (1976). Family configuration and intelligence. *Science*, **192**, 227–236.

Zelazo, P. R., Kearsley, R. B. & Ungerer, J. A. (1984). *Learning to speak: a manual for parents.* Hillsdale, NJ: LEA.

10

Interviewing Prepubertal Children about Suicidal Ideation and Behavior

Leslie K. Jacobsen, Ilene Rabinowitz, Michele S. Popper,
Robert J. Solomon, Mae S. Sokol,
and Cynthia R. Pfeffer
The New York Hospital-Cornell Medical Center,
Westchester Division, White Plains, New York

Objective: *Much of the literature on assessment of suicidal children has focused on identifying risk factors associated with suicidal ideation and behavior in this population. Unique problems encountered in interviewing prepubertal children about suicidal ideation and behavior are examined in this paper.* **Method:** *Observations of problems encountered in interviewing prepubertal children about suicidal ideation and behavior were gleaned in the context of interviews of children admitted to a child psychiatry inpatient unit and interviews of the parents of these children.* **Results:** *Unique problems include difficulties in assessment of suicidal intent, impact of cognitive development, particularly of the concept of death, interaction between current emotional state and memory of previous suicidal episodes, characteristics of play associated with suicidal states, effects of parents' attitudes toward assessment on information gathering, and the impact of certain risk factors on cognition and behavior during the interview.* **Conclusion:** *Interviewing children about suicidal ideation and behavior necessitates that the clinician attend to multiple elements of the interview simultaneously. These interviews are further complicated by the stressful thoughts and feelings that can be raised in both clinician and child in reaction to exploring the child's suicidal*

Reprinted with permission from the *Journal of the American Academy of Child and Adolescent Psychiatry*, 1994, Vol. 33(4), 439–452. Copyright © 1994 by the American Academy of Child and Adolescent Psychiatry.

This work was performed at The New York Hospital-Westchester Division.

ideation and behavior. Additional research is needed to refine the process of reliable interviewing of children about suicidal ideation and behavior and to develop instruments both to quantitate the different elements of these interviews and to guide the clinicians conducting them.

The growing incidence of suicide and attempted suicide among young people is concerning. In 1991, 266 children between 5 and 14 years old committed suicide in the United States (National Center for Health Statistics, 1993). This reflects an age-specific mortality rate for suicide of 0.7 per 100,000. The incidence of suicidal ideation and suicide attempts among children has been found to be even higher, however. Investigators studying community samples of normal children and adolescents have observed rates of suicidal ideation ranging between 6.6% (Kashani et al., 1989) and 26% (Velez and Cohen, 1988) and rates of suicide attempts ranging between 2.8% (Kashani et al., 1989) and 3.4% (Velez and Cohen, 1988). Among children undergoing psychiatric treatment the prevalence of suicidal ideation and the prevalence of suicide attempts has been found to be 20.5% and 12.8%, respectively, in outpatients (Pfeffer et al., 1980) and 52.3% and 26.2% in inpatients (Pfeffer et al., 1982).

These numbers indicate that many clinicians who work with children will encounter children who are suicidal. That detection of suicidal ideation and behavior is fundamental to suicide prevention underscores the importance of the clinician's ability to elicit these symptoms from children and to talk about them with the children and their parents. Much of the literature on assessment of suicidal children has focused on identifying risk factors associated with suicidal ideation and behavior in this population (Brent, 1987; Carlson and Cantwell, 1982; Cohen-Sandler et al., 1982; Kazdin et al., 1983b; Kovacs et al., 1993; Pfeffer, 1989; Pfeffer et al., 1992, 1993a; Robbins and Alessi, 1985). Yet, to date, few papers have gone beyond this to discuss the unique problems encountered in interviewing children about suicidal ideation and behavior, such as the problem of assessing suicidal intent; the impact of the child's level of cognitive development, particularly his or her concept of death, on the interview; the interaction between the child's current emotional state and what the child recalls of previous suicidal episodes; the role of specific characteristics of the child's play associated with suicidal ideation and behavior; the effects of parents' attitudes toward the assessment on information gathering; and the impact that certain risk factors can have on the child's cognition and behavior during the interview. The potential complexity and difficulty of these interviews is perhaps best suggested by the following vignette.

Mark, an 11-year-old depressed boy, was transferred to a child psychiatry inpatient unit from a pediatric intensive care unit after he made a serious suicide attempt by ingesting his 1-week supply of imipramine tablets. His outpatient psychiatrist and family reported no known history of suicidal behavior. Upon review of his pediatric record, however, it was learned that at age 3 years he drank some Clorox bleach "which he mistook for water." Recently he had taped several GI Joe dolls at their necks to the wall of his bedroom at home. Over the course of several interviews, the boy gradually began to talk about long-standing suicidal thoughts.

The goal of this paper is to discuss some fundamental complexities of interviewing prepubertal children about suicidal ideation and behavior. The importance of these complexities was highlighted in a study involving multiple semistructured interviews of 39 prepubertal children aged 6 to 12 years admitted to the child psychiatry inpatient unit of The New York Hospital-Westchester Division, and interviews of the parents of these children. These interviews focused on identifying and characterizing previous and current suicidal ideation and behavior in the children.

ASSESSMENT OF SUICIDAL INTENT

In the assessment of suicidal ideation and behavior, establishing the presence and quantifying the degree of suicidal intent is essential, yet complex. Degree of suicidal intent reflects a balance between the wish to die and the wish to live (Beck et al., 1974). The importance of suicidal intent as a measurable component of suicidal episodes in adults has been suggested by its positive correlation with medical lethality (Beck et al., 1975) and its value as a prognosticator of future completed suicide (Pierce, 1977, 1981). In children, suicidal intent has been found to be positively correlated with hopelessness (Kazdin et al., 1983b).

Linehan (1986) highlighted the variability with which suicidal intent is measured. Some authors (Dorpat and Boswell, 1963) have used the medical consequences of individuals' suicidal acts as an indirect measure of their intent to die. However, suicidal intent and medical lethality have been shown to be two distinct dimensions of suicidal behavior (Beck et al., 1975).

Scales developed by Beck et al. (1974) to quantify suicidal intent in adults take into account the intensity and duration of the individual's wish to die and the degree to which that wish exceeds the wish to live, as well as the circumstances, thoughts, and feelings associated with suicidal behavior. Although these scales have been used infrequently in individuals below the age of 18, one study (Brent, 1987) in which the charts of 107 adolescent and 23 child psychiatric inpatients who had made suicide attempts were reviewed, found a significant positive correlation between the level of suicidal intent and the lethality of suicide attempt. This was similar to the relationship between level of suicidal intent and lethality of suicide attempt that Beck et al. (1975) observed in adults. Alternatively, a recent study conducted by Kingsbury (1993), in which adolescents 13 to 18 years of age were interviewed using the Beck Suicide Intent Scale shortly after they attempted suicide, found that the adolescents' reports about their suicidal intent were only weakly correlated with the lethality of their actions. Kingsbury (1993) suggested that this low correlation may reflect deficiencies in adolescents' ability to accurately assess potential consequences of different suicidal behaviors in the context of the heightened affect surrounding a suicide attempt. This finding indicates that if Brent (1987) had interviewed his child and adolescent subjects at the time of their suicide attempts, rather than gleaning his data from charting done over the course of his subjects' hospitalizations, he too might have observed a lower correlation between suicidal intent and lethality of suicide attempt.

Direct clinical observation of children has suggested that they also may vary in their level of understanding of the potential lethality of different suicidal acts, even in the absence of heightened affective states (Pfeffer, 1986). Thus, failure of a child to perform a highly lethal suicide attempt could occur even in the presence of significant suicidal intent. For example, it is not unlikely that a 5-year-old child with intent to die might also believe that ingesting two aspirins would be lethal.

Another complexity in understanding suicidal intent is the related but distinct concept of motivation. Wishful thoughts motivating suicidal intent in children have been amply described. These include the wish to gain more attention or otherwise effect change in the environment as a result of committing suicide, the wish for reunion with a lost loved person, the wish to escape from an intolerable situation, and the wish for revenge (Ackerly, 1967; Bender and Schilder, 1937; Lukianowicz, 1968).

The following vignette is an example of a child who had intent to die, as well as motivation both propelling and inhibiting her intent to end her life.

Judith was an 8-year-old girl who was admitted to a psychiatric inpatient unit after she threatened to kill herself with a butter knife. She was found by her mother standing alone in the kitchen one evening with a knife held up to her chest, emphatically stating "I want to kill myself." Later, when asked about her understanding of the potential lethality of her actions, Judith indicated her conviction that she could kill herself with a butter knife. She added, "I couldn't tell people that I wanted to kill myself, then I would be a bad girl. My family loves me, I would break their hearts. I'm the oldest. I'm supposed to take care of my sister and brother. My mother would be worried too. I took care of her."

Judith's home environment was a stressful one. She was the eldest child living at home with her mother, who was depressed and unable to care for her children. Her desire to escape from this situation motivated Judith to think of suicide. Judith provides an example of a child who was able to talk about her suicidal intent as well as the factors mitigating that intent, such as her strong sense of familial obligation and her desire to avoid hurting her family.

Thus, the assessment of suicidal intent in children necessitates an understanding of three components: the child's understanding of the potential lethality of a given suicidal act, the actual medical lethality of the suicidal act, and the motives for the suicidal act.

IMPACT OF THE CHILD'S LEVEL
OF COGNITIVE DEVELOPMENT ON THE INTERVIEW

Communicating with prepubertal children about suicidal ideation and behavior requires an appreciation of the complexity and diversity of their cognitive development. In particular, the degree of development of children's verbal skills and concepts of time, causality, and death significantly impacts what they communicate to clinicians. The 6- to 12-year age group potentially includes children in the following Piagetian stages of cognitive development: preoperations, concrete operations, and formal operations (Piaget and Inhelder, 1969). In addition to the broad range of levels of cognitive development that may be encountered in this age group, clinicians must contend with the fact that children acquire specific cognitive skills over a range of ages, such that normal children of a given age can exhibit different levels of cognitive development (Lewis and Volkmar, 1990). Thus, clinicians assessing children for the presence of suicidal ideation and behavior cannot rely on age alone to tell them how and what a child will be able to communicate.

Further complicating the clinician's task, children's grasp of cognitive skills may fluctuate in the context of emotional distress or physical illness. A dramatic example of this effect was reported by Anna Freud (1951), who noted that some children, particularly those with recently developed verbal skills, lost their ability to speak when separated from their mothers. More recently, Terr (1985) has observed a loss of developmental achievements, such as basic trust of others and the ability to be autonomous, in children stressed by trauma. Communicating with a clinician about previous or current suicidal ideation or behavior can be highly stressful for children and may thus render them susceptible to temporary loss of cognitive skills. Children whose cognitive skills are temporarily compromised or are poorly developed to begin with may have difficulty communicating about suicidal ideation and behavior, raising the risk that their suicidal ideation and behavior may go undetected. To address this risk, clinicians may choose to act conservatively, to ensure the safety of the child, when making disposition and treatment decisions involving developmentally delayed or regressed children who do not report suicidal ideation or behavior.

The following vignette illustrates an interview with a child whose verbal skills were limited, as was her mastery of the concept of time. Implications for the clinicians are discussed.

Brenda was a 6-year-old girl who was admitted to a psychiatric inpatient unit after she injured her brother with a sharp toy and cut herself twice with a knife. Verbal communication was limited not only as a result of her young age, but also by the fact that her first language was not the same as that of the interviewer's. Despite this, after several sessions Brenda was able to refer to her self-destructive behavior.

When asked whether she ever thought about killing herself, Brenda replied, "No. Yes. When I'm angry I do like this." Brenda hit her head softly with her fist. The interviewer then asked Brenda whether she thought about killing herself often, and Brenda answered, "Yes. No. Sometimes."

Although Brenda's undeveloped verbal skills limited the degree to which she could respond to the interviewer in words, her behavior during the interview offered much information. For example, her ability to use hand motions in response to the question about thoughts of killing herself was an important substitute for verbal communication, and it belied her tendency toward self-directed aggression. The importance of asking direct questions about suicidal ideation and behavior even in the context of interviewing children with abnormal cognitive development is highlighted by this vignette: such questions are often readily understood by children and can elicit important information about their potential for suicidal states.

Brenda's answer to the question about the frequency of her thoughts about killing herself suggests that she does not yet understand the concept of frequency, a complete understanding of which is part of a mature concept of time (Piaget, 1969). While Piaget (1969) and Piaget and Inhelder (1971) found evidence that children develop a mature concept of time at approximately the age of 9, other investigators (Fraisse, 1963; Friedman, 1978; Voyat, 1977) have found that important elements of this concept are not consistently mastered until later ages. Determining the frequency of suicidal ideation and behavior enables the clinician to make the important distinction between stable, persistent symptoms and transient ones. Obtaining reliable information from children about the frequency of their symptoms can be facilitated by formulating questions in a more concrete fashion, such as, "Do you think about killing yourself more than once or twice a day?" Similarly, using events as references may help children provide information about the temporal order and duration of their symptoms. For example, children may more easily respond to the question, "Have you tried to hurt yourself since last summer?" rather than to the question, "Have you tried to hurt yourself in the last 6 months?" Ultimately, some prepubertal children will not be able to provide information about the frequency of their suicidal ideation and behavior, in which case obtaining information from multiple informants becomes particularly important.

Children's mastery of the concept of causality, relating events with their causes, also impacts on the interview. Children who have not mastered this concept may have difficulty linking their behavior with antecedent emotional states, as well as identifying causal events that have led to certain emotional states. Such difficulties can significantly hamper children's ability to communicate about suicidal episodes. In the example above, Brenda was able to link the emotional state of anger with self-directed aggressive behavior and with thoughts of wanting to kill herself. This understanding of the concept of causality stands in stark contrast to her poor grasp of the concept of frequency and her poorly developed verbal skills.

Although even preschool-age children have been found to exhibit some grasp of these concepts, evidence indicates that children's mastery of these concepts continues to develop beyond the preschool years (Masters and Carlson, 1984; Schwartz and Trabasso, 1984). Indeed, Piaget and Inhelder (1969) observed that children in the preoperational stage of cognitive development (approximately ages 2 or 3 through 7 or 8 years) exhibited "finalism," or the belief that all phenomena have causes and nothing occurs by chance. In this stage, contiguity of events tends to be an important factor in the child's deduction of a causal relationship. Thus, children in the preoperational stage may be more vulnerable to becoming confused about the relationship between their emotional states and subsequent behavior when these do not occur in close temporal proximity. Such confusion not only renders communication about suicidal episodes more difficult for children, but it makes prediction of future suicidal ideation and behavior more complex because the potential precipitants of suicidal states cannot be clarified. Later, as children reach the concrete operational and formal operational stages of cognitive development, they become capable of rational thought and of abstract thought and thus are more able to accurately deduce a causal relationship between emotional states and behavior separated in time.

Finally, children's conceptualization of death also exists on a developmental continuum and influences how children think about suicide. Studies have suggested that only at the age of 9 to 10 years do children begin to understand death as the permanent cessation of life (Anthony, 1971; Nagy, 1959). Before this age, death may be conceived as a temporary state or as a person.

Children who are suicidal can have high levels of intent to die irrespective of their conceptualization of death. Thus, clinicians interviewing children who are suicidal may encounter significant suicidal intent and life-threatening behavior in children who believe that their death would be temporary and reversible, as well as in children who believe that death represents a permanent exit from life. In a study of 10- to 12-year-old children, an age group in which death is usually understood to be irreversible, Orbach and Glaubman (1978) found that, when asked to think about their own death, suicidal children were significantly more likely to exhibit a belief in life after death either aggressive or normal children. This finding suggests that suicidal children may tend to regress in terms of their conceptualization of death.

In summary, preparedness on the part of clinicians for the diversity of verbal abilities and levels of maturity with which the concepts of time, causality, and death are understood by the children they are interviewing about suicidal ideation and behavior is essential to gleaning accurate and reliable information from these interviews.

IMPACT OF THE CHILD'S EMOTIONAL STATE
ON THE INTERVIEW

The emotional state of children at the time of interview may influence greatly what they communicate about both current and previous suicidal episodes. Although, to date, there have been few published attempts to quantify the magnitude or quality of the effect of current emotional state on children's communications about current or previous suicidal states during psychiatric evaluation, studies of the effect of mood on memory in children and adults have yielded findings that may be relevant to this question. For example, Bower (1981) demonstrated that hypnotized adults in whom happy or sad moods are induced recall word lists learned while in the same hypnotically induced mood significantly more accurately than word lists learned in a different hypnotically induced mood. Similarly, hypnotized adults induced into pleasant or unpleasant moods tend to recall mood-congruent incidents that occurred over the preceding week and mood-congruent episodes from childhood (Bower, 1981). Mood state-dependent recall was also demonstrated in 8- and 10-year-old schoolchildren in whom happy or sad moods were induced by means of video-film sequences (Forgas et al., 1988).

In the vignette that follows, the information a child communicated about a past suicidal episode changed significantly with changes in his current emotional state.

Steven was a 12-year-old boy who was admitted to a psychiatric inpatient unit after threatening to kill himself by taking an overdose of his mother's cardiac medication. During interviews that followed admission, Steven discussed the suicidal episode that had preceded admission in great detail and openly expressed his current despondency, saying "I can't wait 80 or 90 years to die." He maintained that he was "75%" sure that taking an overdose before admission would have led to an immediate death from cardiac arrhythmia.

Two weeks later another boy Steven's age was admitted to the unit (at this time most of the unit patients were much younger than Steven), with Steven's mood brightening considerably as a consequence. During an interview at this time he reported that, at the time of his suicide threat, he did not believe that taking the overdose would be lethal and was highly ambivalent about wanting to die.

The dramatic changes in Steven's statements about the level of his suicidal intent raised the question of which statement was accurate. The findings of Bower (1981) and Forgas et al. (1988) on mood state-dependent recall, together with the probability that Steven was highly dysphoric at the time of his suicide threat, suggest that Steven's earlier report of his suicidal episode was most accurate. Thus, despite his later comments, Steven would be viewed as having had a high level of intent at the time of his suicide threat.

In summary, although few published data exist to inform clinicians about the effect of current emotional state on children's communications about suicidal ideation and behavior, studies of adults and of children suggest that recall of past events may be more accurate if the child's current mood state is similar to his or her mood state during the past events. Thus, attempts to estimate the accuracy of a child's report about past suicidal ideation or behavior can be aided by determining what differences exist between the child's mood state during the interview and his or her mood state during the suicidal episode.

ROLE OF PLAY IN INTERVIEWING CHILDREN
ABOUT SUICIDAL IDEATION AND BEHAVIOR

Play is intrinsic to childhood, in part because of the means it provides children of assimilating piecemeal experiences that are too large to be assimilated at once (Waelder, 1933). By observing the play of prepubertal children, clinicians can glean information about experiences or events that are too overwhelming for them, or are beyond their verbal capabilities, to describe in words. Furthermore, children who have engaged in suicidal behavior may have a proclivity toward enacting their feeling states and thus may more readily express their suicidal ideation and propensity toward suicidal behavior in play themes rather than in language.

Pfeffer (1979) described several aspects of play that may predict suicide potential: (1) play dealing with developmental issues of separation, loss, and autonomy; (2) repetitive dangerous and reckless play; (3) themes of repeated misuse and destruction; (4) life-endangering, unrealistic repetitive acting out of omnipotent fantasies such as being a superhero like Superman. Such play themes may reflect states of aggression, depression, hopelessness, or preoccupation with death. Attention to these elements can facilitate the decision whether to include suicidal ideation or behavior in the differential diagnosis.

The case of Nancy is an example of the value of play observation in a child for whom verbal communication in an interview setting was impaired because of hyperactivity, thought disorder, and developmental language delay.

Nancy, a 10-year-old girl, was admitted to a psychiatric inpatient unit after she swallowed a staple and stated "I want to die." On several occasions her caretaker had to stop Nancy from holding her head under the bathtub water for dangerously long periods of time.

During the play sessions, Nancy became deeply enveloped in angry and aggressive affects as she enacted the following play scenarios: fires in people's homes, children getting hurt and killed, ambulances picking up children and leaving them on the side of the road along the way to the hospital. She played out roles of dying victims—first of a hit-and-run car accident, and then that of a drowning child. She stated: "That car drove over my face, and now I'm dead. . . . I'm drowning; someone has to save me or I'll die."

Nancy eagerly enacted scenes with puppets: "This guy Joey is out of it. He is real upset. . . . I'm not sure why 'cause he's very sad. He's grouchy today, too . . . he's angry . . . when he's angry he fights for his life." When asked whether she ever felt so angry or upset as to want to end her life, she quickly responded, "I swallowed a staple once." Upon further questioning, she denied that this act was intended for self-harm, and focused instead on another toy in the room, ignoring the interviewer's questions.

The themes in Nancy's play of children carrying out dangerous acts, children being harmed and dying, and children being rescued only to then be abandoned suggest the possibility of suicidal ideation that Nancy was not capable of describing in words. In addition, Nancy's intense immersion in dysphoric, aggressive, and irritable affects during her play further suggests risk for suicidal behavior (Pfeffer, 1986). Thus, this vignette illustrates how both distinct play themes and quality of play may suggest the presence of suicidal ideation and behavior.

In summary, play is a normative medium of expression in prepubertal children. By using play in the assessment of prepubertal children for suicidal ideation and behavior, the clinician enhances the likelihood of observing themes and affective states associated with suicidal risk beyond what is often possible in verbal interaction with such children.

ROLE OF PARENTS IN EVALUATING SUICIDAL IDEATION AND BEHAVIOR IN CHILDREN

Gathering data from multiple informants, including each person who has held a parenting role in relationship to the child in question, is an important element of the evaluation for suicidal ideation and behavior, particularly, as noted above, with children whose level of cognitive development renders them unable to communicate accurately about their suicidal episodes. In addition to contributing information to the evaluation of their children, parents themselves need to be assessed in terms of the adequacy of their response to their children's suicidal ideation or behavior. Studies demonstrating a lack of agreement between parents and children on the nature, extent, and severity of the children's psychopathology underscore the importance of obtaining information from multiple informants when assessing children, although the basis for these discrepancies remains unresolved. (Angold et al., 1987; Herjanic and Reich, 1982; Kazdin et al., 1983a; Lobovits and Handal, 1985; Orvaschel et al., 1981; Reich et al., 1982; Weissman et al., 1987).

Similar discrepancies have been observed between parent and child reports of children's suicidal ideation and behavior. Kashani et al. (1989), Velez and Cohen (1988), and Walker et al. (1990) each conducted studies in which parents and children were interviewed regarding the children's suicidal ideation and acts. Results from each of these studies indicated that parents are significantly less likely to report the presence of suicidal ideation, or a history of suicide attempts, in their children than are the children themselves. In all three studies, failure of parents to report suicidal ideation or behavior reported by their children was interpreted as lack of awareness of these symptoms on the part of the parents.

The assumption that parental underreporting of their children's suicidal ideation and acts reflects parental unawareness fails to take into account the complex and powerful forces, both societal and psychological, that impinge upon the parents of suicidal children. Calhoun et al. (1980) illustrated the tremendous social stigma that these parents must contend with when they found that persons reading a newspaper article about a child who committed suicide were significantly more likely to dislike and to blame the child's parents than when reading an article about a child whose death was caused by viral illness. These findings reflect societal attitudes that are likely to amplify feelings of guilt experienced by families of suicidal children and thus to contribute to any tendency family members may have to deny, distort, and conceal information regarding the child's suicidal behavior.

While the findings of Kashani et al. (1989), Velez and Cohen (1988), and Walker et al. (1990) suggest that asking parents about suicidal ideation and behavior in their children would tend not to yield valid or reliable data, parents can be a source of critical, and otherwise unavailable, information about suicidal children.

Ellen was an 11-year-old girl who was admitted to a psychiatric inpatient unit after an episode during which she assaulted her father, damaged much of her and her father's property with a wrench, and attempted to jump out of a second-floor window.

Over the preceding year, Ellen had frequently threatened verbally to commit suicide. As the psychosocial stressors in Ellen's life mounted, her suicide threats began to involve action. On two occasions, for example, she stood before her father and threatened to cut herself with a kitchen knife that she held to her wrist. Yet in all these incidents Ellen did not exhibit the total loss of behavioral control and lack of concern for her belongings that so alarmed her father during the episode before admission. On route to the hospital Ellen's father sat next to Ellen, physically restraining her lest she attempt to jump from the car.

The behavior of Ellen's father toward Ellen before her admission reflected a firm conviction of Ellen's suicidal intent. Yet when Ellen's father was later questioned explicitly about this, he expressed the belief that Ellen never really intended to harm or kill herself, and the underlying sentiment that such ideation and intent is incompatible with childhood.

In contrast to her father, Ellen's denial of the events necessitating hospitalization was profound; she remained unable to discuss these events, or the intent of her behavior during them, in any meaningful way throughout the interviews with her.

In the preceding vignette, the suicidal child's parent was better able to provide information needed to assess the suicidal intent of the child than the child herself. Yet this information could be elicited only via obtaining a detailed description from Ellen's father of the behavior and statements of both parent and child during each episode in question. In contrast, asking Ellen's father explicitly whether he thought his daughter had been suicidal increased both his anxiety and his need to minimize the seriousness of his daughter's actions.

Further complicating the evaluation of some suicidal children is the presence of parental psychopathology. Suicidal behavior in children has been associated with a family history of psychopathology, suggesting the importance of this problem (Carlson and Cantwell, 1982; Garfinkel et al., 1982; Livingston, 1993; Pfeffer et al., 1979, 1980, 1984; Shaffer, 1974; Tishler and McKenry, 1982; Weissman et al., 1984, 1992). Examining the impact of parental psychopathology on variance between parent and child reports of child symptomatology, Kashani et al. (1985) found that parents with major affective illness tended to report symptoms of attention-deficit and oppositional behavior in their children with greatest frequency, whereas the children themselves reported symptoms of depression and anxiety with greatest frequency.

The following vignette describes a child whose parents, themselves troubled, strongly disagreed about the presence of suicidal intent in their child.

Robert was an 11-year-old boy who was admitted to a psychiatric inpatient unit after he attempted to jump out of a moving car. He had suffered from numerous vegetative symptoms of depression over the preceding year and had made two suicide threats several months before admission, one in which he held a knife to his wrist and another in which he had prepared to hang himself. Both threats were made in his father's presence.

Robert's father was a chronically overwhelmed, anxious, and highly dysphoric man who was undergoing outpatient psychiatric treatment at the time of Robert's hospitalization. He was intensely preoccupied with

Robert's physical and mental health and had begun to diagnose many of Robert's behaviors, like his abruptly running out of the house during an argument, as suicidal. In stark contrast, Robert's mother, who was chronically suspicious, saw all of Robert's behaviors, including his attempt to jump from a car moving at high speed, merely as efforts to "get attention."

In this vignette the importance of actively seeking a detailed description of each suicidal episode is again underscored. Robert's parents each had interpreted Robert's behavior through the prism of their own long-standing psychiatric symptoms. These interpretations colored the information they volunteered during our interviews. Ultimately, careful interviews of Robert, who was both bright and articulate, seemed to yield the least distorted description of his suicidal episodes.

The cases of Ellen and Robert illustrate both the complexity of the data arising from interviews of the parents of suicidal children and the importance of bearing in mind the social and emotional pressures to which these parents are subject.

In summary, interviewing the parents of suicidal children can be challenging, particularly in the context of parental psychopathology or when the veracity of parent reports is not clear. Yet parents remain a potential source of crucial information about suicidal children. In all cases, avoiding the use of highly stigmatized language with parents can reduce their need to distort and conceal information about their children. Eliciting detailed descriptions from parents of what they have observed in their children is more likely to yield a rich and accurate picture of the children's symptoms than asking parents to diagnose their children (e.g., "Has your child been suicidal?").

IMPACT OF THE PRESENCE OF RISK FACTORS ON THE INTERVIEW

The presence of certain risk factors for suicidal ideation and behavior in prepubertal children can significantly impact their behavior and cognition during the interview. To be prepared to deal with the potential effects of the presence of such risk factors in children being interviewed, clinicians must be able to identify risk factors for suicidal ideation and behavior in children and understand how these risk factors can influence children's cognitive, behavioral, and psychosocial functioning. In this section, research identifying risk factors for suicidal ideation and behavior in children is reviewed. This review is followed by a discussion of the potential impact that the presence of risk factors can have on interviews of prepubertal children about suicidal ideation and behavior.

Particularly in the last decade, increasing numbers of studies have attempted to identify risk factors for suicidal ideation and behavior in children and adolescents. A recent longitudinal follow-up study comparing prepubertal inpatients who had made suicide attempts, prepubertal inpatients with suicidal ideation, prepubertal inpatients who were not suicidal, and prepubertal nonpatient controls found that inpatients who had made suicide attempts were six times more likely to report at least one more suicide attempt during the 6- to 8-year follow-up period than were nonpatient controls (Pfeffer et al., 1991, 1993a). Prepubertal inpatients with suicidal ideation were nearly four times more likely to report a suicide attempt during the follow-up period than were nonpatient controls. Strikingly, impaired social adjustment, stressful life events, and mood and substance abuse disorders, when occurring within the year before the suicide attempt during the follow-up period, were stronger risk factors than whether the child had a history of suicidal ideation or attempts (Pfeffer et al., 1991, 1993a).

Of these factors, Pfeffer et al. (1993a) observed that the strongest risk factors for occurrence of a suicide attempt during the follow-up period were poor social adjustment and the presence of a mood disorder before the suicide attempt. This replicates and expands upon the findings of studies and case reports which have illustrated an association between suicidal behavior in children and adolescents and various indices of poor social adjustment, including dysfunction in the relationships the child or adolescent has to family members (Asarnow et al., 1987; King et al., 1990, 1993; Lewinsohn et al., 1993; Pfeffer, 1981), poor social skills (Asarnow et al., 1987; Barter et al., 1968), and poor leisure skills (King et al., 1990). The observation that the presence of a mood disorder was an important risk factor for suicide attempts during the follow-up period also replicates and expands upon findings of studies demonstrating a relationship between mood disorders, especially depression, and suicidal behavior in children and adolescents (Andrews and Lewinsohn, 1992; Brent et al., 1990; Carlson and Cantwell, 1982; Garfinkel et al., 1982; Hoberman and Garfinkel, 1988; King et al., 1993; Kovacs et al., 1993; Levy and Deykin, 1989; Lewinsohn et al., 1993; Myers et al., 1985; Pfeffer et al., 1979, 1980, 1982, 1984, 1991; Robbins and Alessi, 1985; Shaffer, 1988; Swanson et al., 1992; Weiner and Pfeffer, 1986), and between depression and completed suicide in adolescents and young adults (Brent et al., 1993b; Rao et al., 1993).

Pfeffer et al. (1993a) did not find assaultive behavior or disruptive behavior disorders to be significant risk factors for suicide attempts during the follow-up period. This finding concurs with that of Myers et al. (1985) who, in a chart review study of preadolescent psychiatric inpatients, found similar rates of conduct disorder among suicidal and nonsuicidal subjects. In contrast, other cross-sectional studies of children and adolescents have revealed an association between conduct disorder and suicidal ideation and behavior (Andrews and Lewinsohn, 1992; Apter et al., 1988; Kashani et al., 1989; Kovacs et al., 1993), conduct disorder and completed suicide (Brent et al., 1993b; Hoberman and Garfinkel, 1988), antisocial behavior and completed suicide (Marttunen et al., 1992), and aggression and suicidal behavior (Cohen-Sandler, 1982; Pfeffer et al., 1986). The presence of a substance abuse disorder was noted by Pfeffer et al. (1993a) to be a risk factor for suicide attempts during the follow-up period, when the subjects were entering adolescence. However, in that study, no subjects reported substance or alcohol abuse at the initial assessment, when they were in the prepubertal age range. Cross-sectional studies have found substance and alcohol abuse to be a risk factor for suicidal ideation and behavior and completed suicide in samples of adolescents (Andrews and Lewinsohn, 1992; Brent et al., 1993b; King et al., 1993; Levy and Deykin, 1989; Swanson et al., 1992), and in mixed samples of preadolescents and adolescents (Brent, 1987; Hoberman and Garfinkel, 1988).

A high rate of stressful life events, identified by Pfeffer et al. (1993a) as an important risk factor for suicide attempts at initial assessment and during the follow-up period, has also been identified as a risk factor for suicidal behavior in children aged 5 to 14 (Cohen-Sandler et al., 1982). Cohen-Sandler et al. (1982), in a retrospective study, found that suicidal children experienced stressful life events significantly more frequently both over their lifetimes and in the 12 months preceding the episode of suicidal ideation or behavior than either depressed or psychiatric control children. These stressful events often involved parental loss due to separation, divorce, illness, or death. A similar relationship was recently observed in adolescents 13 to 18 years of age by Brent et al. (1993a), who noted a greater frequency of loss of a relative to death in suicide attempters compared with nonattempters. Relatedly, environmental and family factors such as family violence, abuse, and neglect have also been associated with suicidal behavior in children (Paulson et al., 1978; Rosenthal and Rosenthal, 1984) and adolescents (Deykin et al., 1985; Pfeffer et al., 1988).

Several studies have demonstrated that the presence of a family history of psychopathology is significantly more common in suicidal than in nonsuicidal children (Carlson and Cantwell, 1982; Garfinkel et al., 1982; Kashani et al. 1989). More specifically, significant correlations have been observed between suicidal ideation and behavior in children and depression and suicidal ideation and behavior in first-degree relatives (Pfeffer et al., 1979, 1980, 1984; Weissman et al., 1984, 1992), particularly mothers (Pfeffer et al., 1993b).

Although Pfeffer et al. (1993a) noted that demographic factors such as age at initial assessment, gender, race/ethnicity, religion, and social status were not significantly associated with suicidal behavior during the follow-up period, Mattsson et al. (1969), in a retrospective study of children and adolescents presenting to a child psychiatry clinic with suicidal behavior, observed that all patients engaging in suicidal behavior who were under the age of 12 were boys. Other cross-sectional studies of prepubertal children have not found significant differences between the frequency or severity of suicidal behavior in boys and girls (Pfeffer et al., 1982, 1986). In contrast, a recent longitudinal follow-up study of depressed children and nondepressed psychiatric controls found that, although there were no gender differences in the rate of suicidal ideation and attempts at initial assessment, girls were significantly more likely to experience suicidal ideation and make suicide attempts than boys during follow-up, regardless of psychiatric diagnosis (Kovacs et al., 1993). The authors of this longitudinal study noted that many of the children entered puberty during the follow-up period, which ranged between 1 and 12 years, suggesting that this effect of gender may emerge during adolescence. Many studies of both clinical and nonclinical populations have pooled data from children and adolescents, rendering the demographic findings difficult to interpret in terms of their specific relevance to prepubertal children (Garfinkel et al., 1982; Kashani et al., 1989; Velez and Cohen, 1988). Regarding completed suicide, epidemiological data indicate that white male children and adolescents are at greatest risk (National Center for Health Statistics, 1993; Shaffer, 1974).

All the risk factors described above may exert effects on the behavior and cognition of children and thus complicate interviews of prepubertal children about suicidal ideation and behavior. In the following vignette, a child with a number of factors increasing her risk for suicidal behavior is described. In addition, the impact that these factors had on the interviewer's efforts to assess her suicide attempt is illustrated.

Sally was an 8-year-old girl who was admitted to a psychiatric inpatient unit after she attempted to jump from a 10th-floor window during an altercation with her brother. Sally had been experiencing increasing difficulties in many spheres of her life for years. Her relationship with her parents was strained to the point that she rarely talked and frequently argued with them. Because of her argumentativeness and social awkwardness Sally was rejected by most of her peers and played with much younger children. During the year preceding her hospitalization, Sally had become progressively more depressed. She began to lose weight, spent most of her free time in her room, and heard a voice instructing her to jump out of the window.

During an interview after admission Sally sat motionless, stared at the floor, and answered the interviewer's questions in a soft voice, slowly, and in short sentences. At times Sally refused to answer questions and ignored the interviewer. Encouragement and reassurance that the purpose of the interview was to help her feel better enabled Sally to begin to respond to the interviewer's queries. With the interviewer's use of simple questions, which often had to be repeated because of Sally's cognitive slowness and poor concentration, Sally was eventually able to describe her sadness, her wish to die to escape her troubles, and her frightening auditory hallucinations, which commanded her to jump out of the window.

In this vignette a child whose risk for suicidal behavior was heightened by the presence of poor social adjustment, as evidenced by her chronically conflictual relationship with her parents and poor peer relations, together with a severe mood disturbance, characterized by depression, social withdrawal, weight loss, irritability, auditory hallucinations, and psychomotor retardation, presented unique challenges to the interviewer. The impact of Sally's mood disturbance on her behavior and her cognition necessitated that the interviewer word questions simply, be prepared to repeat questions that were not understood, and allow Sally more time than a cognitively intact child would require to answer questions. Although Sally's poor eye contact, irritability, social withdrawal, and delayed response to questions were associated with her depression, the extent to which her poor social adjustment also contributed to these symptoms could not be distinguished.

In summary, studies have identified a number of important risk factors for suicidal ideation and behavior in children. To determine whether a given risk factor is present, often the clinician must gather information about such things as the child's current psychiatric symptoms, whether the child has experienced suicidal ideation or has attempted suicide in the past, the status of the child's relationships with family members and peers, the child's use of free time, the occurrence of stressful life events (particularly events that threaten or disrupt family integrity), and whether there is any family history of psychiatric illness or suicidal ideation or behavior. In addition, the clinician must be prepared for the impact that the presence of certain risk factors can have during the interview, particularly on children's level of psychomotor activation, cognitive function, irritability, compliance, and relatedness to the interviewer, so that appropriate adjustments in the interview process can be made.

DISCUSSION

In the preceding six sections a number of important aspects of the process of interviewing children about suicidal ideation and behavior have been elaborated and discussed. Each of these elements of the interview is complex and this can present a challenge to the clinician. The fact that these elements must be considered simultaneously in the context of such interviews further complicates the clinician's task. Thus, while attempting to assess a child's level of suicidal intent, and to distinguish intent from motivation and the medical lethality of any previous suicide attempts, the clinician must also bear in mind limitations that the child's level of cognitive development may place on his or her ability to communicate verbally. In addition, the clinician must be attuned to the child's current emotional state and its effect on what the child recalls of previous suicidal episodes, and to important information about suicidal ideation and behavior which the child may convey in his or her play. The clinician needs to be aware of the extent to which parents are able to provide accurate information about suicidal ideation and behavior in their children and needs to help parents share this information by avoiding the use of stigmatized language and by eliciting detailed descriptions of what the parents have observed in their children. Finally, the clinician must be alert to the presence of risk factors for suicidal ideation and behavior and the impact that these may be having on the child's behavior and cognition during the interview.

Clinicians may organize the process of interviewing prepubertal children about suicidal ideation and behavior by using key questions. Table 1 contains examples of questions that can be used as a scaffold by clinicians conducting such interviews. The questions are provided to illustrate an approach to the aspects of interviewing prepubertal children about suicidal ideation and behavior which have been discussed in each of the sections of this paper, with the exception of the section on the role of play in these interviews. In addition, examples of questions that can be used to determine whether or not a prepubertal child has previously been or is currently suicidal, the most important goal of the interview, are provided at the top of Table 1. These questions do not represent an exhaustive list of questions that should be asked of prepubertal children who may be suicidal. Furthermore, rather than being asked in the particular order in which they are listed in Table 1, these questions should be inserted where they most naturally fit in the flow of the interview. Examples of questions illustrating an approach to interviewing parents about suicidal ideation and behavior in their children are also provided. In fact, depending on the clinical situation, all ques-

TABLE 1

Sample Questions for Interviewing Prepubertal Children
about Suicidal Ideation and Behavior

Ascertaining the Presence of Previous or Current Suicidal Ideation or Behavior
1. Did you ever feel so upset that you wished you were not alive or wanted to die?
2. Did you ever do something that you knew was so dangerous that you could get hurt or killed?
3. Did you ever hurt yourself or try to hurt yourself?
4. Did you ever try to kill yourself?

Assessment of Suicidal Intent
1. Did you tell anyone that you wanted to die or were thinking about killing yourself?
2. Did you do anything to get ready to kill yourself?
3. Was anyone near you or with you when you tried to kill yourself?
4. Did you think that what you did would kill you?
5. After you tried to kill yourself did you still want to die, or did you want to live?

Interviewing Children Whose Grasp of the Concepts of Time, Causality, and Death May Not Be Mature
1. Do you think about killing yourself more than once or twice a day?
2. Have you tried to kill yourself since last summer/since school began?
3. What did you think would happen when your tried to jump out of the window?
4. What would happen if you died; what would that be like?

Assessing the Potential Impact of the Child's Current Emotional State upon Recall of Suicidal Ideation and Behavior
1. How do you remember feeling when you were thinking about or trying to kill yourself?
2. How is the way you feel then different from the way you feel now?

Interviewing Parents about Suicidal Ideation and Behavior in Their Children
1. What exactly happened (step by step) on the day that your child spoke of wanting or tried to hurt him/herself?
2. How did you find out that your child was thinking about or trying to hurt him/herself?
3. What were you doing when your child was thinking about or trying to hurt him/herself?
4. What happened after your child thought about or tried to hurt him/herself?

Determining the Presence of Risk Factors for Suicidal Ideation and Behavior
1. Have you ever thought about or tried to kill yourself before?
2. How have you been getting along with your friends and family?
3. Has anything happened recently which has been upsetting to you or your family?
4. Have you had a problem with feeling sad, having trouble sleeping, not feeling hungry, losing your temper easily, or feeling tired all of the time recently?
5. Have you used alcohol or drugs recently?

tions in Table 1 can potentially be used with the parents of children who may be suicidal.

While the goal of this paper has been to address fundamental aspects of interviewing children about suicidal ideation and behavior, its scope has made the exclusion of some important issues necessary. That such interviews can be highly stressful to both the clinician and the child involved is one such issue. For clinicians with children of their own, fears of their own children becoming suicidal can be aroused in the context of interviewing suicidal children. In addition, many clinicians experience both disbelief that children are capable of being suicidal and tremendous anxiety about clinical decision-making involving suicidal children, particularly with regard to the decision whether to hospitalize them or not. Furthermore, the clinician may fear that asking a child about suicidal ideation and behavior may induce or intensify suicidal states in the child. Given the significant stress that exploring current or previous suicidal ideation and behavior can represent to a child, the clinician's sensitivity and ability to shift the focus of discussion or play to a less stressful subject to protect the child from becoming overwhelmed is essential. Finally, saving less stressful topics unrelated to suicide for the latter part of the interview can help to ensure that the child does not leave the interview in a highly stressed or overwhelmed state.

Interviewing children about suicidal ideation and behavior is both complex and demanding in ways that will differ with children of different developmental levels and with different risk factors. In addition, these interviews can be highly stressful to both clinician and child. Therefore, thorough assessment of any given child's suicidal state will often require multiple interview sessions. Considering the importance of these interviews, along with the opportunity they can present to clinicians to help children learn to think about difficult feelings and to problem solve more effectively, this is a worthwhile investment of time. In addition, a semistructured interview format which allows clinicians to introduce specific questions when the child appears clinically ready to address the issues embodied in the questions is recommended.

Finally, research is needed to further clarify the optimal means of interviewing children about suicidal ideation and behavior and to develop instruments both to quantitate the different elements of these interviews and to guide the clinicians conducting them.

REFERENCES

Ackerly WC (1967), Latency-age children who threaten or attempt to kill themselves. *J Am Acad Child Psychiatry* 6:242-261

Andrews JA, Lewinsohn PM (1992), Suicidal attempts among older adolescents: prevalence and co-occurrence with psychiatric disorders. *J Am Acad Child Adolesc Psychiatry* 31:655-662

Angold A, Weissman MM, John K et al. (1987), Parent and child reports of depressive symptoms in children at low and high risk of depression. *J Child Psychol Psychiatry* 28:901-915

Anthony S (1971), *The Discovery of Death in Childhood and After.* London: The Penguin Press

Apter A, Bleich A, Plutchik R, Mendelsohn S, Tyano S (1988), Suicidal behavior, depression, and conduct disorder in hospitalized adolescents. *J Am Acad Child Adolesc Psychiatry* 27:696-699

Asarnow JR, Carlson GA, Guthrie D (1987), Coping strategies, self-perceptions, hopelessness, and perceived family environments in depressed and suicidal children. *J Consult Clin Psychol* 55:361-366

Barter JT, Swaback DO, Todd D (1968), Adolescent suicide attempts: a follow-up study of hospitalized patients. *Arch Gen Psychiatry* 19:523-527

Beck AT, Beck R, Kovacs M (1975), Classification of suicidal behaviors: 1. Quantifying intent and medical lethality. *Am J Psychiatry* 132:285-287

Beck AT, Schuyler D, Herman I (1974), *The Prediction of Suicide.* Bowie, MD: Charles Press

Bender L, Schilder P (1937), Suicidal preoccupations and attempts in children. *Am J Orthopsychiatry* 7:225-235

Bower GH (1981), Mood and memory. *Am Psychol* 36:129-148

Brent DA (1987), Correlates of the medical lethality of suicide attempts in children and adolescents. *J Am Acad Child Adolesc Psychiatry* 26:87-91

Brent DA, Kolko DJ, Allan MJ, Brown RV (1990), Suicidality in affectively disordered adolescent inpatients. *J Am Acad Child Adolesc Psychiatry* 29:586-593

Brent DA, Kolko DJ, Wartella ME et al. (1993a), Adolescent psychiatric inpatients' risk of suicide attempt at 6-month follow-up. *J Am Acad Child Adolesc Psychiatry* 32:95-105

Brent DA, Perper JA, Moritz G et al. (1993b), Psychiatric risk factors for adolescent suicide: a case-control study. *J Am Acad Child Adolesc Psychiatry* 32:521-529

Calhoun LG, Selby JW, Faulstich ME (1980), Reactions to the parents of the child suicide: a study of social impressions. *J Consult Clin Psychol* 48:535-536

Carlson GA, Cantwell DP (1982), Suicidal behavior and depression in children and adolescents. *J Am Acad Child Psychiatry* 21:361-368

Cohen-Sandler R, Berman AL, King RA (1982), Life stress and symptomatology:

determinants of suicidal behavior in children. *J Am Acad Child Psychiatry* 21:178–186

Deykin EY, Alpert JJ, McNamarra JJ (1985), a pilot study of the effect of exposure to child abuse or neglect on adolescent suicidal behavior. *Am J Psychiatry* 142:1299–1303

Dorpat TL, Boswell JW (1963), An evaluation of suicidal intent in suicide attempts. *Compr Psychiatry* 4:117–125

Forgas JP, Burnham DK, Trimboli C (1988), Mood, memory, and social judgments in children. *J Pers Soc Psychol* 54:697–703

Fraisse P (1963), *The Psychology of Time.* New York: Harper and Row

Freud A (1951), Observations on child development. *Psychoanal Study Child* 6:18–30

Friedman WJ (1978), Development of time concepts in children. *Adv Child Dev Behav* 12:267–298

Garfinkel BD, Froese A, Hood J (1982), Suicide attempts in children and adolescents. *Am J Psychiatry* 139:1257–1261

Herjanic B, Reich W (1982), Development of a structured psychiatric interview for children: agreement between child and parent on individual symptoms. *J Abnorm Child Psychol* 10:307–324

Hoberman HM, Garfinkel BD (1988), Completed suicide in children and adolescents. *J Am Acad Child Adolesc Psychiatry* 27:689–695

Kashani JH, Goddard P, Reid JC (1989), Correlates of suicidal ideation in a community sample of children and adolescents. *J Am Acad Child Adolesc Psychiatry* 28:912–917

Kashani JH, Orvaschel H, Burk JP, Reid JC (1985), Informant variance: the issue of parent-child disagreement. *J Am Acad Child Psychiatry* 24:437–441

Kazdin AE, French NH, Unis AS, Esveldt-Dawson K (1983a), Assessment of childhood depression: correspondence of child and parent ratings. *J Am Acad Child Psychiatry* 22:157–164

Kazdin AE, French NH, Unis AS, Esveldt-Dawson K, Sherick RB (1983b), Hopelessness, depression, and suicidal intent among psychiatrically disturbed inpatient children. *J Consult Clin Psychol* 51:504–510

King CA, Hill EM, Naylor M, Evans T, Shain B (1993), Alcohol consumption in relation to other predictors of suicidality among adolescent inpatient girls. *J Am Acad Child Adolesc Psychiatry* 32:82–88

King CA, Raskin A, Gdowski CL, Butkus M, Opipari L (1990), Psychosocial factors associated with urban adolescent female suicide attempts. *J Am Acad Child Adolesc Psychiatry* 29:289–294

Kingsbury SJ (1993), Clinical components of suicidal intent in adolescent overdose. *J Am Acad Child Adolesc Psychiatry* 32:518–520

Kovacs M, Goldston D, Gatsonis C (1993), Suicidal behaviors and childhood-onset depressive disorders: a longitudinal investigation. *J Am Acad Child Adolesc Psychiatry* 32:8-20

Levy JC, Deykin EY (1989), Suicidality, depression, and substance abuse in adolescence. *Am J Psychiatry* 146:1462-1467

Lewinsohn PM, Rohde P, Seeley JR (1993), Psychosocial characteristics of adolescents with a history of suicide attempt. *J Am Acad Child Adolesc Psychiatry* 32:60-68

Lewis M, Volkmar F (1990), *Clinical Aspects of Child and Adolescent Development.* Philadelphia: Lea & Febiger

Linehan MM (1986), Suicidal people: one population or two? *Ann NY Acad Sci* 487:16-34

Livingston R (1993), Children of people with somatization disorder. *J Am Acad Child Adolesc Psychiatry* 32:536-544

Lobovits DA, Handal PJ (1985), Childhood depression: prevalence using *DSM-III* criteria and validity of parent and child depression scales. *J Pediatr Psychol* 10:45-54

Lukianowicz N (1968), Attempted suicide in children. *Acta Psychiatr Scand* 44:415-435

Marttunen MJ, Aro HM, Lönnqvist JK (1992), Adolescent suicide: endpoint of long-term difficulties. *J Am Acad Child Adolesc Psychiatry* 31:649-654

Masters JC, Carlson CR (1984), Children's and adults' understanding of the causes and consequences of emotional states. In: *Emotions, Cognition, and Behavior,* Izard CE, Kagan J, Zajonc R, eds. New York: Cambridge University Press, pp 438-463

Mattsson A, Seese LR, Hawkins JW (1969), Suicidal behavior as a child psychiatric emergency. *Arch Gen Psychiatry* 20:100-109

Myers KM, Burke P, McCauley E (1985), Suicidal behavior by hospitalized pre-adolescent children on a psychiatric unit. *J Am Acad Child Psychiatry* 24:474-480

Nagy MH (1959), The child's view of death. In: *The Meaning of Death,* Feifel H, ed. New York: McGraw-Hill Book Company, pp 79-98

National Center for Health Statistics (1993), Advance report of final mortality statistics, 1991. *Monthly Vital Statistics Report,* Vol 42, No 2. Hyattsville, MD: US Public Health Service

Orbach I, Glaubman H (1978), Suicidal, aggressive, and normal children's perception of personal and impersonal death. *J Clin Psychol* 34:850-857

Orvaschel H, Weissman MM, Padian N, Lowe TL (1981), Assessing psychopathology in children of psychiatrically disturbed parents: a pilot study. *J Am Acad Child Psychiatry* 20:112-122

Paulson MJ, Stone D, Sposto R (1978), Suicide potential and behavior in children ages 4 to 12. *Suicide Life Threat Behav* 8:225-242

Pfeffer CR (1979), Clinical observations of play of hospitalized suicidal children. *Suicide Life Threat Behav* 9:235–244

Pfeffer CR (1981), The family system of suicidal children. *Am J Psychother* 35:330–341

Pfeffer CR (1986), *The Suicidal Child.* New York: The Guilford Press

Pfeffer CR (1989), Assessment of suicidal children and adolescents. *Psychiatr Clin North Am* 12:861–872

Pfeffer CR, Conte HR, Plutchik R, Jerrett I (1979), Suicidal behavior in latency-age children: an empirical study. *J Am Acad Child Psychiatry* 18:679–692

Pfeffer CR, Conte HR, Plutchik R, Jerrett I (1980), Suicidal behavior in latency-age children: an outpatient population. *J Am Acad Child Psychiatry* 19:703–710

Pfeffer CR, Klerman GL, Hurt SW, Kakuma T, Peskin JR, Siefker CA (1993a), Suicidal children grow up: rates and psychosocial risk factors for suicide attempts during follow-up. *J Am Acad Child Adolesc Psychiatry* 32:106–113

Pfeffer CR, Klerman GL, Hurt SW, Lesser M, Peskin JR, Siefker CA (1991), Suicidal children grow up: demographic and clinical risk factors for adolescent suicide attempts. *J Am Acad Child Adolesc Psychiatry* 30:609–616

Pfeffer CR, Newcorn J, Kaplan G, Mizruchi MS, Plutchik R (1988), Suicidal behavior in adolescent psychiatric inpatients. *J Am Acad Child Adolesc Psychiatry* 27:357–361

Pfeffer CR, Normandin L. Kakuma T (1993b), Suicidal children grow up: family psychopathology. Presented at American Academy of Child and Adolescent Psychiatry, annual meeting, 1993

Pfeffer CR, Peskin JR, Siefker CA (1992), Suicidal children grow up: psychiatric treatment during follow-up period. *J Am Acad Child Adolesc Psychiatry* 31:679–685

Pfeffer CR, Plutchik R, Mizruchi MS, Lipkins R (1986), Suicidal behavior in child psychiatric inpatients and outpatients and in nonpatients. *Am J Psychiatry* 143:733–738

Pfeffer CR, Solomon G, Plutchik R, Mizruchi MS, Weiner A (1982), Suicidal behavior in latency-age psychiatric inpatients: a replication and cross validation. *J Am Acad Child Psychiatry* 21:564–569

Pfeffer CR, Zuckerman S. Plutchik R, Mizruchi MS (1984), Suicidal behavior in normal school children: comparison with child psychiatric inpatients. *J Am Acad Child Psychiatry* 23:416–423

Piaget J (1969), *The Child's Conception of Time.* London: Routledge and Kegan Paul Ltd

Piaget J, Inhelder B (1969), *The Psychology of the Child.* New York: Basic Books, Inc

Piaget J, Inhelder B (1971), *The Child's Conception of Space.* London: Routledge and Kegan Paul Ltd

Pierce DW (1977), Suicidal intent in self-injury. *Br J Psychiatry* 130:377–385

Pierce DW (1981), The predictive validation of a suicide intent scale: a five year follow-up. *Br J Psychiatry* 139:391–396

Rao U, Weissman MM, Martin JA, Hammond RW (1993), Childhood depression and risk of suicide: a preliminary report of a longitudinal study. *J Am Acad Child Adolesc Psychiatry* 32:21–27

Reich W, Herjanic B, Welner Z, Gandhy PR (1982), Development of a structured psychiatric interview for children: agreement on diagnosis comparing child and parent interviews. *J Abnorm Child Psychol* 10:325–336

Robbins DR, Alessi NE (1985), Depressive symptoms and suicidal behavior in adolescents. *Am J Psychiatry* 142:588–592

Rosenthal PS, Rosenthal S (1984), Suicidal behavior by preschool children. *Am J Psychiatry* 141:520–525

Schwartz RM, Trabasso R (1984), Children's understanding of emotions. In: *Emotions, Cognition, and Behavior*, Izard CE, Kagan J, Zajonc R, eds. New York: Cambridge University Press, pp 409–437

Shaffer D (1974), Suicide in childhood and early adolescence. *J Child Psychol Psychiatry* 15:275–291

Shaffer D (1988), The epidemiology of teen suicide: an examination of risk factors. *J Clin Psychiatry* 49(suppl):36–41

Swanson JW, Linskey AO, Quintero-Salinas R, Pumariega AJ, Holzer CE (1992), A binational school survey of depressive symptoms, drug use, and suicidal ideation. *J Am Acad Child Adolesc Psychiatry* 31:669–678

Terr LC (1985), Psychic trauma in children and adolescents. *Psychiatr Clin North Am* 8:815–835

Tishler CL, McKenry PC (1982), Parental negative self and adolescent suicide attempts. *J Am Acad Child Psychiatry* 21:404–408

Velez CN, Cohen P (1988), Suicidal behavior and ideation in a community sample of children: maternal and youth reports. *J Am Acad Child Adolesc Psychiatry* 27:349–356

Voyat G (1977), Perception and concept of time: a developmental perspective. In: *The Personal Experience of Time*, Gorman BS, Wessman AE, eds. New York: Plenum Press, pp 135–160

Waelder R (1933), The psychoanalytic theory of play. *Psychoanal Q* 2:208–224

Walker M, Moreau D, Weissman MM (1990), Parents' awareness of children's suicide attempts. *Am J Psychiatry* 147:1364–1366

Weiner AS, Pfeffer CR (1986), Suicidal status, depression, and intellectual functioning in preadolescent psychiatric inpatients. *Compr Psychiatry* 27:372–380

Weissman MM, Fendrich M, Warner V, Wickramaratne P (1992), Incidence of psychiatric disorder in offspring at high and low risk for depression. *J Am Acad Child Adolesc Psychiatry* 31:640–648

Weissman MM, Prusoff BA, Gammon GD, Merikangas KR, Leckman, JF, Kidd KK (1984), Psychopathology in the children (ages 6-18) of depressed and normal parents. *J Am Acad Child Psychiatry* 23:78-84

Weissman MM, Wickramaratne P, Warner V et al. (1987), Assessing psychiatric disorders in children: discrepancies between mother's and children's reports. *Arch Gen Psychiatry* 44:747-753

11

Prediction of Eating Problems: An 8-Year Study of Adolescent Girls

Julia A. Graber and Jeanne Brooks-Gunn
Teachers College, Columbia University, New York

Roberta L. Paikoff
University of Illinois, Chicago

Michelle P. Warren
College of Physicians and Surgeons, Columbia University, New York

Little prospective work has charted the onset and predictors of subclinical or clinical eating problems. Eating problems were studied in 116 adolescent girls drawn from a normal population of students enrolled in private schools in a major metropolitan area who have been followed longitudinally over an 8-year period from young adolescence to young adulthood. Over a quarter of the sample scored above the level identifying a serious eating problem at each of the 3 times of assessment (mean ages = 14.3, 16.0, and 22.3 years). Examination of the adolescent pattern of eating problems over young and mid-adolescence indicated that pattern was associated with (a)

Reprinted with permission from *Developmental Psychology*, 1994, Vol. 30, 823–834. Copyright © 1994 by the American Psychological Association, Inc.

Portions of this article were presented in a symposium, "The Development and Course of Eating Disorders Across Adolescence and Young Adulthood," at the biennial meeting of the Society for Research in Child Development, March 1993, New Orleans, Louisiana.

This project was supported by grants from the National Institute of Child Health and Development and the W. T. Grant Foundation to Jeanne Brooks-Gunn and was conducted under the aegis of the Adolescent Study Program, codirected by Jeanne Brooks-Gunn and Michelle P. Warren.

We acknowledge the contributions of Ilana Attie for her work on previous phases of the study; Richard Fox, Claire Holderness, Alice Michael, and Jamie Traegger for their assistance with the follow-up project; the staff at Educational Testing Service, Princeton, New Jersey; and the staff of the Adolescent Study Program for their assistance over the course of the project. We also acknowledge the influence of Anne Petersen's work on behavioral trajectories on the present conceptual framework. We are especially grateful to the young women and their mothers for their continued participation and support in this research.

> *earlier pubertal maturation and higher body fat, (b) concurrent psychological disturbances, (c) subsequent eating problems, and (d) other long-term adjustment outcomes such as depressive affect in young adulthood.*

Adolescents face numerous challenges during the transition from childhood to adulthood (Feldman & Elliott, 1990; Gunnar & Collins, 1988; Lerner & Foch, 1987). These include physical, cognitive, and social changes altering every domain of the individual's life. Many of these transitions are sources of risk to physical and mental well-being for adolescents. Although adolescents in developed countries are healthy in that they experience a low incidence of disease, the World Health Organization (WHO; 1981) reported that adolescents are increasingly experiencing new health risks leading to mortality and morbidity. Even though morbidity has declined over the past 20 years in other age groups, it has increased by 11% for adolescents (U.S. Congress, 1991). Threats to adolescent health and well-being include injury from accidents, suicide, substance abuse, sexually transmitted diseases, dieting, eating problems, and eating disorders, which are more common in girls (Millstein, Petersen, & Nightingale, 1993).

Eating disorders and unhealthy eating behaviors such as restricted eating are problems experienced by many adolescent girls. Estimates of anorexia and bulimia nervosa using the *Diagnostic and Statistical Manual of Mental Disorders* (3rd ed., rev., *DSM-III-R*; American Psychiatric Association, 1987) diagnostic criteria range from 0.2% or 1 in every 500 girls for anorexia (Robins et al., 1984) to 1%–2.8% (Fairburn & Beglin, 1990; Kendler et al., 1991) of adolescent girls and young women for bulimia. Subclinical problems are even more prevalent, with sources (e.g., Schwartz, Thompson, & Johnson, 1985) estimating that at least 20% of girls in this age range (nearly 2½ million girls) will exhibit bulimic behaviors. Although most evidence has suggested that bulimia nervosa is more prevalent in middle- and upper-middle-class White girls, some evidence suggests that rates are increasing in other ethnic and social class groups (Hsu, 1987), especially for girls who experience more pressure to acculturate to White, middle-class standards (Pumariega, 1986).

These figures do not include the additional numbers of adolescent girls who will engage in less extreme but still unhealthy dieting behaviors (perhaps another 20% of all girls). Unhealthy eating practices in and of themselves have been linked to serious physical and psychological disturbances for adolescent girls (e.g., Sallis, 1993). Our investigation focuses on a nonclinical group of adolescent girls who exhibit a range of behaviors from problematic and unhealthy eating behaviors to healthy eating habits.

Adolescent girls are increasingly concerned with weight and thinness (Attie & Brooks-Gunn, 1987). Cultural ideals for beauty emphasize a slender body shape typical of prepubertal development that is unattainable for most adolescents and women after puberty (Faust, 1983). Adolescent girls may engage in excessive dieting in an attempt to meet these unattainable cultural ideals even though they are not overweight. When attempting to lose weight, these girls often use unhealthy practices such as fad diets or purging behaviors including induced vomiting and laxative use rather than adhering to a balanced diet and engaging in appropriate amounts of physical activity (Killen et al., 1986; Storz & Greene, 1983).

Several correlates of subclinical eating problems have been identified. (Many of these correlates have also been associated with eating disorders.) As the adolescent transition is characterized by biological, psychological, and social changes, correlates of eating problems have been reported in each of these domains. Pubertal maturation and the concomitant increases in body fat have been associated with increased dieting and unhealthy behaviors in early adolescence (Attie & Brooks-Gunn, 1989; Killen et al., 1992). Negative body image, which has a close association with weight, has been predictive of problematic eating behaviors during the mid-adolescent years as well (Attie & Brooks-Gunn, 1989).

Additional personality characteristics such as perfectionist striving and depressive symptoms have also been linked to the development of eating problems (Garner, Olmsted, & Polivy, 1983; Johnson & Maddi, 1986). Given that the incidence of both depression and eating disorders increases across the adolescent decade and given that both disorders and the subclinical behaviors associated with them are more frequently reported in girls, depressive affect and eating problems would appear to be linked developmentally, although causal links have yet to be determined. Associations with stressful life events and general psychological distress have also been linked to concurrent eating problems but have not been strongly predictive of changes in eating behaviors over a 4-month interval (Rosen, Compas, & Tracy, 1993). With the exception of a few researchers (Attie & Brooks-Gunn, 1989; Patton, Johnson-Sabine, Wood, Mann, & Wakeling, 1990; Rosen et al., 1993) who have examined eating problems across early and mid-adolescence, investigations of these correlates have frequently been lacking a developmental perspective, with most nonclinical studies reporting on samples of college-age women (e.g., Drewnowski, Yee, & Krahn, 1988; Striegel-Moore, Silberstein, Frensch, & Rodin, 1989).

Family relationships and environment, especially maternal beliefs about weight and dieting, have been suggested as important factors in eating behaviors and attitudes of adolescent girls (Orbach, 1986; Strober, Morrell, Burroughs, Salkin, & Jacobs, 1985). Pike and Rodin (1991) not only found higher levels of disorderd eating in mothers of adolescent girls with disordered eating, but the mothers of girls with disordered eating patterns were also more critical of their daughters' weight and physical appearance. Families with adolescents who have an eating disorder are characterized by enmeshment, overprotectiveness, rigidity, and a lack of conflict resolution (Minuchin, Rosman, & Baker, 1978; Sargent, Liebman, & Silver, 1985). Familial correlates of eating disorders have predominantly been examined in clinical samples (Crisp, Harding, & McGuinness, 1974; Minuchin et al., 1978), with little attention to developmental family processes.

Eating problems and disorders in girls tend to emerge coincidentally with developmental challenges occurring during two adolescent transition periods (Levine, 1987). The transition into adolescence as marked by pubertal development has been associated with the occurrence of anorexia nervosa, whereas the transition out of adolescence into young adulthood has been associated with the occurrence of bulimia nervosa, especially in girls moving away from home to attend college. Subclinical behaviors such as excessive dieting, weight concerns, and bingeing are pervasive across adolescence for girls (Story et al., 1991).

Despite a burgeoning literature on the aforementioned correlates of eating disorders and subclinical disrupted eating patterns (over 800 articles published in the previous 2 years), prospective longitudinal investigations using a developmental psychopathology framework are lacking (Attie, Brooks-Gunn, & Petersen, 1990). Developmental psychopathology has focused on the interconnections of normal development and the development of maladaptive behaviors and processes across the life span (Sroufe & Rutter, 1984).

The few studies that have examined eating disorders and subclinical behaviors longitudinally have predominantly studied late adolescents in college (Drewnowski et al., 1988; Striegel-Moore et al., 1989) or large survey samples of adults (King, 1989; Vollrath, Koch, & Angst, 1992). Despite differences among studies, of note is that certain commonalities exist across these projects. First, all of the studies report on a single follow-up of their respective samples from 6 months to 2 years after initial participation. Second, all define subgroups of the sample who in some cases have clinical disorders but in most have serious disturbances in behavior. These may be individuals who binge but do not meet *DSM-III-R* criteria for bulimia nervosa or who report high rates of dieting or weight concerns. Thus, while most individuals in each of these samples reported healthy eating attitudes, individuals who reported clinical and subclinical behaviors formed unique subgroups. Finally, of particular note is that these studies all report that, within the follow-up period, some individuals experience persistent problems, others have a lessening of symptoms, whereas others experience an increase in symptoms. For this last group, it is not uncommon for these individuals to have already been dieters who began to engage in bulimic behaviors. Individuals who have persistent problems also report higher rates of other forms of psychopathology, that is, depression (Vollrath et al., 1992) or personality disturbances (King, 1989). In addition, in those studies in which reports of onset of unhealthy practices were obtained (Vollrath et al., 1992; Yager, Landsverk, & Edelstein, 1987), mean age of onset was between 14 and 15 years of age.

Hence, the existing longitudinal investigations of eating problems have generally considered serious but subclinical behaviors, have found changes in symptoms over the course of a few years, and have often noted greater pathology in individuals with recurrent eating problems. As yet, despite the suggestion that these behaviors are likely to begin earlier in development, little prospective work has examined patterns of disturbed eating across the adolescent decade. It is hypothesized that early patterns of disturbed eating during adolescence may set adolescents on a trajectory for continued eating problems as well as alternative forms of psychopathology. What is lacking in the literature is an understanding of who experiences transient versus recurrent problems during adolescence and what the long-term outcomes of such patterns of disturbance might be. Both Rutter (1989) and Elder (1985) have discussed the use of trajectories to delineate developmental patterns across the life span. This approach has been particularly valuable in the identification of continuities and discontinuities in the development of psychopathology (Rutter, 1989) and the understanding of correlates of both.

This study examined the pattern of eating behaviors and attitudes, identifying factors associated with the development of maladaptive behaviors and protective factors associated with healthy behaviors in a sample of girls followed from young adolescence through young adulthood. The specific goals of this study were to examine (a) change in eating attitudes over the adolescent decade, (b) whether girls enter onto trajectories for the development of eating problems as young adolescents, and (c) the biological, psychological, and social correlates of entry onto a particular trajectory, the short-term outcomes, and the long-term outcomes of these adolescent behavior patterns.

METHOD

Participants and Procedure

The participants in this study are 116 young women who have been followed longitudinally as part of the Adolescent Study Program. These women were initially seen when they were in 7th, 8th, or 9th grade (Time 1) and again 2 years later in 9th, 10th, or 11th grade (Time 2). Most recently, they have been interviewed and have completed questionnaires during the transition to young adulthood when they were between the ages of 21 and 23 (Time 3). The mean age of the sample for each time of assessment was 14.31 (SD = 1.05), 16.03 (SD = 1.00), and 22.3 (SD = 1.14) years.

Participants were recruited from private girls' schools in a major North-eastern metropolitan area. The sample was predominantly White and from middle- to upper-middle-class well-educated families. At Time 1, girls participated in a large cross-sectional study of adolescent development. Consent from schools was obtained first, followed by letters to parents soliciting the participation of mothers and their daughters. Girls completed questionnaires in small groups at their schools and were weighed and measured by a nurse employed by the research program. At Time 2, only the girls who were mid-adolescents (Grades 9–11) were recontacted to participate in the present longitudinal project (N = 193). Girls again completed questionnaires and were weighed and measured at school, if possible. At Time 3, the young women completed questionnaires through the mail and completed phone interviews to ascertain additional information about their current situations and affective adjustment. Adolescents were paid for their participation at all times of measurement.

Given that 6 years had passed from Time 2 to Time 3, 12% of girls and their families could not be located at Time 3. An additional 18% failed to respond to our mail and telephone requests. This resulted in a final participation rate of 70% of the original Time 2 sample (N = 134). The present analyses included only those girls who had complete item data on the measure of eating attitudes at all three times of measurement. Analysis of Time 2 measures found no consistent differences between girls who did and did not go on to participate in the study at Time 3 on any of the 12 variables used in this study. One significant difference was that girls who did not continue to participate in the study reported less family cohesion than girls who did continue to participate (p < .05). Bonferroni-type adjustments in the alpha level based on the number of comparisons were not made; such adjustments would have resulted in the elimination of this difference. No differences were found for the measures of eating behaviors, depressive affect, or other measures of family relations.

Measures

Measures have been selected on the basis of their pertinence to the development of eating problems. These cover the domains of attitudes about eating, physical development, personality, psychopathology, and family relationships. Cronbach's alpha was calculated for each measure. Overall, measures were quite reliable in this sample of adolescent girls, with alphas ranging from .67 to .94; 65% of alphas were greater than .80 and only two were below .70.

Assessment of eating problems. Eating attitudes were measured by using the EAT-26, an abbreviated version of the 40-item Eating Attitudes Test (EAT; Garner & Garfinkel, 1979), at all three times of measurement (α = .77, .88, and .91, respectively). (An abbreviated version was administered at the first time of measurement.) The EAT-26 is rated on a 6-point Likert-type scale from *describes me not at all* (1) to *describes me very well* (6) and covers the areas of pathological avoidance of fattening foods and preoccupation with a thin body shape (dieting behaviors), thoughts about food and bulimic behaviors such as bingeing and purging, and the respondent's self-control of eating and perceived social pressures to gain weight. The EAT-26 has demonstrated validity with both clinical and nonclinical samples (Garner & Garfinkel, 1980; Schwartz, Thompson, & Johnson, 1982).

We used the scoring system developed by Garner and his colleagues (Garner, Olmsted, Bohr, & Garfinkel, 1982), which identifies individuals who are likely to have clinical levels of anorexia or food control problems. This scoring method collapses item responses of 1, 2, or 3 to 0 and recodes 4, 5, and 6 to 1, 2, and 3, respectively; item scores are summed. A cutoff score of 20 was established (Garner et al., 1982) that differentiates potential clinical from subclinical reports.[1] Although questionnaire methods for diagnosing clinical eating disorders are less conclusive than are diagnostic interviews

---

[1] Because the first assessment in young adolescence used an abbreviated form of the EAT-26, the standard scoring system (Garner, Olmsted, Bohr, & Garfinkel, 1982) could not be applied. Instead, mean scores were calculated at Times 1 and 2 on the original 1–6 scale. Then, the two scoring methods were compared such that the mean score associated with the cutoff score of 20 was identified from the mid-adolescence time of measurement. Extrapolating from this score, we determined a cutoff score for the young-adolescent time of measurement (3.00). Given that the range, mean, and standard deviation for the EAT-26 were similar across times of measurement, we decided that this approach provided comparable scoring across time. In addition, previous comparisons conducted on the abbreviated and long versions of the SIQYA have verified the comparability of short and long forms in the assessment of self-image in a related sample of early adolescents (Brooks-Gunn, Rock, & Warren, 1989).

(Szmukler, 1985), this approach is accepted as a method of screening samples and clearly identifies girls with serious eating problems (King, 1989; Patton et al., 1990). Because the present study examines a normal sample of girls, reports of clinical levels of eating disorders were expected to be low; hence, the EAT-26 was not expected to identify "cases." However, we used the cutoff score of 20 to categorize those girls who have serious eating problems as seen in other studies (King, 1989).

Correlates of eating problems

PHYSICAL DEVELOPMENT. As weight is considered an important influence on eating attitudes and behavior, and as weight has meaning in relation to height, we expected that increased body fat would be associated with greater impulses to diet and to engage in unhealthy eating practices. Height and weight were reported by the participants at each time of measurement. The percentage of body fat was estimated on the basis of equations developed by Mellits and Cheek (1970). Although these formulas have been criticized because of concerns about the representativeness of the sample on which they were developed, body fat is used in our research as a relative measure within the sample or within subject over time rather than as an absolute measure.

At Time 3, when all participants were expected to be postmenarcheal, the young women were asked to report their age at menarche. It has been demonstrated that women and adolescent girls are accurate in reporting their age of menarche for researchers and health professionals (Bean, Leeper, Wallace, Sherman, & Jagger, 1979; Rierdan & Koff, 1985). Age at menarche was used as a continuous variable.

BODY IMAGE. On the basis of the literature on correlates of eating problems discussed previously, poor body image was expected to be related to eating problems whereas positive body image was expected to be associated with healthy behaviors. Body image and satisfaction with body parts and appearance were assessed by using the Satisfaction With Body Parts scale (Padin, Lerner, & Spiro, 1981) and the Body Image subscale of the Self-Image Questionnaire for Young Adolescents (SIQYA; Petersen, Schulenberg, Abramowitz, Offer, & Jarcho, 1984). The SIQYA has nine subscales tapping various dimensions of self-image nad has established reliability and validity with adolescents of these ages (Brooks-Gunn, Rock, & Warren, 1989; Petersen et al., 1984). The Body Image subscale of the SIQYA asks subjects to rate on a 1- to 6-point Likert-type scale how much each statement describes themselves. Items include "I am proud of my body" and "I frequently feel ugly and unattractive." In addition to standard items addressing satisfaction with appearance, the Body Image subscale of the SIQYA also includes items addressing satisfaction with one's pubertal development, such as "I am uncomfortable with the way my body is developing." This scale was administered at Times 1 and 2 (α = .74 and .71, respectively). As this measure is designed for young and early adolescents, it was not included in the young-adult follow-up assessment. At Times 2 and 3, the Satisfaction With Body Parts scale (Padin et al., 1981) was given (α = .85 and .82, respectively). This scale asks for ratings of the attractiveness of 13 body parts (e.g., thighs, hips, hair, and breasts) and overall appearance on a 1- to 5-point scale; the scale has established reliability and stability in samples of young adult women and older adolescents. At Time 2, the two body image measures were highly correlated (r = .72, p < .0001), indicating that the measures were tapping the same construct.

SELF-IMAGE AND PSYCHOLOGICAL WELL-BEING. A variety of personality measures were administered at each time of testing. Again, each of the measures analyzed were chosen on the basis of the previously discussed literature that has identified several psychological correlates of eating problems in short-term longitudinal or cross-sectional studies. We expected that internalizing behaviors such as depressive affect or feelings of ineffectiveness would be more highly associated with the development of eating problems than would externalizing behaviors (e.g., aggressive affect). At the first time of testing, girls completed the Psychopathology subscale (α = .67) of the SIQYA (Petersen et al., 1984). At the second time of testing, this scale was replaced by measures chosen to assess specific aspects of psychopathology or psychological adjustment instead of the more global construct. The Perfectionistic (α = .85) and Ineffectiveness (α = .90) subscales of the Eating Disorders Inventory (EDI; Garner et al., 1983) were administered at Time 2 to assess psychological functioning associated with eating problems. The EDI has been validated for use with both clinical and nonclinical samples (Garner et al., 1983). Because of the time constraints of the participants in young adulthood, these scales were deleted from the test battery.

The Youth Self-Report (YSR; Achenbach & Edelbrock, 1986) was also given at Time 2. This measure assesses a range of affective states and related constructs. In the present investigation, we used the Aggressive Affect (α = .84), Delinquency (α = .80), and Hyperactivity (α = .69) subscales as indicators of mood and behavior regulation problems that may be associated with disturbed eating. In particular, these scales tap externalizing behaviors indicative of "acting out" and disturbances with impulse control that may be related to difficulty regulating eating behavior (e.g., bingeing). These scales have demonstrated validity in the assessment of externalizing behaviors. The Internalizing scales of the YSR were not used in these analyses: As these scales are highly correlated with measures of depressive affect, their inclusion in analyses would have been redundant.[2] At Time 3, the YSR was not administered because it would no longer have been an age-appropriate measure for most of the participants in the study.

The Emotional Tone subscale of the SIQYA was administered at Times 1 and 2 (α = .77 and .85, respectively) and has been used as an indicator of depressive affect in young adolescents (Ebata, 1987). The Center for Epidemiological Studies Depression Scale (CES-D; Radloff, 1977) was used at Times 2 (α = .88) and 3 (α = .88) because it is a well-validated and reliable measure of depressive affect with adolescents and young adults (Radloff, 1991). Because the CES-D can be used as an indicator of clinical levels of depression in addition to depressive affect, it was added at Time 2. Emotional Tone was discontinued at Time 3 because it was considered to be less appropriate for young women (it was developed for adolescents rather than young adults) and was subsumed by the CES-D. The Emotional Tone scale and the CES-D are highly related in this sample, with $r = -.64$ at Time 2, indicating that they tap similar constructs for girls in late adolescence. (As high scores on the SIQYA reflect better adjustment and self-image, the correlation is negative as expected.)

FAMILY RELATIONSHIPS. We assessed family relationships using several measures over time designed to target developmentally salient family interactions. We expected that family conflict and low warmth would be associated with eating problems and that high family warmth and low conflict might act as protective factors for the development of problems. The Family Relations subscale of the SIQYA (Petersen et al., 1984) was used to assess relationships with parents at Times 1 and 2 (α = .76 and .82, respectively). At Time 2, family organization and functioning were also measured by using the Family Environment Scale (FES; Moos, 1974). The FES has demonstrated validity for discriminating relevant groups such as clinical and non-clinical families (Billings & Moos, 1982). Girls completed the Cohesiveness and Conflict subscales of the FES to assess closeness and conflict in the family system (α = .87 and .78, respectively). The true–false format of the

---

[2]The scoring of the YSR was conducted before the release of the present method of scoring developed by Achenbach and Edelbrock (1986); the YSR was scored with the system recommended at that time. Although it is possible to rescore the subscales by using the present system, results of analyses on the Time 1 and Time 2 data, using the earlier method, have been published. Thus, for the sake of consistency, we continued to use the same scale scores in our analyses. As examinations of the two approaches indicate few substantial differences (e.g., a few items removed from a scale and included on a related scale) and as the present scales have good reliabilities (α ranging from .69 to .84), we felt that it was more important to retain comparability for the present analyses.

FES was altered to a 4-point Likert-type scale. Other research (e.g., Plomin, McClearn, Pedersen, Nesselroade, & Bergeman, 1988) has found this scoring approach to be a useful and reliable adaptation of the scale.

As most young women at Time 3 no longer lived at home, the FES was not considered an appropriate measure of family relations. Instead, at Time 3, we asked these young adults to complete the Relationship With Mother and the Relationship With Father scales (Hoffman, 1984) to assess conflictual independence (α = .92 for relationship with mothers and α = .94 for relationship with fathers).

Risk trajectories and correlates of trajectories. Because some of the girls had recurrent or chornic problems whereas others exhibited only transitory problems across the adolescent years, the pattern of eating problems was examined. Cutoff scores on the EAT-26 from both of the first two times of measurement were used to identify four subgroups of girls. Girls with chronic eating problem were above the cutoff at both times. Girls who were below the cutoff at both times were classified as *low risk*, where risk refers to risk of having or developing a serious eating problem (as tapped by the EAT-26). Being above the cutoff at either of the first two times of measurement but not at the other is classified as *transient risk* for having a serious, potentially clinical disturbance. Girls who were below the cutoff as young adolescents and above the cutoff as mid-adolescents were classified as *late-transient risk*, and girls who were initially above the cutoff but were subsequently below it were classified as *early-transient risk*. We analyzed the two transient groups as distinct groups to test whether mental health trajectories of eating problems were different depending on the timing of the onset of the problem (i.e., early vs. late in adolescence). Because the difference between a score of 19, 20, or 21 may not represent a substantial difference in attitudes and behaviors, we reran analyses using two alternative cutoff scores for classifying girls into groups on the basis of slightly higher ($\geqslant$ 22) versus slightly lower ($\geqslant$ 18) cutoff scores. In both sets of analyses, overall effects were the same, although F values were somewhat lower or higher, depending on the analysis, than those reported.

By grouping girls on the basis of their attitudes or behaviors over time, it was possible to identify correlates of group membership (Times 1 and 2) and the short-term (Time 2) and long-term (Time 3) outcomes of these trajectories. Categorizing individuals by pattern of psychological disturbance is a commonly used practice in clinical studies and has been recommended as a useful methodological strategy for understanding the development of psychopathology (Rutter, 1989).

RESULTS

Change in Eating Attitudes Over Time

The means and standard deviations for the EAT-26 at each time of measurement were 2.43 (*SD* = 0.86) in young adolescence, 13.11 (*SD* = 10.3) in mid-adolescence, and 14.05 (*SD* = 10.66) in late adolescence or the transition to adulthood. Means for the EAT-26 remained virtually the same across time despite necessary differences in scoring at Time 1. However, the percentages of girls whose scores were indicative of having a serious eating problem (possibly clinical disorder) suggest that disturbed eating attitudes and behaviors were a problem for a quarter of the sample at each period of adolescence, with 31 young adolescent girls (26.7%), 32 mid-adolescent girls (27.6%), and 29 late-adolescent girls (25.9%) above the cutoff on the EAT-26. The cross-time correlation for the EAT-26 scores between young and mid-adolescence scores was .43 (*p* < .05) and .37 (*p* < .05) between mid- and late adolescence and .12 (*ns*) between young and late adolescence. As expected, scores that were closer in time exhibited higher correlations. The correlations also suggest that girls did not maintain their rank ordering within the sample; hence, at any one time, it was a somewhat different subgroup of girls who were experiencing highly disturbed eating behaviors. This confirmed the necessity of classifying girls into subgroups on the basis of the pattern of their behaviors (as previously described) rather than viewing the sample as a developmentally homogeneous group.

Traditional regression techniques were not considered appropriate for analyzing change over time, because it was clear from the descriptive analyses that girls exhibited different patterns of disturbances (e.g., *r* = .37 between mid- and late-adolescent EAT-26 scores). Using regression analyses of the whole group to ascertain the correlates of behavior would have been unsuccessful given that girls' behaviors were heterogeneous; the regression approach would not have adequately accounted for behavioral change over time (Rogosa & Willett, 1985; Willett, 1988), especially for distinguishing correlates that may only be related to very high or very low scores. Our goal was to test whether homogeneous subgroups existed on the basis of pattern of adolescent eating behavior and to identify the correlates of these different patterns to understand healthy and potentially pathologic development. As noted, similar approaches that have defined subgroups of behaviors have been used by researchers studying eating behaviors in college students (Striegel-Moore et al., 1989) and adults (King, 1989; Vollrath et al., 1992).

Risk Trajectories Based on EAT-26 Scores

On the basis of EAT-26 scores in young and mid-adolescence, 70 girls (60.3%) were in the low-risk group for having or developing a serious eating problem, 14 (12.1%) were in the early-transient-risk group, 15 (12.9%) were in the late-transient-risk group, and 17 (14.7%) were in the chronic group. We conducted an analysis of variance (ANOVA) to examine group differences on a variety of psychological and physical constructs at each time of measurement. For similar measures, multivariate analysis of variance (MANOVA) was conducted; Pillais multivariate tests are reported. We conducted follow-up tests on significant univariate effects by using Fisher's least-significant-difference (LSD) test to assess specific group differences. Because girls were of different ages at any one time of measurement, we conducted analyses using age as a covariate within a time period. Age was either not a significant covariate or did not influence main effects in any of the analyses. Intercorrelations among measures are shown by time period (e.g., Table 1). Note that strong associations among like constructs are not common and are usually accounted for by the multivariate analyses. Table 2 lists the main effects and means by risk group for each analysis.

Entry onto risk-group trajectories (young adolescence). During young adolescence, several correlates of group membership were identified from the physical and psychological measures. The percentage of body fat differentiated the chronic group from all other girls, with girls in the chronic group having the highest percentage of fat. This is particularly striking as this group differed at Time 1 from girls in the early-transient-risk group who were also identified as having scores suggestive of a disorder or serious problem but who did not continue to have high scores. Multivariate and

TABLE 1

Correlation Matrix: Eating Attitudes and Correlates of Behavior
in Young Adolescence

Measure	1	2	3	4	5
1. EAT-26	—				
2. % of body fat	.39**	—			
3. Body Image[a]	−.50**	−.14	—		
4. Psychopathology[a]	.48**	.12	−.48**	—	
5. Family Relations[a]	−.35**	−.11	.33**	−.19*	—

Note. EAT-26 = an abbreviated version of the 40-item Eating Attitudes Test.
[a] Assessed with the Self-Image Questionnaire for Young Adolescents.
$*p < .05.$ $**p < .001.$

univariate effects were also found for the Body Image, Psychopathology, and Family Relations subscales. Multivariate effects would be expected on the basis of the moderate correlations among the three scales from the SIQYA as shown in Table 1. For Body Image, low-risk girls reported the most positive feelings about their bodies and differed from girls in the chronic and early-transient-risk groups who had the lowest scores; girls in the early-transient-risk group also differed from girls in the late-transient-risk group. For Psychopathology, low-risk and late-transient-risk groups had the least psychopathology and differed from chronic and early-transient-risk groups who reported the most. For Family Relations, again, low-risk and late-transient-risk groups reported the most positive family relations differing from the early-transient-risk group.

In summary, during young adolescence, correlates of group membership could be identified with (a) positive family relations and body image and low psychopathology associated with a low-risk trajectory for the development or occurrence of eating problems, and (b) poorer family relations and body image and higher psychopathology and a higher percentage of body fat associated with a chronic trajectory for eating problems, and temporarily disturbed eating attitudes typical of the early-transient-risk group girls.

Correlates of risk-group trajectories (mid-adolescence). During mid-adolescence, similar analyses identified immediate outcomes of these trajectories. Unfortunately, as height was not obtained from several girls during mid-adolescence, results for the physical measure, percentage of body fat, are reported for a reduced sample size. However, results are significant and similar to those for Time 1. Chronic girls have a higher percentage of body fat than all other girls. Age at Time 2 was a significant covariate but did not influence the nature of the main effect for risk group.

Psychological differences among groups also persisted into mid-adolescence. At Time 2, additional measures of personality and psychopathology were administered to assess more thoroughly the nature of the correlates of disturbed eating behaviors. Intercorrelations among measures are shown in Table 3 and again confirm the need to conduct multivariate analyses among like measures. Whereas the correlations with eating behaviors and other measures were predominantly weak, correlations among similar constructs were moderate to strong, with the strongest associations between the most similar constructs (e.g., the two measures of body image, ineffectiveness and depressive affect). As indicated in Table 2, risk-group effects were found for nearly all measures, including multivariate effects for (a) the two body image measures with univariate effects on both scales, (b) the two scales of the EDI with a univariate effect for Ineffectiveness, (c) the three

TABLE 2
Correlates of Young and Mid-Adolescence Risk-Group Trajectories as Determined from Eat-26 Scores

Measure	Effect		Risk group			
	Multivariate $F(df)$	Univariate $F(df)$	Low	Early-transient	Late-transient	Chronic
Young adolescence						
% of body fat		7.45*** (3, 107)				
M			31.75b	32.65b	31.83b	39.58a
SD			6.01	7.26	3.75	7.52
SIQYA scales	6.57*** (9, 291)					
Body Image		15.65*** (3, 109)				
M			4.12a	2.78b,x	3.74y	3.22b
SD			0.74	0.63	0.81	0.90
Psychopathology		12.10*** (3, 109)				
M			2.74a	3.35b	2.48a	3.76b
SD			0.66	0.96	0.69	0.85
Family Relations		6.10*** (3, 101)				
M			5.04b	4.13a	5.11b	4.59
SD			0.69	1.22	0.74	0.60
Mid-adolescence						
% of body fat		5.42** (3, 82)				
M			35.13b	36.20b	34.05b	41.89a
SD			5.34	7.64	4.28	7.84
Body image	5.43*** (6, 216)					
Body Image (SIQYA)		11.87*** (3, 112)				
M			4.49a	3.63b	4.14x	3.49b,y
SD			0.69	0.56	0.72	1.01
Satisfaction With Body Parts		4.70** (3, 108)				
M			3.55a	3.04b	3.46	3.12b
SD			0.50	0.61	0.53	0.80
Perfectionism (EDI)	5.42*** (6, 224)	2.54 (3, 112)				
M			3.48	3.82	3.17	4.20
SD			1.12	1.27	1.42	1.13

	F				
Ineffectiveness (EDI)	11.34*** (3, 112)				
M		1.82$_a$	2.39	2.05$_a$	3.02$_b$
SD		0.69	0.81	0.77	1.11
CES-D (Depressive Affect)	12.64*** (3, 109)				
M		13.81$_b$	16.86$_b$	15.86$_b$	27.94$_a$
SD		8.40	8.06	9.66	8.06
Youth Self-Report	2.90** (9, 336)				
Delinquency	5.61** (3, 112)				
M		6.14$_a$	8.07	8.07	10.65$_b$
SD		3.70	4.29	5.04	5.40
Aggression	6.97*** (3, 112)				
M		10.54$_a$	12.79	10.67$_a$	17.41$_b$
SD		5.22	5.94	6.34	6.78
Hyperactive	3.70* (3, 112)				
M		5.59$_a$	6.57	4.87$_a$	8.41$_b$
SD		3.29	2.14	3.76	4.72
Late adolescence					
EAT-26 (total score)	4.86** (3, 108)				
M		10.41$_a$	17.23$_b$	19.27$_b$	15.81
SD		8.85	12.28	12.60	8.55
% of body fat	4.32** (3, 98)				
M		28.61$_b$	28.62$_b$	27.70$_b$	32.51$_a$
SD		3.88	3.88	3.59	5.37
Age at menarche	3.45* (3, 108)				
M		13.04$_a$	12.85	12.60	11.94$_b$
SD		1.42	1.28	1.12	0.75
CES-D (Depressive Affect)	3.42* (3, 107)				
M		12.71$_a$	14.00	13.47	20.47$_b$
SD		8.18	6.16	10.99	9.01

Note. Pillais value is reported for the multivariate F test. Subscripts denote significant differences between groups. Groups with the same subscript are not significantly different and groups without a subscript are not different. EAT-26 = an abbreviated version of the 40-item Eating Attitudes Test; SIQYA = Self-Image Questionnaire for Young Adolescents; EDI = Eating Disorders Inventory; CES-D = Center for Epidemiological Studies Depression Scale.

* $p < .05$.   ** $p < .01$.   *** $p < .001$ and $.0001$.

337

TABLE 3
Correlation Matrix: Eating Attitudes and Correlates of Behavior in Mid-Adolescence

Measure	1	2	3	4	5	6	7	8	9	10	11	12
1. EAT-26	—											
2. % of body fat	.18	—										
3. Body Image (SIQYA)	-.30**	-.21*	—									
4. Satisfaction with Body Parts	.19	-.27**	.71***	—								
5. Perfectionism (EDI)	.12	.13	-.25*	-.09	—							
6. Ineffectiveness (EDI)	.31**	.18	-.76***	-.49***	.40***	—						
7. Aggression (YSR)	.17	.12	-.37***	-.01	.43***	.51***	—					
8. Delinquency (YSR)	.20*	.09	-.32**	-.01	.33**	.34**	.64***	—				
9. Hyperactive (YSR)	.03	.01	-.51***	-.32**	.24*	.61***	.60***	.48***	—			
10. CES-D (Depressive Affect)	.38***	.22*	-.52***	-.25*	.29**	.62***	.52***	.34**	.46***	—		
11. Family Cohesion (FES)	-.07	.00	.24*	.03	-.24*	-.42***	-.32**	-.41***	-.20*	-.19	—	
12. Family Conflict (FES)	.07	.08	-.28**	-.06	.26**	.45***	.43***	.25*	.10	.33**	-.55***	—

Note. EAT-26 = an abbreviated version of the 40-item Eating Attitudes Test; SIQYA = Self-Image Questionnaire for Young Adults; EDI = Eating Disorders Inventory; YSR = Youth Self-Report; CES-D = Center for Epidemiological Studies Depression Scale; FES = Family Environment Scale.
*p < .05. **p < .01. ***p < .001.

scales of the YSR with univariate effects on each subscale, and (d) family relations as assessed by two scales of the FES, F (6, 206) = 2.21, $p < .05$ (value not shown in Table 2); this was a weak effect, with neither univariate reaching significance. A univariate effect was found for the CES-D measure of depressive affect. In all of the cases, girls in the chronic group had lower functioning and greater psychopathology than girls in the low-risk group. For Body Image, Ineffectiveness, Aggressive Affect, and Hyperactivity, girls in the late-transient-risk group also differed from girls in the chronic group. This is particularly interesting because girls in the late-transient-risk group reported high EAT-26 scores at this time but did not also have the higher levels of psychopathology that were reported by girls in the high-chronic group. Also of note is that girls in the early-transient group appeared to have intermediate levels of psychopathology even though the level of disturbance in eating attitudes had declined (i.e., their EAT-26 scores were below the cutoff score and were indistinguishable from scores of low-risk girls during mid-adolescence).

Long-term outcomes of risk-group trajectories (young adulthood). Long-term outcomes of adolescent trajectories were assessed at Time 3, the young adulthood assessment. We examined scores on the EAT-26 to see if earlier disturbances corresponded to subsequent eating attitudes; in this analysis, only girls in the late-transient-risk group differed from girls in the low-risk group, with girls in the early-transient and chronic groups exhibiting intermediate scores.

As all of the young women in the sample were postmenarcheal at Time 3, it was possible to determine if the risk groups differed on their timing of pubertal maturation. The chronic and the low-risk groups were differentiated by their age at menarche, with girls in the chronic group having the earliest age of menarche and girls in the low-risk group having the latest age of menarche. Percentage of body fat, calculated from self-reports of adult height and weight, again demonstrated physical differences among the groups, with girls in the chronic group continuing to have a higher percentage of body fat than other girls. This indicates that chronic eating disturbances were associated with a particular body type rather than being associated with the pubertal process. That is, earlier maturing girls would have higher rates of body fat because their development is more advanced than that of other girls.

As in earlier assessment, psychological differences were also found in young adulthood. Girls in the chronic group reported higher rates of depressive affect than any other group of girls. However, no group differences were found for the satisfaction with body parts or on the family relations measures. Intercorrelations among measures, shown in Table 4, were weak,

TABLE 4
Correlation Matrix: Eating Attitudes and Correlates of Behavior in Young Adulthood

Measure	1	2	3	4	5	6	7
1. EAT-26	—						
2. % of body fat	.21*	—					
3. Age at menarch	.01	-.12	—				
4. Satisfaction with Body Parts	-.27**	-.29**	.15	—			
5. CES-D (Depressive Affect)	.29**	-.03	-.24*	-.29**	—		
6. Conflict with mother	.26**	.05	-.04	-.12	.34***	—	
7. Conflict with father	.01	-.15	-.13	.12	.25**	.57***	—

Note. EAT-26 = an abbreviated version of the 40-item Eating Attitudes Test. CES-D = Center for Epidemiological Studies Depression Scale.

*$p < .05$. **$p < .01$. **$p < .001$.

with only a few correlations showing stronger associations (e.g., the measures of relationship with each parent).

To determine if risk trajectories based on EAT-26 scores in young and mid-adolescence were related to subsequent serious eating problems in young adulthood, we ran cross-tabulations between the risk groups and whether or not girls were above the cutoff score for having a serious eating problem during the transition to adulthood. An association was found between risk group and subsequent maladaptive eating at Time 3, $\chi^2(3, N = 112) = 15.47$, $p < .01$, $\eta = .37$. Specifically, of the 17 girls in the chronic group, 7 (46.7%) were above the cutoff for having a serious eating problem. However, similar rates of disturbed eating were observed in both the transient groups (early and late), with 46.7% and 46.2%, respectively, of young women in these risk groups also reporting elevated scores. It is interesting to note that only 13% of girls in the low-risk group had elevated scores in young adulthood. This is noteworthy given the high incidence of eating problems during the college years.

In summary, it is clear that girls began on different mental health trajectories in the young adolescent years and that risk trajectory was associated with their pubertal maturation, was linked to particular physical characteristics as well as psychological functioning, and was associated with the subsequent development of eating problems. More important, these young adolescent trajectories are predictive of young adult adjustment outcomes.

DISCUSSION

The rates and patterns of eating problems in this sample confirm that eating problems pose a serious health problem for adolescent girls, many of whom are still experiencing physical growth. The percentage of girls who experience a serious and possibly clinical disorder before the college years suggests that the eating problems and disorders are occurring at exactly the time when they are likely to result in lifelong consequences both for physical and psychological development. At this time, there is little research that has examined the physiological and lasting physical effects of brief periods of disturbed behavior as reported by girls in this study.

Perhaps the most significant result of this examination is that the development of eating problems follows different trajectories during the adolescent decade. It was possible to identify physical and psychological characteristics of girls who would have not only long-term eating problems but also other adjustment disturbances as indicated by depressive affect.

Use of longitudinal analyses clarified these paths in ways that could not have been achieved with cross-sectional examinations.

For example, girls in the chronic group had earlier ages at menarche. However, at any one time of measurement, the girls reporting elevated EAT-26 scores included some girls who were on-time or later maturers. Pubertal timing effects would have been obscured in a cross-sectional examination. Instead, these findings suggest that early maturation is a risk factor for not simply an episodic eating problem but also chronic problems.

The psychological correlates of the trajectories are also noteworthy. Depressive affect was highest in the chronic group. This is in line with existing research on clinical samples that has reported comorbidity of eating disorders and depression in adults (Herzog, Keller, Sacks, Yeh, & Lavori, 1992). Figure 1 depicts the means for the CES-D by risk group at both mid-adolescence and the transition to young adulthood. The fact that girls with chronic eating problems appear to experience elevated depressive affect in subsequent years (i.e., prevalence of group differences in later times of measurement rather than earlier times) lends support to the assertion that the etiology of the disorders is distinct (Strober & Katz, 1987). In addition, the mean CES-D score for the girls in the chronic risk group during mid-adolescence is over the cutoff for identifying a clinical depressive episode (see Figure 1). It should be remembered that girls in the late-transient-risk group also have elevated EAT-26 scores at this time of measurement; however, only the chronic group is distinct in the level of depressive affect reported. This group continued to experience higher levels of depressive affect than other girls into young adulthood, although the group mean dropped below the clinical cutoff. This suggests that girls with recurrent eating problems experience more comorbidity than girls with transient problems, a finding that is comparable with the clinical literature (e.g., Hatsukami, Eckert, Mitchell, & Pyle, 1984; Lancelot, Brooks-Gunn, & Warren, 1991).

It is possible that girls in the late-transient group are on a similar trajectory as girls in the chronic group but have started on this path somewhat later and that they will develop greater pathology over time. However, the present findings suggest that recurrent problems in adolescence are more closely linked to physical development and other psychopathology. Even though girls in the late-transient group had more disturbed eating in young adulthood, they did not have the same physical or psychological characteristics; this appears to be a different behavioral pattern that merits further investigation.

The fact that eating problems had only a minimal association with family relations in this sample is surprising, although this may be attribut-

Mid-Adolescence

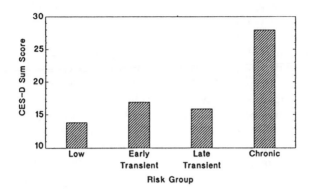

Late Adolescence

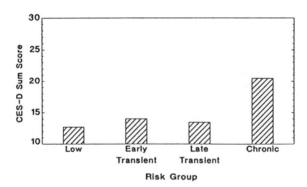

Figure 1. Risk-group means for the Center for Epidemiological Studies Depression (CES-D) scale at mid-adolescence and the late-adolescence transition to young adulthood. Girls in the chronic-risk group report significantly higher rates of depressive affect than any other group of girls at both times of measurement, although overall scores for the sample decrease over time.

able to the use of only questionnaire reports of family relations rather than more in-depth assessment strategies. There was some indication that positive family relations were associated with the low-risk trajectory group and may have acted as a protective factor for the development of eating problems. In contrast, entry onto a chronic-risk trajectory was associated with biological or physical factors such as higher rates of body fat, early maturational timing, and psychological factors such as higher psychopathology and poorer body image. This is consistent with other research that finds that early-maturing girls experience higher rates of family conflict and greater persistence of that conflict across adolescence than do other girls and boys (Paikoff & Brooks-Gunn, 1991; Steinberg, 1987). Earlier maturational timing may represent the interplay between psychological development and social pressures in that early-maturing girls have had less time to develop coping strategies for dealing with the physical changes of puberty (e.g., weight gain) and experience those changes before other girls and boys, leading to a different social context for their development (Brooks-Gunn, Petersen, & Eichorn, 1985; Graber & Brooks-Gunn, in press).

The generalizability of these results is constrained by certain aspects of this study. As the sample was predominantly White and upper-middle class, results may be different in adolescent girls from other ethnic and socioeconomic backgrounds. As previously noted, rates of eating disorders are increasing in other ethnic and socioeconomic groups (e.g., Hsu, 1987; Pumariega, 1986). Striegel-Moore and her colleagues (Striegel-Moore, Pike, Rodin, Schreiber, & Wilfley, 1993) reported that associations among dieting behavior and pressures, weight and body fat, and body image were similar in White and African American prepubertal girls. Although such findings are suggestive of potential common processes, further investigation is required before the findings from this study can be applied to a broader range of adolescent girls and young women.

An additional limitation of this investigation is the reliance on questionnaire data by the same respondent (i.e., the adolescent rather than a parent or clinician). Studies have commonly reported convergence of self-report data and low correspondence between reporters as in the case of parent-child agreement on reports of depression (Kendall, Cantwell, & Kazdin, 1989). Kendall and his colleagues noted that it is impossible to say which reporter is "better" because each may be assessing behavior in different contexts. They suggested the use of measures with established normative databases and cutoff scores when clinical conditions are being assessed.

In the case of our primary measure, the EAT-26 does not have a high predictive value for identifying clinical "cases" (King, 1989; Szmukler, 1985). This is partly because the predictive value of a questionnaire usually drops when the prevalence of the disorder is below 20%, as is the case with eating disorders (Szmukler, 1985; Williams, Hand, & Tarnopolosky, 1982). It is clear that if we wanted to focus only on clinical levels of eating disorders rather than subclinical problems, it would have been necessary to use the suggested practice of screening with the EAT-26 followed by a diagnostic interview of all individuals over the cutoff score of 20. However, prior research (King, 1989) found that "false positives" identified along with clinical cases by the EAT-26 were not healthy individuals but instead were individuals who exhibited subclinical problems, psychological distress, and excessive weight concerns and dieting. Given that these behaviors pose significant health risks in and of themselves, we deemed it appropriate to investigate all girls above the cutoff and to refer to them as experiencing serious eating problems. In addition, predictive value has been found to increase in adolescent samples from private versus public schools (Szmukler, 1985). Although all cutoff scores represent, to some extent, an arbitrary numerical distinction between groups of individuals, the score of 20 is well established as being likely to differentiate serious problems.

Eating problems such as dieting, preoccupation with weight, and bingeing emerge during the adolescent years and have been associated with several serious health problems over and above frank eating disorders (Sallis, 1993). Dieting prior to puberty can result in the delay of pubertal development, whereas dieting and weight loss postpubertally have been associated with amenorrhea and the reversion to prepubertal hormonal functioning (Warren, 1983). As skeletal growth continues across adolescence into young adulthood in most women, dieting practices that result in inadequate calcium intake or disrupted hormonal functioning have been associated with skeletal problems such as scoliosis and increased likelihood of bone injuries during adolescence and young adulthood (Akella, Warren, Jonnavithula, & Brooks-Gunn, 1991; Warren, Brooks-Gunn, Hamilton, Hamilton, & Warren, 1986) and subsequent development of osteoporosis in adulthood (Warren et al., 1991).

The ability to identify risk groups is perhaps the first step in developing prevention and intervention programs to offset the health risks of disturbed eating behaviors. In the case of eating disorders and serious subclinical problems, primary prevention is indicated for all girls in early adolescence given the rates and timing of onset of eating problems reported in this sample. In addition, secondary prevention should be targeted to "at-risk" adolescents such as early-maturing girls with higher percentages of body fat because these are the girls who are at the highest risk for experiencing recurrent problems. The development of primary and secondary prevention programs that encompass the psychological, social, and physical correlates of eating problems providing both nutrition education and social skills enhancement is essential at this time to offset the consequences of girls' developing more serious problems during the adolescent decade.

REFERENCES

Achenbach, T. M., & Edelbrock, C. S. (1986). *Youth self-report profile for girls aged 11-18.* Burlington: University of Vermont Press.

Akella, P., Warren, M. P., Jonnavithula, S., & Brooks-Gunn, J. (1991). Scoliosis in ballet dancers. *Medical Problems of Performing Artists, 6*, 84–86.

American Psychiatric Association. (1987). *Diagnostic and statistical manual of mental disorders* (3rd ed., rev.). Washington, DC: Author.

Attie, I., & Brooks-Gunn, J. (1987). Weight concerns as chronic stressors in women. In R. C. Barnett, L. Biener, & G. K. Baruch (Eds.), *Gender and stress* (pp. 218–254). New York: Free Press.

Attie, I., & Brooks-Gunn, J. (1989). Development of eating problems in adolescent girls: A longitudinal study. *Developmental Psychology, 25*, 70–79.

Attie, I., Brooks-Gunn, J., & Petersen, A. C. (1990). A developmental perspective on eating disorders and eating problems. In M. Lewis & S. Miller (Eds.), *Handbook of developmental psychopathology* (pp. 409–420). New York: Plenum Press.

Bean, J. A., Leeper, J. D., Wallace, R. B., Sherman, B. M., & Jagger, H. J. (1979). Variations in the reporting of menstrual histories. *American Journal of Epidemiology, 109*, 181–185.

Billings, A. G., & Moos, R. H. (1982). Family environments and adaptation: A clinically applicable typology. *American Journal of Family Therapy, 10*, 26–38.

Brooks-Gunn, J., Petersen, A. C., & Eichorn, D. (1985). The study of maturational timing effects in adolescence. *Journal of Youth and Adolescence, 14*, 149–161.

Brooks-Gunn, J., Rock, D., & Warren, M. P. (1989). Comparability of constructs across the adolescent years. *Developmental Psychology, 25*, 51–60.

Crisp, A. H., Harding, B., & McGuinness, B. (1974). Anorexia nervosa, psychoneurotic characteristics of parents: Relationship to prognosis. *Journal of Psychosomatic Research, 18*, 167–173.

Drewnowski, A., Yee, D. K., & Krahn, D. D. (1988). Bulimia in college women: Incidence and recovery rates. *American Journal of Psychiatry, 145*, 753–755.

Ebata, A. T. (1987). *A longitudinal study of psychological distress during early adolescence.* Unpublished doctoral dissertation, Pennsylvania State University.

Elder, G. H., Jr. (1985). Perspectives on the life course. In G. H. Elder, Jr. (Ed.), *Life course dynamics: Trajectories and transitions, 1968–1980* (pp. 23–49). Ithaca, NY: Cornell University Press.

Fairburn, C. G., & Beglin, S. J. (1990). Studies of the epidemiology of bulimia nervosa. *American Journal of Psychiatry, 147*, 401–408.

Faust, M. S. (1983). Alternative constructions of adolescent growth. In J. Brooks-Gunn & A. C. Petersen (Eds.), *Girls at puberty: Biological and psychosocial perspectives* (pp. 105–126). New York: Plenum.

Feldman, S., & Elliott, G. (Eds.). (1990). *At the threshold: The developing adolescent.* Cambridge, MA: Harvard University Press.

Garner, D. M., & Garfinkel, P. E. (1979). The Eating Attitudes Test: An index of the symptoms of anorexia nervosa. *Psychological Medicine, 9*, 1–7.

Garner, D. M., & Garfinkel, P. E. (1980). Socio-cultural factors in the development of anorexia nervosa. *Psychological Medicine, 10*, 547–556.

Garner, D. M., Olmsted, M. P., Bohr, Y., & Garfinkel, P. E. (1982). The Eating Attitudes Test: Psychometric features and clinical correlates. *Psychological Medicine, 12*, 871–878.

Garner, D. M., Olmsted, M. P., & Polivy, J. (1983). Development and validation of a multidimensional eating disorder inventory for anorexia nervosa and bulimia. *International Journal of Eating Disorders, 2*, 15–34.

Graber, J. A., & Brooks-Gunn, J. (in press). Biological and maturational factors in development. In V. B. Van Hasselt & M. Hersen (Eds.), *Handbook of adolescent psychopathology: A guide to diagnosis and treatment.* New York: Macmillan.

Gunnar, M., & Collins, W. A. (Eds.). (1988). *Development during transition to adolescence: Minnesota symposia on child psychology* (Vol. 21). Hillsdale, NJ: Erlbaum.

Hatsukami, D., Eckert, E., Mitchell, J., & Pyle, R. (1984). Affective disorder and substance abuse in women with bulimia. *Psychological Medicine, 14*, 701–704.

Herzog, D. B., Keller, M. B., Sacks, N. R., Yeh, C. J., & Lavori, P. W. (1992). Psychiatric comorbidity in treatment-seeking anorexics and bulimics. *Journal of the American Academy of Child and Adolescent Psychiatry, 31*, 810–818.

Hoffman, J. A. (1984). Psychological separation of late adolescents from their parents. *Journal of Counseling Psychology, 31*, 170–178.

Hsu, L. K. G. (1987). Are the eating disorders becoming more common in Blacks? *International Journal of Eating Disorders, 6*, 113–124.

Johnson, C., & Maddi, K. L. (1986). The etiology of bulimia: Biopsychosocial perspectives. *Adolescent Psychiatry, 13*, 253–274.

Kendall, P. C., Cantwell, D. P., & Kazdin, A. E. (1989). Depression in children and adolescents: Assessment issues and recommendations. *Cognitive Therapy and Research, 13*, 109–146.

Kendler, K. S., MacLean, C., Neale, M., Kessler, R., Heath, A., & Eaves, L. (1991). The genetic epidemiology of bulimia nervosa. *American Journal of Psychiatry, 148*, 1627–1637.

Killen, J. D., Hayward, C., Litt, I., Hammer, L. D., Wilson, D. M., Miner, B., Taylor, B., Varady, A., & Shisslak, C. (1992). Is puberty a risk factor for eating disorders? *American Journal of Diseases in Children, 146*, 323–325.

Killen, J. D., Taylor, C. B., Telch, M. J., Saylor, K. E., Maron, D. J., & Robinson, T. N. (1986). Self-induced vomiting and laxative and diuretic use among teenagers. *Journal of the American Medical Association, 255*, 1447–1449.

King, M. B. (1989). Eating disorders in a general practice population. Prevalence, characteristics and follow-up at 12 to 18 months. *Psychological Medicine* (Monograph Suppl. 14), 1–34.

Lancelot, C., Brooks-Gunn, J., & Warren, M. P. (1991). A comparison of DSM-III and DSM-III-R bulimia classifications. *International Journal of Eating Disorders, 10*, 57–66.

Lerner, R. M., & Foch, T. T. (Eds.). (1987). *Biological–psychosocial interactions in early adolescence: A life-span perspective.* Hillsdale, NJ: Erlbaum.

Levine, M. P. (1987). *Student eating disorders: Anorexia nervosa and bulimia.* Washington, DC: National Education Association.

Mellits, E. D., & Cheek, D. B. (1970). The assessment of body water and fatness from infancy to adulthood. *Monographs of the Society for Research in Child Development, 35* (No. 7, Serial No. 140), 12–26.

Millstein, S. G., Petersen, A. C., & Nightingale, E. O. (Eds.). (1993). *Promotion of health behavior in adolescence.* New York: Oxford University Press.

Minuchin, S., Rosman, B. L., & Baker, L. (1978). *Psychosomatic families: Anorexia nervosa in context.* Cambridge, MA: Harvard University Press.

Moos, R. H. (1974). *Family Environment Scale.* New York: Consulting Psychologists Press.

Orbach, S. (1986). *Hunger strike: The anorectic's struggle as a metaphor for our age.* New York: Norton.

Padin, M. A., Lerner, R. M., & Spiro, A. (1981). Stability of body attitudes and self-esteem in late adolescents. *Adolescence, 16,* 371–384.

Paikoff, R. L., & Brooks-Gunn, J. (1991). Do parent–child relationships change during puberty? *Psychological Bulletin, 110,* 47–66.

Patton, G. C., Johnson-Sabine, E., Wood, K., Mann, A. H., & Wakeling, A. (1990). Abnormal eating attitudes in London schoolgirls—a prospective epidemiological study: Outcome at twelve month follow-up. *Psychological Medicine, 20,* 383–394.

Petersen, A. C., Schulenberg, J. E., Abramowitz, R. H., Offer, D., & Jarcho, H. D. (1984). a Self-Image Questionnaire for Young Adolescents (SIQYA): Reliability and validity studies. *Journal of Youth and Adolescence, 13,* 93–111.

Pike, K. M., & Rodin, J. (1991). Mothers, daughters, and disordered eating. *Journal of Abnormal Psychology, 100,* 198–204.

Plomin, R., McClearn, G. E., Pedersen, N. L., Nesselroade, J. R., & Bergeman, C. S. (1988). Genetic influence on childhood family environment perceived retrospectively from the last half of the life span. *Developmental Psychology, 24,* 738–745.

Pumariega, A. J. (1986). Acculturation and eating attitudes in adolescent girls: A comparative and correlational study. *Journal of the American Academy of Child and Adolescent Psychiatry, 25,* 276–279.

Radloff, L. S. (1977). The CES-D scale: A self-report depression scale for research in the general population. *Applied Psychological Measurement, 1,* 385–401.

Radloff, L. S. (1991). The use of the Center for Epidemiologic Studies Depression Scale in adolescents and young adults. *Journal of Youth and Adolescence, 20,* 149–166.

Rierdan, J., & Koff, E. (1985). Timing of menarche and initial menstrual experience. *Journal of Youth and Adolescence, 14,* 237–244.

Robins, L. N., Helzer, J. E., Weissman, M. M., Orvaschel, H., Gruenberg, E. M., Burke, J. D., & Regier, D. A. (1984). Lifetime prevalence of specific psychiatric disorders in three sites. *Archives of General Psychiatry, 41,* 949–958.

Rogosa, D., & Willett, J. B. (1985). Understanding correlates of change by modeling individual differences in growth. *Psychometrika, 50,* 203–228.

Rosen, J. C., Compas, B. E., & Tacy, B. (1993). The relation among stress, psychological symptoms, and eating disorder symptoms: A prospective analysis. *International Journal of Eating Disorders, 14,* 153–162.

Rutter, M. (1989). Pathways from childhood to adult life. *Journal of Child Psychology and Psychiatry, 30,* 23–51.

Sallis, J. F. (1993). Promoting healthful diet and physical activity. In S. P. Millstein, A. C. Petersen, & E. Nightingale (Eds.), *Promotion of health behavior in adolescence* (pp. 209–241). New York: Oxford University Press.

Sargent, J., Liebman, R., & Silver, M. (1985). Family therapy for anorexia nervosa. In D. M. Garner & P. E. Garfinkel (Eds.), *Handbook of psychotherapy for anorexia nervosa and bulimia* (pp. 257–279). New York: Guilford Press.

Schwartz, D. M., Thompson, M. G., & Johnson, C. L. (1982). The socio-cultural context. *International Journal of Eating Disorders, 1,* 20–36.

Schwartz, D. M., Thompson, M. G., & Johnson, C. L. (1985). Anorexia nervosa and bulimia: The sociocultural context. In S. W. Emmett (Ed.), *Theory and treatment of anorexia nervosa and bulimia* (pp. 95–112). New York: Brunner/Mazel.

Sroufe, L. A., & Rutter, M. (1984). The domain of developmental psychopathology. *Child Development, 55,* 17–29.

Steinberg, L. (1987). Impact of puberty on family relations: Effects of pubertal status and pubertal timing. *Developmental Psychology, 23,* 451–460.

Story, M., Rosenwinkel, K., Himes, J. H., Resnick, M., Harris, L. J., & Blum, R. W. (1991). Demographic and risk factors associated with chronic dieting in adolescents. *American Journal of Diseases in Children, 145,* 994–998.

Storz, N. S., & Greene, W. H. (1983). Body weight, body image, and perception of fad diets in adolescent girls. *Journal of Nutrition Education, 15,* 15–18.

Striegel-Moore, R. H., Pike, K., Rodin, J., Schreiber, G., & Wilfley, D. (1993, March). *Predictors and correlates of drive for thinness: A comparison of 600 Black and White pre-pubertal girls.* Paper presented at the biennial meeting of the Society for Research in Child Development, New Orleans, LA.

Striegel-Moore, R. H., Silberstein, L. R., Frensch, P., & Rodin, J. (1989). A prospective study of disordered eating among college students. *International Journal of Eating Disorders, 8,* 499–509.

Strober, M., & Katz, J. L. (1987). Do eating disorders and affective disorders share a common etiology? A dissenting opinion. *International Journal of Eating Disorders, 6,* 171–180.

Strober, M., Morrell, W., Burroughs, J., Salkin, B., & Jacobs, C. (1985). A controlled family study of anorexia nervosa. *Journal of Psychiatric Research, 19,* 239–246.

Szmukler, G. I. (1985). The epidemiology of anorexia nervosa and bulimia. *Journal of Psychiatric Research, 19,* 143–153.

U.S. Congress, Office of Technology Assessment. (1991, April). *Adolescent health: Vol. I. Summary and policy recommendations* (Publication No. OTA-H-4468). Washington, DC: U.S. Government Printing Office.

Vollrath, M., Koch, R., & Angst, J. (1992). Binge eating and weight concerns among young adults: Results from the Zurich cohort study. *British Journal of Psychiatry, 160,* 498–503.

Warren, M. P. (1983). Effects of undernutrition on reproductive function in the human. *Endocrine Reviews, 4,* 363–377.

Warren, M. P., Brooks-Gunn, J., Fox, R. P., Lancelot, C., Newman, D., & Hamilton, W. G. (1991). Lack of bone accretion and amenorrhea in young dancers: Evidence for a relative osteopenia in weight bearing bones. *Journal of Clinical Endocrinology and Metabolism, 72,* 847–853.

Warren, M. P., Brooks-Gunn, J., Hamilton, L. H., Hamilton, W. G., & Warren, L. F. (1986). Scoliosis and fractures in young ballet dancers: Relationships to delayed menarcheal age and secondary amenorrhea. *New England Journal of Medicine, 314,* 1348–1353.

Willett, J. B. (1988). Questions and answers in the measurement of change. In E. Z. Rothkopf (Ed.), *Review of research in education* (Vol. 15, pp. 345–422). Washington, DC: American Educational Research Association.

Williams, P., Hand, D., & Tarnopolosky, A. (1982). The problem of screening for uncommon disorders—a comment on the Eating Attitudes Test. *Psychological Medicine, 12,* 431–434.

World Health Organization. (1981). *Global strategy for health by the year 2000.* Geneva, Switzerland: World Health Organization.

Yager, J., Landsverk, J., & Edelstein, C. K. (1987). A 20-month follow-up study of 628 women with eating disorders: I. Course and severity. *American Journal of Psychiatry, 144,* 1172–1177.

12

A Clinical Picture of Child and Adolescent Narcolepsy

Ronald E. Dahl, John Holttum, and Laura Trubnick

Western Psychiatric Institute and Clinic,
University of Pittsburgh School of Medicine, Pittsburgh

Although narcolepsy is rarely diagnosed before adulthood, symptoms often begin much earlier and can easily mimic psychiatric disorders in children and adolescents. Clinical experience from a pediatric sleep center is reviewed in 16 consecutive cases of polysomnographically proven narcolepsy with onset of symptoms by age 13 years. Only 1 of the 16 patients presented with the classic clinical tetrad of symptoms (sleepiness, cataplexy, hypnagogic hallucinations, and sleep paralysis). Behavioral and emotional disturbances were present in 12 of 16 cases, with four patients appearing to have been misdiagnosed with a psychiatric disorder before recognition of the narcolepsy. Obesity appeared as an unexpected association in this case series, with 11 of the 16 narcoleptic patients found to be overweight at the time of diagnosis. The varied clinical presentations, polysomnographic findings, family history, and associated psychiatric symptoms are described. The importance of considering narcolepsy in the differential diagnosis of any child or adolescent with excessive sleepiness is emphasized.

Reprinted with permission from the *Journal of the American Academy of Child and Adolescent Psychiatry*, 1994, Vol. 33(6), 834–841. Copyright © 1994 by the American Academy of Child and Adolescent Psychiatry.

From the Department of Psychiatry, Western Psychiatric Institute and Clinic, University of Pittsburgh School of Medicine, Pittsburgh, PA.

The authors thank Beverly Nelson, B.S.N., and the staff of the child and adolescent sleep laboratory for their skillful work obtaining polysomnographic studies in these patients, as well as Deborah Small for her administrative assistance with these patients, their families, and manuscript preparation.

Narcolepsy is a neurological disorder with considerable relevance to the practice of child and adolescent psychiatry for at least three reasons: (1) core symptoms of narcolepsy (sleepiness, cataplexy, and hallucinations) can easily mimic psychiatric disorders; (2) young narcoleptic patients often have significant behavioral and emotional changes; and (3) adult narcoleptics frequently report that their diagnosis was missed for years as children or adolescents.

The chance of encountering a young narcoleptic in a clinical mental health setting is not remote. The prevalence of narcolepsy in the United States has been estimated as 4 to 10 per 10,000 individuals (Dement et al., 1973). Although it has been written that narcolepsy rarely occurs in children, studies indicate that whereas the *diagnosis* is not usually made until adulthood, the onset of symptoms in most cases begins by adolescence (Navelet et al., 1976; Yoss and Daly, 1960). The "classic" clinical picture of narcolepsy includes a tetrad of symptoms: severe daytime sleepiness, cataplexy (sudden loss of muscle tone), hypnagogic hallucinations (vivid dream-like visual images before falling asleep), and sleep paralysis (persistence of rapid eye movement [REM] sleep muscle paralysis after awakening). However, only a minority of patients present with the complete tetrad of symptoms (Aldrich, 1992), and there is a great deal of heterogeneity in clinical descriptions of young narcoleptics (Allsopp and Zaiwalla, 1992; Kotagal et al., 1990; Navelet et al., 1976; Reimao and Lemmi, 1991; Yoss and Daly, 1960; Young et al., 1988).

The similarities between the symptoms of narcolepsy and those of major psychiatric disorders fueled years of debate concerning pathogenesis (Zarconi and Fuchs, 1976). Although current understanding indicates a neurological basis for narcolepsy, the core symptoms can easily be confused with psychiatric illness, particularly in children and adolescents. Hypnagogic hallucinations, especially in a young or frightened child, can mimic a psychosis. Cataplexy was described in the early psychiatric literature as an hysterical phenomenon based on its occurrence in moments of high emotional tension (Zarconi and Fuchs, 1976), and this phenomenon can be mistaken for conversion in children (Yoss and Daly, 1960). Hypersomnia can be a common manifestation of major depressive disorder, particularly in adolescents (Ryan, 1987). Thus, if mood disturbances are present, excessive sleepiness could be misattributed to depression. Furthermore, sleepiness in children is often associated with irritability, impulsivity, and difficulties with focused attention, which can exacerbate or be mistaken for behavioral disorders (Allsopp and Zaiwalla, 1992; Dahl et al., 1991; Dahl, 1992). Navelet and colleagues (1976) reported that among a sample of 88 adults with narcolepsy, 13% had been given a diagnosis of attention deficit disorder as children based on symptoms that were, in retrospect, believed to be an early manifestation of narcolepsy. Diagnostic confusion may also result from the fact that common pharmacological treatments for depression and attention-deficit hyperactivity disorder (tricyclic antidepressants and stimulants) can also improve narcolepsy symptoms.

In addition to the potential for misdiagnosis as a psychiatric disorder, a significant percentage of children with narcolepsy are overlooked entirely or have their symptoms attributed to temperament. One clinical series of 400 narcoleptic patients found that 59% of subjects experienced the onset of symptoms before age 15 years, but only 4% received the diagnosis by that age (Yoss and Daly, 1960). Similarly, Navalet found that among 88 adult narcoleptics, 43 (49%) reported symptoms by age 15 but none were diagnosed before age 19 (Navalet et al., 1976). Clinical experience in many large sleep centers is consistent with the concept that many narcolepsy patients experience early onset of significant symptoms, which go unrecognized and untreated in the early phases of the illness. Delayed and mistaken diagnosis in early-onset narcolepsy may contribute significantly to adult psychosocial dysfunction associated with the disorder (Aldrich, 1992; Broughton et al., 1981; Kales et al., 1982).

METHOD

Subjects

We describe 16 consecutive cases of polysomnographically confirmed narcolepsy with definite onset of symptoms in childhood or early adolescence (each case had well-documented symptoms by age 13 years). Our pediatric sleep center is part of a university hospital system, is directed by a pediatrician certified in sleep disorders medicine, and is physically located in a psychiatric institute within the Division of Child Psychiatry. Subjects were referred for evaluation of a suspected sleep disorder by the following sources: child psychiatrist ($n = 4$); pediatrician ($n = 4$); neurologist ($n = 4$); school health official ($n = 2$); or self-referral ($n = 2$). Patients and their families underwent thorough clinical evaluations including interviews, physical examinations, completion of sleep/wake diaries and, when indicated, medical evaluations.

Sleep Studies and Diagnostic Criteria

Each subject had all-night EEG sleep recordings and daytime nap studies (multiple sleep latency test; MSLT). The MSLT consists of five standardized nap opportunities to quantify daytime sleep tendency (Carskadon, 1989). The diagnosis of narcolepsy required a mean sleep latency of 7 minutes or less on the MSLT *and* at least two naps containing REM sleep.

CASE STUDIES

A clinical summary of the 16 cases is shown in Table 1. Clinical vignettes are briefly presented for four of these cases (using fictional initials).

Case 1: Classic clinical presentation initially misdiagnosed as a conversion disorder. S.Y., a 13-year-old white female, developed increasing hypersomnolence over 3 months, with progressively earlier bedtimes, frequent after-school naps, and falling asleep in school. Her parents' first concern, however, was the onset of abrupt "spells" of leg weakness lasting 1 to 5 minutes, accompanied by tremulousness, slurred speech, ptosis, and head sagging. S.Y. typically used walls or furniture to prevent falling at these times. After these incidents, she recovered immediately with no sequelae. Her parents had also noted a distinct personality change: usually a calm and cheerful child, she had become argumentative, easily frustrated, and occasionally aggressive.

Evaluation by the family's pediatrician resulted in a referral to a pediatric neurologist to rule out a seizure disorder. The neurologist performed blood chemistry analyses, thyroid function tests, magnetic resonance imaging scan, and a sleep-deprived EEG; all results were reportedly normal. A long-term video EEG recorded two of the "spells" with no evidence of an ictal event. The neurologist concluded that the symptoms were nonorganic because the patient could be "talked out of the episodes." A diagnosis of a conversion disorder was given and referral was made to a child psychiatrist. The psychiatrist did not find sufficient evidence for a major psychiatric disorder (despite the recent personality changes), and because of the prominent hypersomnolence, referred the family to our pediatric sleep center.

Clinical evaluation in our center was highly suggestive of narcolepsy with a definite history of sudden episodes of muscle weakness when she laughed or experienced anxiety, and a dramatic, unexplained increase in total sleep requirements. The sleep study confirmed the diagnosis of narcolepsy, with a mean sleep latency of 2 minutes in the MSLT and REM sleep in four of the five naps. She showed a very good clinical response to treat-

TABLE 1

Clinical Summary of 16 Cases of Child and Adolescent Narcolepsy

Subject	Age at Onset	Age at Dx	Sex	Core Symptoms				Comorbidity at Diagnosis			Source of Referral to Sleep Eval	Family History of Narcolepsy
				Excessive Sleepiness	Cataplexy	Sleep Paralysis	Hypnagogic Hallucination	Obesity	Behavior/ Emotional Disturbances	Psychiatric Disorder		
S.Y.	13	13	F	++	++	−	±	++	++	−	Child psychiatrist	−
K.T.	4	11	F	++	−	−	−	+	−	−	Pediatric neurologist	+
S.M.	3	6	F	++	+	−	−	+	++	−	Pediatrician	−
M.Z.	12	14	M	++	++	−	++	+	++	+	Child psychiatrist	+
D.F.	9	11	M	++	−	−	+	+	+	−	Pediatric neurosurgeon	−
R.G.	10	13	F	++	+	−	+	++	+	−	Neurologist	−
T.K.	11	12	M	++	−	−	+	−	−	−	Pediatric neurologist	−
N.G.	10	13	F	++	+	−	++	−	+	−	Pediatrician	−
J.L.	10	19	F	++	−	−	−	+	+	−	School official	−
T.E.	11	13	M	++	+	−	++	+	+	+	Child psychiatrist	+
G.M.	9	12	M	++	+	−	−	+	+	+	Child psychiatrist	+
P.L.	12	14	F	++	+	−	−	++	+	+	Pediatrician	−
B.W.	11	13	F	++	−	−	+	++	+	−	School official	−
L.T.	11	15	M	++	+	++	+	−	−	−	Self/parents	±
M.M.	11	18	M	++	+	−	+	−	−	−	Pediatrician	−
W.I.	13	17	F	++	−	−	−	−	+	−	Self/parents	−

Note: Ages are given in years. − = absent; + = present; ++ = prominent or severe.

ment with methylphenidate for sleepiness and protriptyline for cataplexy.
Case 2: Absence of any accessory core symptoms and significant delay in diagnosis. The parents of K.T. reported that since infancy she required substantially more sleep than her twin sister. Throughout toddler and preschool ages, despite getting considerably more night sleep than her twin, K.T. required multiple daytime naps and was frequently found asleep in unusual circumstances. Her excessive need for sleep became a major family concern when she began school, resulting in medical evaluation. The family's pediatrician noted enlarged tonsils and adenoids and a history of mild snoring and made a presumptive diagnosis of obstructive sleep apnea. Although a sleep study had not been performed, her tonsils and adenoids were removed at age 7 because of the sleepiness. However, the sleepiness persisted, and at age 11 years, the family sought out another opinion from a pediatric neurologist, who found no evidence of a neurological disorder and referred the patient to our center.

Our clinical interview indicated no depression, mood lability, difficulty falling asleep, or sleep continuity disturbances. Despite 10½ to 12 hours of sleep each night, K.T. was intermittently sleepy throughout the day and fell asleep during any quiet activity such as car rides or watching television, as well as one to three times per day in school. Her academic and social functioning was thought to be below her capacity, but remained good. There were no symptoms of sleep paralysis, cataplexy or hypnagogic hallucinations. Initial family history was negative for sleep disorders (however, it was later discovered that a paternal great-aunt had been diagnosed with narcolepsy). Sleep studies showed definite narcolepsy syndrome, with mean sleep latency of 1 minute on the MSLT and REM in all five naps. The subject's twin sister also was evaluated, and histocompatibility studies revealed the DR2 and DQw1 genotype (each shows strong associations with narcolepsy) in *both* children; however, the other twin showed no clinical or laboratory signs of narcolepsy. Treatment (including methylphenidate and scheduled daytime naps at school) resulted in a dramatic decrease in the sleepiness as well as improved academic and social function.

Case 3: Initial diagnosis as psychotic depression. M.Z. presented at age 13 with a 2-year history of hypersomnolence, depressed mood, irritability, fighting with peers, opposition at home, and academic failure. He was observed to have excessive daytime sleepiness with very disturbed nighttime sleep. Before falling asleep, he would see people staring at him and things floating in his room. M.Z. stated that at bedtime, he perceived a "dead man" under his bed that he could sometimes feel touching him at night. He did not experience psychosis or hallucinations at other times. His mental status examination revealed intense distress, depressed affect, and periodic suicidal ideation (he had a plan to take an overdose of pills). Between ages 13 and 14, M.Z. underwent several psychiatric evaluations, outpatient treatment, and one psychiatric hospitalization; diagnoses were major depression with psychosis and oppositional defiant disorder. Schizophrenia was considered a possible diagnosis. He had been treated with desipramine, amitriptyline, and perphenazine, with variable improvement of symptoms.

During his second psychiatric hospitalization, referral to the pediatric sleep center was made when his hallucinations were recognized as hypnagogic. Our clinical evaluation was consistent with narcolepsy syndrome as M.Z. gave a clear history of hypnagogic hallucinations, excessive sleepiness, and cataplexy. (In retrospect, inpatient medical charts also had documented numerous episodes of abrupt limp unresponsiveness that had been erroneously attributed to either conversion or willful refusal to respond.) M.Z. expressed that at night, he experienced intense fear of going to bed due to his hypnagogic hallucinations. The hypnagogic hallucinations and daytime sleepiness had become worse since discontinuing amitripryline. M.Z.'s polysomnographic studies revealed REM sleep in all five naps, with a mean sleep latency of 2 minutes. Although M.Z. showed a good clinical response to treatment of his narcolepsy in the hospital, he continued to have numerous psychosocial and family problems, erratic compliance with treatment as an outpatient, and multiple out-of-home placements; he was lost to follow-up.

Case 4: Significant school and social impairment. R.G. was 13 years old when she presented with complaints of excessive sleepiness with sleep attacks at school since the fifth grade (age 10). She was falling asleep 4 to 10 times a day in school, even when highly interested. R.G. had an early bedtime with immediate sleep onset, but her sleep was often disrupted by hypnagogic and hypnopompic hallucinations, which she described as vivid images "left over" from her dreams. Despite her insight that these images were not real, she was compelled to turn on the light and examine the room to reassure herself. She had mild but definite symptoms of cataplexy: suddenly feeling her body become weak for a few seconds when she laughed or was surprised. She had become socially withdrawn and showed a significant deterioration in school performance. There were no significant medical problems or evidence of a psychiatric disorder. Sleep studies showed definite narcolepsy. Treatment resulted in a significant improvement in all domains; however, some sleepiness and social withdrawal have persisted.

DISCUSSION

Many of the patients in this series struggled for years (misdiagnosed or undiagnosed) with severe school and social difficulties during important maturational stages of their lives. Although recognition and treatment of narcolepsy did not abolish all symptoms in most young patients, it did result in significant academic and social improvement in every case, as well as an altered interpretation of symptoms by teachers, friends, family members, and the patients themselves. Resolving suspicions of substance abuse, accusations of laziness, and derogatory nicknames was often as significant to some young patients as the correction of inappropriate medical or psychiatric diagnoses.

In this series, the classic presentation of all four core symptoms (sleepiness, cataplexy, sleep paralysis, and hypnagogic hallucinations) was the exception rather than the rule, with only one subject showing the complete tetrad. The core symptoms of narcolepsy appear to represent a dysregulation of normal REM sleep. During normal REM sleep, there is a postsynaptic inhibition of skeletal muscles in humans and other mammals (presumably preventing body movements during dreams). Cataplexy and sleep paralysis appear to be *inappropriate* activation of this muscle paralysis while the patient is awake (Siegel et al., 1991). Similarly, hypnagogic hallucinations are believed to be closely related to normal REM dream imagery, which in narcolepsy occurs before the patient is fully asleep. Thus, these core symptoms appear to represent a blurring of the boundaries normally containing REM sleep physiology to specific times of the night. Each of these core symptoms will be discussed briefly in relation to this case series.

Sleepiness

Although excessive sleepiness was a prominent symptom in all 16 cases, only 3 of the young narcoleptics showed the classic pattern of sleep attacks. In several cases, the only manifestation of sleepiness was an increase in the total number of hours out of 24 spent asleep. In some patients, the family members believed the child just needed much more sleep than siblings or peers. In other cases, the excessive need for sleep was attributed to depression or temperament, or it was not a source of concern. In some cases, if the patient was able to obtain 12 or more hours of sleep per night, daytime sleepiness was minimal. In other patients, however, daytime sleepiness was prominent no matter how much night sleep was obtained. In the majority of cases, daytime sleepiness was significantly exacerbated (or began) near the onset of pubertal changes. It should also be emphasized that all of these patients demonstrated *true sleepiness* (episodes of inability to remain awake), not simply fatigue or a subjective sense of tiredness. Furthermore, in all cases, it was established that the *sleepiness was not the consequence of inadequate hours in bed, nor of erratic sleep/wake schedules.*

Cataplexy

Cataplexy episodes were dramatic in two subjects, symptoms were subtle or mild in seven patients, and they were absent in seven. In some patients with definite cataplexy, however, the symptoms were missed by academic physicians, who at times mistook the behaviors for willful unresponsiveness or conversion symptoms. In other cases, the cataplexy was easily missed because it was quite subtle, consisting of mild weakness in the legs, torso, head, or neck, associated with sudden emotional changes such as laughter, surprise, or anger. One young girl initially denied all cataplexy-like symptoms in our interview, but later was directly observed to have dramatic loss of muscle tone when she laughed. She and her family acknowledged that for years she had "turned into a bowl of jello" when she laughed, but they had just regarded it as her way of laughing. Another young girl had a very limited version of cataplexy: her head would droop forward, her jaw would become limp, and her tongue would hang slightly out of her mouth; however, this girl had learned to hide these episodes by quickly propping her jaw in her hand when she felt an episode beginning. In two cases of cataplexy, the children initially described their episodes as "dizziness." On careful questioning, however, it was clear that the dizzy spells were simply loss of balance secondary to muscle weakness, with no sense of vertigo or change of consciousness.

Hypnagogic Hallucinations

Hypnagogic hallucinations were dramatic and disturbing in three cases, mild or subtle in six, and absent in seven. In three of the young narcoleptic subjects the hypnagogic hallucinations were so frightening that they significantly interfered with sleep. This pattern occasionally resulted in vicious cycles of sleep deprivation due to avoiding bed (because of associated fears), resulting in increased sleepiness. In most of the cases, the hypnagogic hallucinations were strictly visual, typically consisting of a transformation of real images (such as light coming under the door or shadows from hanging clothes) turning into fantastic, dream-like visual images. In younger children, it was sometimes difficult to discriminate early hypnagogic hallucinations from normal childhood bedtime fears or vivid imaginations. In a few cases, hypnagogic hallucinations recurred after middle-of-the-night arousals and significantly interfered with sleep continuity. In at least two patients, hypnagogic hallucinations also occurred with daytime naps or when the patient fell asleep at school. There was considerable variation with respect to the interpretation of these images: some children had a clear understanding that these "images" were essentially dreams, whereas in other cases, youngsters had great difficulty being reassured that these perceptions were not real. Two patients reported tactile hallucinations as well as visual, and one patient described auditory hallucinations as she fell asleep which she described as "dream-like voices."

Sleep Paralysis

Sleep paralysis was present in only 1 of the 16 patients with narcolepsy. Sleep paralysis is the continuation of normal REM sleep paralysis after morning awakening. Although it can occur occasionally in up to 10% of the normal population, it is a frequent symptom among many adult narcoleptics. The one boy in this case series with sleep paralysis had very significant symptoms, often waking up with a complete inability to move. Although this was initially extremely frightening, he had learned to "break the spell" by concentrating on wiggling one finger as well as learning that he had control over his eye movements and breathing.

Sleep Study Results

Polysomnographic studies yielded results similar to those reported in adult narcoleptics: (1) Nocturnal sleep, particularly REM sleep, was often fragmented by movements and brief unexplained arousals (9 of 16 patients had sleep efficiencies below 90%). (2) Patients showed severe daytime sleepiness in objective nap studies (15 of 16 patients achieved sleep in all five nap opportunities, with an average latency less than 5 minutes). (3) REM sleep occurred during daytime naps. Seven patients had REM sleep in all five naps, four patients had four REM naps, two had three REM naps, and three had two REM naps.

Within the narcoleptic group there was no apparent relationship between the severity of clinical symptoms and the degree of EEG sleep findings. For example, the patient with the most dramatic polysomnographic results (all sleep latencies less than 1 minute with immediate REM sleep at night and every nap) had *no* cataplexy, hypnagogic hallucinations, or sleep paralysis whatsoever, and no behavioral or emotional disturbances. In contrast, the one patient with the complete clinical tetrad of core symptoms had sleep findings that barely met criteria for narcolepsy (mean sleep latency of 7 minutes and only two sleep-onset REM periods). None of these patients (including the severely obese children) showed evidence of obstructive sleep apnea syndrome.

Family History

Family history was positive for narcolepsy in four of the cases, although in one case, it was not discovered until after the child's narcolepsy was diagnosed. In one case, multiple family members gave convincing clinical histories of narcolepsy but refused formal polysomnographic studies. Genetic studies of narcolepsy reveal a very strong association with HLA type DR2 and DQw1 (Langdon et al., 1986; Matsuiki et al., 1992). Evidence supports a model of autosomal dominant transmission with incomplete penetrance (Singh et al., 1990). Current understanding suggests that penetrance is very low and/or environmental factors also play a critical role. In a well-controlled study, only 3% to 5% of patients had a first-degree relative with narcolepsy, although 40% had a family member with some symptoms of excessive sleepiness (Guilleminault et al., 1989).

Comorbid Obesity

An unexpected observation in these cases was the prominence of obesity. This was initially evident in the case of K.T., who was one of twins. Although the family had been told at the children's birth that they were identical twins, K.T. had always been heavier and needed considerably more sleep. Family records before 2 years of age clearly document the twins' marked disparity in both physical size and sleep needs. This association prompted assessments of weight and growth in subsequent narcoleptic patients. Four of the 16 patients in this case series were severely obese. These four female patients, aged 13 to 14 at the time of diagnosis, weighed 200 to 250 lb and had body mass indices of 35 to 37. Seven other patients were moderately obese at the time of diagnosis, with a body mass index of 25 to 30. Only 5 of the 16 patients were normal weight or thin at the time of diagnosis. One of the nonobese patients had the onset of narcolepsy after a 15-lb weight gain at the end of an athletic season when she went from thin to average weight. Also, as stated earlier, several of these patients had the onset (or significant exacerbation) of sleepiness in association with the onset of pubertal growth spurt—a time of rapid change in body mass and proportion.

Although, to our knowledge, obesity has never been reported as having a significant association with adult narcolepsy, a review of the pediatric literature reveals clear precedents. Kotogal et al. (1990) found three of their four narcoleptic children were obese, and Allsopp and Zaiwalla (1992) reported obesity in two of their three young narcoleptics, including a 9-year-old boy in whom narcolepsy symptoms were accompanied by the development of "voracious appetite and binging."

There are at least three possible sources of association between weight gain and narcolepsy: (1) narcoleptic children may have decreased caloric expenditure secondary to increased sleep; (2) narcolepsy could be associated with dysregulation of both sleep and appetite in some patients; and (3) children with *both* obesity and narcolepsy may be more severely symptomatic and more likely to be identified at an early age. In two patients in our series and in one case reported by Allsopp and Zaiwalla, there was a definite clinical history of increased appetite. However, there is also support for the concept that weight gain may exacerbate hypersomnia (Kurtz et al., 1976). In our sample the time course of weight gain and hypersomnia could not be reliably disentangled.

Psychiatric and Emotional/Behavioral Changes

In four cases it appears that a psychiatric diagnosis was inappropriately given before the diagnosis of narcolepsy was recognized, including one major depressive disorder, one major depressive disorder with psychosis, one conversion disorder, and one attention deficit disorder. In these cases, once narcolepsy was recognized and treated, there was no evidence for a separate psychiatric disorder. In four other cases, however, patients continued to meet criteria for a psychiatric disorder after the recognition and treatment of narcolepsy. In one case, the psychiatric disorder (schizophrenia) seemed clearly independent of the narcolepsy. In that case, the patient had one first-degree relative with schizophrenia and another with narcolepsy, and there were independent symptoms for each diagnosis (e.g., both hypnagogic hallucinations as well as daytime auditory hallucinations). In three other cases (one major depressive disorder, a dysthymia, and one attention-deficit hyperactivity disorder/oppositional defiant disorder), the overlap between psychiatric symptoms and narcolepsy symptoms made it impossible to establish the independence of the disorders in the opinions of the treating physicians.

In 12 of the 16 cases in this series parents reported significant emotional or behavioral disturbances with social and academic impairment at or near the time of onset of symptoms of narcolepsy. Furthermore, in the other four cases, in which the clinical evaluation had initially indicated no behavioral/emotional symptoms or school or social difficulties, the families noted an improvement in these domains after treatment of narcolepsy.

There are at least four possibilities to explain the strong associations between early-onset narcolepsy and behavioral and emotional disturbances in this series:

1. Emotional/behavioral changes may reflect the *sequelae* of chronic sleep disturbances in narcolepsy.

2. The pathophysiology of narcolepsy may involve dysregulation of emotion and arousal, as well as also of sleep.

3. Because our sleep center is located in a psychiatric institute, referral bias may have contributed to the association.

4. Children and adolescents with both narcolepsy and an underlying behavioral or emotional disorder may be more likely to come to medical attention, reflecting a "Berkson's bias" (Berkson, 1946).

The relative likelihood of these possibilities could not be formally evaluated by our data. In the future, careful longitudinal studies, as well as basic research in these areas, may help to disentangle these relationships.

Medical Disorders

At least three cases were initially misdiagnosed as a medical disorder, including two patients who underwent surgical procedures (one ventriculoperitoneal shunt and one tonsillectomy) in unsuccessful attempts to treat the hypersomnia. In several cases, expensive medical workups, including magnetic resonance imaging scans, endocrinological tests, and video EEG recordings, were performed before narcolepsy syndrome had been considered in the differential diagnosis.

Treatment

To our knowledge there are no controlled studies examining treatment issues specifically in young narcoleptics. Our general approach to treatment is based on adult experience with narcolepsy and follows four basic principles:

1. Education, counseling, and support (working closely with both the family and school officials).

2. Establishing regular sleep/wake schedules, often including scheduled daytime naps, as well as promoting good sleep/wake habits and hygiene.

3. Stimulant medication for sleepiness. (Although there are differing opinions and a lack of empiric data, we favor short-acting stimulants such as methylphenidate with "drug holidays" on weekends and vacations to avoid tolerance and minimize dosage increases.)

4. In cases with significant cataplexy or hypnagogic hallucinations, REM suppressant medications (such as protriptyline) are used to control symptoms.

As sketched in the cases, treatment often resulted in dramatic improvements in major symptom domains. It is important to emphasize, however, that education, counseling, and optimizing sleep habits and schedules appear to be at least as important as the pharmacotherapy. It is also important to point out the chronic nature of this disorder and its recurrent exacerbations and symptoms throughout adulthood.

Summary

The central clinical message is that narcolepsy should be considered in the differential diagnosis of any patient with an unexplained excessive need for sleep. Neither the absence of accessory core symptoms of narcolepsy nor the presence of emotional or behavioral disturbances should prevent consideration of narcolepsy. Irritability, mood disturbances, nonspecific personality changes, social and academic impairment, and obesity should, if anything, raise the suspicion of narcolepsy. Polysomnographic studies are required to confirm the diagnosis. It seems likely that early recognition and optimal treatment of narcolepsy holds at least some promise in minimizing the psychosocial dysfunction associated with narcolepsy.

REFERENCES

Aldrich MS (1992), Narcolepsy. *Neurology* 42(suppl 6):34–43

Allsopp MR, Zaiwalla Z (1992), Narcolepsy. *Arch Dis Child* 67:302–306

Berkson J (1946), Limitations of the application of fourfold table analysis to hospital data. *Biometrics* 2:47–51

Broughton R, Ghanem Q, Hishikawa Y, Sugita Y, Nevsimalova S, Roth B (1981), Life effects of narcolepsy in 180 patients from North America, Asia and Europe compared to matched controls. *Can J Neurol Sci* 10:100–104

Carskadon MA (1989), Measuring daytime sleepiness. In: *Principles and Practice of Sleep Medicine*, Kryger MH, Roth T, Dement WC, eds. Philadelphia: WB Saunders Company, pp 684–688

Dahl RE (1992), Child and adolescent sleep disorders. In: *Neurology For Child Psychiatrists*, Kaufman DM, ed. Baltimore: Williams & Wilkins, pp 169–194

Dahl RE, Pelham WB, Wierson MC (1991), The role of sleep disturbance in attention deficit disorder symptomatology. *J Pediatr Psychol* 16:229–239

Dement WC, Carskadon MA, Ley R (1973), The prevalence of narcolepsy. *Sleep Research* 2:147

Guilleminault C, Mignot WC, Grumet FC (1989), Familial patterns of narcolepsy. *Lancet* 335:1376–1379

Kales A, Soldatos CR, Bixler EO et al. (1982), Narcolepsy-cataplexy. II. Psychosocial consequences and associated psychopathology. *Arch Neurol* 39:169–171

Kotagal S, Hartse KM, Walsh JK (1990), Characteristics of narcolepsy in preteenaged children. *Pediatrics* 85:205–209

Kurtz D, Lambert E, Krieger J (1976), Hormones, endocrine disease and daytime sleepiness In: *Narcolepsy*, Guilleminault C, Dement W, Passouant P, eds. New York: Spectrum, pp 367–384

Langdon N, Welsh KI, Van Dam M, Vaugham RW, Parkes JD (1986), Genetic markers in narcolepsy. *Lancet* 2:1178–1180

Matsuiki K, Grumet FC, Lin X, Guilleminault C, Dement WC, Mignot E (1992), DQ (rather than DR) marks susceptibility for narcolepsy. *Lancet* 339:1052

Navelet Y, Anders T, Guilleminault C (1976), Narcolepsy in children. In: *Narcolepsy*, Guilleminault C, Dement W, Passouant P, eds. New York: Spectrum, pp 171–177

Reimao R, Lemmi H (1991), Narcolepsy in childhood and adolescence. *Arq Neuropsiquiatr* 49:260–264

Ryan ND, Puig-Antich J, Rabinovich H et al. (1987), The clinical picture of major depression in children and adolescents. *Arch Gen Psychiatry* 44:854–861

Siegel JM, Nienhuis R, Fahringer HM et al. (1991). Neuronal activity in narcolepsy: identification of cataplexy-related cells in the medial medulla. *Science* 252:1315–1318

Singh SM, George CFP, Kryger MH, Jung JH (1990), Genetic heterogeneity in narcolepsy. *Lancet* 335:726–727

Yoss RE, Daley DD (1960), Narcolepsy in children. *Pediatrics* 25:1025–1030

Young D, Zorick F, Wittig R, Roehrs T, Roth T (1988), Narcolepsy in a pediatric population. *Am J Dis Child* 142:210–213

Zarconi VP, Fuchs HE (1976), Psychiatric disorders and narcolepsy. In: *Narcolepsy*, Guilleminault C, Dement W, Passouant P, eds. New York: Spectrum, pp 231–256

13

Urban Poverty and the Family Context of Delinquency: A New Look at Structure and Process in a Classic Study

Robert J. Sampson

University of Chicago

John H. Laub

Northeastern University and Henry A. Murray Research Center, Boston

This paper reanalyzes data from the Gluecks' classic study of 500 delinquents and 500 nondelinquents reared in low-income neighborhoods of central Boston. Based on a general theory of informal social control, we propose a 2-step hypothesis that links structure and process: family poverty inhibits family processes of informal social control, in turn increasing the likelihood of juvenile delinquency. The results support the theory by showing that (1) erratic, threatening, and harsh discipline, (2) low supervision, and (3) weak parent-child attachment mediate the effects of poverty and other structural factors on delinquency. We also address the potential confounding role of parental and childhood disposition. Although difficult children who display early antisocial tendencies do disrupt family management as do antisocial and unstable parents, mediating processes of informal social control still explain a large share of variance in adolescent delinquency. Overall, the results underscore the indirect effects of structural contexts like family poverty on adolescent delinquency within disadvantaged populations. We note implications for current debates on race, crime, and the "underclass" in urban America.

Reprinted with permission from *Child Development*, 1994, Vol. 65, 523–540. Copyright © 1994 by the Society for Research in Child Development, Inc.

We thank three anonymous reviewers and the guest editor of *Child Development*, Vonnie C. McLoyd, for constructive criticisms of a previous draft. We also thank Sandra Gauvreau for research assistance. The data were derived from the Sheldon and Eleanor Glueck archives of the Harvard Law School Library, currently on long-term loan to the Henry A. Murray Research Center of Radcliffe College.

In 1950, Sheldon and Eleanor Glueck published their now classic study, *Unraveling Juvenile Delinquency.* In one of the most frequently cited works in the history of delinquency research, the Gluecks sought to answer a basic and enduring question—what factors differentiate boys reared in poor neighborhoods who become serious and persistent delinquents from boys raised in the same neighborhoods who do not become delinquent or antisocial? To answer this question, the Gluecks studied in meticulous detail the lives of 500 delinquents and 500 nondelinquents who were raised in the same slum environments of central Boston during the Great Depression era.

The research design of the Gluecks' study provides a unique opportunity to address anew poverty and its sequelae in adolescence. Namely, what is the *process* by which family poverty leads to delinquency within structurally disadvantaged urban environments? It is our contention that sociological explanations of delinquency have too often focused on structural background (e.g., poverty) without an understanding of mediating family processes, especially informal social control. Competing explanations based on behavioral predispositions (e.g., early conduct disorder) have also been neglected in structural accounts of delinquency. On the other hand, developmental models in psychology tend to emphasize family process and early antisocial behavior to the neglect of structural context and social disadvantage.

Based on our reconstruction and reanalysis of the Gluecks' original data, this article rejects a bifurcated strategy by uniting structure and process in an integrated theoretical framework. Our major thesis is that poverty and structural disadvantage influence delinquency in large part by reducing the capacity of families to achieve effective informal social controls. In this sense, we argue that scholars of child and adolescent development must come to grips with structural contexts of disadvantage and not just focus on families "under the roof."

The historical context of the Gluecks' data also serves as a baseline for assessing current research on children and poverty. The boys in the Glueck sample were born in the Depression era and grew to young adulthood in the context of a rapidly changing economy after World War II (1945–1965). This context raises interesting questions relevant to an understanding of how poverty influences developmental patterns of delinquency. For example, are the risk factors associated with crime similar across different structural contexts? Were characteristics of today's "underclass" (e.g., chronic joblessness, poverty) found among these earlier Boston families? Current debates, especially in public policy circles, seem to imply that criminal behavior is inevitably linked to race and drugs. Yet the delinquency problem in the historical context we are analyzing was generated not by blacks, but by white ethnic groups in structurally disadvantaged positions. And though drugs were not pervasive, delinquency and antisocial behavior were. Indeed, the boys in the Gluecks' delinquent sample were persistent and serious offenders, many of whom can be labeled "career criminals" using contemporary language. By analyzing a white sample that is largely "underclass" by today's economic definition (see Jencks, 1992; Wilson, 1987), we provide an alternative perspective to current thinking about race, crime, and poverty.

FAMILY PROCESS AND INFORMAL SOCIAL CONTROL

The hypotheses guiding our analysis are derived from a general theory of age-graded informal social control over the life course (see Sampson & Laub, 1993). Our general organizing principle is that the probability of deviance increases when an individual's bond to society is weak or broken (Hirschi, 1969). In other words, when ties that bind an individual to key societal institutions (e.g., attachment to family, school, work) are loosened, the risk of crime and delinquency is heightened. Unlike formal sanctions, which originate in purposeful efforts to control crime, informal social controls "emerge as by-products of role relationships established for other purposes and are components of role reciprocities" (Kornhauser, 1978, p. 24).

Our theoretical conceptualization on the family is drawn in part from "coercion theory" as formulated by Patterson (1980, 1982). Unlike most sociological theories, coercion theory places a prominent etiological role on direct parental controls in explaining delinquency. In particular, the coercion model assumes that less skilled parents inadvertently reinforce their children's antisocial behavior and fail to provide effective punishments for transgressions (Patterson, 1982; see also Gottfredson & Hirschi, 1990, p. 99). Based on research designed to assess this perspective, Patterson argues that "parents who cannot or will not employ family management skills are the prime determining variables. . . . Parents of stealers do not track; they do not punish; and they do not care" (1980, pp. 88–89).

The emphasis on parent-child interaction in coercion theory shares much in common with Hirschi's (1969) social control theory. The model of Patterson differs mainly in the mediating mechanisms it emphasizes—that is, direct parental controls as found in discipline and monitoring practices. By contrast, Hirschi's (1969) original formulation of control theory emphasized indirect controls in the form of the child's attachment to parents. On balance, however, Patterson's model is consistent with social control theory because direct parental controls are likely to be positively related to relational, indirect controls (Larzelere & Patterson, 1990, p. 305). Moreover, Gottfredson and Hirschi (1990) include direct parental controls in a recent statement of control theory that relies heavily on Patterson's coercion model. Their reformulated theory of effective parenting includes monitoring the behavior of children, recognizing their misdeeds, and punishing (correcting) those misdeeds accordingly in a consistent and loving manner (Gottfredson & Hirschi, 1990, p. 97). In addition, Hirschi (1983) argues that parental affection and a willingness to invest in children are essential underlying conditions of good parenting, and hence, the prevention of misbehavior.

This view of families also corresponds to Braithwaite's (1989) notion of "reintegrative shaming," whereby parents punish in a consistent manner and within the context of love, respect, and acceptance of the child. The opposite of reintegrative shaming is stigmatization, where parents are cold, authoritarian, and enact a harsh, punitive, and often rejecting regime of punishment (1989, p. 56). When the bonds of respect are broken by parents in the process of punishment, successful child rearing is difficult to achieve.

Given their theoretical compatibility, we draw on the central ideas of social control and coercion theory along with the notion of reintegrative shaming to develop a model of informal family social control that focuses on three dimensions—*discipline, supervision*, and *attachment*. In our view, the key to all three dimensions of informal social control lies in the extent to which they facilitate linking the child to family, and ultimately society, through emotional bonds of attachment and direct yet socially integrative forms of control, monitoring, and punishment. These dimensions of informal family control have rarely been examined simultaneously in previous research. Hence our theoretical model permits assessment of the relative and cumulative contributions of family process to the explanation of delinquency.

Poverty and Family Process

The second part of our theory posits that structural background factors influence delinquency largely through the mediating dimensions of family process (see also Laub & Sampson, 1988). Our specific interest in this article is the indirect effect of family poverty on delinquency among those children living in disadvantaged communities. Although examined in the developmental psychology literature (for a recent review see McLoyd, 1990), it is ironic that sociological research on delinquency often fails to account for how structural disadvantage influences parenting behavior and other aspects of family life. As Rutter and Giller (1983, p. 185) have stated, "serious socio-economic disadvantage has an adverse effect on the parents, such that parental disorders and difficulties are more likely to develop and good parenting is impeded" (see also McLoyd, 1990, p. 312). Furthermore, Larzelere and Patterson (1990, p. 307) have argued that many lower-class families are marginally skilled as parents, in part because they experience more stress and fewer resources than do middle-class parents. McLoyd (1990, p. 312) has also expressed the view that "poverty and economic loss diminish the capacity for supportive, consistent, and involved parenting." In reviewing the extant literature, she found that economically disadvantaged parents and those parents who experience economic stress are more likely to use punitive, coercive parenting styles, that is, use of physical punishment, as opposed to reasoning and negotiation. Low-income parents also face heightened risks of spousal violence, drug and alcohol abuse, and criminal involvement (McLoyd, 1990), behaviors that undermine socially integrative parent-child relationships and interactions.

Equally important and relevant here is the large body of literature establishing the effects of stressors such as economic crises and divorce on parenting behavior. For example, Patterson (1988) has shown that stressful experiences increase the likelihood of psychological distress, which in turn leads to changes in parent-child management practices. Specifically, Patterson (1988) found that distressed mothers are more likely to use coercive discipline, thereby contributing to the development of antisocial behavior in children (see also Patterson, DeBaryshe, & Ramsey, 1989, p. 332). Elder and Caspi (1988) examined the effects of stressful economic circumstances on parents and their children. They found that in times of economic difficulty, aversive interactions between parents and children increase while the ability of parents to manage their children diminishes. Using more recent data, Conger et al. (1992) confirmed that economic hardship was indirectly linked to adolescent development largely through its effect on parenting behavior.

It seems clear that poverty and the accompanying stresses resulting from economic deprivation influence parent-child relationships and interactions within the family. Integrating this viewpoint with our general theory of informal social control, we thus hypothesize that the effect of poverty and disadvantaged family status on delinquency is mediated in large part through parental discipline and monitoring practices.

ANTISOCIAL CHILDREN: RECONSIDERING FAMILY EFFECTS

Two research findings raise questions regarding unidirectional models that attribute the development of delinquency as flowing solely from parental influence. The first is empirical research establishing the early onset of many forms of childhood misbehavior (Robins, 1966; West & Farrington, 1973; White, Moffitt, Earls, Robins, & Silva, 1990). In one of the best studies to date, White et al. (1990) examined the predictive power of behavior measured as early as age 3 on antisocial outcomes at ages 11 and 13. They found that teacher and/or parent-reported behavioral measures of hyperactivity and restlessness as a young child (age 3), difficulty in management of the child at age 3, and early onset of problem behaviors at 5 predicted later antisocial outcomes. White et al.'s (1990) research shows the extent to which later delinquency is foreshadowed by early misbehavior and general difficulty among children.

Second, there is evidence that styles of parenting are in part a reaction to these troublesome behaviors on the part of children. Lytton (1990) has written an excellent overview of this complex body of research, which he subsumes under the theoretical umbrella of "control systems theory." This theory argues that parent and child display reciprocal adaptation to each other's behavior level (see also Anderson, Lytton, & Romney, 1986), leading to what Lytton calls "child effects" on parents. One reason for these child effects is that reinforcement does not work in the usual way for conduct-disordered children. As Lytton (1990, p. 688) notes, conduct-disordered children "may be underresponsive to social reinforcement and punishment." Hence, normal routines of parental child rearing become subject to disruption based on early antisocial behavior—that is, children themselves differentially engender parenting styles likely to further exacerbate antisocial behavior.

The behavior that prompts parental frustration is not merely aggressiveness or delinquency, however. Lytton (1990, p. 690) reviews evidence showing a connection between a child being rated "difficult" in preschool (e.g., whining, restlessness, inadaptability to change, strong-willed resistance) and the child's delinquency as an adolescent—a relation that holds independent of the quality of parents' child-rearing practices. For example, Olweus (1980) showed by a longitudinal path analysis that mothers of boys who displayed a strong-willed and hot temper in infancy later became more permissive of aggression, which in turn led to greater aggressiveness in middle childhood. Moreover, there is intriguing experimental evidence that when children's inattentive and noncompliant behavior is improved by administering stimulant drugs (e.g., Ritalin), their mothers become less controlling and mother-child interaction patterns are nearly normalized (Lytton, 1990, p. 688). All of this suggests that parenting, at least in part, is a reaction to the temperament of children, especially difficult ones.

Further evidence in favor of "child effects" from the criminological literature is found in West and Farrington's (1973) well-known longitudinal study. They showed that boys' "troublesomeness" assessed at ages 8 and 10 by teachers and peers was a significant predictor of later delinquency, independent of parental supervision, parental criminality, and family size. However, the reverse was not true—parental effects on delinquency disappeared once early troublesomeness was taken into account. As Lytton observes, this finding "suggests the primacy of child effects" (1990, p. 690).

In short, there is a sound theoretical and empirical basis for expanding our model by introducing early childhood effects. Lytton's review suggests a strategy to ascertain the relative importance of parent and child influences. Namely, one can test the effects of early childhood factors on later delinquency, with parent factors held constant, against the prediction of parents' effects on delinquency, with early childhood factors held constant. The relative strength of each set of variables would be an index of the importance of the main independent variables—child or parent (1990, p. 694). Put more simply, the key question is whether our family process model holds up after we consider early childhood difficulty and antisocial predispositions. If parenting or family effects on delinquency are spurious, then our model should collapse once childhood behaviors are controlled. On the other hand, if control systems theory is correct, we are liable to see both child *and* parent effects on the outcome of adolescent delinquency. We assess our theoretical model of structure and family process by employing this strategy.

METHOD

The present article is based on data from the first wave of the Gluecks' original study of juvenile delinquency and adult crime among 1,000 Boston males born between 1924 and 1935 (Glueck & Glueck, 1950, 1968). As part of a larger, long-term project we have reconstructed and computerized these data, a process that included the validation of key measures found in the original files. For a full description of these efforts and other procedures taken to address prior criticisms of the Gluecks' study, see Sampson and Laub (1993).

The Gluecks' delinquent sample comprised 500 10–17-year-old white males from Boston who, because of their persistent delinquency, had been recently committed to one of two correctional schools in Massachusetts (Glueck & Glueck, 1950, p. 27). The nondelinquent or "control-group" sample was made up of 500 white males age 10–17 chosen from the Boston public schools. Nondelinquent status was determined on the basis of official record checks and interviews with parents, teachers, local police, social workers, recreational leaders, and the boys themselves. The Gluecks' sampling procedure was designed to maximize differences in delinquency, an objective that by all accounts succeeded (Glueck & Glueck, 1950, pp. 27–29).

A unique aspect of the *Unraveling* study was the matching design. The 500 officially defined delinquents and 500 nondelinquents were matched case-by-case on age, race/ethnicity (birthplace of both parents), measured intelligence, and neighborhood deprivation. The delinquents averaged 14 years, 8 months, and the nondelinquents 14 years, 6 months when the study began. As to ethnicity, 25% of both groups were of English background, another fourth Italian, a fifth Irish, less than a tenth old American, Slavic, or French, and the remaining were Near Eastern, Spanish, Scandinavian, German, or Jewish. As measured by the Wechsler-Bellevue Test, the delinquents had an average IQ of 92 and nondelinquents 94. The matching on neighborhood ensured that both delinquents and nondelinquents grew up in disadvantaged neighborhoods of central Boston. These areas were regions of poverty, economic dependency, and physical deterioration, and were usually adjacent to areas of industry and commerce (Glueck & Glueck, 1950, p. 29).

A wealth of information on social, psychological, and biological characteristics, family life, school performance, work experiences, and other life events was collected on the delinquents and controls in the period 1939–1948. These data were collected through an elaborate investigation process that involved interviews with the subjects themselves and their families as well as interviews with key informants such as social workers, settlement house workers, clergymen, schoolteachers, neighbors, and criminal justice and social welfare officials. The home-interview setting also provided an opportunity to observe home and family life (Glueck & Glueck, 1950, pp. 41–53).

Interview data and home investigations were supplemented by field investigations that meticulously culled information from the records of both public and private agencies that had any involvement with a subject or his family. These materials verified and amplified the materials of a particular case investigation. For example, a principal source of data was the

Social Service Index, a clearinghouse that contained information on all dates of contact between a family and the various social agencies (e.g., child welfare) in Boston. Similar indexes from other cities and states were utilized where necessary. For *Unraveling*, the Gluecks employed two case collators to sift through the several thousand entries over the 7½-year project.

The Gluecks also searched the files of the Massachusetts Board of Probation, which maintained a central file of all court records from Boston courts since 1916 and from Massachusetts as a whole from 1924. These records were compared and supplemented with records from the Boys' Parole Division in Massachusetts. Out-of-state arrests, court appearances, and correctional experiences were gathered through correspondence from equivalent state depositories. Of equal importance was the Gluecks' collection of self-reported, parental-reported, and teacher-reported delinquency of the boy.

Measures

Descriptive statistics and intercorrelations for the full set of measures are displayed in Table 1. To tap the central concept of *family poverty*, we created a scale from information on the average weekly income of the family and the family's reliance on outside aid. The latter measures whether the family was living in comfortable circumstances (having enough savings to cover 4 months of financial stress), marginal circumstances (little or no savings but only occasional dependence on outside aid), or financially dependent (continuous receipt of outside aid for support). The resulting standardized scale of poverty was scored so that a high value represents the combination of low income and reliance on public assistance. Although the Gluecks' matching design controls for neighborhood deprivation, there is still considerable variation among families in poverty (see Table 1).

Five additional features of the structural background of families are introduced as control variables.[1] *Residential mobility* is an interval-based measure of the number of times the boy's family moved during the childhood and ranges from none or once to 16 or more times. *Family size* is the number of children in the boy's family and ranges from one to eight or more. *Family disruption* is coded one when the boy was reared in a home where one or both parents were absent because of divorce, separation, desertion, or death. *Maternal employment* is a dichotomous variable where housewives were coded 0 and working mothers (full time or part time) were

---

[1] Controls were selected on both theoretical grounds (see also Sampson & Laub, 1993, chap. 4) and empirical significance in preliminary analysis.

TABLE 1

Descriptive Statistics and Correlations

Variable	Mean	SD	Minimum	Maximum	Valid N
Structural context:					
Family poverty[a]	.00	1.64	-3.64	3.45	998
Residential mobility	6.75	4.72	1	16	999
Family size	5.08	2.21	1	8	999
Family disruption	.47	.50	0	1	1,000
Maternal employment	.40	.49	0	1	993
Foreign born	.60	.49	0	1	987
Parent/child disposition:					
Parental deviance	1.45	1.27	0	4	1,000
Parental instability	.62	.72	0	2	972
Child difficult/antisocial	.72	.80	0	3	884
Family process:					
Erratic/harsh discipline[a]	-.02	1.73	-3.24	3.14	856
Maternal supervision	1.97	.86	1	3	989
Parent-child attachment	3.72	1.21	1	5	960
Adolescent delinquency:					
Official status	.50	.50	0	1	1,000
Self-parent-teacher reported	8.44	6.67	1	26	1,000

PAIRWISE PEARSON CORRELATION COEFFICIENTS

	2	3	4	5	6	7	8	9	10	11	12	13	14
1. Family poverty	.40	.26	.21	-.04	-.07	.38	.25	.20	.35	-.32	-.34	.34	.33
2. Residential mobility		.05	.40	.18	-.18	.50	.35	.27	.28	-.44	-.43	.41	.41
3. Family size			-.09	-.20	.13	.08	.02	.01	.23	-.11	-.02	.16	.17
4. Family disruption				.19	-.13	.38	.24	.15	.13	-.27	-.46	.26	.28
5. Mother's employment					-.02	.17	.16	.08	.10	-.28	-.16	.14	.16
6. Foreign born						-.21	-.10	-.03	.07	.05	.04	-.04	-.07
7. Parental deviance							.35	.22	.36	-.48	-.44	.41	.41
8. Parental instability								.25	.30	-.39	-.31	.36	.34
9. Child difficult/antisocial									.35	-.30	-.30	.45	.45
10. Erratic/harsh discipline										-.51	-.40	.52	.50
11. Maternal supervision											.49	-.63	-.62
12. Parent-child attachment												-.50	-.49
13. Official status													.86
14. Self-parent-teacher reported													

[a] Standardized scale based on z scores.

coded 1. *Foreign-born* indexes whether one or both parents were born outside the United States.

It is possible, of course, that the poverty status and other structural characteristics of families resulted from prior differences among parents that are correlated with dysfunctional family management (Patterson & Capaldi, 1991). To address this possible confounding, we control for the criminality and drinking habits of mothers and fathers as determined from official statistics and interview data. Criminality refers to official records of arrest or conviction, excluding minor auto violations and violation of license laws. Alcoholism/drunkenness refers to intoxication and includes frequent, regular, or chronic addiction to alcohol, and not to very occasional episodes of overdrinking in an atmosphere of celebration. Not surprisingly, there were strong relations between crime and heavy drinking and between mother's and father's crime/drinking. Hence we formed a summary scale ranging from 0 to 4 that measures the extent of what we term *parental deviance* (see Table 1). For example, a subject whose mother and father both had a criminal record and a history of excessive drinking received a score of 4.

The Gluecks also collected data on each parent's mental condition and temperament from official diagnoses and medical reports from hospitals and clinics, and on occasion from unofficial observations made by social workers (Glueck & Glueck, 1950, p. 102). The ordinal variable labeled *parental instability* reflects whether none (0), one (1), or both (2) of the boy's parents were diagnosed with "severe mental disease or distortion" including "marked emotional instability," "pronounced temperamental deviation," or "extreme impulsiveness." Taken together, the parental deviance and instability measures capture key dispositional characteristics that have been argued to underlie family poverty and other disadvantaged outcomes.[2]

Family process. The three intervening dimensions of family process are style of discipline, supervision, and parent-child attachment. Parenting style was measured by summing three variables describing the discipline and punishment practices of mothers and fathers. The first constituent variable concerns the use of physical punishment and refers to rough handling, strappings, and beatings eliciting fear and resentment in the boy—not to casual or occasional slapping that was unaccompanied by rage or hostility. The second constituent variable measures threatening or scolding be-

---

[2] Evidence of the validity of the instability measure is suggested by its significant positive correlation with parental deviance (.35, see Table 1) and also an indicator of low parental IQ (data not shown). By comparison, low IQ was weakly related to our family-process measures, and thus we control for the more direct indicator of volatile and impulsive parental temperament.

havior by mothers or fathers that elicited fear in the boy. The third component taps erratic and negligent discipline, for example, if the parent vacillated between harshness and laxity and was not consistent in control, or if the parent was negligent or indifferent about disciplining the boy.

The summation of these constituent variables resulted in two ordinal measures tapping the extent to which parents used inconsistent disciplinary measures in conjunction with harsh physical punishment and/or threatening or scolding behavior. In Braithwaite's (1989) scheme, these measures tap the sort of punitive shaming and negative stigmatization by families that engender delinquency. The validity of measures is supported by the high concordance between mother's and father's use of erratic/harsh discipline (gamma = .60). For example, of fathers who employed harsh physical punishment, threatening behavior, and erratic discipline (code 3), 44% of the mothers were also coded 3. By contrast, less than 1% of boys' fathers coded 0 on the erratic/harsh scale had mothers coded high (3) in erratic/harsh discipline. For reasons of both theoretical parsimony and increased reliability, we created standardized scales that combined mother and father's *erratic/harsh discipline.*

Maternal supervision is an ordinal variable coded 3 if the mother provided supervision over the boy's activities at home or in the neighborhood. If unable to supervise the boys themselves, mothers who made arrangements for other adults to watch the boy's activities were also assigned a 3. A code of 2 was assigned to those mothers providing partial or fair supervision. Supervision was considered unsuitable (code = 1) if the mother left the boy on his own, without guidance or in the care of an irresponsible person.[3]

As the Gluecks originally observed, attachment is a "two-way street"— parent to child and child to parent (Glueck & Glueck, 1950, p. 125). Accordingly, the Gluecks gathered interview-based information from both the parents and boys themselves on emotional attachment and rejection. For example, the Gluecks developed a three-point ordinal indicator of the extent to which the boy had a warm emotional bond to the father and/or mother as displayed in a close association with the parent and in expressions of admiration. Similarly, the Gluecks measured whether the parents were loving and accepting of the child or were rejecting in emotional attention—that is, whether parents were openly hostile or did not give the child much emotional attention. Because the parent-child and child-parent indicators of attachment were strongly related (gamma = .58),

---

[3]The Gluecks did not collect data on father's supervision. This focus reflects the era in which the Gluecks' study was conceived, wherein mothers assumed primary responsibility for the supervision of children.

we combined them into a single ordinal scale labeled *parent-child attachment* that ranges from 1 (low) to 5 (high).

Child effects. Although the *Unraveling* study was not longitudinal, there are retrospective data on three key dimensions of troublesome childhood behavior. From the parent's interview there is an indicator distinguishing those children who were overly restless and irritable from those who were not. A second measure reflects the extent to which a child engaged in violent temper tantrums and was predisposed to aggressiveness and fighting. The Gluecks collected data only on habitual tantrums—when tantrums were "the predominant mode of response" by the child to difficult situations growing up (1950, p. 152). This measure corresponds closely to one validated by Caspi (1987).[4] The third variable is the boy's self-reported age of onset of misbehavior. We created a dichotomous variable where a 1 indexes an age of onset earlier than age 8. Those who had a later age of onset *and* those who reported no delinquency (and hence no age of onset) were assigned a zero.

As expected, all three measures are significantly correlated. For example, of those children rated difficult in childhood, 34% exhibited tantrums, compared to 13% of those with no history of difficultness. Similarly, for those with an early onset of misbehavior, 47% were identified as having tantrums, compared to 20% of those with no early onset (all p's < .05). To achieve theoretical and empirical parsimony, we summed the three indicators to form an ordinal scale that measures *child difficult/antisocial behavior*. The scale ranges from 0, indicating no signs of early conduct disorder or difficulty in child rearing, to a score of 3, indicating that a child was difficult and irritable, threw violent temper tantrums, and engaged in antisocial behavior prior to age 8.

There is evidence of the predictive validity of our child-effects measure derived from self, parent, and teacher reports. Fully 100% of those scoring high on child antisocial behavior were arrested in adolescence, compared to 25% of those scoring low (gamma = .69). More importantly, the child-effects measure predicts criminal behavior well into adulthood. Using data on adult crime collected by the Gluecks as part of a follow-up study (Glueck & Glueck, 1968), 60% of those scoring high on childhood antisocial behavior were arrested at ages 25–32, compared to less than 25% with no signs of early disorder. Perhaps most striking, there is a rather strong monotonic relation between childhood antisocial disposition and arrests even at ages

---

[4]The tantrum measure is taken from a combined parent/teacher-reported interview. As Lytton (1990) notes, the fact that it is typical to derive ratings of a child's early temperament and of parental practices from the parent interview alone makes for methodological confounding. We avoid this through multiple sources of measurement (self, parent, and teacher).

32–45 (gamma = .37). Hence, although early antisocial behavior was determined by retrospective reports, the techniques used by the Gluecks appear valid (see also Sampson & Laub, 1993, pp. 47–63).

Delinquency. The outcome of adolescent delinquency is measured using both the official criterion of the Gluecks' research design (1 = delinquent, 0 = control group) and "unofficial" delinquency derived by summing self, parent, and teacher reports. In preliminary analysis we also examined measures for particular offenses (e.g., truancy as reported by parents, teachers, and self) and the total amount of delinquency for all crime types reported by a particular source (e.g., self-report total, parent-report total). Because the results were very similar, the present analysis is based on the sum of all delinquent behaviors that were measured consistently across reporters. That is, we eliminated incorrigibility (e.g., vile language, lying) and other behaviors that were only asked of one source (e.g., teacher reports of school vandalism). The unofficial measure thus reflects adolescent delinquency measured by parents, teachers, and the boys themselves.

Reliability and Validity

Because of their strategy of data collection, the Gluecks' measures pertain to multiple sources of information that were independently derived from several points of view and at separate times. The level of detail and the range of information collected by the Gluecks will likely never be repeated given contemporary research standards on the protection of human subjects. As Robins et al. (1985, p. 30) also point out in their analysis of social-science data from an earlier era analogous to the Gluecks: "In conformity with the precomputer era of data analysis, the coding was less atomized than it would have been today. Consequently, we have only the coders' overall assessment based on a variety of individual items."

This method of data collection limits the extent to which reliability can be determined by traditional criteria (e.g., intercoder reliability). As described above, however, our basic measurement strategy uses multiple indicators of key concepts and composite scales whenever possible and theoretically appropriate. Note also that the Glueck data are different in kind from survey research where measurement error, especially on attitudes, is large. That is, the Glueck data represent the comparison, reconciliation, and integration of multiple sources of information even for individual items (see Glueck & Glueck, 1950, pp. 70–72; 1968, pp. 205–255). Moreover, our measures refer to behavior (e.g., discipline, supervision) and objective structural conditions (e.g., poverty, broken homes)—not attitudes.

To verify the coding of the family-process variables, we also conducted a validation test for the purposes of this article. Selecting a 10% random sample of the delinquent subjects ($N = 50$), we coded from the original interview narratives the three key elements of family process—supervision, parenting style, and parental attachment—blind to the actual codes of the Gluecks. We then compared our scores with those of the Gluecks and in general found excellent correspondence. For example, the correlation (gamma) between our coding and the Gluecks' for parental supervision, father's rejection, and mother's rejection was .87, .92, and .98, respectively. We found significant levels of agreement for other key indicators of family process as well, using both gamma and kappa statistics on percent agreement corrected for chance.

Finally, the correlations in Table 1 reveal that our key measures are related in a manner consistent with theory and past research. In particular, erratic/harsh discipline is negatively related to supervision and parent-child attachment ($-.51$ and $-.40$, respectively, $p < .05$), whereas maternal supervision is positively related to parent-child attachment (.49, $p < .05$). These and other significant correlations in the predicted and expected direction (see Table 1) support standard criteria for construct validation.

RESULTS

Our analysis begins in Table 2 with an overview of the bivariate association between family process and delinquency as measured by official records and total unofficial delinquency. The magnitude and direction of relationships support the informal social-control model. All relationships are in the expected direction, quite large, and maintain whether one considers official or unofficial delinquency. For example, both official and unofficial delinquency increase monotonically as erratic/harsh discipline increases (gammas = .70 and .59., respectively). Delinquency also declines monotonically with increasing levels of supervision and attachment. In fact, 83% of those in the low supervision category were delinquent, compared to only 10% of those in the high category (gamma = $-.84$). The unofficial criterion shows an even greater differential. Parental attachment is similarly related to both official and unofficial delinquency.

We next consider the extent to which the three dimensions of informal social control potentially mediate the effect of more distal, structural fac-

TABLE 2
Bivariate Association between Family Process and Delinquency

	Discipline Erratic/Harsh			Maternal Supervision			Parent-Child Attachment		
	Low (288)	Medium (224)	High (334)	Low (382)	Medium (252)	High (355)	Low (414)	Medium (194)	High (352)
Officially delinquent (%)	18	51	74	83	58	10	77	47	21
Gamma		.70*			−.84*			−.73*	
Unofficially delinquent[a] (%)	10	39	53	60	39	5	57	32	13
Gamma		.59*			−.72*			−.62*	

[a] Percent unofficially delinquent refers to the trichotomized "high" category.

*$p < .05$.

tors. To accomplish this goal, Panel A of Table 3 displays the results of ordinary-least-squares (OLS) models of family process variables regressed on structural background factors and parental disposition. The results support the theoretical prediction that structural poverty has significant effects on informal social control. For example, the data in columns 1 and 2 show that poverty, in addition to large families, parental deviance, parental instability, and foreign-born status, contributes significantly to erratic use of harsh/punitive discipline (β = .17, t ratio = 4.66).[5]

The results for maternal supervision are also consistent with our general social control framework—poverty significantly reduces effective monitoring (t ratio = -2.84). In addition to parental disposition, other features of structural context are salient too, especially residential mobility, family size, and employment by mothers. There has been much debate about the effect of mother's employment outside of the home on delinquency, but relatively little on how supervision might mediate this structural factor (see Hoffman, 1974; Laub & Sampson, 1988; Maccoby, 1958). In the Glueck data and time era (circa 1940), employment by mothers outside of the home appears to have a significant negative effect on mother's supervision.[6] This is exactly the pattern supportive of a social control framework and confirmed by other empirical research (see Maccoby, 1958; Wilson, 1980). It remains to be seen whether employment outside of the home by mothers has any direct effect on delinquency. It is also worth noting that mother's employment has no discernible effect on erratic/harsh discipline and parent-child attachment.

In columns 5 and 6 we turn to the relational dimension of family social control—emotional attachment and bonding between parent and child. Substantively, the results suggest that in families experiencing marital disruption, frequent residential moves, disadvantaged financial/ethnic position, and a pattern of deviant or unstable parental conduct, parents and children are more likely to exhibit indifference or hostility toward each other. Interestingly, these effects are rather substantial and much larger than those associated with family size and maternal employment.

Panel B displays the replication models that add "child effects" to the

---

[5] Statistical significance tests—including the use of one-tailed hypothesis tests appropriate for theoretical predictions—are not strictly applicable given the Gluecks' nonprobability sampling scheme. As a general rule of thumb, we thus focus on coefficients that are greater than twice their standard errors, which approximates a .05 level of significance. Among "significant" coefficients, our interest is the relative magnitude of effects.

[6] Bearing in mind this historical context, the Gluecks' concern with working mothers and single parents was that children would be deprived of maternal supervision (see Glueck & Glueck, 1950, p. 112). Again, such views reinforce traditional gender roles of women as housewives and mothers by defining their primary role as nurturing children.

TABLE 3

OLS Linear Regression Models of Family Process on Structural Context
and Parent/Child Disposition

	FAMILY PROCESS					
	Erratic/Harsh Discipline		Maternal Supervision		Parent-Child Attachment	
A. Structural Context and Parental Disposition (N = 800)	β	t ratio	β	t ratio	β	t ratio
Family poverty	.17	4.66*	−.09	−2.84*	−.15	−4.28*
Residential mobility	.07	1.81	−.21	−5.85*	−.17	−4.59*
Family size	.16	4.90*	−.13	−4.30*	−.01	−.29
Family disruption	−.05	−1.35	−.04	−1.16	−.22	−6.75*
Maternal employment	.05	1.54	−.20	−7.04*	−.03	−1.04
Foreign born	.13	4.30*	−.07	−2.60*	−.11	−3.81*
Parental deviance	.23	6.01*	−.24	−7.12*	−.18	−4.86*
Parental instability	.17	4.96*	−.19	−6.26*	−.10	−3.21*
Adjusted R^2	.26		.41		.32	

	FAMILY PROCESS					
	Erratic/Harsh Discipline		Maternal Supervision		Parent-Child Attachment	
B. Adding Child Effects (N = 716)	β	t ratio	β	t ratio	β	t ratio
Family poverty	.16	4.38*	−.06	−1.64	−.17	−4.58*
Residential mobility	.03	.73	−.18	−5.06*	−.15	−3.94*
Family size	.18	5.41*	−.16	−5.26*	−.02	−.58
Family disruption	−.06	−1.56	−.01	−.42	−.19	−5.55*
Maternal employment	.07	2.12*	−.22	−7.29*	−.02	−.70
Foreign born	.13	4.09*	−.08	−2.70*	−.12	−3.77*
Parental deviance	.20	4.90*	−.24	−6.80*	−.19	−4.83*
Parental instability	.13	3.79*	−.16	−5.01*	−.05	−1.44
Child diff./antisocial	.22	6.67*	−.15	−4.94*	−.13	−3.96*
Adjusted R^2	.30		.43		.34	

* $p < .05$.

explanation of family process.[7] The results suggest that difficult and anti-social childhood behavior disrupts effective parenting. Specifically, children who were rated difficult, habitually engaged in violent tantrums, and exhibited early misbehavior tended to generate lower levels of supervision by their mothers during adolescence. Consistent with a control-systems perspective, troublesome childhood behavior also significantly predicts

---

[7] Because of missing data on child effects, there are almost 100 fewer cases available for analysis in Panel B. Changes in parameter estimates from Panel A may thus reflect in part a slightly different sample composition.

the erratic/harsh use of discipline by parents and weakened attachment between parent and child. These results support Lytton's (1990) arguments regarding the endogeneity of parental styles of discipline and control of children, especially direct controls. Simply put, parents appear responsive to early behavioral difficulties—angry temperamental children who misbehave provoke in their parents a disrupted style of parenting and control.

Considering the central role of childhood behavior, the finding that the effects of structural context remain largely intact becomes all the more impressive. Indeed, the rationale for introducing child effects was not to establish conclusively the validity of "control systems" theory, but rather to test the validity of our theoretical conceptions about the indirect effects of poverty on adolescent delinquency. In this regard, note that family poverty, independent of child disposition, continues to exert significant and relatively large effects on erratic/harsh discipline and parent-child attachment. Moreover, it is possible that the reduced effect of poverty on supervision in Panel B (t ratio $= -1.64$, $p < .10$) reflects in part an indirect effect whereby poverty increases early antisocial behavior, which further disrupts parenting. In any case, the data support a structure-process model—poverty and structural context explain informal social control by families, regardless of parental disposition and childhood antisocial behavior.

Explaining Delinquency

Panel A of Table 4 displays the effects of structural context, parental disposition, and family process on adolescent delinquency.[8] The first two columns of data list the ML logistic results for the official delinquency criterion. Columns 3 and 4 list the OLS results for the summary measure of unofficially reported delinquency. In general the results are invariant across method and measurement of delinquency. The majority of structural context and parental disposition factors have insignificant direct effects on delinquency, operating instead through the family process variables. The main exception is family size, which has a direct positive effect on both official and self-parent-teacher-reported delinquency. Residential mobility and family disruption also have small direct effects on unofficial delinquency.

---

[8]The dichotomous nature of official delinquency violates the assumptions of OLS regression. Maximum-likelihood (ML) logistic regression is thus used, preserving the ordinal and interval-based nature of predictor variables. The unstandardized logistic coefficients in Table 4 represent the change in the log-odds of official delinquency associated with a unit change in the exogenous variable. Because the units of measurement of the independent variables are not uniform, we also present the ML t ratios of coefficients to standard errors. The self-parent-teacher summary index of delinquency ranges from 1 to 26, and is estimated with OLS regression.

TABLE 4

OLS Linear and ML Logistic Regression of Delinquency on Structural Context, Family Process, and Parent/Child Disposition

	DELINQUENCY			
	Official Status		Self-Parent-Teacher Reported	
A. Structural Context and Parental Disposition (N = 800)	ML Logistic[a]		OLS Linear	
	b	t ratio	β	t ratio
Family poverty	.10	1.36	.04	1.46
Residential mobility	.03	1.20	.07	2.21*
Family size	.14	2.63*	.08	2.82*
Family disruption	.32	1.36	.06	2.10*
Maternal employment	−.14	−.62	−.02	−.64
Foreign born	.04	.18	−.03	−1.32
Parental deviance	−.00	−.04	.01	.23
Parental instability	.21	1.36	.05	1.60
Erratic/harsh discipline	.38	5.26*	.17	5.25*
Maternal supervision	−1.27	−8.15*	−.36	−9.89*
Parent-child attachment	−.47	−4.51*	−.15	−4.70*
	ML Model χ^2 = 485, 11 df		OLS R^2 = .48	

	DELINQUENCY			
	Official Status		Self-Parent-Teacher Reported	
B. Adding Child Effects (N = 716)	ML Logistic[a]		OLS Linear	
	b	t ratio	β	t ratio
Family poverty	.09	1.18	.02	.64
Residential mobility	.01	.33	.07	1.97*
Family size	.18	3.04*	.10	3.59*
Family disruption	.33	1.24	.07	2.23*
Maternal employment	−.00	−.00	.01	.26
Foreign born	.01	.04	−.03	−1.25
Erratic/harsh discipline	.35	4.22*	.13	3.87*
Maternal supervision	−1.21	−7.06*	−.33	−8.77*
Parent-child attachment	−.50	−4.24*	−.15	−4.54*
Parental deviance	.03	.25	.01	.28
Parental instability	.10	.61	.02	.76
Child difficult/antisocial	1.09	6.35*	.19	6.72*
	ML Model χ^2 = 475, 12 df		OLS R^2 = .52	

[a] Entries for ML Logistic "b" are the raw maximum-likelihood coefficients; "t ratios" are coefficients divided by SE.

* $p < .05$.

On the other hand, the three family-process variables exhibit significant effects on delinquency in the predicted theoretical direction. Several of these effects are quite large, especially the negative effect of maternal supervision on delinquency (OLS β = $-.36$, ML t ratio = -8.15). At the same time, erratic/punitive discipline and parent-child attachment have independent effects on delinquency of similar magnitudes (β = .17 and -.15, respectively). Net of background variables and parental disposition, then, both direct family controls (discipline and monitoring) and indirect social control (affective bonding between child and parent) distinguish nondelinquents from serious, persistent delinquents.

The initial results support the predictions of our theoretical strategy— when an intervening variable mediates the effect of an exogenous variable, the direct effects of the latter should disappear. For the most part that is what Table 4 yields. Moreover, when OLS and ML logistic regression models are estimated without the hypothesized mediating variables, virtually all structural context factors have large, significant effects on delinquency in the expected manner. In particular, the reduced-form t ratio for the effect of poverty on unofficial delinquency is 4.96 (further underscoring the between-family variations in poverty). But, as seen in Table 4, the significant effect of poverty on delinquency is eliminated when discipline, supervision, and attachment are controlled. The calculation of indirect effect estimates reveals that of the total effect of all structural context and parental disposition factors on delinquency, approximately 67% is mediated by family process. The results thus demonstrate the importance of considering indirect effects of poverty and other dimensions of structural background.[9]

Panel B of Table 4 displays two replication models of structural background, parental disposition, family process, and child effects on delinquency. The results suggest three substantive conclusions. First, much like earlier models, family poverty and most other structural background factors influence delinquency largely through the mediating dimensions of family process. Second, the child-effects measure has a significant direct effect on delinquency that is unaccounted for by family process and structural context. Third, and most important from our perspective, are the robust results regarding family process. Despite controlling for childhood and parental disposition, the dimensions of parental discipline, attachment, and supervision all continue to influence delinquent conduct in the

---

[9] Even when the unofficial delinquency measure is broken down by reporter (self, parent, teacher) and offense types, the same general pattern emerges (data not shown). Consistent with Table 4, for example, mother's supervision has the largest effect on truancy, runaway, larceny, smoking/drinking, vandalism, and motor-vehicle theft.

manner predicted by our informal social-control model. Mother's supervision has by far the largest effect on self-parent-teacher-reported delinquency, with a standardized coefficient almost double the child effect (β = −.33).

On balance, then, our theoretical model remains intact, surviving a test that controls for early childhood antisocial behavior. Hence one way of interpreting Table 4 is that variations in adolescent delinquency unexplained by early propensity to deviance are directly explained by informal processes of family social control in adolescence. The magnitude of the family-process effects is especially noteworthy—for example, independent of all other factors including childhood antisocial behavior, a one-unit increase in mother's supervision (on a three-point scale) is associated with over a 50% decrease in official delinquency. The magnitudes of the standardized effects on unofficial delinquency tell the same story.[10]

Structural Equation Models

To this point in the analysis it is clear that structural context, parental disposition, and child antisocial behavior have similar effects on supervision, attachment, and erratic/harsh discipline. This pattern suggests that the three family-process measures are tapping the same latent construct. Further evidence for this specification was seen earlier in Table 1—all three indicators are highly intercorrelated—in fact, the smallest correlation is −.40 between attachment and erratic/harsh discipline. Thus, even though supervision, attachment, and erratic/harsh discipline exhibited independent effects in the OLS regression models, there are both theoretical and empirical reasons to consider an alternative strategy that specifies all three measures as underlying a latent construct of informal social control.

To estimate this alternative conception, we take advantage of recent advances in Jöreskog and Sörbom's (1989) LISREL 7.20 and PRELIS 1.20 programs for maximum-likelihood (ML) estimation of linear covariance-structure models with data that are non-normally distributed. The basic specification of our covariance structure model is shown in Figure 1 (for a similar specification see Larzelere & Patterson, 1990). Both delinquency

---

[10]To assess the robustness of results, we introduced additional control variables and examined mean-substitution and pairwise-deletion models where we entered a dichotomous variable for missing cases. For example, we controlled for residual differences in the matching variables of age and IQ, along with mesomorphy and extroversion. two "constitutional" variables emphasized by the Gluecks. Family-process effects retained their significant predictive power. We also examined attachment to delinquent peers and ethnic group differences in family process (using dichotomous variables for Italian, English, and Irish background). Again, the major substantive results remained intact (see also Sampson & Laub, 1993, pp. 94–95, 118–121).

and informal social control are specified as latent constructs. The former is measured with official delinquency and self-parent-teacher reports, whereas the latent construct of informal social control is hypothesized to generate the correlations among erratic/harsh discipline, parent-child attachment, and maternal supervision. The direction and magnitude of factor loadings support the validity of specified variables as indicators of the latent constructs. As before, structural context and child/parent disposition are treated as exogenous observed variables. However, family disruption was insignificant in the initial LISREL estimation, and was thus dropped to improve the model fit.

Figure 1 presents the ML weighted-least-squares LISREL estimates of all significant path coefficients. The model fits the data very well, yielding a chi-square of 30 with 28 degrees of freedom ($p = .35$). Indeed, as seen in the adjusted goodness-of-fit index (.99), there is an excellent match between the observed covariances and our theoretical specification of family process. Informal social control also has a large and significant negative effect on the latent construct of delinquency (t ratio $= -4.06$). Perhaps most striking,

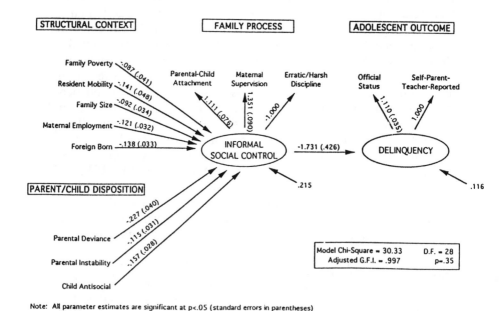

Note: All parameter estimates are significant at p<.05 (standard errors in parentheses)

Figure 1. ML weighted-least-squares covariance-structure model of structural context, parent/child disposition, informal social control, and delinquency ($N = 716$).

the latent family construct now mediates all prior effects of structural context and parent/child disposition. Calculating indirect effect estimates, we find that 68% of the total effect of exogenous factors on delinquency is mediated by informal social control. Note, for example, that poverty has a significant negative effect on informal social control (t ratio = -2.12) net of other context variables and parent/child disposition. This finding substantiates earlier OLS analyses. Similarly, both parental deviance and instability independently reduce informal social control, in turn increasing delinquency.

Interestingly, however, note that the child-disposition measure has a large negative effect (t ratio = -5.61) on informal social control but no direct effect on delinquency. This is the only major finding that does not comport with earlier regression analyses—once a family-process measurement model is specified, the influence of childhood antisocial behavior on delinquency works solely through attenuated informal social control. Although this finding needs to be replicated in future analysis, it does support the control-systems hypothesis (Lytton, 1990) that child effects are important primarily for their influence on family management. Similarly, the lack of a direct effect on delinquency suggests that the correlation between childhood and adolescent delinquency is less an indication of a latent antisocial trait than a *developmental process* whereby delinquent children systematically undermine effective strategies of family social control, in turn increasing the odds of later delinquency. In any case, the more general message in Figure 1 is that the latent construct of informal social control is the primary factor in explaining adolescent delinquency.

DISCUSSION

Our major finding is that family process mediated approximately two-thirds of the effect of poverty and other structural background factors on delinquency. Whether analyzed with standard regression techniques or covariance structure models, the data paint a consistent picture. Namely, poverty appears to inhibit the capacity of families to achieve informal social control, which in turn increases the likelihood of adolescent delinquency.

The data thus support the general theory of informal social control explicated at the outset. We believe that this theory has significance for future research by positing how it is that poverty and structural disadvantage influence delinquency in childhood and adolescence. A concern with only direct effects conceals mediating relations and may thus lead to misleading conclusions regarding the theoretical importance and policy relevance of more distal structural factors such as poverty (see also Conger et al., 1992; Larzelere & Patterson, 1990; McLoyd, 1990). More generally, families do not exist in isolation (or just "under the roof") but instead are systematically embedded in social-structural contexts—even taking into account parental predispositions toward deviance and impulsive temperament.

The data further point to the complex role of social selection and social causation in the genesis of delinquency. Although difficult children who display early antisocial tendencies do appear to self select or sort themselves into later states of delinquency, family processes of informal social control still explain a significant share of variance in adolescent delinquency. Moreover, the covariance structure analyses further suggest that the effect of childhood antisocial/difficult behavior is mediated by family process. Although "child effects" are clearly present, a full understanding of delinquency thus requires that we also come to grips with the socializing influence of the family as reflected in disciplinary practices, supervision and direct parental controls, and bonds of attachment.

Not only do our results point to the indirect effects of poverty on adolescent delinquency, they simultaneously suggest that strong family social controls may serve as an important buffer against structural disadvantage in the larger community. Recall that all boys were reared in economically deprived neighborhoods of central Boston in the Great Depression era, conditions similar to disadvantaged "underclass" communities in many inner-city areas today (see Wilson, 1987). Yet there were marked variations in both family poverty and delinquency risk within these structurally deprived areas of Boston in the 1930s and 1940s, just as there are in the worst inner cities of today. Cohesive families characterized by consistent, loving, and reintegrative punishment, effective supervision, and close emotional ties appear to have overcome these disadvantaged conditions in producing a low risk of adolescent delinquency. In this sense it is mistaken to assume that residents of concentrated poverty areas (e.g., the "underclass") face homogeneous odds—whether it be for negative *or* positive outcomes.

Despite the consistency of results, we recognize that limitations of the data preclude definitive conclusions. Because the Gluecks used a sample of institutionalized delinquents and neighborhood socioeconomic status as one of the matching variables, our conclusions are limited to the relative effects of family poverty on serious and persistent delinquency within a disadvantaged sample (for a critique of this aspect of the Gluecks' research design, see Reiss, 1951). Whether our results hold for adolescents (including noninstitutionalized delinquents) drawn from a wider range of socioeconomic positions is an important issue for future research. Many of the measures we used in the present analysis were also retrospective in nature and may have been confounded by the original coders' global impressions. Issues of temporal order and discriminant validity thus cannot be resolved with certainty (see Bank, Dishion, Skinner, & Patterson, 1990). In particular, a richer set of prospective child-effects and parental-disposition measures is needed to assess more rigorously the role of individual differences. Whether child effects are fully mediated by family processes of informal social control (see Fig. 1) would seem to be an especially salient question for future work.

Nevertheless, it bears emphasis that our findings on family process are consistent with much previous research—including key observations of the Gluecks some 40 years ago. Note also the recent meta-analysis by Loeber and Stouthamer-Loeber (1986, p. 37) where they found that aspects of family functioning involving direct parent-child contacts are the most powerful predictors of delinquency and other juvenile conduct problems. Apparently, the fundamental causes of delinquency are consistent across time and rooted not in race (e.g., black inner-city culture) but generic family processes—such as *supervision, attachment,* and *discipline*—that are systematically influenced by family poverty and structural disadvantage. We hope that future research will address further the connections we have emphasized between poverty and mediating family processes, especially as they bear on both risk and avoidance of adolescent delinquency in disadvantaged communities.

REFERENCES

Anderson, K., Lytton, H., & Romney, D. (1986). Mothers' interactions with normal and conduct-disordered boys: Who affects whom? *Developmental Psychology,* **22,** 604–609.

Bank, L., Dishion, T., Skinner, M., & Patterson, G. (1990). Method variance in structural equation modeling: Living with "glop." In G. Patterson (Ed.), *Depression and aggression in family interaction* (pp. 248–279). Hillsdale, NJ: Erlbaum.

Braithwaite, J. (1989). *Crime, shame, and reintegration.* Cambridge: Cambridge University Press.

Caspi, A. (1987). Personality in the life course. *Journal of Personality and Social Psychology,* **53,** 1203–1213.

Conger, R., Conger, K., Elder, G. H., Jr., Lorenz, F., Simons, R., & Whitbeck, L. B. (1992). A family process model of economic hardship and adjustment of early adolescent boys. *Developmental Psychology,* **63,** 526–541.

Elder, G. H., & Caspi, A. (1988). Economic stress in lives: Developmental perspectives. *Journal of Social Issues*, **44**, 25–45.

Glueck, S., & Glueck, E. (1950). *Unraveling juvenile delinquency*. New York: Commonwealth Fund.

Glueck, S., & Glueck, E. (1968). *Delinquents and nondelinquents in perspective*. Cambridge, MA: Harvard University Press.

Gottfredson, M., & Hirschi, T. (1990). *A general theory of crime*. Stanford, CA: Stanford University Press.

Hirschi, T. (1969). *Causes of delinquency*. Berkeley: University of California Press.

Hirschi, T. (1983). Crime and the family. In J. Wilson (Ed.), *Crime and public policy* (pp. 53–68). San Francisco: Institute for Contemporary Studies.

Hoffman, L. W. (1974). Effects of maternal employment on the child: A review of the research. *Developmental Psychology*, **10**, 204–228.

Jencks, C. (1992). *Rethinking social policy: Race, poverty, and the underclass*. Cambridge, MA: Harvard University Press.

Jöreskog, K., & Sörbom, D. (1989). *LISREL VI: A guide to the program and applications*. Chicago, IL: Scientific Software.

Kornhauser, R. (1978). *Social sources of delinquency*. Chicago: University of Chicago Press.

Larzelere, R., & Patterson, G. (1990). Parental management: Mediator of the effect of socioeconomic status on early delinquency. *Criminology*, **28**, 301–323.

Laub, J. H., & Sampson, R. J. (1988). Unraveling families and delinquency: A reanalysis of the Gluecks' data. *Criminology*, **26**, 355–380.

Loeber, R., & Stouthamer-Loeber, M. (1986). Family factors as correlates and predictors of juvenile conduct problems and delinquency. In M. Tonry & N. Morris (Eds.), *Crime and justice* (Vol. 7, pp. 29–150). Chicago: University of Chicago Press.

Lytton, H. (1990). Child and parent effects in boys' conduct disorder: A reinterpretation. *Developmental Psychology*, **26**, 683–697.

Maccoby, E. (1958). Children and working mothers. *Children*, **5**, 83–89.

McLoyd, V. C. (1990). The impact of economic hardship on black families and children: Psychological distress, parenting, and socioemotional development. *Child Development*, **61**, 311–346.

Olweus, D. (1980). Familial and temperamental determinants of aggressive behavior in adolescent boys: A causal analysis. *Developmental Psychology*, **16**, 644–660.

Patterson, G. (1980). Children who steal. In T. Hirschi & M. Gottfredson (Eds.), *Understanding crime: Current theory and research* (pp. 73–90). Beverly Hills, CA: Sage.

Patterson, G. (1982). *Coercive family process*. Eurgene, OR: Castalia.

Patterson, G. (1988). Stress: A change agent for family process. In N. Garmezy & M. Rutter (Eds.), *Stress, coping, and develoment in children* (pp. 235–264). Baltimore: Johns Hopkins University Press.

Patterson, G., & Capaldi, D. (1991). Antisocial parents: Unskilled and vulnerable. In P. Cowan & M. Hetherington (Eds.), *Family transitions* (pp. 195–218). Hillsdale, NJ: Erlbaum.

Patterson, G., DeBaryshe, B., & Ramsey, E. (1989). A developmental perspective on antisocial behavior. *American Psychologist*, **44**, 329–335.

Reiss, A. J., Jr. (1951). Unraveling juvenile delinquency: II. An appraisal of the research methods. *American Journal of Sociology*, **57**, 115–120.

Robins, L. N. (1966). *Deviant children grown up.* Baltimore: Williams & Wilkins.

Robins, L. N., Schoenberg, S., Holmes, S., Ratcliff, K., Benham, A., & Works, J. (1985). Early home environment and retrospective recall: A test for concordance between siblings with and without psychiatric disorders. *American Journal of Orthopsychiatry*, **55**, 27–41.

Rutter, M., & Giller, H. (1983). *Juvenile delinquency: Trends and perspectives.* New York: Guilford.

Sampson, R. J., & Laub, J. H. (1993). *Crime in the making: Pathways and turning points through life.* Cambridge, MA: Harvard University Press.

West, D., & Farrington, D. P. (1973). *Who becomes delinquent?* London: Heinemann.

White, J., Moffitt, T., Earls, F., Robins, L., & Silva, P. (1990). How early can we tell? Predictors of childhood conduct disorder and adolescent delinquency. *Criminology*, **28**, 507–533.

Wilson, H. (1980). Parental supervision: A neglected aspect of delinquency. *British Journal of Criminology*, **20**, 203–235.

Wilson, W. J. (1987). *The truly disadvantaged: The inner city, the underclass, and public policy.* Chicago: University of Chicago Press.

Part IV

INSTITUTIONAL ISSUES

This section brings together two papers that address very different aspects of institutional care and treatment. The first paper by Blacher and Baker (Chapter 14) directs attention to the question of whether and to what degree families maintain an attachment to their mentally retarded children following out-of-home placement. Thirty years ago, prevailing professional opinion encouraged early placement of retarded and otherwise severely handicapped children. Such children were considered to be a source of stress for all family members, and familial involvement, both pre- and post-placement, was viewed as ill-advised. However the content of professional advice has changed markedly in recent years. Increasing acceptance and broad dissemination of normalization as a guiding principle in the organization of services for children encourages the maintenance of a continuing and developmentally appropriate relationship with the child regardless of place of residence.

In this longitudinal study, semistructured interviews designed to assess the behavioral and emotional dimensions of family involvement and detachment over time and families' post-placement adjustment were conducted with 55 families approximately one and two years following placement of their retarded child. The development of specific questions was guided by a conceptual model of the "psychological tasks of detachment" parallel to the "psychological tasks of divorce" proposed by Wallerstein and colleagues (Annual Progress, 1987). Steps in this process include: (1) acknowledging the reality of the need to place; (2) placing; (3) disengaging from pre-placement stress and resumption of daily activities; (4) experiencing loss of the placed child; (5) experiencing resurgence of attachment; (6) resolving guilt; (7) resolving loss and accepting the permanency of placement; (8) achieving realistic hopes for the child and family.

The results indicated little evidence of behavioral detachment. Although parents reported experiencing reduced stress and greater freedom to pursue personal interests and family activities following placement, they continued to visit and call their children with a high degree of regularity. Respondents also reported feelings of loss, along with a resurgence of complex emotions, including happiness, stress, sadness, and guilt, most particularly in association with visiting. Blacher and Baker consider whether the development of strong attachments during a long period of residence at home contributed to the ability of these families to maintain meaningful contact with their children following placement. The experience of close involvement with service providers during the pre-placement period may also have provided a model for continued close interaction with the staff of residential facilities. Although examination of the effects of placement on behavioral, emotional, and cognitive aspects of the functioning of retarded children awaits further study, the results of the present investigation underscore the importance of individualizing "conventional wisdom" when endeavoring to assist families of severely handicapped children reconcile the sometimes conflicting needs of their handicapped children and other family members.

The "quiet room" is a ubiquitous component of most inpatient psychiatric units, and the importance of this feature of the milieu to staff charged with the responsibility of insuring the safety of the inpatient environment has rarely been questioned. It is generally agreed that quiet room is a useful and effective tool in managing agitated or aggressive children, helping them to calm down rapidly, minimizing the need for chemical or mechanical restraints. Traditionally, institutional quiet rooms are drab and unattractive, frequently without windows, painted white or gray, furnished only with a mattress on a vinyl floor. Yet, little is known about the effects of quiet room design on therapeutic efficacy in either children or adults. Glod, Teicher, Butler, Savino, Harper, Magnus, and Pahlavan remedy this gap by examining whether altering the design of a quiet room resulted in more rapid calming of agitated or aggressive hospitalized children. In the study reported in Chapter 15, one of five traditional quiet rooms was altered by painting the white walls pink, installing carpeting, and painting a 6×6 mural depicting playful dolphins, fish, and crabs that gave an illusion of movement. Effectiveness of the changes was studied in two phases separated by a year. In all, 19 patients (mean age = 9.6 years) were studied using a within-subjects, repeated-measures design. The Overt Aggression Scale was used to rate patients at the time of quiet room placement, and at 5-minute intervals thereafter, until the child was removed. Children were not aware that a study was being conducted, although staff were.

The results were highly significant. A striking reduction in total aggression scores was observed in children placed in the redesigned quiet room within 5 minutes of entry. Simple modifications in the design of the room appeared to enhance calming and diminish aggression as well as the need for PRN medication. The authors urge caution in interpreting the findings because the study design did not permit adequate control of all possible confounding factors. Although replication is desirable, it is clear from the data that no adverse effect attached to the introduction of these modifications of design. This challenge to traditional institutional practice should not go unheeded by those responsible for the care and treatment of children in hospital settings.

14

Family Involvement in Residential Treatment of Children with Retardation: Is There Evidence of Detachment?

Jan Blacher and Bruce L. Baker
University of California, Riverside

Family involvement could be critical for successful residential treatment. Historically, however, out of home placement for children with mental retardation meant a severing of meaningful ties with their families. Today, families have greater involvement with pre-placement services and might be more involved in residential treatment as well. Families (N = 55) were interviewed twice, approximately one and two years after placement, to assess their involvement with the child and their reactions to placement. Contrary to previous findings, family involvement was high and stable; there was no evidence of behavioral detachment. Moreover, respondents primarily reported post-placement benefits to the family. Family emotional reactions were considered within a framework of "psychological tasks of placement."

INTRODUCTION

"A parent who long ago placed his special child in an institution told us that within a week we'll be wondering why we had not done so sooner. He's wrong. I won't wonder. I know precisely

Reprinted with permission from the *Journal of Child Psychology and Psychiatry*, 1994, Vol. 35, 505–520. Copyright © 1994 by the Association for Child Psychology and Psychiatry.

This paper was supported by Grant No. HD21324 from the National Institute on Child Health and Human Development to the first author. The authors appreciate the assistance of Barbara Bromley, Paula Eberhard, Kathy Mattson, Robin Steinback and Loretta Winters of the U.C. Riverside Families Project.

why. Because out of sight [is] not only out of mind but also beyond responsibility."

(Greenfeld, 1986, p. 269)

Josh Greenfeld wrote these thoughts soon after placing Noah, his son with autism and severe retardation, into a group home. They reflect three critical questions about families and residential treatment that have received surprisingly little empirical study. First, do families stay involved after placement—or are they really beyond responsibility? Second, how do families continue to think and feel about the placed child—is he really out of mind? And third, how do families adjust to the dramatic change in the family system represented by placing a member—do families indeed experience such relief that they wonder why they had not made this momentous decision sooner? The present study is the first longitudinal examination of these questions, based on interviews with families at two timepoints after their placement of a child with retardation.

From the moment a child with severe retardation or handicaps is born, the possibility of out-of-home placement exists. Many families do place at some time during the family lifecycle, but families differ greatly in the relationship they maintain with the placed child. Only a generation or so ago, professionals tended to discourage attachment to the child with retardation or other handicaps, recommending that parents place him or her at birth and try to forget. Involvement, pre- or post-placement, was ill-advised, as the presence of such a child in the family was regarded as a source of stress for everyone. Yet the widely accepted normalization philosophy of recent years would argue otherwise—for maintaining a continuing and developmentally appropriate relationship with the child, regardless of where he or she is living (Turnbull, Turnbull, Bronicki, Summers & Roeder-Gordon, 1989). There are many important roles that families can play in the often isolated lives of sons and daughters living in residential settings (Blacher & Baker, 1992). Moreover, for families who ultimately want to bring their child back home, residential settings should be viewed as a support system and not as substitute placements for families who have failed (Jensen & Whittaker, 1987).

Post-Placement Behavioral Involvement and Detachment

What do we know about post-placement family involvement with children who are mentally retarded? Is there a process of "detachment," a disengaging or loosening of ties or attachment to the child? Bowlby (1980) used the term detachment to refer to a *child's* disengaging from his mother, shown by an almost complete absence of attachment behavior after spending a week or more out of his mother's care. Here we use the term to refer to a mother's behavior after the child has been placed. With children who have severe mental retardation and/or other impairments, the mother's behavior appears especially important in determining the course of mother-child attachment (Blacher, 1984; Blacher & Meyers, 1983). Having a child in residential placement is likely to disrupt the natural bond between family and child, facilitating detachment (Willer *et al.*, 1981). Fisher and Tessler (1986) inferred detachment from behavioral indicators: visitations to a residential facility or child visits home. Regular and frequent involvement or contact would be suggestive of interest in and concern for the child, and a sense of attachment. Conversely, lack of visitation or behavioral contact with the child would be viewed as a form of "detachment."

Most studies of post-placement involvement have focused on visitation patterns, typically with placed adults, and have consistently found that families maintained little contact with their son or daughter once placed (Baker & Blacher, 1988). This near isolation is not limited to institutional placements; recent studies of community residences have found low family involvement as well (Anderson, Lakin, Hill & Chen, 1992; Grimes & Vitello, 1990; Stoneman & Crapps, 1990). Hill, Rotegard and Bruininks (1984) interviewed direct care staff about family visitation with over 900 individuals in community residences. They reported that for every five residents, one had no personal contact with family members, three were visited from one to three times a year, and only one was visited more frequently. A common assumption, albeit untested, has been that family contacts are more frequent at first but diminish sharply over time.

These reports of post-placement involvement, however, primarily studied families who raised their child before the passage in the United States of Public Law 94-142, The Education For All Handicapped Children Act. This law heralded new service provisions and opportunities for parent involvement while the child still lived at home. Indeed, studies of parent involvement with retarded children living at home have indicated high rates of involvement in schooling (Meyers & Blacher, 1987). Thus, parents raising their child in the post 94-142 era have been primed for higher rates of behavioral involvement, and one might expect these parents to continue involvement even if they place their child out of the home (Blacher & Baker, 1992; Fisher & Tessler, 1986).

A recent cross-sectional study involving interviews with 62 families who had placed their child within the previous two years found high rates of post-placement involvement (Baker & Blacher, 1993). Behavioral components of involvement included visits to the facility, visits home, phone calls, and involvement in the child's Individualized Habilitation Plan (IHP). Most families had at least a monthly visit with the child, half called weekly, and three quarters had attended the most recent educational planning meeting. One purpose of the present study was to follow involvement in this sample of families longitudinally, looking for evidence of detachment.

Emotional and Cognitive Involvement

"We think of Noah constantly. He is the unspoken thought that fills all the silences" (Greenfeld, 1986, p. 269). A second purpose of the present study was to broaden our conceptualization of family involvement and detachment beyond its behavioral components (actions like visitation and calling) to include emotions (feelings in reference to the placed child) and cognitions (thoughts about the placed child), two components that are, in the present context, not easily separated. Decreasing feelings of attachment toward the child and of guilt about placement, thinking and talking less often about the child, and less desire to bring the child home may reflect detachment.

Several earlier studies indicated continued emotional involvement post-placement (e.g. Hewett, 1970), and one found that where a strong pre-placement bond had been formed the level of parental interest in the child after institutionalization was high (Downey, 1965). Attachment between parents and child appeared to be stronger in older children who had remained at home longer prior to institutionalization. Others have hypothesized that strong pre-placement bonds between parent and child will help to overcome obstacles to post-placement involvement, such as distance (Fisher & Tessler, 1986), and will make it more likely that the child will eventually return home (Willer, Intagliata & Wicks, 1981).

In Baker and Blacher's (in press) cross-sectional study attachment was also considered. Professed attachment was still high during the first two years post-placement. Evidence for emotional detachment was mixed. While respondents indicated some lessening of attachment since placement, neither attachment at present nor perceived change in attachment related to time since placement. Some parents may have already "detached" back when they anticipated making the placement, or during the placement process itself. In the present study we examined attachment longitudinally in these same families, and explored additional thoughts and feelings.

Post-Placement Adjustment

The third purpose of this study was to examine family adjustment or well-being following out-of-home placement of the child with mental retardation. Studies about readjustment following other traumatic events—death of a spouse (Parkes & Weiss, 1983), rape (Kilpatrick, Veronen & Best, 1985; Koss & Burkhart, 1989), and birth (Blacher, 1984) or adoption of a child with handicaps (Glidden, 1991)—are informative. This literature suggests that there are stages of readjustment that the person goes through, that the process is a lengthy one, and that initial reactions in many cases predict long-term outcomes. The literature on divorce, in particular, may be useful for the study of detachment posed herein. Both divorce and out-of-home placement are usually traumatic processes that involve the removal of one family member from the home.

As a theoretical framework for understanding what families experience emotionally after they place their child with retardation, we designed interview questions for parents to parallel the "psychological tasks" of divorce proposed by Wallerstein (1983; Wallerstein & Kelly, 1980) in her longitudinal study of divorce outcome. Although Wallerstein's focus was more on the consequences to the child, broader family relationships are implicitly involved—e.g. reactions to loss of the divorced parent, visitation patterns, changes in attachment or emotional bonds. We adapted these to describe parental adjustment to child placement and will refer to them as the psychological tasks of detachment, as follows: 1. Acknowledging the reality of the need to place; 2. Placing; 3. Disengaging from pre-placement stress and resumption of daily activities; 4. Experiencing loss of the placed child; 5. Experiencing resurgence of attachment (e.g. upon visitation); 6. Resolving guilt or other negative cognitions or feelings; 7. Resolving loss and accepting the permanency of placement; 8. Achieving realistic hopes for the child and family. The families in the present sample had already accomplished the first two tasks, as their children were already placed. We will consider issues related to psychological tasks 3–8.

To summarize, this study of families with a retarded child in residential treatment explored: (1) Behavioral dimensions of family involvement and detachment over time; (2) Emotional dimension of family involvement and detachment over time; and (3) Families' post-placement adjustment.

METHOD

Overview

Parents with a mentally retarded child living outside of the home were interviewed twice following placement. The first interview took place on average of 10.9 months after placement and the second interview took place an average of 10.6 months following the first interview. The interviews investigated parental involvement with the placed child and family post-placement adaptation.

Subjects

Subjects were 55 families with a child in out-of-home placement. Inclusion criteria were that the child was between the ages of 2 and 18 years, was designated by the referral agency as having moderate, severe, or profound mental retardation, and had been placed within two years of the initial interview. Placement was defined as living outside of the home for at least one month before the initial interview. Twelve families had been followed in a longitudinal study of families with children who have severe handicaps (Blacher, 1990) and the additional 43 families were recruited from lists of families that had recently placed, maintained by California Regional Centers, central agencies for persons with developmental disabilities.

Table 1 summarizes parent reports about selected characteristics of the placed child, the family, and the facility. At the Time 1 interview children ranged in age from 2.5 to 17.2 years and had resided in the placement from 1 to 22 months. Although all children were designated by Regional Centers to have at least moderate mental retardation, parent designations shown in Table 1 were somewhat higher, with some children categorized as mildly retarded. Most of the families were intact and had other children living at home; the parents were generally well educated, with about three quarters having attended college. Over half of the facilities were small, with seven or fewer residents; may of these were foster care homes, a dominant model of community placement in California. The larger facilities were comprised of medium sized and large group homes, large private residential schools, and state developmental centers. About half of the facilities were more than 30 miles away from the family home.

Procedures

Interviews were conducted in the home and lasted from 1.5 to 2 hours. For both Time 1 and Time 2 interviews, 53 respondents were mothers and 2 were fathers, although fathers were present in some other interviews. Interviews were conducted by one of two interviewers, each women with considerable experience with mental retardation, families, and interviewing.

The Time 1 interviews ranged from 1 to 22 months after the placement (Mean = 10.9, *SD* = 5.8). The Time 2 interviews ranged from 5 months to 27 months after the initial one (Mean = 10.6), although all but four were completed within 6–16 months.

TABLE 1

Child, Family and Facility Characteristics at Time 1 Interview (N = 55)

Child			
Age in years	$X = 10.7$	$SD =$	4.0
Months in placement at Time 1	$X = 10.9$	$SD =$	5.8
Months in placement at Time 2	$X = 21.5$	$SD =$	7.3
		N	$\%$
Sex (boys)		32	58.2
Birth order			
First born		27	49.1
Second		16	29.1
Third +		12	21.8
Ethnicity			
Anglo		39	70.9
Black		6	10.9
Hispanic		2	3.6
Asian–American		1	1.8
Other		7	12.7
Level of mental retardation (parent report)			
Mild		14	25.5
Moderate		12	21.8
Severe, profound		29	52.8
Level of behavior problems (parent report)			
No behavior problems		10	18.2
Mild		10	18.2
Moderate		18	32.7
Severe		17	30.9

Parent and Family			
Mother's age in years at T1 ($N = 53$)	$X = 37.6$	$SD =$	7.5
Father's age in years at T1 ($N = 42$)	$X = 41.6$	$SD =$	9.1
Family socioeconomic status* ($N = 51$)	$X = 54.1$	$SD =$	22.3
Siblings living at home ($N = 54$)	$X = 1.4$	$SD =$	1.0

Education	Father ($N = 42$)		Mother ($N = 53$)	
	N	$\%$	N	$\%$
High school or less	9	21.4	14	26.4
College, 2 years or less	16	38.1	22	41.5
College 4 years	10	23.8	10	18.9
MA or beyond	7	16.7	7	13.2
Mother employed ($N = 53$)			35	66.0

Facility		
Proximity of placement to parents' home		
Less than 30 miles away	28	50.9
30–60 miles away	15	27.3
More than 60 miles away	12	21.8
Size of the placement facility		
Small (7 or fewer)	33	60.0
Medium (8–15)	5	9.1
Large (16–49)	2	3.6
Very large (50+)	15	27.3

*Note: Socioeconomic status is represented by Duncan occupation score for mother or father, whichever was higher.

For another purpose, interviews were conducted with staff at a sub-set ($N = 26$) of the placement facilities; staff provided an estimate of how often parents visited. These interviews can provide a check on the validity of parent interview reports. This is limited, however, because facility interviews were reports by clinical staff, not actual counts, and they were conducted an average of 10 months after the Time 2 interviews.

Measures

At Time 1, respondents completed a *Demographic Questionnaire* about characteristics of the child, parent and family. The Time 1 and Time 2 *Post-Placement Interviews* consisted primarily of questions with specific response categories; the few open-ended questions were coded by the interviewer according to predetermined categories. Most of the variables derived from the interview were based on single items. The Time 1 and Time 2 interviews asked some questions in common, particularly about behavioral involvement and emotional attachment. The Time 2 interview asked a number of additional questions about thoughts, feelings, activities and plans since placement.

Behavioral involvement. Respondents at both timepoints were asked about three types of family contacts with the child in placement: *child visits home, visits to the facility,* and *phone calls* to the facility. The scales are shown in Table 2. They also rated how often they *discuss their child* with someone, and this is shown in Table 4.

Emotional involvement. Respondents at both timepoints were asked about two aspects of attachment to the child: *present attachment,* and *change in attachment* since placement (see Table 2). These questions were prefaced by an explanation that we were interested in how close, emotionally, parents get to children with handicaps. The interviewer went on to say that some parents feel close to their child, emotionally "bonded," while other parents have difficulty feeling close to their child, and that we use attachment to mean that emotional closeness or bond that may be established between a parent and child.

At Time 2, respondents were also asked two questions about guilt: *guilt at present* and *change in guilt* since placement. These scales are shown in Table 4. Respondents were also asked a number of questions about positive and negative feelings during contacts with the child.

Thoughts and beliefs. Respondents at both timepoints were asked whether they viewed *placement as permanent* for their child (see Table 2). At Time 2, respondents were also asked how often they *thought about the child* in placement, on average and during the past week (see Table 4).

Family life post-placement. Respondents at Time 2 were asked about specific changes in their lives in six areas (recreation, social life, job related stresses, marriage, their relationships with other children, and relationships with relatives and friends), and they rated their life in each area since placement as worse (-1), unchanged (0) or better ($+1$). If the respondent was unmarried or did not have other children, the relevant variables were coded 0 for no change. Respondents also rated whether their other children were much worse off (-2) to much better off ($+2$) following placement. Scores from these seven items were summed into a Life Change Index, with a possible range of -8 (worse in every area) to $+8$ (better in every area); the scale alpha = .62.

Respondents were asked whether and how having the child at home had affected *long range plans*, and whether and how family goals and/or *plans had changed* since placement. Finally, respondents were asked whether *bringing the child home* would make family life worse or better (Table 4).

RESULTS

We first report family involvement over time, using *t*-tests and Pearson correlation coefficients to compare scores on variables assessed at both Time 1 and Time 2. Then we examine descriptively additional dimensions of post-placement adjustment that were assessed only at Time 2. Next, we correlate months since placement with Time 2 involvement scores, as an alternative way of examining changes over time in placement. Finally, we examine correlations among the primary variables of interest: post-placement involvement, adjustment, and child and family demographics.

Family Involvement Over Time: Time 1 to Time 2

Involvement variables assessed at both timepoints included visits, phone calls, feelings of attachment, and beliefs about the permanency of placement.

Visits. Table 2 shows frequencies of visits home and visits to the child at the facility. At each timepoint scores on these two types of visits were uncorrelated; families who choose one type of involvement were not any more or less likely to choose the other. We collapsed visits into a combined visits score. At Time 1 involvement was very high, with 81% of families reporting a visit with their son or daughter at least monthly. At Time 2, this comparable figure remained high, at 80%. Parent estimates were corroborated by the facility interviews, which yielded slightly higher combined visits scores and correlated significantly with parent scores, $r(24) = .51$, $p < .01$.

TABLE 2
Involvement Variables Assessed at Time 1 and Time 2
Post-Placement Interviews (*N* = 55, Except as Noted)

	Time 1		Time 2	
	N	%	N	%
Visits home (N = 54)				
0. My child has not come home	4	7.4	5	9.3
1. For holidays and birthdays only	9	16.7	7	13.0
2. 3–6 times a year	3	5.6	10	18.5
3. Every other weekend (1 or 2/month)	35	64.8	26	48.1
4. Every weekend	3	5.6	6	11.1
Visits at facility				
0. Only to pick child up for home visits	19	34.5	23	41.8
1. Holidays and birthdays only	9	16.4	2	3.6
2. 3–6 times a year	5	9.1	16	29.1
3. Every other weekend	15	27.3	9	16.4
4. Every weekend	7	12.7	5	9.1
Combined visits: home and facility (N = 54)				
0. None	1	1.9	0	0.0
1. Birthdays, special holidays	5	9.3	5	9.3
2. 3–6 times a year	4	7.4	6	11.1
3. 1 per month	21	38.9	19	35.2
4. More than 1 per month	13	24.1	13	24.1
5. Weekly	5	9.3	9	16.7
6. More than weekly	5	9.3	2	3.7
Phone calls (N = 52)				
0. Never	4	7.7	0	0
1. Special occasions or if problems	4	7.7	3	5.8
2. About 3–6 times a year	0	0	3	5.8
3. About once a month (1–3/month)	18	34.6	13	25.0
4. About once a week (1–6/week)	20	38.5	25	48.1
5. Every day (1/day or more)	6	11.5	8	15.4
Present attachment				
0. No, not at all	1	1.8	2	3.6
1. A little/not very strong	3	5.5	2	3.6
2. Somewhat	10	18.2	10	18.2
3. Much attached/quite strong	15	27.3	20	36.4
4. A great deal/very strong	26	47.3	21	38.2
Change in attachment since placement				
1. Attachment is lessening	20	36.4	20	36.4
2. Same as before placement	23	41.8	27	49.1
3. Attachment is stronger	12	21.8	8	14.5
Placement permanency				
0. Temporary	17	31.5	11	20.4
1. Undecided	8	14.8	14	25.9
2. Permanent	29	53.7	29	53.7

Table 3 shows Time 1 and Time 2 correlations and mean scores. Scores for the two timepoints were highly correlated for visits home, visits to the facility, and combined visits. Mean changes over time were small and not statistically significant; indeed, the mean combined visits score was identical at the two timepoints.

Phone calls. Frequency of phone calls to the residential facility was a less direct measure of involvement with the child, as these were most likely to involve contact with staff. Table 2 indicates a high level of phone contact: at Time 1, calls were reported at least weekly by 50% of families and on some occasion by almost all families (92%). At Time 2, these percentages had increased to 63.5% and 100%. As shown in Table 3, Time 1 and Time 2 scores for phone calls were highly correlated. The mean phone call score increased significantly from Time 1 to Time 2.

Attachment. Table 2 shows frequencies of present attachment and changes in attachment. At both timepoints 75% of respondents reported strong present attachment. Present attachment scores at Time 1 and Time 2 were significantly correlated and the mean change over time was small and not significant. At each timepoint, about a third of respondents indicated that attachment had lessened since placement. However, the change in attachment variable did not elicit a stable response; the Time 1–Time 2 correlation was small and non-significant.

Permanency of placement. Table 2 also shows beliefs about the permanency of placement. At both timepoints about half of the respondents indicated that placement was permanent. Scores at Time 1 and Time 2 were significantly correlated and the changes were slight and non-significant.

TABLE 3
Family Involvement Variables, at Time 1 and Time 2

Variable	N	r (T1T2)	X T1	X T2	t
Visits to facility	55	.59$	1.67	1.47	– 1.12
Visits home	54	.73$	2.44	2.39	– .50
Combined visits	54	.67$	3.39	3.39	.00
Phone calls to facility	52	.55$	3.23	3.62	2.40*
Present attachment	55	.62$	3.13	3.02	– .90
Change in attachment	55	.19	1.85	1.78	– .59
Placement permanency	54	.42†	1.22	1.33	.88

*$p < .05$.
†$p < .01$.
$$p < .0001$.

Dimensions Assessed Only at Time 2

Additional dimensions of post-placement involvement and adjustment that were assessed only at Time 2 included: feelings of guilt, resurgence of feelings with visitation, thoughts of the child, discussions about the child, thoughts about consequences of the child returning home, family life changes, and family future goals and plans.

Guilt. Table 4 shows respondents' reports of guilt feelings and changes in guilt since placement. Fifteen parents (27%) reported that they had never felt guilty about placing their child. Forty parents (73%) reported some feelings of guilt, and guilt was a daily or constant feeling for half of them. Nonetheless, guilt was decreasing with time; 27 of the 40 parents (68%) reported feeling less guilty at the Time 2 interview than right after placing the child.

Feelings at visitation. Visitation clearly leads to a resurgence of feelings: positive, negative, and mixed. The child's visit home induces more stress (54% of respondents) but at the same time feelings of happiness (64%). The visit ends with feelings of relief (64%) as well as guilt (44%) and sadness (58%) over leaving the child. Visits to the child at the facility reflect a comparable mix of emotions.

Thinking and talking about the placed child. All but two respondents reported missing the child. Table 4 indicates how often parents reported thinking about and talking about their child. Over three in four respondents reported thinking about the child at least daily, both when this was asked "on average" and "for the past week." These two highly correlated items ($r = .87$) were combined into a "thoughts of child" variable for further analyses. Similarly, three in four respondents discussed their child with someone at least once a week. These talks were primarily with spouse (40%), other family member (27%) or friends (22%), but were rarely with professionals.

Family life after placement. Life Change Index items are shown in Table 5; the great majority of parents reported life to be better following placement, especially in recreation, social life, and relationships with and adjustment of their other children. Life Change total scores ranged from 0 to 8, ($M = +4.9$, $SD = 2.2$) with no respondents scoring worse on average.

Family goals and plans. Fully 58% of respondents indicated that having a handicapped child at home had previously led the family to reconsider long range plans, such as where they lived, what jobs mother and/or father took, or whether they pursued further education. Placement clearly had an impact, as many respondents indicated that long-range plans (53%) and goals for the family (56%) had now changed.

Consequences of bringing the child home. All but one respondent reported having thought about what life would be like if they were to bring the child

TABLE 4
Variables Assessed Only at Time 2 Post-Placement Interview

	N	%
Discuss child with someone (N = 54)		
0. Never	1	1.9
1. Special occasions/when facility calls	1	1.9
2. About once or twice a month	11	20.4
3. About once a week	23	42.6
4. Every day	18	33.3
Guilt (N = 55)		
0. Don't feel guilty	15	27.3
1. Not very often, less than weekly	20	36.4
2. A lot, daily, constantly	20	36.4
Change in guilt since placement (N = 40)		
1. Less guilty now	27	67.5
2. About the same	10	25.0
3. More guilty now	3	7.5
Think about child (N = 55)		
0. Never	0	0
1. Monthly	2	3.6
2. Weekly	10	18.2
3. Daily	25	45.5
4. Constantly	18	32.7
Think about child past week (N = 55)		
0. Not at all	2	3.6
1. Once	5	9.1
2. 2 or 3 times	6	10.9
3. Once a day	20	36.4
4. Several times a day	22	40.0
Consequence of bringing child home (N = 54)		
1. A lot worse	27	50.0
2. A little worse	17	31.5
3. About the same	4	7.4
4. A little better	4	7.4
5. A lot better	2	3.7

back home to stay. As shown in Table 4, there was little variability in their conclusions: fully 81.5% indicated that life would be worse.

Cross-Sectional Analyses

At the Time 2 interview children had been placed an average of 21.5 months, but this varied from 7 to 35 months. To address the question of detachment over time further, correlations were run between months in the placement and the Time 2 scores for all of the behavioral, emotional, and cognitive variables considered above. All but one of these correlations was non-significant; thoughts of child decreased with greater time in the placement, $r(53) = -.27$, $p = .05$. Life Change Index scores also tended to decrease with greater time in the placement, $r(44) = -.28$, $p = .06$.

Relationships Among Involvement Variables

Correlations were run between the following key involvement variables: visits home; visits at the facility; present attachment; guilt, thoughts of child, placement permanency, and consequences of bringing child home. Of the 21 correlations, six were significant at $p < .05$. These relationships among the involvement variables were logical but modest; they were not strong enough to suggest that variables should be combined further. Respondents who reported thinking about their child more frequently also reported higher attachment [$r(53) = .42$, $p < .01$], and higher guilt [$r(53) = .37$, $p < .01$]. Belief that placement was permanent related to more visits at the facility [$r(53) = .34$, $p < .05$], fewer visits home [$r(53) = -.28$, $p < .05$], and worse consequences expected if the child returned home to live [$r(52) = -.34$, $p < .05$]. Perceived worse consequences also related to fewer visits home [$r(52) = .28$, $p < .05$].

Predictors of Involvements

There was considerable variability in the child, family, and facility characteristics. Correlations were run between the seven involvement variables above and the following 10 variables: child age, sex, birth order, level

TABLE 5
Life Changes for Better or Worse in Specific Areas Since Placement of the Child

| | % of respondents | | |
	Worse	Same	Better
Siblings' adjustment ($N = 47$)	0.0	10.6	89.4
Recreation ($N = 55$)	1.8	20.0	78.2
Social Life ($N = 54$)	1.9	22.2	75.9
Relationships with other children ($N = 51$)	3.9	25.5	70.6
Marriage ($N = 35$)	17.1	31.4	51.4
Relationships with relatives and friends ($N = 55$)	3.6	45.5	50.9
Job related stresses ($N = 55$)	12.7	45.5	41.8

of retardation, and behavior problems, mother age, mother education, family socioeconomic status, facility distance and facility size. We recognize that with this many correlations some will reach significance by chance. The following relationships, therefore, should be interpreted cautiously; applying a Bonferoni correction to these correlations, and thereby adjusting the alpha to $p < .001$, results in none reaching significance.

Behavioral involvement. Behavioral indicators of visits home and visits to the facility are of primary interest; there were 20 correlations with demographics and 10 correlations with cognitive and emotional indicators; of these 30 correlations, eight were significant at $p < .05$ two-tailed. Table 6 shows these relationships. We have noted that these two types of visitation represent different and unrelated types of involvement. This is further supported by the pattern of predictors. Home visits were more frequent when the child was less retarded, the facility was less far away, and parents were less likely to view the placement as permanent and the consequences of the child's eventual return home as negative. Facility visits were more likely when children were more retarded, the family was of higher socioeconomic status, and the facility was larger and tended to be further away; these children were more likely to be permanently placed and the consequences of their eventual return home tended to be deemed more negative.

Stepwise multiple regressions were conducted for visits home and visits to the facility, using the set of variables that correlated with each at $p < .05$

TABLE 6

Significant Correlations Between Demographic Variables
and Behavioral Involvement

	Visits home	Visits to facility
Level of retardation	$-.37^{\ddagger}$	$.35^{\ddagger}$
Socioeconomic status	$-.04$	$.31^{\dagger}$
Distance from placement	$-.31^{\dagger}$	$.24^{*}$
Size of placement	$-.09$	$.43^{\ddagger}$
Permanent placement	$-.28^{\dagger}$	$.34^{\dagger}$
Worse if child returned home	$.28^{\dagger}$	$-.23^{*}$

Stepwise Multiple Regression for Visits Home				
Step	Mult R.	Rsq	RsqCh	FCh
1. Level of retardation	.37	.14	.14	$7.52^{\ddagger}$
2. Distance from placement	.48	.23	.09	$5.32^{\dagger}$

$^{*}p < .10.$
$^{\dagger}p < .05.$
$^{\ddagger}p < .01.$

and setting p to enter at .05. The predictor equation for home visits is shown in Table 6. Level of retardation and distance from the facility combined to account for 23% of the variance in home visits. The predictor equation for visits to the facility had only one variable, size of the placement, which explained 18% of the variance. Larger facilities tended to have more severely retarded children, permanently placed by families with higher socioeconomic status, so after facility size was accounted for, no other variable independently related to visits.

Emotional and cognitive involvement. There were 50 correlations between the demographic variables and the involvement variables of attachment, guilt, thoughts of child, permanency of placement, and perceived consequences of bringing the child home; of these, nine were significant at $p < .05$. As above, with this many correlations some may have occurred by chance; all, however, were logical relationships. Attachment and thoughts of child were not related to any demographic variable. Guilt was expressed more by younger mothers [r (51) = $-.29$, $p < .05$] who had placed children who were younger [r (53) = $-.29$, $p < .05$] and later born [r (53) = $-.35$, $p < .01$]. Placement was more likely to be viewed as permanent when the child had greater retardation [r (53) = .36, $p < .01$], was first born [r (53) = $-.39$, $p < .01$], and was placed in a large facility [r (47) = .31, $p < .05$]. The consequences of bringing the child home were viewed as worse with children who were older [r (52) = .39, $p < .01$], more retarded [r (52) = $-.32$, $p < .05$] and later born [r (52) = .31, $p < .05$].

Predictors of Life Change

Life Change Scale score was correlated with the 10 demographic and seven involvement variables considered above. There were only three significant relationships. In families experiencing more positive post-placement life change the placed child had more severe behavior problems [r (44) = .31, $p < .05$]. Life Change related positively to visiting the child at the facility [r (44) = .31, $p < .05$], but negatively to expecting benefits if the child were to return home to live [r (43) = $-.37$, $p < .01$]. It is interesting that the experience of more positive life change post-placement did not relate to other indices of involvement, such as bringing the child home for visits, to feelings of attachment or guilt, or to a view of the placement as permanent.

DISCUSSION

This longitudinal study examined family involvement during the first several years after placing a child with mental retardation out of the natural home. The primary questions asked whether there was evidence of detachment, a lessening of involvement over time. Findings indicated that these families were maintaining high involvement, in contrast with families who raised their retarded children in previous generations. Four in five families had at least a monthly visit with their child, and two in three families called weekly. There was no evidence for detachment on behavioral indices of involvement. Visitation, to the facility or at home, remained highly stable, and phone calls actually increased significantly. Although involvement was likely higher in this volunteer sample than it would have been for randomly selected families, selection bias probably does not account for all of the difference from previous studies, since most of them also used volunteer samples.

Changes in parents' thoughts and feelings since placement also were not consistent with a simple linear hypothesis of detachment. As a unifying framework, we posited psychological tasks of detachment for the family (adapted from Wallerstein, 1983). The families we studied had already met the tasks of acknowledging the need to place and securing a residential placement for their child with mental retardation. We do not argue that the remaining tasks will be faced in order or that all will be relevant for any given family—only that these represent an ongoing process of family adjustment that is little recognized after the clear behavioral indicator of placement itself.

There was striking evidence that families *disengaged from pre-placement stress and resumed daily activities* (Task #3). Respondents reported almost exclusively positive effects on their lives of the decision to place. Primarily, they experienced reduced stress and greater freedom to pursue personal interests and family activities. There is, perhaps, a "honeymoon effect," as reports of positive changes are highest in the early months of placement. It appears that improvements in family well-being did not negatively affect post placement involvement with the child; in fact, these may allow families to maintain higher contact. We have noted elsewhere the consistent finding that families believe the current placement is best and resist changes, even when professionals feel it is in the best interest of their members, and we invoked the theory of cognitive dissonance to help explain this phenomenon (Baker & Blacher, 1988). This same process may be operating when parents who have finally placed then report very positive life changes following placement and predict that life will be much worse if the child were to return home.

Despite the perceived benefits of placement, however, respondents reported *experiencing loss of the child* (Task #4). Out of sight is definitely not out of mind, with most parents reporting daily thoughts and at least weekly conversations about the child. The frequency of thinking about the child did drop with time, and many parents indicated that attachment was lessening. Yet some parents indicated that attachment was increasing, and when respondents were asked about their absolute level of attachment, a consistent three in four reported very high present attachment to the child at both timepoints. It may be that our effective time period of up to three years post-placement is too short a period within which to see marked decline in attachment, if, indeed, such an outcome will occur. The slight decrease in thoughts about the child may be a precursor to a subsequent decline in feelings and or behavioral involvement.

A linear conceptualization of adaptation is complicated, however, by the *resurgence of attachment with contacts* (Task #5) and *resolution of guilt and other negative feelings* (Task #6). Negative emotions, such as sadness or guilt, are likely chronic and never far from the surface (Blacher, 1984; Olshansky, 1962). The majority of parents reported feelings of guilt about placement, a reaction that is in part engendered by present societal and professional opposition to placement. Nonetheless, such feelings are diminishing with time. Visitation is accompanied by a resurgence of emotions, with happiness, stress, sadness, and guilt all frequently voiced. It is important to note that although most respondents readily admitted to negative emotions, the predominant picture was one of decreased stress, positive feelings, and positive outlooks.

Placement of the child was viewed as permanent by slightly over half of the families and as temporary by another quarter; presumably these families had *decided about the permanency of placement* (Task #7). We do not know, however, to what extent families will ultimately change their decision about placement, for, unlike divorce, placement is a readily reversible process. It is notable, though, that most respondents said that life would be worse if the child returned home to stay, so it seems likely that some of the families who view placement as temporary or are undecided will not make moves to end it soon.

We cannot be certain about whether families *achieved realistic goals for the child and the family* (Task #8) during these first years post-placement. Yet more than half of the respondents reported changes in long-range plans for themselves and their families (e.g. mother returns to school), suggesting changes within the family system that may further denote a lasting decision about placement.

In conclusion, there was not much evidence for detachment in these families. The construct of detachment may have several component parts: behavioral, emotional and cognitive, with changes in these dimensions occurring at different paces. Families seem to determine a type and level of behavioral involvement that they will have and to maintain this for some time; this may be the last area to diminish. In any event, the lack of immediate detachment is a promising finding, given the importance of continuing family involvement in the success of residential placement (Schalock & Lilley, 1986).

It may be that some emotional distancing already took place during the long process of deciding about placement (Blacher, 1990; Blacher & Hanneman, 1993). Still, within the first years following placement involvement was high and consistent, although patterns differed. Parents who lived closer to the facility and whose child was less retarded were more likely to maintain contact through home visits. Visits to the facility, however, were more frequent with larger programs, an interesting finding considering the predominant professional argument that individuals with mental retardation are best served in small "homelike" facilities. Policies about service delivery have paid scant attention to family preferences.

We would note several possible reasons for high involvement generally. Families today are not as likely to place children with severe handicaps at birth, but, rather, keep them at home for longer periods; this likely allows attachment to build and perhaps buffer against subsequent detachment. Moreover, this cohort of families had very high preplacement involvement in their child's schooling and other services (Meyers & Blacher, 1987) and the zeitgeist gives prominence to an enduring relationship with families (Taylor, Lakin & Hill, 1989).

These are resilient families. They have lived through the difficult years of having a child with severe handicaps at home and the requisite sacrifices. They have struggled with making a professionally unpopular decision to place. And they have placed. But with it all, rather than experiencing family dissolution, parents can at the same time report an increase in well-being, the maintenance of meaningful contact, and a positive outlook.

REFERENCES

Anderson, D. J., Lakin, K. C., Hill, B. K. & Chen, T. (1992). Social integration of older persons with mental retardation in residential facilities. *American Journal on Mental Retardation*, **96**, 488–501.

Baker, B. L. & Blacher, J. (1988). Family involvement with community residential programs. In M. P. Janicki, M. W. Krauss & M. M. Seltzer (Eds), *Community residences for persons with developmental disabilities: here to stay*, pp. 173–188. Baltimore: Brookes.

Baker, B. L. & Blacher, J. (1993). Out-of-home placement for children with mental retardation: dimensions of family involvement. *American Journal of Mental Retardation*, **98**, 368.

Blacher, J. (1984). A dynamic perspective on the impact of a severely handicapped child on the family. In J. Blacher (Ed.), *Severely handicapped young children and their families: research in review*, pp. 3–50. Orlando, FL: Academic Press.

Blacher, J. (1990). Assessing placement tendency in families with children who have severe handicaps. *Research in Developmental Disabilities*, **11**, 341–351.

Blacher, J. & Baker, B. L. (1992). Toward meaningful family involvement in out-of-home placements. *Mental Retardation*, **30**, 35–43.

Blacher, J. & Hanneman, R. (1993). Out of home placement of children and adolescents with severe handicaps: behavioral intentions and behavior. *Research in Developmental Disabilities*, **14**, 145–160.

Blacher, J. & Meyers, C. E. (1983). A review of attachment formation and disorder in handicapped children. *American Journal of Mental Deficiency*, **87**, 359–371.

Bowlby, J. (1980). *Attachment and loss. Volume III. Loss, sadness, and depression.* London: The Hogarth Press.

Downey, K. J. (1965). Parents' reasons for institutionalizing severely mentally retarded children. *Journal of Health and Human Behavior*, **6**, 147–155.

Fisher, G. A. & Tessler, R. C. (1986). Family bonding of the mentally ill: an analysis of family visits with residents of board and care homes. *Journal of Health and Social Behavior*, **27**, 236–249.

Glidden, L. M. (1991). Adopted children with developmental disabilities: postplacement family functioning. *Children and Youth Services Review*, **13**, 363–377.

Greenfield, J. (1986). *A client called Noah: a family journey continued.* San Diego: Harcourt Brace Jovanovich.

Grimes, S. K. & Vitello, S. J. (1990). Follow-up study of family attitudes toward deinstitutionalization: three to seven years later. *Mental Retardation*, **28**, 219–225.

Hewett, S. (1970). *The family and the handicapped child.* London: Allen & Unwin.

Hill, B. K., Rotegard, L. L. & Bruininks, R. H. (1984). The quality of life of mentally retarded people in residential care. *Social Work*, **29**, 275–280.

Jensen, J. M. & Whittaker, J. K. (1987). Parental involvement in children's residential treatment: from preplacement to aftercare. *Children and Youth Services Review*, **9**, 81–100.

Kilpatrick, D. G., Veronen, L. J. & Best, C. L. (1985). Factors predicting psychological distress among rape victims. In C. R. Figley (Ed.), *Trauma and its wake: the study of treatment of post-traumatic stress disorder* (pp. 113–141). New York: Brunner/Mazel.

Koss, M. P. & Burkhart, B. R. (1989). A conceptual analysis of rape victimization: long-term effects and implications for treatment. *Psychology of Women Quarterly*, **13**, 27–40.

Meyers, C. E. & Blacher, J. (1987). Parents' perception of schooling for severely handicapped children: Home and family variables. *Exceptional Children*, **53**, 441–449.

Olshansky, S. (1962). Chronic sorrow: a response to having a mentally defective child. *Social Casework*, **43**, 191–194.

Parkes, C. M. & Weiss, R. S. (1983). *Recovery from bereavement.* New York: Basic Books.

Schalock, R. L. & Lilley, M. A. (1986). Placement from community-based mental retardation programs: how well do clients do after 8 to 10 years? *American Journal of Mental Deficiency*, **90**, 669–676.

Stoneman, Z. & Crapps, J. M. (1990). Mentally retarded individuals in family care homes: relationships with the family-of-origin. *American Journal on Mental Retardation*, **94**, 420–430.

Taylor, S. J., Lakin, K. C. & Hill, B. K. (1989). Permanency planning for children and youth: out-of-home placement decisions. *Exceptional Children*, **55**, 541–549.

Turnbull, H. R., Turnbull, A. P., Bronicki, G. J., Summers, J. A. & Roeder-Gordon, C. (1989). *Disability and the family: a guide to decisions for adulthood.* Baltimore: Brookes.

Wallerstein, J. S. (1983). Children of divorce: the psychological tasks of the child. *American Journal of Orthopsychiatry*, **53**, 230–243.

Wallerstein, J. S. & Kelly, J. B. (1980). *Surviving the breakup: how children and parents cope with divorce.* New York: Basic Books.

Willer, B., Intagliata, J. & Wicks, N. (1981). Return of retarded adults to natural families: issues and results. In R. H. Bruininks, C. E. Meyers, B. B. Sigford & K. C. Lakin (Eds), *Deinstitutionalization and community adjustment of mentally retarded people* (Monograph No. 4, pp. 207–216). Washington, DC: American Association on Mental Deficiency.

15

Modifying Quiet Room Design Enhances Calming of Children and Adolescents

Carol A. Glod and Martin H. Teicher
McLean Hospital, Belmont, Massachusetts;
and Harvard Medical School, Boston

Martha Butler
St. Elizabeth's Hospital, Brighton, Massachusetts

Margaret Savino, David Harper, and Eleanor Magnus
McLean Hospital

Kambiz Pahlavan
Charter Hospital, Milwaukee

Objective: *To determine whether altering design of a quiet room (QR) produced more rapid calming of agitated or aggressive hospitalized children.* **Method:** *One of five similar QRs was modified by painting the white walls tea rose, carpeting the vinyl floor, and painting a picturesque mural on one wall. The effects of these modifications were assessed in 19 patients (mean age 9.6 years), using a within-subjects, repeated-measures design. Overt Aggression ratings were made at the time of placement, and at 5-minute intervals thereafter, until the child*

Reprinted with permission from the *Journal of the American Academy of Child and Adolescent Psychiatry*, 1994, Vol. 33(4), 558–566. Copyright © 1994 by the American Academy of Child and Adolescent Psychiatry.

From the Hall-Mercer Snider Developmental Biopsychiatry Research Program, McLean Hospital, Belmont, MA (Ms. Glod, Dr. Teicher, Mr. Harper, and Ms. Magnus), Department of Psychiatry, Harvard Medical School, Boston, MA (Ms. Glod and Dr. Teicher), St. Elizabeth's Hospital, Brighton, MA (Ms. Butler), Hall-Mercer Center for Children and Adolescents, McLean Hospital (Ms. Savino), and Charter Hospital, Milwaukee, WI (Dr. Pahlavan). Ms. Glod was a Ph.D. candidate at the time this study was done.

This study was supported in part by awards from the Snider family, the Hall-Mercer Foundation, and NIMH grants MH-43743 (M.H.T.) and MH-36224. We thank Jan Wise, RN., for designing and painting the mural.

Presented at the American Psychiatric Association Annual Meeting, May 4, 1992.

was dismissed. Children were blind to the fact that a study was being conducted; raters and staff were not. **Results:** *Total aggression ratings were 45% lower in the modified QR than in the standard QR (p < .03), and initial aggression scores fell by 50% during 5 minutes of placement in the modified QR, but only after 20 minutes of placement in the standard QR (p < .0001). Motor excitement and verbal aggression were the two component factors most strongly influenced by QR design.* **Conclusion:** *This preliminary report suggests that it may be possible to modify QRs to facilitate calming of aggressive, agitated children and provides preliminary support for redesign of QRs.*

Quiet rooms are a ubiquitous component of most inpatient psychiatric units and are a valuable tool in the management of agitation and assaultive behavior. Psychiatric staff are confronted daily with the need to use a variety of management techniques, including quiet room placement, to prevent further escalation of dangerous behavior and to maintain the safety of the patient and hospital environment. As the severity and acuity of the child inpatient population increases, quiet rooms become an important management tool that can potentially reduce the need for more controversial measures such as seclusion or restraint. Although quiet rooms are an important and frequently used inpatient intervention, a computerized literature search failed to reveal any published studies that scientifically evaluated the effects of quiet room design on therapeutic efficacy in either adults or children. Cotton and Geraty (1984), however, published design recommendations for a therapeutic milieu for children which include specific design criteria for quiet rooms. Their suggestions were based on the theoretical premise that conventional hospital architecture and interior design frequently conveyed a negative antitherapeutic message and that it should be possible to redesign aspects of the milieu to exert a more therapeutic effect, while still following formal design codes. In regard to the quiet room, they specifically proposed that warm color tones should be used to allow for a change in mood, that carpeting should be used instead of tile, and that children should be able to observe a pleasant scene. Overall they suggested, without experimental validation, that quiet rooms should be attractive, nonpunitive, and cozy (Cotton and Geraty, 1984). In contrast, quiet rooms at our facility were designed years earlier in a more conventional manner, with blank white walls without windows, grey-speckled vinyl floors, and only a thin mattress for comfort. The goal of this study was to empirically ascertain whether modifying quiet room design, along the lines suggested by Cotton and Geraty (1984), would enhance therapeutic efficacy.

Myriad reports exist on interventions available to control aggressive, disruptive, or self-injurious behavior of children. Much of the literature centers on the controversy surrounding the use of seclusion or restraint versus less restrictive measures (Cotton, 1989; Irwin, 1987). Several studies have noted the positive effects of seclusion on adult psychiatric patients (Mattison and Sacks, 1978; Soloff and Turner, 1981). Although different philosophies exist regarding the use of these techniques, most have been used with children and adolescents. Several studies have explored the frequency of different interventions, including seclusion, restraint, chemical restraint, quiet room use, and holding techniques in children and adolescents. Seclusion generally refers to locked-door seclusion, where the patient is involuntarily locked in a room until his or her behavior comes under control. Conversely, quiet rooms are not locked, and at our institution they are without doors. Garrison (1984) found that seclusion or restraint was used in 33% to 35% of all patients, with younger boys most likely to require seclusion and restraint. Other patient groups may also be at high risk for restraint or seclusion, e.g., adolescents diagnosed with borderline personality disorder, psychotic disorders, conduct disorder, or attention-deficit hyperactivity disorder (Erickson and Realmuto, 1983). Millstein and Cotton (1990) reported that children who frequently were placed in seclusion had a strong history of physical abuse, neurological impairment, poor verbal ability, assaultive behavior, and a suicide attempt in the 6 months before admission. Joshi and colleagues (1988) investigated the characteristics associated with quiet room use by prepubertal children. In their sample, the frequency and duration of quiet room use decreased significantly over time, with children most often using this intervention on a voluntary basis.

The American Psychiatric Association Task Force Report on Seclusion and Restraint (American Psychiatric Association, 1985) specified that the indications and procedures for seclusion of children be similar to those used for adults; however, little systematic study has been performed. With initiative from political leaders, many states have attempted to limit the use of seclusion for young children, and retrospective studies have examined the effect of these laws. Antoinette and colleagues (1990) found that after legislation prohibited the use of locked seclusion, use of tranquilizing medications in hospitalized children increased significantly. They concluded that locked seclusion may be a necessary therapeutic intervention and should be considered as an alternative intervention. In a similar study in children and adolescents, Swett et al. (1989) failed to find an increased use of *chemical* restraint, but instead reported a significant increase in the overall number of patients, episodes and hours spent in *mechanical* restraint. Thus, while attempts have been made to limit the use of seclusion, to promote more humane treatment, the outcome may be to increase the use of chemical or mechanical restraints, which pose problems and risks of their own.

To date, the majority of published studies have endeavored to delineate the indications, risk factors, or alternatives to the use of quiet rooms, seclusion rooms, and restraints, or have studied the impact of legislation preventing the use of locked seclusion. While it is difficult to draw firm conclusions from these reports, it appears that many respected authorities in child psychiatry believe that these interventions are, at times, useful and necessary, and it is likely that some combination of quiet rooms, seclusion rooms, or restraints will remain an integral, yet controversial, intervention on many psychiatric units. This is particularly true as managed health care strives to ensure that only the most seriously disturbed and hard-to-manage children receive inpatient treatment.

Although opinions in the field are divided regarding the justification or need for restraints or seclusion with children or adolescents, it appears that there is reasonable consensus that less restrictive interventions are often necessary to help agitated or aggressive children calm down quickly, while minimizing the need for chemical or mechanical restraints. In many facilities quiet rooms are used as one intervention to help children calm down and regain control. As Cotton and Geraty (1984) have stated, quiet rooms are often crucial to an institution's overall commitment to treat extremely disturbed children while striving to avoid the use of mechanical restraints or overreliance on psychotropic medications for relief of temporary behavioral crises. It is likely that quiet rooms work, in part, by reducing some forms of stimulation while providing alternative sensory cues. Parameters such as color, texture, and overall visual gestalt should therefore influence the effectiveness of the quiet room. Ulrich (1984) had previously observed, in a retrospective chart review, that merely being able to view a pleasant natural scene from a hospital window (versus a brick wall) significantly reduced the need for analgesic medications, and diminished length of stay, in patients recovering from cholecystectomies. Thus, a preliminary study was conducted to ascertain whether altering quiet room design, along the lines proposed by Cotton and Geraty (1984), influenced the behavior of children and adolescents. This was viewed as the first step in the progressive redesign of the quiet room, to help make it into a safe, nonpunitive environment that would facilitate rapid recovery of agitated or aggressive children and would minimize the need for chemical or mechanical restraints.

METHOD

Quiet Room Design

A committee consisting of the Director of Inpatient Psychiatry, Clinical Nursing Supervisor, a staff nurse, a research psychiatrist and research nurse met to review design alterations that could be made within hospital regulations. A decision was made to modify one of five similar quiet rooms. The walls were painted pastel pink (tea rose), with a picturesque mural (6 feet × 6 feet) of playful dolphins, fish, and crabs, which gave an illusion of movement. The mural was painted on one wall, and the room was carpeted with short-pile, tightly woven, dark-plum synthetic material. The four standard quiet rooms had white walls and grey-speckled vinyl tiles. No quiet room had windows or doors, and each had a nearly opaque skylight. The standard quiet rooms were 10 feet × 12 feet, and the modified one was 10 feet × 10 feet. We then sought to determine whether the newly designed quiet room differentially affected the behavior of child and adolescent inpatients.

Quiet Room Assignment

In the therapeutic milieu of our institution, quiet rooms are one of many interventions in an overall behavioral treatment program. Children are engaged in a point system based on positive reward to reinforce acceptable and appropriate behavior. When children and adolescents become increasingly agitated, a series of interventions (staff talks, time out, chair time, etc.) are first used to help the child regain control. If these less restrictive interventions fail, holding techniques or quiet room placement may be necessary. The quiet room is used to remove the child from others and to reduce stimulation in order to help promote control, rather than as punitive treatment. Quiet room placement was determined by the clinical staff based on availability of rooms, placement of other children in adjacent rooms, and ease of view of the patient. All five rooms (the modified and four standard rooms) are situated in close proximity. As each room has no doors, locked-door seclusion is never an alternative (doors were removed after legislation restricted the use of seclusion with children). The most restrictive measures used are chemical and/or mechanical restraint, as the last steps to help protect the child and others and to prevent or diminish dangerous behavior. At least one nursing staff member continuously monitors all children placed into quiet rooms. If mechanical restraints are used, a staff person is assigned to observe that child continuously during the entire time restraints are used (one-to-one observation). Thus, for the purposes of this study, our raters sat with the staff person who was assigned quiet room observation. Children were removed from the quiet rooms once their behavior calmed, based on clinical assessment by the nursing staff.

Experimental Design

During two 6-week periods (approximately 1 year apart), on Monday through Friday between 3 and 7 P.M., we rated all children assigned to quiet rooms for clinical reasons by nursing staff. During this period 40 children were placed in quiet rooms, and 214 sessions were rated. We selected for analysis all children who had been placed at least once in both the modified quiet room and a standard quiet room for threatening or assaultive behavior or for failure to respond to less restrictive interventions. Patients who voluntarily requested quiet room placement in order to spend time alone, and those using the quiet room as a "time out," were excluded. A within-subject design was used so that each patient served as his or her own control.

Patients were evaluated by one of four raters using a time-sample approach, with ratings made at the time of quiet room placement and at 5-minute intervals thereafter, until the child was removed from the quiet room. The assessment instrument was the Overt Aggression Scale of Yudofsky et al. (1986), with slight modification to be more apropos to children and adolescents in quiet rooms. Five variables were derived from this scale: verbal aggression, physical aggression toward self, physical aggression toward others, motor excitement, and disorganization. Each variable was rated on a 0 (absence of behavior) to 4 (extreme) scale, with the exception of physical aggression toward others (rated 0 to 3). Additional interventions (p.r.n. medications, restraint), used at the discretion of the clinical staff, were recorded. A total aggression score was calculated as the sum of the ratings on the five variables, plus the score for additional interventions (holding = 1, p.r.n. medication = 2, restraint = 3). Interrater reliability for the total instrument was based on the average Pearson correlation between the six cross-comparisons of four different raters ($r = .89$, range .81 to .93).

The Institutional Review Board of our facility concluded that informed consent was not required, because the study was purely observational. Hence, patients were unaware that a study was being conducted. The final subject pool consisted of 19 inpatients: 14 males and 5 females, mean age 9.6 $\pm$ 3 years (range 4 to 15), representing a wide range of diagnoses. These subjects had been placed in the modified quiet room 30 times and in the standard quiet room 46 times. When patients had more than one placement in either the modified or standard quiet room, results were averaged to derive mean values for each subject in each type of quiet room.

Statistical Analyses

Data were analyzed using a repeated-measures analysis of variance (Systat), with quiet room placement and time as the two factors. As length of time in the quiet room varied widely between subjects and placements, the first six periods were used for analysis, as almost all subjects spent at least 25 minutes in the quiet room. In those rare instances when a child was released from the quiet room before the sixth period, his or her final ratings were carried through to the end of the analysis period.

RESULTS

Assignment Bias

The data were first analyzed to determine whether there was any degree of initial bias in the placement of children in the modified quiet room (e.g., were children excluded from the modified quiet room during their most severe episodes?). There were no significant differences in the initial ratings of total aggression as a function of quiet room placement (F [1,18] = 1.67, p = .213), nor were there any effects of initial quiet room placement on any aggression factor (motor excitement F [1,18] = 1.71, p = .208; verbal aggression F [1,18] = .60, p = .81; aggression toward others F [1,18] = 1.99, p = .175; aggression toward self F [1,18] = .783, p = .388; disorganization F [1,18] = .298, p = .592). Hence, it appeared that there was no significant bias in the severity of symptoms of these children when they were placed in the modified quiet room versus a standard quiet room.

Overall Aggression Levels

The data were then analyzed to determine whether there were any differences in aggression scores during the 25-minute assessment period as a function of quiet room placement. Total aggression scores were 45% lower in the modified quiet room than in the standard quiet room (F [1,18] = 6.09, p < .03). The component aggression factors were analyzed to identify which specific aggression factors may have been influenced by quiet room placement (Figure 1). Motor activity was 37% lower in the modified quiet

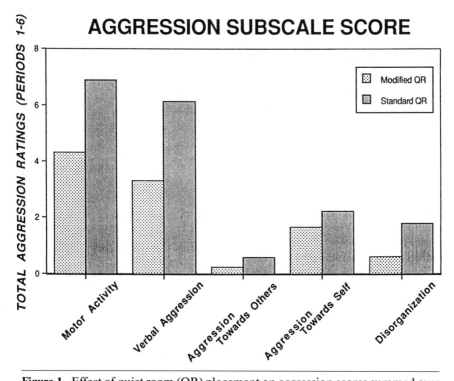

Figure 1. Effect of quiet room (QR) placement on aggression scores summed over the first six periods (25 minutes) of quiet room placement. Motor excitement, disorganization, and physical aggression toward self were rated on a scale of 0 (absence of behavior) to 4 (extreme). Physical aggression toward others was rated on a scale of 0 to 3 (extreme).

room than in the standard quiet room (F [1,18] = 8.49, $p < .01$), and verbal aggression was 46% lower (F [1,18] = 9.36, $p < .007$). A trend emerged for a 60% reduction in scores of physical aggression against others in the modified quiet room (F [1,18] = 3.78, $p < .07$). Quiet room design did not exert a statistically significant differential effect on either physical aggression toward self or disorganization. Aggression toward self scores were 26% lower in the modified quiet room (F [1,18] = 0.41, not significant [NS]). Disorganization factor scores were 66% lower in the modified quiet room than in the standard quiet room; however, this difference (due largely to one patient) failed to reach significance (F (1,18] = 0.82, NS).

Replication

The study was conducted in two phases separated by a year. This was done to minimize the possible effects of a novel change (Hawthorne Effect) on either patients or raters. The data were thus analyzed to determine whether the effects of quiet room placement on total aggression scores were the same after replication a year later. Ten children were studied during the first phase of the study, and nine subjects were studied, a year later, during the second phase. Total severity scores were 54% lower in the modified quiet room than in the standard quiet room during the first phase of the study and were 38% lower in the modified quiet room than in the standard quiet room during the second phase. Analysis of variance indicated that there were no significant differences in overall severity levels between the two phases (F [1,17] = 2.30, p = .15) and, more importantly, that quiet room modification had the same effect on severity during both phases of the study (F [1, 17] = 0.0018, p = .97, quiet room × phase interaction). Hence, it appeared that the influence of quiet room modification on total aggression scores was not a short-term artifact of novelty.

Time Course of Effect

Data were analyzed at each rating period to ascertain when significant differences emerged between quiet rooms on measures of total severity, and for the aggression factor scores in which there were significant effects of quiet room placement. Differences emerged in total aggression scores between the modified and standard quiet rooms after 5 minutes of placement (period 2; p < .04) and were most significant after 10 minutes of placement (p < .001; Figure 2). Motor excitement scores differed significantly between quiet rooms after 5 to 10 minutes of placement and were again significantly different after 20 minutes (Figure 3). Verbal aggression scores in the two types of quiet rooms were significantly different during the first 10 to 20 minutes of placement (Figure 3). Thus, the modified quiet room appeared to exert a greater calming effect than did the standard quiet room during the first 5 to 20 minutes of exposure, with maximal differences emerging approximately 10 minutes after placement.

Rate of Improvement

To ascertain whether the modified and standard quiet rooms differed in the rate of improvement of aggressive symptoms, the data were analyzed to determine the *half-time* of improvement, defined as the time from entrance

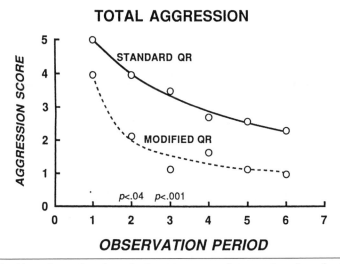

Figure 2. Alterations of total aggression scores over time as a function of quiet room (QR) placement. Ratings began immediately after quiet room placement and occurred at 5-minute intervals thereafter. Significant differences between quiet rooms occurred after 10 and 15 minutes of placement. Time course regression lines were determined by nonlinear fit to a two-parameter (slope, half-time) logistic decay equation.

into the quiet room until the initial aggression score was reduced by 50%. Half-time was calculated from the mean group data obtained at 5-minute intervals, using iterative nonlinear regression to a logistic decay equation (DeLean et al., 1978). The best-fitting regression functions are illustrated in Figures 2 and 3. Analysis of variance F values were calculated to ascertain whether half-time measures differed between quiet room placements. This statistical measure was calculated using simultaneous constrained curve fitting, with the F ratio derived from the degradation in goodness-of-fit when the two curves were forced to share the same half-time (DeLean et al., 1978).

Dramatic and significant differences in half-time between the modified and standard quiet rooms were evident in total aggression and in three of the component factors: motor excitement, verbal aggression, and disorganization (Table 1). Total aggression scores fell by 50% after only 5.1 ± 1.9 minutes in the modified quiet room versus 20.4 ± 1.1 minutes in the standard quiet room (F [1,9] = 52.47 p < .00001; Figure 2). Similarly, motor

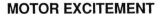

MOTOR EXCITEMENT

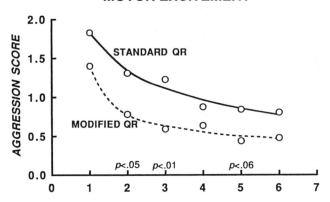

VERBAL AGGRESSION

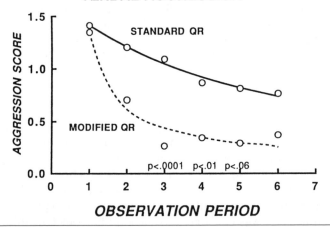

OBSERVATION PERIOD

Figure 3. Alterations of motor excitement and verbal aggression scores over time as a function of quiet room (QR) placement. Ratings began immediately after quiet room placement and occurred at 5-minute intervals thereafter. Motor scores differed significantly between quiet rooms after 5 and 10 minutes of placement and again after 20 minutes. Significant differences in verbal aggression scores were evident during the first 10, 15, and 20 minutes of placement.

TABLE 1
Rate of Improvement in Aggressive Symptoms in Modified Versus Standard Quiet Rooms

Measures	Modified QR		Standard QR		Significance	
	Half-Time[a]	r[b]	Half-Time[a]	r[b]	F Value[c] (df 1,9)	p
Total aggression	5.1 ± 1.9	.976	20.4 ± 1.1	.995	52.47	<.00001
Motor excitement	7.2 ± 1.3	.990	17.2 ± 1.8	.985	23.77	<.001
Verbal aggression	4.1 ± 1.9	.964	27.2 ± 2.2	.99	88.78	<.00001
Disorganization	6.2 ± 1.7	.953	34.2 ± 10.1	.922	28.34	<.001
Aggression toward self	7.1 ± 11.4	.795	4.2 ± 3.9	.976	0.06	NS
Aggression toward others	3.8 ± 0.05	.999	3.3 ± 0.4	.999	0.1	NS

Note: QR = quiet room; NS = not significant.
[a] Half-time is measured (in minutes) for the entire group, as the time from entrance into the QR until initial ratings was reduced by 50%. Half-time is calculated from mean data at 5-minute intervals, using iterative nonlinear regression to a logistic decay equation.
[b] *r* refers to the degree of correlation between the actual mean group measures and the estimated measures based on the fitted logistic decay equation.
[c] *F* values were calculated based on simultaneous constrained curve fitting, with the *F* ratio based on degradation in goodness-of-fit when the two curves were forced to share the same half-time.

excitement, verbal aggression, and disorganization were reduced by half approximately 15 minutes sooner in the modified quiet room than in the standard quiet room (Table 1; Figure 3). In contrast, aggression toward self scores and aggression toward others scores rapidly abated in both the modified and standard quiet rooms, and there were no statistically significant differences in response times between these conditions (Table 1).

PRN Medications and Restraints

The greater calming effect of placement into the modified quiet room was also reflected in the behavior of the clinical staff. In the standard quiet room, 10 of the 19 patients required p.r.n. medications after quiet room placement, whereas in the modified quiet room only 4 required p.r.n. medications ($\chi^2 = 4.07$, $p < .05$). This finding, however, was complicated by the fact that patients had more sessions in the standard quiet room. Thus, the likelihood of receiving a p.r.n. medication was calculated for each patient. Overall, patients had a 16% likelihood of receiving p.r.n. medication during each placement in the modified quiet room and a 38% likelihood of receiving p.r.n. medication in the standard quiet room (Sign-Rank Test: $p = .065$, two-tailed). Patients also seemed to require less time in the modified quiet room (36 versus 46 minutes); however, this difference failed to reach statistical significance ($p > .20$). Use of restraint did not differ with quiet room placement. Only two children required restraint in the modified quiet room, and three children in the standard quiet room.

DISCUSSION

This is the first study of its kind to investigate the effects of modifying quiet room design on the behavior of children and adolescents. A repeated-measures, within-subjects design was used to determine whether differential effects could be observed between standard and modified quiet rooms. Simple modifications of an existing quiet room, along the guidelines suggested by Cotton and Geraty (1984), appeared to enhance calming and diminish aggression. Effects of quiet room placement occurred rapidly and were most marked during the first 5 to 10 minutes. The most significant effects of quiet room placement occurred on measures of motor excitement and verbal aggression. Measures of total aggression, motor excitement, verbal aggression, and disorganization declined much more rapidly in the modified quiet room than in the standard quiet room. There was also approximately a 50% reduction in the need for p.r.n. medications in the modified quiet room. Thus, it appeared that the modified quiet room was associated with more rapid reduction in aggression scores in this child psychiatric sample.

These findings should, however, be interpreted cautiously as a number of limitations exist in this study. First, a single-blind design was used. Raters were seated, and behaved, in such a manner as to appear to be part of the staff observing children in the quiet rooms, and the children appeared to be unaware that an investigation was under way. Nursing staff and raters, however, were aware of the purpose of this study, and ratings and interventions may have been biased by their preconceptions. To minimize the effect of novel change (Hawthorne effect), we collected half of the data 1 year after the quiet room was redesigned. After this period of time, the novelty of the modified quiet room and any initial belief about its properties should have dissipated. Even after a full year of use, the modified quiet room still had the same differential effect on aggression as it did initially, suggesting that this modification had an enduring effect and was not merely a novelty.

Second, this study was limited by use of a nonrandom assignment to quiet rooms, and there may have been a bias to place less agitated children in the modified quiet room. This did not appear to be the case in the subjects we studied, as there were no significant differences in aggression scores between quiet rooms during the first rating period. Moreover, the most robust statistical difference observed between quiet rooms was apparent in the half-life analyses, and this measure was corrected for initial differences in severity. It is possible that certain children were never placed in the modified quiet room during the course of the study, either because they were too out of control or were too likely to defecate or urinate on the carpet. As we only studied children who had been placed in both the standard and modified quiet rooms, any child routinely excluded from the modified quiet room would have been eliminated from this study. We also evaluated the ratings from 20 subjects who during the course of the study were rated only in a standard quiet room. Overall, their initial rating of total aggression in the standard quiet room was nonsignificantly lower than the standard quiet room ratings of the group studied in both quiet rooms (4.03 ± 2.95 versus 4.99 ± 2.55). Only one subject who was evaluated in only the standard quiet room had an initial total aggression score greater than two standard deviations from the mean of the children studied in both quiet rooms. Hence it does not appear that a significant number of children were excluded from study in the modified quiet room because of unusually aggressive behavior.

Third, while children were placed into the quiet room, a number of prior or concomitant variables may have influenced the outcome, and these factors were not controlled. Decisions to use the quiet room were made clinically, without any a priori protocol, although the philosophy and practice of the milieu required use of the least restrictive measures as a first intervention. Children in this sample received a wide array of interventions before, and during, quiet room placement. Use of p.r.n. medications, holding techniques, and chemical or mechanical restraint were all at the discretion of the staff. Control of intervening variables, such as escalation of behavior by other children in surrounding rooms or the type of interactions with staff members during placement, could have differentially affected outcome. The fact that p.r.n. medications were administered during twice as many sessions in the standard quiet room is of concern, as greater use of medication may have caused the standard quiet room to appear more effective than it actually was.

Duration of time spent in the quiet room was determined in part by the child's behavior, the therapeutic philosophy and bias of individual members of the nursing staff, and the demands and level of acuity on the inpatient units. Although each patient's need for quiet room placement was continuously reassessed by clinical staff, there appeared to be a great deal of variability and capriciousness in the duration of placement. Thus, our major outcome measures were based on the repeated objective assessment of levels of motoric excitement, disorganization, and verbal and physical aggression, rather than duration of quiet room placement.

Finally, another limitation of this study was the lack of baseline determination of the equivalence of the quiet rooms before modification. Initial studies were not conducted to demonstrate that the "modified quiet room" was equivalent to the standard quiet rooms before it was modified. Hence, some other factor, such as the location, geometry, or size of the selected room, may have also contributed to its differential efficacy.

In this first empirical study of quiet room design, it appears that the design of the quiet room may have influenced its therapeutic efficacy, and it seemed feasible to objectively evaluate the effects of design modifications. Rater-based assessment of verbal aggression, motor excitement, and total aggression showed statistically significant differences between placement in a standard or modified quiet room. Initial levels of motor excitement, verbal aggression, and disorganization abated more quickly in the modified quiet room. Additional studies are necessary to determine whether these effects persist under more rigorous experimental conditions, with random assignment to quiet rooms, with baseline determination of equivalence and with ratings conducted by observers blind to purpose of the study. Although we focused on a few simple modifications, based on the work of Cotton and Geraty (1984), to make the quiet room more "pleasing" and comfortable, many other modifications could be considered, including the use of music or the presence of soft, safe objects. Additional studies are necessary to ascertain how quiet room design may affect children with different diagnoses and to evaluate how it affects children at different stages of development.

Quiet rooms exist for the purpose of providing a safe place for children to calm down and to regain control over their aggressive behavior or feelings. As such, the quiet room represents one tool in our armamentarium of instruments. The purpose of this study was largely to demonstrate that calming effects of the quiet room can be measured and to suggest that we should not assume that quiet rooms have been designed for optimal efficacy or that design factors such as color, texture, and visual interest are irrelevant to children. Empirical efforts to optimize quiet room design may prove even more effective in future studies, and it is conceivable that attention to this factor will improve clinical care by providing a nonpunitive intervention that may reduce the need for p.r.n. medications, mechanical restraints, or locked seclusion.

Clinical Implications

This preliminary report suggests that altering quiet room design may have beneficial effects on the agitated and aggressive behavior of children and adolescents. This challenges an institutional tradition that quiet rooms should have bare white walls, with little color or comfort. Redesign of a quiet room along theoretical guidelines to use warmer tones, visual interest (e.g., a mural), and more comfortable floor material appeared to enhance therapeutic efficacy. In this preliminary study, it appeared that motoric excitement, verbal aggression, and disorganization were much more rapidly brought under control with these modifications. These results provide preliminary support for recommendations for redesign of the quiet rooms as suggested by Cotton and Geraty (1984). Their recommendations were based on an overall therapeutic philosophy that the inpatient milieu should be cheerful, comfortable, and adaptive. To this end, striking color schemes were recommended, as opposed to traditional institutional colors, along with a variety of noninstitutional textures (Cotton and Geraty, 1984). Thus, environmental modification may serve as an alternative strategy to diminish agitated or aggressive behavior. Further research is necessary to test more carefully the hypothesis that these design modifications can promote more rapid calming or reduce the need for p.r.n. medications. The potential of hospital design factors to influence behavior should not be surprising. Previous research has shown that merely being able to view a natural scene, versus a brick wall, through a hospital window, reduced the need for p.r.n. analgesics, diminished the number of negative evaluative comments by nursing staff, and decreased length of stay of patients recovering from cholecystectomies (Ulrich, 1984). With careful objective research, it may be possible, over time, to identify specific environmental factors that can significantly augment the therapeutic efficacy of the hospital environment for child psychiatry patients. Appropriate use of these design modifications may decrease the need for more restrictive and dangerous interventions, decrease the need for tranquilizing medications, and effectively reduce duration of hospitalization.

REFERENCES

American Psychiatric Association (1985), *Task Force Report 22. Seclusion and Restraint: The Psychiatric Uses*. Washington, DC: American Psychiatric Association

Antoinette T, Iyengar S, Puig-Antich J (1990), Is locked seclusion necessary for children under the age of 14? *Am J Psychiatry* 147:1283–1289

Cotton NS (1989), The developmental-clinical rationale for the use of seclusion in the psychiatric treatment of children. *Am J Orthopsychiatry* 59:442–450

Cotton NS, Geraty RG (1984), Therapeutic space design: planning an inpatient children's unit. *Am J Orthopsychiatry* 54:624–636

DeLean AP, Munson PJ, Rodbard D (1978), Simultaneous analysis of families of sigmoidal curves: application to bioassay, radioligand, and physiological dose-response curves. *Am J Physiol* 235:E97–E102

Erikson WD, Realmuto G (1983), Frequency of seclusion in an adolescent psychiatric unit. *J Clin Psychiatry* 44:238–241

Garrison WT (1984), Aggressive behavior, seclusion and physical restraint in an inpatient child population. *J Am Acad Child Psychiatry* 23:448–452

Irwin M (1987), Are seclusion rooms needed on child psychiatric units? *Am J Orthopsychiatry* 57:125–126

Joshi PT, Capozzoli JA, Coyle JT (1988), Use of a quiet room on an inpatient unit. *J Am Acad Child Adolesc Psychiatry* 27:643–644

Mattison MR, Sacks MH (1978), Seclusion: uses and complications. *Am J Psychiatry* 135:1210–1213

Millstein KH, Cotton NS (1990), Predictors of the use of seclusion on an inpatient child psychiatric unit. *J Am Acad Child Adolesc Psychiatry* 29:254–256

Soloff PH, Turner SM (1981), Patterns of seclusion: a prospective study. *J Nerv Ment Dis* 169:37–44

Swett C Jr, Michaels AS, Cole JO (1989), Effects of a state law on rates of restraint on a child and adolescent unit. *Bull Am Acad Psychiatry Law* 17:165–169

Ulrich RS (1984), View through a window may influence recovery from surgery. *Science* 224:420–421

Yudofsky SC, Silver JM, Jackson W, Endicott J, Williams D (1986), The overt aggression scale for the objective rating of verbal and physical aggression. *Am J Psychiatry* 143:35–39

Part V

CLINIC AND SCHOOL-BASED INTERVENTIONS

The papers in Part V address a range of interventions for children who present with behavioral, emotional, and developmental difficulties. The initial paper (Chapter 16), by Fonagay and Target, describes a chart review of 763 cases of child psychoanalysis and psychotherapy at the Anna Freud Centre. In this report, the first of a series exploiting this data base, the authors examine predictors of treatment outcome in children with disruptive behavior disorders. Despite the frequency with which children and adolescents are engaged in insight-oriented treatments, studies of the effectiveness of this approach are almost nonexistent. The records of the Anna Freud Centre over the past 40 years are a unique source of information about children in the course of analysis and psychotherapy.

The following categories of information were reliably extracted from the clinical records: (1) demographic measures including biographical and social information on the child and his/her family (e.g., cultural background, socioeconomic status, current size, and structure); (2) diagnostic information including DSM-III-R Axis I and II diagnoses, made separately for the past, the time of referral, and termination; (3) presenting symptomatology recorded retrospectively using the Child Behavior Checklist; (4) level of functioning rated at the beginning and at the end of treatment on the Children's Global Assessment Scale; (5) clinical information, including losses and separations, medical history and hospitalizations, behavior and performance in school, and psychiatric histories, treatment, and current functioning of parents; as well as (6) information about treatment; (referral, session frequency, length of treatment, change of therapist, reason for termination, and the gender and years of experience of the therapist were recorded on a standardized form with operational definitions).

For this paper, 135 children were identified for whom the primary diagnosis was disruptive behavior disorder, including 58% with oppositional defiant disorder, 8% with attention-deficit hyperactivity disorder, 23% with conduct disorder, and 10% with a V code of antisocial behavior. Sixty-seven percent were offered and accepted intensive psychoanalytic treatment (four or five times weekly); the remainder were seen one or two times per week. These children were individually matched with 135 children treated for emotional disorders, including anxiety, depressive and obsessive disorders at the clinic during the same period. Treatment outcomes for the two groups were assessed using ratings of maladjustment, changes in adaptive levels, and presence of diagnosis.

As the authors point out, there are no measures available for assessing the structural changes purported to occur during psychoanalytic treatment. Rates of improvement were significantly higher for the group with emotional disorders than for the disruptive group. In addition, the percentage of children with disruptive behavior disorders who returned to a level of functioning within the normal range falls short of recent reports of the rates of improvement for conduct-disordered children who receive a combination of parent-management training and problem-solving–skills training.

Nevertheless, within the disruptive group it was possible to identify predictors of good outcome. Significant improvement was more frequent among those children with comorbid anxiety disorders who were without significant learning difficulties, whose mothers were not in concurrent treatment, and who themselves remained in intensive treatment for more than one year. Children younger than 9 years appeared to be especially likely to benefit from intensive treatment. For older children, four or five times weekly treatment did not significantly improve outcome. Even for this group, however, intensive treatment significantly reduced the likelihood of early termination. This pattern of findings is interpreted by the authors as suggesting that the efficacy of nonintensive psychodynamic treatment of disruptive behavior disorders might be maximized if treatment were initially offered relatively intensively and reduced when the likelihood of premature termination had passed.

A thoughtful discussion highlights both the strengths and limitations of the data base in identifying groups of children for whom dynamically oriented therapy may be most effective. The value of a rigorously operationalized, clinically based data set in addressing questions of the effectiveness of treatment interventions is well demonstrated, and provides a model for future investigations of therapeutic efficacy.

As increasing attention is paid to health care costs, the need to demonstrate the efficacy of psychotherapeutic techniques, particularly short-term techniques, is increasingly important. The next paper (Chapter 17) is particularly timely, providing both a model for conducting a treatment-outcome study and data supporting a specific treatment. Kendall uses a randomized clinical trial to study the effects of intervention on children diagnosed with anxiety disorders. Although behavioral treatments are known to be effective with specific fears or phobias, little is known about treatment of generalized anxiety disorders (e.g., separation anxiety) in children. Kendall used a wait-list control condition to assess the effects of a cognitive-behavioral treatment compared to no treatment.

Children were assessed by multiple reporters at baseline, at the treatment conclusion, and at one-year follow-up. The author describes a 16-

session treatment that combines behavioral techniques, such as exposure, relaxation, and role play, with cognitive retraining, such as identification and modification of anxious self-talk.

The study demonstrated effectiveness of the intervention. Both child self-report (anxiety and depression measures) and parent data (symptomatology checklist) provided clinically and statistically significant effects. Although treatment studies of externalizing problems have found teacher data informative, in this study teachers did not appear to be good observers of internalizing behaviors. The child-therapist relationship may have accounted for the differences between the treatment and control groups. Children who rated the relationship more highly indicated more improvement on the self-report scales. However, parental change scores were independent of the child's rating of the therapist. Thus, Kendall concludes that treatment gains can be obtained independent of therapist-specific variables. Treatment gains were maintained at one-year follow-up.

This study provides support for using a manualized cognitive-behavioral treatment for anxious preadolescents (8- to 13-year-olds). Further studies are needed to replicate the results and to determine the extent to which a related parent training would be efficacious—some evidence is cited—and to which younger children might be able to utilize some of the cognitive-behavioral principles.

The third paper (Chapter 18) in Part V is a comprehensive review of the efficacy of lithium in the treatment of child and adolescent psychopathology. Allessi and colleagues review 58 published reports, including 22 case reports, 26 case series (open clinical trials), and 9 double-blind placebo-controlled studies. Lithium was most effective for treating aggression and bipolar illness. There is less conclusive evidence for the efficacy of treating a variety of other disorders, including the behavioral problems associated with mental retardation and developmental disorders. The authors also review the mechanisms of action, including second-messenger systems and serotonin and adrenergic receptors. In a discussion of medication management they describe three methods for achieving a therapeutic steady-state blood level of lithium. Potential adverse effects, including mild symptoms as well as CNS, neuromuscular and endocrinological side effects, are reviewed. This paper is a useful review of the use of lithium, one effective treatment for aggression and manic-depressive illness, in children and adolescents.

The increasing need to demonstrate therapeutic efficacy leads us to an interesting critique of sensory integration therapy. In Chapter 19, Hoehn and Baumeister describe the theoretical underpinnings of this widely used therapy and then review the few studies assessing its effectiveness. *Sensory integration* is a term used to describe the organization of sensory input, proprioceptive, vestibular, and tactile. Ayres proposed that reading and writing as well as motor acts are dependent on sensory integration, and therefore children with learning disabilities could be helped by focusing on the sensory-integration difficulty. The therapy reportedly alters sensorimotor neural organization. According to these authors, Ayres focused on assessing postrotary nystagmus; however, the primary measure she developed has questionable reliability and validity.

Despite the measurement difficulty, the authors proceed to address two questions: Do children with learning disabilities show problems in sensory integration? And does sensory-integration therapy help children with learning disabilities? The reviewed studies provided multiple sessions per week of occupational therapy for 6 to 12 months. The majority found no improvement on visual-motor or academic tasks compared to control groups. Perceptual-motor training and no treatment at all were as effective as sensory-integration therapy in increasing nystagmus duration. This suggests that factors nonspecific to treatment, such as placebo or Hawthorne effects, and the instability of the measure are accounting for the occasional significant results. Reviewing only well-designed studies, the authors conclude that there is no evidence that sensory-integration therapy has an effect on academic abilities or on theoretically prerequisite sensorimotor, perceptual, and motor functions.

This article reiterates and supports a statement made by the American Academy of Pediatrics in 1985 about the lack of value of neurophysiological retraining programs, including optometric training, patterning, and sensory-integration training. Parents have to choose from a wide array of therapies offered to treat specific developmental disorders. Professionals should be aware of the scientific methods available for evaluating the efficacy of therapies. This will enable them to help parents make informed decisions so that children are not spending much of their time in unproven treatments.

The following two papers deal with effective educational interventions. Reynolds' paper, "Effects of a Preschool Plus Follow-On Intervention for Children at Risk" (Chapter 20), discusses early intervention for disadvantaged children. In economic times in which social and educational programs are susceptible to budget cuts, it becomes increasingly important to carefully design and conduct program evaluations.

Reynolds presents the results of a quasi-experiment; children were not randomly assigned to groups. Rather, children differentially participated in a comprehensive school-based service program. The participants were over 1,000 inner-city Chicago black children. One group was not enrolled in any of the programs. Another group received only preschool and kindergarten. Other groups received no preschool but primary-school services, or both preschool, kindergarten, and one to three years of primary-grade intervention. The Child Parent Center and Expansion Program was designed to improve school readiness and adjustment by providing health, social, academic, and school support services. Parent involvement, small class sizes, and a large staff were important aspects of the program.

A variety of outcomes were assessed in grades 3 through 5. These were reading and math achievement, teacher ratings of adjustment, parental involvement in school, special education placement, and grade retention. There were differences between the intervention and comparison group on achievement that were maintained up to two years post-intervention. The gap narrowed over time as a result of the comparison group catching up. The results indicate that the combination of preschool, kindergarten, and elementary school was most beneficial. Starting early—that is, having a preschool program—was an important influence on social adjustment. Providing ongoing service through the early elementary years significantly reduced grade retention. The duration of the program was unrelated to parent involvement.

Results of this study indicate that a preschool program alone, such as Head Start, can impact initial school adjustment. However, an ongoing intervention to grade 2 or 3 is needed to maintain those gains and to impact achievement. School achievement is affected more by the duration of intervention than the early enrollment. The broader follow-on services appear critical to helping children stay in school and at grade level. Although the services are moderately costly, cost-benefit analyses can be done to demonstrate the impact of not providing such services and having poorer social adjustment and a higher school dropout rate.

The next paper (Chapter 21) considers an intervention for children with learning disabilities. One particular group of reading-disabled children show difficulty in the early stages of learning to read. Hatcher, Hulme, and Ellis propose that training in phonological skills along with training in reading (e.g., phonically-based reading training) and spelling are critical to improving reading ability. Previous studies have not assessed the impact of reading training only, phonological training only, and a combination of the two.

The intervention occurred over 20 weeks from fall to spring. Children's academic and phonological skills were assessed before the beginning of school and after the intervention (7 months apart). A third follow-up assessment was conducted 9 months after the intervention was completed. Four groups of 32 7-year-old children matched for IQ, age, and reading ability were selected. Reading ability was defined as single-word reading, where children had to underline one of a group of words to match a word spoken by the tester. All of the children were approximately 1 standard deviation below average on this measure. Children were administered an extensive battery of tests prior to intervention. The tests measured reading comprehension, spelling, and phonological skills (e.g., sound deletion, sound blending, nonword segmentation, and sound categorization). Each training group received 40 half-hour sessions two times per week for 20 weeks. Numerous teachers provided the training. Groups were provided with reading with phonological training, phonological training only, and reading only. The fourth group received no special training. Children's progress in each training activity was monitored and used to determine when a child was ready to move to the next section. The reading training including reading and writing letters and words, and reading in context.

Results of the study support differential effectiveness of the three teaching methods. The group who received reading and phonological analysis showed significantly more progress than the control group on reading and spelling measures. The group who received only phonological training actually showed the greater improvement in phonological skills. Thus the improvement in literacy cannot be attributed solely to improvement in phonological skills. That is, phonological skills are necessary but not sufficient for learning to read well.

This study has several implications for educational practice. Often, when children are doing poorly in an academic subject, additional teaching is provided in that subject. This study demonstrates that a more systematic program of teaching phonological skills and reading is an effective approach to treating children with early reading difficulties. Whether this type of approach will be successful with older children who have reading difficulties will require further studies. It appears, however, that the gains diminish somewhat and that children with reading difficulty may need ongoing support to maintain the gains. Although this intervention was provided on an individual basis, many elements of the program can be applied in small groups.

16

The Efficacy of Psychoanalysis
for Children with Disruptive Disorders

Peter Fonagy and Mary Target

University College London and The Anna Freud Centre, London

Objective: *This paper describes a chart review of 763 cases of child psychoanalysis and psychotherapy at the Anna Freud Centre, and illustrates its usefulness by examining predictors of treatment outcome in children with disruptive disorders.* **Method:** *135 children and adolescents with a principal diagnosis of disruptive disorder were individually matched with others suffering from emotional disorders. Outcome was indicated by diagnostic change and change in overall adaptation (clinically significant improvement or return to normal functioning).* **Results:** *Improvement rates were significantly higher for the emotional than for the disruptive group. Within the disruptive group, significant improvement was more frequent among children with oppositional defiant disorder (56%) than those with attention deficit hyperactivity disorder (36%) or conduct disorder (23%). However, 31% of the children terminated treatment within 1 year. Of those disruptive children who remained in treatment more than 1 year, 69% were no longer diagnosable on termination. Fifty-eight percent of the variance in outcome ratings could be accounted for within this group.*

Reprinted with permission from the *Journal of the American Academy of Child and Adolescent Psychiatry*, 1994, Vol. 33(1), 45–55. Copyright © 1994 by the American Academy of Child and Adolescent Psychiatry.

This paper is dedicated to George Moran, late Director of the Anna Freud Centre, who established this study. We gratefully acknowledge the guidance of Professors Donald Cohen and Alan Kazdin, Yale University; also our research team, especially Maureen Parr and Maria Branagan. Linda Mayes, M.D., William Young, M.D., Alison Westman, M.D., and Anna Higgitt, M.D., provided independent validation of psychiatric diagnoses. James Hampton, Ph.D., advised on the statistical analysis.

The crucial variables in predicting attrition and symptomatic im-provement were found to be quite different in the disruptive and emotional groups. **Conclusion:** *Although the study has several methodological limitations, it does suggest demographic, clinical, and diagnostic characteristics of those disruptive children most likely to benefit from intensive and nonintensive psychodynamic treatment.*

Many clinical reviews have addressed the efficacy of psychoanalytic treatment for diverse pathology (e.g., S. Freud, 1937; A. Freud, 1954; Schlessinger, 1984; Tyson and Sandler, 1971). A few systematic studies of analyzability have been conducted with adult patients (most recently, Kantrowitz, 1987; Wallerstein, 1989; Weber et al., 1985). These studies have been reviewed by Bachrach et al. (1991) who are somewhat pessimistic about the extent to which therapeutic benefit can be predicted at initial consultation for cases considered suitable for analysis. Length of treatment, high pretreatment level of functioning, and patient-analyst complementarity repeatedly have emerged as predictors of good outcome.

The literature includes almost no studies of the effectiveness of insight-oriented treatments for children. Heinicke and Ramsey-Klee (1986) evaluated psychoanalytic treatment for latency children referred for learning disturbances. In separate groups, the frequency of treatment sessions was either one or four times per week. Both treatments led to gains in self-esteem, adaptation, and the capacity for relationships, but the gains were significantly greater for the more intensive treatment. Moran and his colleagues (1991) examined the efficacy of child psychoanalytic interventions with children with extremely poorly controlled diabetes. Significant improvements in blood glucose control were observed in a group of 12 patients treated in three or four times weekly psychoanalytic psychotherapy, relative to an untreated control group.

There has, however, never been a major study that has attempted to identify predictors of success in child analytic treatment. At the moment, we have no definite evidence as to which group of children, at what age, with what pathology, and in what kind of family circumstances are most suitable for child analysis. Psychoanalysis is the only psychological treatment that sets itself the ambitious goal of restructuring the components of the individual's adaptation and aims to address all aspects of the patient's personality. Perhaps because of the scope of its ambitions, attempts at operationalizing the process and outcome of child analysis are at very early stages of development. Yet knowledge gained from the work in child analysis remains the primary source of information about the nature of all types of dynamic psychotherapy with children, as well as the foundation of psychodynamic understanding of developmental processes in childhood, adolescence, and adulthood (Cohen, 1992).

Anna Freud was a pioneer in developing methods for accumulating specific information about children during the course of analysis. Because of her commitment to the scientific method and to systematic records, The Anna Freud Centre (AFC) has unique documentation on the children and adolescents who have undergone analyses during the past four decades. Over the past 2 years, we have been working on the first stages of a systematic study of child psychoanalysis. The starting point for this study is the extensive documentation on over 800 cases treated at this center. These cases represent children from the preschool through adolescent phases of development and the major domains of developmental psychopathology (emotional, disruptive, and developmental disorders).

Our database permits us to investigate a number of interesting questions. Here we report a study where the outcomes of the psychoanalysis of children with disruptive and with emotional disorders were compared. Studies of the natural history of these two groups of disorders (see Pepler and Rubin, 1991; Robins and Rutter, 1990) have shown that disruptive behavioral problems have a high level of persistence and frequently predict later antisocial tendencies (e.g., Robins, 1981; Weiss and Hechtman, 1986) even when the childhood disorder takes a less serious form (e.g., Havinghurst et al., 1962). By contrast, children with emotional disorders are almost as likely to be normally adjusted in adulthood as those without psychiatric difficulties in childhood (Kohlberg et al., 1984; Rutter and Sandberg, 1985).

Corresponding with such differences in natural history, treatment responses of these groups also clearly differ, with long-term treatment outcomes tending to be limited for the disruptive disorder group (Dumas, 1989; Kazdin, 1987). Systematic reviews of the relative responsiveness of these groups to psychodynamic treatments have not been reported.

METHOD

Subjects

The sample of closed treatment files available for study numbers 763 cases. This represents approximately 90% of cases treated at the AFC. It excludes cases where treatment was not recommended or did not commence after a diagnostic assessment. It also excludes children of well-known individuals whose files have not been made available for study for reasons of confidentiality and a small number of cases (less than 5% of the total sample) where the documentation of the case was insufficient to enable meaningful analysis.

The sample is unique in several respects, the most important being that the majority of patients (76%) received intensive treatment (four or five times a week). Secondly, the present database includes reports of a large number of psychoanalyses and psychotherapeutic treatments performed by experienced staff as well as by trainees (nearly 40% of the cases were treated by highly experienced analysts).

The Hampstead Disruptive Disorder Sample. There were 135 children with *DSM-III-R* principal diagnosis of disruptive disorder (58% oppositional defiant disorder, 8% attention-deficit hyperactivity disorder (ADHD), 23% conduct disorder, and 10% with a V code of antisocial behavior).

Of these children 67% were offered and accepted intensive psychoanalytic treatment (four or five times weekly), the remainder were seen one or two times per week. Allocation to intensive or nonintensive treatment appeared to be made largely on pragmatic grounds (e.g., distance from the AFC) as opposed to diagnostic considerations. We checked this impression by performing a step-wise discriminant analysis (Jennrich, 1977) to distinguish between intensive and nonintensive cases. We found that only four variables were associated with allocation to intensive treatment: serious marital difficulties between the parents, the child attending the AFC's day-care program, father being relatively well-functioning (GAF score), and father having a history of anxiety symptoms. However, identification of the nonintensive cases, using this discriminant function, was poor; only a slightly above chance number (40%) of nonintensive cases could be correctly predicted on the basis of information available at assessment. We concluded that there were few systematic differences between the groups on the information recorded.

This group was individually matched with 135 children treated for emotional disorder at the clinic during this period. The match included gender, age, socioeconomic status, Children's Global Assessment Scale (CGAS) score (Shaffer et al., 1983), and number of sessions per week. The control sample was selected using a computer algorithm from 368 cases treated for emotional problems. For 95% of cases perfect matches were found. For 5% the stringency of one of two matching criteria (socioeconomic status or CGAS score) was relaxed. The control group comprised children with a principal diagnosis of overanxious disorder or generalized anxiety disorder (28%), separation anxiety disorder (17%), dysthymia or major depressive disorder (18%), phobic or avoidant disorders (17%), sleep disorders (8%), obsessive-compulsive disorder (6%), and post-traumatic or adjustment disorders (6%). The major demographic characteristics of the two groups are shown in Table 1.

There were many differences between the groups of potential relevance to treatment outcome. The disruptive children had fewer mothers with a psychiatric history (F for linear trend = 4.15, df = 1,270, $p < .05$) and more children from foster or residential care, χ^2 = 6.35, (df = 1, N = 270), $p < .02$. They were also more likely to drop out of treatment, χ^2 = 12.14 (df = 3, N = 270), $p < .01$, and therefore their average treatment length was shorter: 2 rather than 2.5 years, F = 5.45, df = 1,266, $p < .02$.

The documentation available for coding charts was: (1) the standard diagnostic profile (A. Freud, 1962). This is based on at least two social history interviews with parents, full (verbatim) report of two interviews with the child, projective and cognitive psychological tests (at least the appropriate Wechsler Intelligence Scale for Children and the Children's or Thematic Apperception Test), and school reports; in addition, in 20% of cases, longitudinal observations also were available from the AFCs preventive services for children with high-risk backgrounds: day care program (10%), toddler group (3%), and pediatric clinic (7%) (these provided a significant proportion of the referrals). (2) Weekly process reports. (3) Reports of regular interviews with parents. (4) Lengthy formal reports of the treatment. (5) Terminal diagnostic profile.

TABLE 1

Demographic Characteristics of Matched Groups of Disruptive and Emotionally Disordered Children in Psychoanalytic and Psychotherapeutic Treatments at the Anna Freud Centre

Variable	Disruptive	Emotional	Statistics
Sample	135	135	
Male	75%	75%	
Mean age in years			
(SD)	9.0 (3.6)	9.0 (3.7)	$F < 1.0$
(Range)	(3.2-17.4)	(2.7-18.0)	
Mean IQ (SD)	111.6 (14.4)	115.8 (17.6)	$F = 3.6$
(Range)	(69-141)	(53-163)	
Social Class I & II	56%	69%	$\chi^2 = 4.7,$ $df = 1$
Mean CGAS[a]			
(SD)	53.6 (8.1)	54.3 (7.0)	$F < 1.0$
(Range)	(32-70)	(38-70)	

[a] CGAS = Children's Global Assessment Scale.

Measures

The measures we report here fall into four categories.

Demographic measures include extensive biographical and social information on the child and on his or her family (e.g., the structure of the family unit, the family's cultural background, socioeconomic status).

Diagnostic information includes *DSM-III-R* Axis I and II psychiatric classifications for the past, the time of referral, and for termination. The reliability of these judgments was checked by three senior child psychiatrists, independent of the chart review, working in the United States and the United Kingdom. The overall reliability was consistently high, κ (Cohen, 1960) ranged between 0.8 and 0.9 for major categories. The reliability for specific diagnoses was somewhat lower but still in the satisfactory to excellent range (0.53 to 1.00). Information on presenting symptomatology was recorded retrospectively using Child Behavior Checklist (CBCL) protocols (Achenbach and Edelbrock, 1986). Coders rated all symptoms clearly identified in assessment material as somewhat or very characteristic of the child. This method of coding on CBCLs does not produce a profile comparable with that derived from parents' ratings. We assessed this by asking parents and therapists to complete the CBCL on 25 current referrals, and these ratings were contrasted with data obtained from the charts by two raters using the procedure above. The level of agreement between the two chart raters was high (mean $r = .85$); however, neither rater showed good agreement with the mother or therapist (mean $r = .55$). The reason appeared to be that the chart raters used stricter criteria, providing conservative symptom profiles relative to parents and therapists. Agreement between all raters for severe symptoms was high ($r > .8$).

Level of functioning was rated at the beginning and at the end of treatment on the CGAS instrument developed by Shaffer and colleagues (1983). This is a 100-point rating scale with anchor points at each decile. Scores higher than 70 are regarded as falling within the normal range. A score less than 30 indicates severe impairment, probably requiring hospitalization. Children rated at 55 or less would be clearly in need of some form of therapeutic help and often special educational provision. The mean CGAS score in each of the matched groups was 54. The interjudge reliability of the CGAS scores at the beginning and end of treatment and the change in CGAS ratings were computed separately on a randomly selected sample of 50 cases. Intraclass *Rs*, computed on the basis of the ratings of four board certified child psychiatrists, were high ($R = .77$ for initial and end of treatment ratings, and $R = .88$ for change scores).

Relevant clinical information on each case includes a limited number of potentially significant etiological factors such as: losses of important figures, separations from the caregivers, significant disturbances in family relationships, medical history, and hospitalizations. We also collected data on the child's behavior and performance at school, previous treatment for psychological disturbance, and psychiatric histories and treatment of the child's parents. Information on the child's treatment covered the referral, the treatment (frequency, duration, interruption, changes of therapist, etc.) and the therapist (e.g., gender, years of experience). We also classified the reasons for termination. The data were recorded on a standardized form that included operational definitions to help raters make judgments on each item. Four raters took part in data collection; each rater's reliability was independently assessed by one of us (M.T.), to a criterion of 95% agreement. Interrater reliability coefficients were calculated for 100 of the charts, and intraclass agreements in excess of .9 were found for all clinical variables used in subsequent analysis. The agreements for psychiatric diagnoses of the parents were somewhat lower than this, and in line with those found for the children.

Outcome Measures

There is no simple way of assessing the outcome of child analysis. Psychoanalysts may feel that the assessment of effectiveness in terms of improved adaptation and reduced symptomatology falls far short of the scope of the psychoanalytic enterprise. Reliable and valid measures of "structural change" (alterations in the child's presumed psychic apparatus) are unavailable for children (but see Wallerstein, 1988). In any case, they could be applied to chart data only with great difficulty. Furthermore, the value of this database may be increased by outcome assessments not unique to it but involving indices in current use in modern psychiatric research.

Three measures of outcome are used in this report. First, diagnostic caseness at the end of treatment, defined as the presence of any diagnosable psychiatric disorder together with an adaptation level rating less than 70.

Second, the child could be considered to be still a case on the ground of maladjustment (i.e., CGAS score at termination). We used the Jacobson and Truax criteria (1991) for clinically significant improvement. These authors propose three methods for determining cutoff points, all of which in our case yielded similar results. We used the Jacobson and Truax formula for calculating the relative likelihood of being in the functional or dysfunctional population, based on the point of equal distance between the means of these two populations, weighted by the distributional properties of each population. The formula for calculating this cutoff is given by Jacobson and Truax as:

$$\text{weighted relative likelihood index} = \frac{s_0 \times M_1 + s_1 \times M_0}{s_0 + s_1}$$

where s_0 is the standard deviation (SD) of the normal group, and M_1 is the central point of the dysfunctional group. We used data from Bird et al. (1987) using the CGAS scale to estimate the SD and mean of the normal population. We used our own sample to estimate population means and SDs for a dysfunctional group. CGAS ratings at termination of fewer than 68 identified cases who still belonged to the dysfunctional group. The two distributions were clearly discrete.

Third, we categorized cases according to the presence of statistically reliable change in adaptation level, based on the method proposed by Jacobson et al. (1984), and modified by Christensen and Mendoza (1986). This uses the SD of the dysfunctional group together with interjudge reliability of the measure to indicate the size of change necessary to identify cases where change could not be owing to measurement error and chance fluctuations. The index of reliable change in CGAS ratings is given by the formula:

$$\text{reliable change} = 1.96 \times \sqrt{2} \times s \times \sqrt{(1 - r_{xx})}$$

where r_{xx} is the best estimate of interrater reliability. In our data, this gives a reliable change index of 7.5 points for the emotionally disordered group and 8.5 for the disruptive disordered children. We took a difference of 8 points or more between ratings at the beginning and end of treatment to indicate a statistically significant change.

We also used the change in CGAS ratings as a continuous variable in predictions of the extent of improvement.

Statistical Analysis

Our statistical analysis commenced with examination of the distributions of our variables; a number of variables showed highly skewed distributions requiring data transformations (Mosteller and Tukey, 1977). Missing data were estimated following the recommendations of Cohen and Cohen (1975) using regression procedures to estimate values. The two groups were contrasted using BMDP2V analysis of variance procedure or

BMDP4F procedure for two-way frequency tables (Dixon, 1988). Stepwise multiple regressions were performed using the BMDP2R procedure, using statistical significance as the criterion for entering and removing variables. Stepwise discriminant function analyses were performed using the BMDP7M procedure, with classifications based on the jackknifed classification matrix, which excludes the case being classified from the computation of the matrix.

RESULTS

Rates of Improvement

Psychoanalysis and psychotherapy were associated with a significant improvement in functioning in both groups. The number of diagnosable cases decreased from 100% at the beginning of treatment to 33% at termination in the total sample. However, this reduction includes 34% of cases from whom insufficient information was available at termination for a conclusive diagnosis. As we had CGAS scores at termination for all but 9% of cases, improvement rates based on adaptation are a better guide to changes during treatment.

There were large differences in improvement rates between the two groups according to all three criteria (Table 2). The number of children without diagnosis was significantly greater in the control group than in the disruptive group, $\chi^2 = 11.0$ ($df = 1,270$), $p < .001$. These diagnoses include disruptive cases with only nondisruptive diagnoses at termination, but excluding these cases would add only about 5% to the undiagnosed disruptive group. The difference in clinically significant improvement rates is also highly significant, $\chi^2 = 15.4$, ($df = 1,270$), $p < .001$. On our third measure of statistically reliable change, we found somewhat higher improvement rates, but again, superior treatment response for the emotional group, $\chi^2 = 20$, ($df = 1,270$), $p < .0001$.

TABLE 2
Improvement Rates According to Different Criteria

	Disruptive (%)	Emotional (%)
No longer case on diagnostic grounds	32.6	52.6
No longer case on grounds of adaptation	32.6	56.3
Reliable improvement in adaptation	45.9	72.6

Among the disruptive group, improvement rates were highest for children with oppositional defiant disorder (e.g., on the measure of reliable change, 56% improved significantly, compared with 36% with ADHD or with a V code of antisocial behavior, and only 23% of conduct disordered children). A 30% to 40% improvement rate in the disruptive group after an average of 2 years of intensive treatment may not seem impressive, but many of these children (31%) terminated treatment within the first year, the majority within the first 6 months. Sixty-nine percent of those who remained in treatment for at least 1 year (and could thus be said to have had an analytic experience) were no longer diagnosable at termination, and 62% showed reliable improvement. These effectiveness rates refer primarily to psychoanalysis, as more than two thirds of the children who dropped out of treatment within the first year were receiving nonintensive help (one or two sessions per week). Forty percent of those in nonintensive therapy dropped out, compared with 25% in analysis, $\chi^2 = 3.46$, ($df = 1, N = 135$), $p < .06$.

We examined the relationship between age and improvement in treatment and found that within the disruptive group there was a strong association: children younger than 9 years ($n = 70$) showed a mean improvement in CGAS of 10.0 points, compared with 5.3 points in the group of older children and adolescents ($n = 65$), $F = 8.47$, $df = 1,133$, $p < .005$. This is not simply owing to lower attrition in younger children as, when only cases continuing beyond 1 year are considered, a comparable difference is found between the younger and older groups, means 11.9 ($n = 51$), and 6.6 ($n = 42$) respectively; $F = 6.48$, $df = 1,91$, $p < .02$. The difference between intensive and nonintensive treatment was particularly marked for the younger age group. A two-way analysis of variance of mean CGAS change yielded a significant interaction term for the age by intensity comparison, $F = 4.98$, $df = 1,131$, $p < .03$. These associations with age were not found within the matched group with primarily emotional disorders.

Mean differences in CGAS ratings between the disruptive and the emotionally disordered groups markedly diminish when we focus on children who had the benefit of full psychoanalytic treatment (Figure 1). The average improvement in CGAS score was 14 in the emotional group and only 7.8 in the disruptive disordered group, $F = 26.12$, $df = 1,268$, $p < .001$. When we exclude children whose treatment ended within the first year, the CGAS change for the disruptive group is 9.5 points ($n = 93$), $F = 20.20$, $df = 1,197$, $p < 0.001$. If we then exclude those in nonintensive treatment, the magnitude of improvement in the disruptive group ($n = 58$) but not in the emotional group ($n = 93$) significantly increases, and the size of the difference between the two groups is reduced, $F = 6.70$, $df = 1,149$, $p < .02$.

When we examine improvement rates for children remaining in intensive treatment for at least 3 years (a realistic basis for judging the effectiveness of full psychoanalytic treatment), then we find that the difference between disruptive ($n = 21$) and emotionally disordered children ($n = 33$) is no longer statistically significant. A very similar pattern emerges if we look at the percentage of children showing reliable improvement. In brief, it appears that psychoanalysis can bring about very substantial improvements in children with disruptive disorders, but children with such disorders are difficult to keep in analysis.

Prediction

A critical question becomes whether we can predict which child is likely to terminate treatment prematurely. Taking the entire disruptive disordered group together, we cannot. A stepwise discriminant analysis was able to identify correctly only 52% of those terminating within 1 year and 88% of those who remained in treatment, approximate $F = 10.32$, $df = 5,129$, $p <$ .001. Significant predictors of remaining in treatment were: being in intensive (four or five times weekly) treatment; having a less well-functioning mother (judged on Axis V of *DSM-III-R*, the GAF score) whose major problem was not anxiety; having specific learning difficulties at school; and continued support to the parents by regular meetings with a social worker.

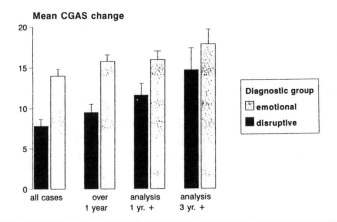

Figure 1. Mean change in Children's Global Assessment Scale (CGAS) scores for the entire sample, children who remained in treatment more than 1 year, children in analysis more than 1 year, and children in analysis more than 3 years.

When we separately examined the children aged 9 years or older (n = 65), among whom the majority (56%) of premature terminations occurred, prediction became more accurate. A stepwise discriminant function analysis correctly identified 74% of dropouts and 87% of those who continued among this older group, on the basis of four variables, approximate F = 13.14, df = 4,57, p < .001. Children who stayed in treatment were relatively likely to be younger, to have specific learning difficulties, to be in intensive treatment, and to have mothers with current psychiatric symptoms. Prediction was less successful for children younger than 9 years (n = 70): only 50% of premature terminators and 90% of those who continued could be identified, approximate F = 5.80, df = 4,63, p < .001. Intensive treatment again emerged as one of the predictive factors for remaining in treatment, along with female gender, and having a less well-functioning mother but not an anxious mother.

It was also difficult to predict the much smaller number (18%) of children terminating within the first year in the emotionally disordered group. A stepwise discriminant analysis identified only 45% of those dropping out, and 92% of those who remained in therapy, approximate F = 7.78, df = 7,127, p < .001. Again, intensive treatment predicted continuation beyond 1 year; other predictors were having a parent with a history of depression, intact parental relationship, no school refusal or truancy, being younger at the beginning of treatment, good peer relationships, and no associated attachment or post-traumatic psychiatric disorder.

We did much better in being able to predict the magnitude of improvement. We examined demographic, diagnostic, and clinical predictors of improvement for both groups in the study using stepwise multiple regression procedure. Overall, treatment outcome was slightly more predictable for children in the emotional group than for disruptive disordered children. Of the variance 40% was accounted for by family, diagnostic, clinical, and treatment variables for the disruptive disordered group, while 52% could be accounted for in the emotional disordered group. Variables that predicted success were, however, different for these two clinical populations. Family and demographic factors (e.g., maternal anxiety disorder or the child having been in foster care) were particularly important predictors for disruptive children but accounted for only 11% of the variance for the emotional disordered group (e.g., parents not divorced or separated). Diagnostic variables were also more important predictors for the disruptive disordered group (e.g., presence of anxiety disorder, absence of other comorbidity, and school-reported problems); for the emotional group, less severe principal diagnoses, better initial adaptation, and the absence of enuresis were the most important diagnostic considerations. However, in total, diagnostic and clinical variables accounted for less than 17% of the variance in out-come as opposed to nearly 25% in the case of the disruptive group. Con-versely, treatment characteristics were the most powerful set of predictors of improvement for the emotionally disordered group (no change of therapist, regular meetings with the parents before the child commenced treatment, as well as length of treatment predicted nearly 20% of the variance). Treat-ment variables were less important in the disruptive disorders group (ac-counted for only 13.8% of variance).

We were able to account for 58% of the variance in treatment outcome for the disruptive group treated for longer than 1 year, $n = 93$, $R^2 = .58$, $F = 12.02$, $df = 9,79$, $p < .001$) (Table 3). There were three especially powerful predictors: the presence of an additional emotional disorder (particularly anxiety), longer treatment, and the absence of other comorbidity (par-ticularly specific developmental disorders). Children were likely to do less well in analysis if they had been in foster care, if the child's mother had a history of anxiety disorder, if the child was underachieving at school rela-tive to his IQ, and if the school expressed serious concerns about the child. Children were likely to do better if their mother was also receiving treat-ment at the Centre, and if the child had been in the Centre's preschool day-care program.

TABLE 3

Prediction of Improvement in Adaptation, Disruptive Group,
Continued Treatment Beyond 1 Year ($n = 93$)

Variable	Regression Coefficient (b)	Standardized Regression Coefficient (β)	F for Variable
Other childhood disorders	−7.47	−.35	21.37***
Length of treatment	21.52	.35	19.49***
Emotional disorder	6.49	.29	15.17***
Underachievement	−5.94	−.25	8.82**
AFC Nursery	8.25	.23	8.63**
Mother anxious	−7.14	−.20	6.29*
Foster care	−6.75	−.19	6.16*
Mother treated (AFC[a])	8.95	.18	5.43*
School/learning difficulties	−4.33	−.19	5.26*
Father anxious	5.83	.15	4.00*

[a] AFC = Anna Freud Centre.
* $p < .05$, ** $p < .01$, *** $p < .001$.

Most of these variables also emerged as significant predictors in a discriminant analysis attempting to distinguish between children who showed significant improvement if treated for at least 1 year. The outcome in 80% of cases could be correctly predicted from a combination of these variables.

We examined whether it was possible to identify those children who were functioning at a lower adaptation level at the end of treatment (9% of those who continued beyond 1 year; 11% of the entire disruptive group). We found that only one third of these children could be predicted on the basis of the information we had collected. Variables significantly associated with worsening of adaptation were: school performance generally below the child's capacity or interfered with by anxiety symptoms, the presence of other childhood disorders with the exception of specific developmental disorders, lower socioeconomic status, and higher paternal GAF score; approximate $F = 9.35$, $df = 6,86$, $p < .001$.

DISCUSSION

The percentage of disruptive disordered children who returned to a level of functioning within the normal range on our measure (33% of all disruptive cases and 36% of those who remained in treatment for more than 1 year) is roughly comparable with those of other studies (Brandt and Zlotnick, 1988; Dumas, 1989). They fall short of recent reports of the rates of improvement for conduct disordered children who receive a combination of parent management training and problem-solving skills training (Kazdin et al., 1992). However, it should be noted that our measure aims to assess the children in all contexts, and even in the latter study, when school and home assessments were combined only 50% of children were functioning within the normal range. Nevertheless, it also should be pointed out that the amount of therapy received was considerably greater in the present study.

The predictors of premature termination of psychoanalytic treatment were found to overlap relatively little with those reported in other studies (Kazdin, 1990). The overall attrition rate was also lower than the normal 45% to 65% (Pekarik and Stephenson, 1988). We found quite consistently that parental psychopathology (with the exception of maternal anxiety) was negatively related to attrition, and other variables found elsewhere to predict dropping out of treatment (such as comorbidity and lower IQ) appeared to make no difference within this group of disruptive children. An additional diagnosis of specific developmental disorder was, in fact, associated with remaining in therapy among children older than 9 years (those most likely to drop out). It may be that associated pathology in both parent and child are more effectively managed within a setting using a psychodynamic approach, where the intervention (for both child and parent) intentionally addresses all areas of personalities and relationships, rather than being focused primarily on the disruptive behavior.

The difference in change scores in children with or without anxiety disorder is highly significant. Where treatment continued for at least 1 year, the magnitude of change for children with both disruptive and anxiety diagnoses was 13, comparable with the average change of nearly 16 in the emotionally disordered group. Sixty-five percent of disruptive children with an additional diagnosis of anxiety showed significant improvements after at least 1 year's treatment, as compared with 50% of those without. This confirms a number of previous observations (Conte et al., 1988) that a history of anxiety is a predictor of good psychotherapy outcome. This observation is in marked contrast to our other finding that all forms of comorbidity other than anxiety reduce the likelihood of successful analytic treatment.

Similarly, specific developmental disorders generally are recognized as aggravating the difficulties of children with disruptive disorders (Rutter, 1989), and they also interfere with the extent to which the child is able to benefit from psychoanalytic treatment. We found that these children generally stayed in treatment but improved significantly less than did others (this relationship was not found in the children with primarily emotional symptoms). Thus there is a complex relationship between comorbidity, attrition, and therapeutic improvement. In brief, anxiety symptoms in disruptive children who stay in treatment are associated with good outcome while all other forms of comorbidity predict relatively poor outcome. It is worth restating that outcome was assessed not just in terms of the disruptive behavior but of overall adaptation and the persistence of diagnosable disorders. Therefore, children with additional symptoms (such as learning disabilities, tics, encopresis) would have been rated as still impaired if these other difficulties had remained while the disruptive behavior improved.

It is reassuring that we were able to demonstrate a dose-effect relationship between treatment length and magnitude of change. This association is one of the more stable findings of the psychotherapeutic literature and has been borne out by meta-analytic investigations (Howard et al., 1986). Howard et al. demonstrated a log-linear relationship between number of sessions and treatment effects over a large number of studies, and these findings are consistent with their observations. It is important to underscore that treatment length in this study is not simply a mediator variable for time between assessment and termination, i.e., spontaneous remission by maturation. Among children in treatment for more than 1 year, those in intensive treatment showed significantly greater improvement than did those treated once or twice a week, over a comparable period. The findings are consistent with Heinicke's classical study of the frequency of child therapy sessions (Heinicke and Ramsey-Klee, 1986). Children younger than 9 years appeared to be especially likely to benefit from intensive treatment. For older children, four or five times weekly treatment did not significantly improve outcome. However, even for this group, assignment to intensive treatment significantly reduced the likelihood of early termination. The pattern of findings suggest that the efficacy of nonintensive psychodynamic treatment of conduct disorder might be maximized if treatment were initially offered relatively intensively (to prevent attrition) and reduced after 6 to 12 months, when the maximum likelihood of premature termination had passed.

The importance of the parents' adjustment also has been shown by previous studies to be a critical predictor in the natural history of disruptive disorders (Patterson et al., 1991; Richman et al., 1982). The finding that children of relatively disturbed mothers were more likely to remain in treatment may be the indirect consequence of the support the mothers themselves gained during the child's treatment, which could have motivated them to continue it. It is also possible the analytic relationship with a better-functioning adult was more valued by children whose primary caregiver showed significant psychiatric disturbance. It is very encouraging that treating the psychological problems of the mother improves the chances of the child benefiting from psychoanalytic treatment, especially in view of the finding that a mother's anxiety related difficulties can hinder it. As in our program all parents receive guidance and support concurrent to the child's treatment, the additional benefit of psychotherapeutic help for the mother is particularly significant. The importance of this component is underscored by findings that maternal stress and depression contribute to (and are exacerbated by) disruptive behavior in children (Dumas and Gibson, 1990; Patterson, 1986). As Kazdin et al. (1992) point out, treatment of parents as well as of children may both enhance the child's gains and help to maintain these in the longer term. A report by Szapocznik and his colleagues (1989) where individual and family based treatments were contrasted points to a somewhat sinister alternative account. In this study, individual treatment, however beneficial it was for the child, could in the medium term lead to a deterioration in family functioning. It is possible that the concurrent treatment of one or both parents preempts such complications.

The importance of contextual factors in psychoanalytic treatment was highlighted by the powerful association between improvement and the child's earlier attendance at the Centre's preschool day-care program. All children who received psychoanalytic help after attending this program stayed in therapy and showed clinically significant improvements. As children are selected for the program on the basis of risk factors (e.g., severe parental pathology, significant economic deprivation), we might have expected a negative association with magnitude of improvement. Our finding illustrates the general need for a multifaceted approach to intervention for children with disruptive disorder if they are to take full advantage of the therapeutic help they are offered. The experience of the day-care program may have provided these children with relationship experiences that sensitized them to the therapeutic encounter. Conversely, the object relations experiences that precede foster care (a negative predictor) may present considerable obstacles in the path of therapeutic improvements.

We found that younger age showed a strong association with good outcome in the disruptive group, even when children terminating within 1 year were excluded. However, this relationship did not emerge in the multivariate analysis of predictors because it was mediated by other variables such as frequency of sessions, comorbidity, and attendance at the Centre's day-care program.

The differences in predictors of good outcome between the matched disruptive and emotional groups emphasize the diagnostic specificity of predictors of analyzability, and may go some way toward explaining why previous studies have failed to predict treatment success in analysis when diagnostic considerations were not part of the design. Not only are different variables relevant for particular diagnostic groups, but also probably different *classes of variables* may need to be considered when making psychoanalytic treatment recommendations for these children. This implication is at odds with the general tendency to regard psychotherapeutic considerations as independent of descriptive nosology at our Centre and, we suspect, at many traditional dynamically oriented institutions (Shapiro, 1989).

In conclusion, let us state some of the limitations of the investigation. The long-term goal of this program of research is to identify groups of children for whom dynamically oriented therapy may be effective. This retrospective investigation obviously did not allow random assignment of children to treatment or control groups. Therefore we cannot conclusively show child analysis to be effective, let alone cost effective, relative to other modes of treatment, or to no treatment. Our grounds for comparison are studies of the natural history of the disorders under scrutiny. The work of other centers, such as the Yale Child Conduct Clinic, has suggested that disruptive children show little or no change during an attention placebo treatment (Kazdin et al., 1992). However, we cannot rule out the possibility of improvements due to spontaneous remission because our recruitment criteria were different.

An additional limitation of the study is its restriction to chart-based information. The validity of archival records is always open to doubt; we cannot be confident that all important aspects of cases were noted and recorded, or that changing scientific interests have not influenced techniques of assessment to a point where phenomena are no longer perceived in comparable ways. An advantage of the AFC data set is that, for historical reasons, both clinical recording and technical approach were relatively consistent, explicit, and standardized. This almost unique psychoanalytic culture may, however, reduce the generalizability of our findings in other ways. British and North American cultures during the past decade have defined a new attitude to psychoanalysis, particularly the psychoanalysis of children, that leads to significant changes in referral patterns. Increasingly, the AFC sees very seriously disturbed children who have failed to respond to alternative, less-intensive, and more cost-effective treatment approaches. Thus while the treatment of the present sample was relatively protected from secular trends and other cultural changes, it is unlikely that a study of the AFC's clinical work over the next 20 years would yield a simple replication of these findings.

Another important limitation is that it was only possible to take measures of improvement at the beginning and end of therapy, rather than at regular intervals throughout the course of the treatment. This means that improvement may be confounded by length of treatment, particularly for disorders which have a high rate of spontaneous remission. Our finding of the relationship of outcome to the amount of therapy received, however, appears to be independent of the simple passage of time.

The unrepresentative sample of subjects relative to other clinics, both in the United Kingdom and in the United States, presents an obstacle to generalizing from this study. Although our cases were higher in socioeconomic status and intelligence than are most similar groups, many other studies of disruptive disordered children have also used atypical samples. In contrast to many studies, the children we studied had clear diagnoses and the study was clinic-based, as opposed to using convenience samples (e.g., recruiting from schools).

Early attrition emerged as the main obstacle to successful psychoanalytic treatment. Parental failure to comply with treatment recommendations has also been found to be a major problem in the implementation of behavioral and cognitive-behavioral programs (Kazdin, 1985). This underlines the importance of reporting success rates on the basis of all cases offered treatment, rather than excluding dropouts, as numerous early behavioral studies did. In our case, starting treatment on a four or five times weekly basis significantly reduced premature termination. It should be noted that beyond the possible value of intensive treatment in reducing the risk of attrition, the willingness to enter such an intensive program indicates high parental motivation. It is possible that certain children were offered intensive treatment because of other factors already suggesting a better prognosis. However, as stated earlier, this possibility was not supported by our attempt to distinguish the two groups using many criteria often associated with treatment outcome.

Attrition presents an additional problem for generalizability. Predictors of outcome identified by the present project can only be considered to apply to those individuals who agree to remain in psychodynamic treatment over a relatively prolonged period.

Nevertheless, the data set yielded powerful and consistent predictions concerning which disruptive disordered child is likely to benefit most from analytic treatment. It appears that treatment is more effective when it lasts longer, is more intensive, with the more anxious subgroup of disruptive children who are without significant learning difficulties and additional diagnoses, whose mother is not notably anxious or is taken into treatment, and who have previous or concurrent experiences likely to establish good object relationships.

The strength of the prediction (58% of the variance in therapeutic outcome accounted for) is considerably better than that reported in most psychotherapy studies with both children and adults, where variables obtained before the start of treatment rarely account for more than 10% to 20% of the variance in outcome (Casey and Berman, 1985; Weisz et al., 1987, 1992). Excluding treatment variables, we were able to specify 40% of this variability, applying predictors similar to those used in other studies.

Several factors may account for this. The most important is the length and relative homogeneity of the treatment offered. Most psychotherapy studies examine brief interventions and therefore identify individuals who benefit from treatment in the short term (Shirk and Russell, 1992). There may have been other children in those samples, with similar demographic and clinical features, who would have benefited from the treatment had it continued. An additional advantage, in terms of prediction, was the heterogeneity of the Hampstead sample, as it was a clinical population rather than one specially drawn up for experimental purposes. It is a less likely, but nevertheless possible, alternative that the superior quality of our raw data and operationalizations gave us a firmer basis from which to predict. One distinction between the present study and others is that the AFC database (for all its limitations) is based on the sophisticated and systematic observations of skilled analysts. In the past, the generally poor reliability of clinical judgments has gradually shifted clinical data collection away from interview data toward far more reliable psychometric instruments. More recently, researchers have become increasingly aware of the limitations, alongside the advantages, of this approach. We feel that the predictive power of this clinically based data set, subjected to rigorous operationalization, may support a paradigmatic shift in research on psychosocial interventions, from a uniquely psychometric tradition to one where such information is supplemented with data collected using traditional clinical skills.

REFERENCES

Achenbach TM, Edelbrock C (1986), *Manual for the Teacher's Report Form and Teacher Version of the Child Behaviour Profile.* Burlington, VT: University of Vermont Department of Psychiatry

Bachrach HM, Galatzer-Levy R, Skolnikoff A, Waldron S (1991), On the efficacy of psychoanalysis. *J Am Psychoanal Assoc* 39:871–916

Bird H, Canino G, Rubio-Stipec M, Ribera J (1987), Further measures of the psychometric properties of the Children's Global Assessment Scale (CGAS). *Arch Gen Psychiatry* 44:821–824

Brandt DE, Zlotnik SJ (1988), *The Psychology and Treatment of the Youthful Offender.* Springfield, IL: Charles C Thomas

Casey RJ, Berman JS (1985), The outcome of psychotherapy with children. *Psychol Bull* 98:388–400

Christensen L, Mendoza JL (1986), A method of assessing change in a single subject: an alteration of the RC index. *Behavior Therapy* 17:305–308

Cohen DJ (1992), From concepts to research and policy. Presentation to American Academy of Child and Adolescent Psychiatry, Institute on Evolving Concepts in Child Psychoanalysis and Psychotherapy. Washington, DC, October 1992

Cohen J (1960), A coefficient of agreement for nominal scales. *Educational and Psychological Measurement* 20:37–46

Cohen J, Cohen P (1975), *Applied Multiple Regression/Correlation Analysis for the Behavioral Sciences.* New York: Lawrence Erlbaum Associates

Conte HR, Plutchik R, Picard S, Karasu TB, Vaccaro E (1988), Self-report measures as predictors of psychotherapy outcome. *Compr Psychiatry* 29:355–360

Dixon WJ (ed) (1988), *BMDP Statistical Software Manual.* Berkeley: University of California Press

Dumas JE (1989), Treating antisocial behavior in children: child and family approaches. *Clinical Psychology Review* 9:197–222

Dumas JE, Gibson JA (1990), Behavioral correlates of maternal depressive symptomatology in conduct-disorder children: II. Systematic effects involving fathers and siblings. *J Consult Clin Psychol* 58:877–881

Freud A (1954), The widening scope of indications for psychoanalysis: discussion. *J Am Psychoanal Assoc* 2:607–620

Freud A (1962), Assessment of childhood disturbances. *Psychoanal Study Child* 17:149–158

Freud S (1937), Analysis terminable and interminable. Standard Edition 23, pp. 209–254

Havinghurst RJ, Bowman PH, Liddle GP, Matthews CV, Pierce JV (1962), *Growing up in River City.* New York: Wiley

Heinicke CM, Ramsey-Klee DM (1986), Outcome of child psychotherapy as a function of frequency of sessions. *J Am Aca Child Psychiatry* 25:247–253

Howard KI, Kopta SM, Krause MS, Orlinsky DE (1986), The dose-effect relationship in psychotherapy. *Am Psychol* 41:159–164

Jacobson NS, Truax P (1991), Clinical significance: a statistical approach to defining meaningful change in psychotherapy research. *J Consult Clin Psychol* 59:12–19

Jacobson NS, Follette WC, Revenstorf D (1984), Psychotherapy outcome research: methods for reporting variability and evaluating clinical significance. *Behav Ther* 15:336–352

Jennrich RI (1977), Stepwise discriminant analysis. In: *Statistical Methods for Digital Computers*, eds K Enslein, A Ralton, HS Wilf. New York: Wiley

Kantrowitz J (1987), Suitability for psychoanalysis. In: *The Yearbook of Psychoanalysis and Psychotherapy.* New York: Guilford Press, pp 403–415

Kazdin AE (1985), *Treatment of Antisocial Behavior in Children and Adolescents.* Homewood, IL: Dorsey Press

Kazdin AE (1987), Treatment of antisocial behavior in children: current status and future directions. *Psychol Bull* 192:187–203

Kazdin AE (1990), Psychotherapy for children and adolescents. *Annu Rev Psychol* 41:21–54

Kazdin AE, Siegel TC, Bass D (1992), Cognitive problem-solving skills training and parent management training in the treatment of antisocial behavior in children. *J Consult Clin Psychol* 60:733–747

Kohlberg L, Ricks D, Snarey J (1984), Childhood development as a predictor of adaptation in adulthood. *Genetic Psychology Monographs* 110:91–172

Moran GS, Fonagy P, Kurtz A, Bolton AM, Brook C (1991), A controlled study of the psychoanalytic treatment of brittle diabetes. *J Am Acad Child Psychiatry* 30:241–257

Mosteller F, Tukey JW (1977), *Data Analysis and Regression.* Reading, MA: Addison-Wesley

Patterson GR (1986), Performance models for antisocial boys. *Am Psychol* 41:432–444

Patterson GR, Capaldi D, Bank L (1991), An early starter model for predicting delinquency. In: *The Development and Treatment of Childhood Aggression*, eds DJ Pepler, KH Rubin. Hillsdale, NJ: Erlbaum, pp 139–168

Pekarik G, Stephenson LA (1988), Adult and child client differences in therapy dropout research. *J Clin Child Psychol* 17:316–321

Pepler DJ, Rubin KH eds (1991), *The Development and Treatment of Childhood Aggression*. Hillsdale, NJ: Erlbaum

Richman N, Stevenson J, Graham PJ (1982), *Pre-School to School: A Behavioural Study*. London: Academic Press

Robins LN (1981), Epidemiological approaches to natural history research: antisocial disorders in children. *J Am Acad Child Psychiatry* 20:566–580

Robins LN, Rutter M, eds (1990), *Straight and Devious Pathways from Childhood to Adulthood*. London: Oxford University Press

Rutter M (1989), Isle of Wight revisited: twenty-five years of child psychiatric epidemiology. *J Am Acad Child Adolesc Psychiatry* 28:633–653

Rutter M, Sandberg S (1985), Epidemiology of child psychiatric disorder: methodological issues and some substantive findings. *Child Psychiatry Hum Dev* 15:209–233

Schlessinger N (1984), On analyzability. In: *Psychoanalysis: The Vital Issues*, eds J Gedo, G Pollock. Madison, CT: International University Press, pp 249–274

Shaffer D, Gould MS, Brasie J et al. (1983), A children's global assessment scale (CGAS). *Arch Gen Psychiatry* 40:1228–1231

Shapiro T (1989), Psychoanalytic classification and empiricism with borderline personality disorder as a model. *J Consult Clin Psychol* 57:187–194

Shirk SR, Russell RL (1992), A reevaluation of estimates of child therapy effectiveness. *J Am Acad Child Adolesc Psychiatry* 31:703–710

Szapocznik J, Rio A, Murray E et al. (1989), Structural family versus psychodynamic child therapy for problematic hispanic boys. *J Consult Clin Psychol* 57:571–578

Tyson A, Sandler J (1971), Problems in the selection of patients for psychoanalysis: comments on the application of concepts of "indications," "suitability," and "analyzability." *Br J Med Psychol* 44:211–228

Wallerstein RS (1988), Assessment of structural change in psychoanalytic therapy and research. *J Am Psychoanal Assoc* 36: Supplement

Wallerstein RS (1989), The psychotherapy research project of the Menninger Foundation: an overview. *J Consult Clin Psychol* 57:195–205

Weber J, Bachrach H, Solomon M (1985), Factors associated with the outcome of psychoanalysis: report of the Columbia Psychoanalytic Center Research Project (II). *International Review of Psychoanalysis* 12:127–141

Weiss G, Hechtman LT (1986), *Hyperactive Children Grown Up*. New York: Guildford Press

Wiesz JR, Weiss B, Alicke MD, Klotz ML (1987), Effectiveness of psychotherapy with children and adolescents: meta-analytic findings for clinicians. *J Consult Clin Psychol* 55:542–549

Weisz JR, Donenberg GR, Han SS (1992), Does one effect size fit all? Child and Adolescent Psychotherapy Outcomes in Experiments and Clinics. Presentation at Workshop on Psychosocial Treatment Research on Child and Adolescent Disorders. National Institute of Mental Health, MD, October 1992

17

Treating Anxiety Disorders in Children: Results of a Randomized Clinical Trial

Philip C. Kendall
Temple University, Philadelphia

In this study a psychosocial treatment for 47 Ss (aged 9–13 years) with anxiety disorders was investigated. A 16-session cognitive-behavioral treatment was compared with a wait-list condition. Outcome was evaluated using child self-report, parent report, teacher report, cognitive assessment, and behavioral observations. Pretreatment-posttreatment changes and maintenance of gains at 1-year follow-up were examined. Results revealed that many treated Ss were found to be without a diagnosis at posttest and at follow-up and to be within normal limits on many measures. The child's perception of the therapeutic relationship and the therapist's perception of parental involvement were measured but were not related to outcome. Discussion focuses on characteristics of effective child therapy and the need for further research on treatment components and alternative treatment methods.

There is tremendous need for research on treatment and preventive strategies in the area of child psychopathology. A President's Commission

Reprinted with permission from the *Journal of Consulting and Clinical Psychology*, 1994, Vol. 62(1), 100–110. Copyright © 1994 by the American Psychological Association, Inc.

This research was supported by National Institute of Mental Health Grant MH 44042 to Philip C. Kendall. I thank Bonnie Howard, Martha Kane, Kevin Ronan, Fran Sessa, Lynne Siqueland, Alan Sockloff, Peter Mikulka, Serena Ashmore Callahan, Erika Brady, Tamar Elisas Chansky, Elizabeth Gosch, Elizabeth Kortlander, Margot Levin, Jennifer Panas MacDonald, Susan Panichelli, Margaret Rowe, Aaron Torrance, and Kimberli Hayden Treadwell. I also extend my appreciation to the cooperating agencies (e.g., CORA) and to the children and families who participated.

A portion of this article was presented as part of Philip C. Kendall's keynote address to the World Congress of Behavior Therapy, Brisbane, Australia, July 1992.

on Mental Health (1978) report suggested that 10–20% of children may require mental health services and called for additional research on child treatment strategies. Recent epidemiological data suggest that 15–22% of children have mental health problems that warrant treatment (Costello, 1990; Tuma, 1989; Zill & Schoenborn, 1990), but fewer than 20% of these children (Tuma, 1989) receive the needed treatment.

Adults seek treatment for the child who acts out or behaves aggressively, yet often overlook the child who withdraws socially. Nevertheless, internalizing problems such as anxiety, isolation, hypersensitivity, depression, and self-consciousness are seen in 10–20% of school-aged children (Johnson, 1979; Orvaschel & Weissman, 1986; Werry, 1986). Fears and anxieties in children are a common part of normal growth, but they are a serious concern when the severity or duration impinges negatively on the routine developmental challenges of childhood (Kendall, Chansky, et al., 1992). Studies have shown the negative impact of anxiety on academic work (e.g., Dweck & Wortman, 1982) and social adjustment (e.g., Strauss, Lease, Kazdin, Dulcan, & Last, 1989).

The limitations that childhood anxiety imposes have long-term implications for adult functioning (Kendall, 1992). A significant number of adults with anxiety disorders reported that they had suffered from separation anxiety or general anxiety symptoms as children (Last, Hersen, Kazdin, Francis, & Grubb, 1987; Last, Phillips, & Statfeld, 1987; Weissman, Leckman, Merikangas, Gammon, & Prusoff, 1974). In addition, older children with anxiety disorders report significantly higher levels of anxiety (and depression) than do younger children with the same diagnoses (Strauss, Lease, Last, & Francis, 1988), which suggests that the symptoms may worsen over time. Given the relationship between childhood anxiety disorders and adult psychological distress, it is essential to address these problems in children (Gittelman, 1986). Three childhood anxiety disorders are identified in the *Diagnostic and Statistical Manual of Mental Disorders* (3rd ed.—rev.; *DSM-III-R*; separation anxiety disorder, avoidant disorder, and overanxious disorder), and there is a pressing need to examine the effectiveness of treatments for children with these diagnoses.

Behavioral techniques have been effective in working with specific childhood fears and phobias (King, Hamilton, & Ollendick, 1988). However, although treatment and assessment of specific fears and phobias appear in the literature, these problems are present in only 3–4% of the population (Ollendick & Francis, 1988) and are rare in clinical referral; in contrast, generally fearful and anxious behavior is often seen (Last, Phillips, et al., 1987). There is no known randomized clinical trial of the effects of psychosocial intervention for children diagnosed as having anxiety disorders.

Outcome research with adults has suggested using specific treatment strategies to address particular problems (e.g., Beutler & Clarkin, 1990; Kiesler, 1971), yet similar research on child therapy is lacking (Institute of Medicine, 1989; Kendall & Morris, 1991). The literature on behavioral techniques with adults has demonstrated efficacy in treating specific fears or phobias, but less research has been conducted on the use of these methods with children (Hatzenbuehler & Schroeder, 1978; Ollendick, 1986; Ollendick & Francis, 1988). Emotive imagery, desensitization, modeling, contingency management, shaping, self-control training, and in vivo exposure are seen as effective and important components of an integrated treatment plan.

Researchers have investigated the role of cognition in anxiety and have suggested implications for treatment. Empirical work suggests that thoughts relating to fear of threat or evaluation by others are common in anxious persons (Beck & Emery, 1986; Ingram, Kendall, Smith, Donnell, & Ronan, 1987; Kendall, Howard, & Epps, 1988). Anxious adults also show excessive self-focused attention (Kendall & Ingram, 1987; MacLeod, Mathews, & Tata, 1986; Sarason, 1975). The literature on adults indicates that there is a need to evaluate cognitive techniques in treating anxiety disorders (Clark & Beck, 1988; Wilson, 1985). Limited research has addressed cognition in childhood anxiety (Kendall & Chansky, 1991), but the need for further investigation is frequently suggested (Barrios, Hartman, & Shigetomi, 1981; Morris & Kratochwill, 1983; Ollendick & Francis, 1988). Zatz and Chassin (1983, 1985) found that in both laboratory and natural test-taking conditions, highly anxious children showed more task-debilitating cognition during testing, including more negative self-evaluation, more off-task thoughts, and less positive self-evaluation. Prins (1986) found that in a natural fear-provoking setting, children's self-speech was significantly related to their reported level of fear. Highly anxious children reported more negative self-speech, including a preoccupation with fear of harm and negative task expectancies.

Studies of cognitive–behavioral treatment for childhood anxiety (for a review see Kendall, Chansky, et al., 1992) have focused on nighttime fears, fear of dental or medical procedures, evaluation anxiety, and a few clinical case studies. Most researchers have reported treatment success over control groups when using a coping-skills approach that combines self-instructional techniques with behavioral techniques such as in vivo exposure, imagery, relaxation, and contingent reward. For example, Kanfer, Karoly, and Newman (1975) used self-control procedures to treat children's nighttime fears. Kanfer et al. compared two types of verbal controlling responses: competence self-statements and stimulus statements. Both groups improved over the neutral group, with the competence group showing the greatest increase in tolerance of the dark. Despite the call for research on a cognitive–behavioral treatment for more generally anxious children (e.g., Strauss et al., 1988), few reports have appeared. Using four diagnosed cases of children with overanxious disorder, Kane and Kendall (1989) reported results from a multiple-baseline design that supported the efficacy of a cognitive–behavioral program. These results are promising.

The present study is the first randomized clinical trial investigating the effectiveness of a cognitive–behavioral therapy with children diagnosed with a childhood anxiety disorder. It was hypothesized that the active treatment condition would produce significant change in the dependent variables in contrast to the wait-list control condition. Improvement was expected to be across measures and maintained at 1-year follow-up.

METHOD

Subjects

Forty-seven children (aged 9–13 years) with anxiety disorders who were referred from multiple community sources served as subjects (27 received active treatment; 20 were wait-list controls). For the 27 treatment subjects, 52% were boys, 48% were girls, 78% were Whites, 22% were African Americans, 52% were aged 11–13 years, and 48% were aged 9–10 years. Control subjects were treated after the wait-list period. For the full sample, 60% were boys, 76% were Whites, and 53% were aged 11–13 years. Treatment and wait-list subjects did not differ significantly on these variables (see Results).

Subjects received a primary anxiety disorder diagnosis (i.e., overanxious disorder, $n = 30$; separation anxiety disorder, $n = 8$; avoidant disorder, $n = 9$) on the basis of separate structured clinical interviews that were conducted separately with both the parent and the subject. When parent and child reports differed, diagnoses were based on parental reports. Children whose primary diagnosis was a specific phobia(s) were not included; children who had diagnosable specific phobias as secondary problems were included. Thirty-two percent of the subjects were comorbid with depression; 15% with attention-deficit hyperactivity disorder, 13% with oppositional defiant disorder, 2% with conduct disorder, and 60% with simple phobias. Children were excluded if they had an IQ below 80, had a disabling physical condition, displayed psychotic symptoms, or were currently using antianxiety medications. Randomization was used in both the assignment of subjects to treatment conditions and the assignment of therapists to clients.

Setting and Personnel

Therapy was provided by seven doctoral candidates (1 man and 6 women) within the Child and Adolescent Anxiety Disorders Clinic of the Division of Clinical Psychology, Temple University.

Measures

Multimethod assessment, as recommended in the child therapy literature (Kazdin, 1986; Kendall & Morris, 1991; Ollendick, 1986), was used. *Structured diagnostic interview.* The Anxiety Disorder Interview Schedule for Children (ADIS; Silverman, 1987) and the ADIS–P (for parents) are structured interview schedules for the diagnosis of childhood anxiety disorders that allow the assessor to screen out other disorders and are consistent with *DSM-III-R* criteria.

Children's self-report measures

REVISED CHILDREN'S MANIFEST ANXIETY SCALES (RCMAS). A measure of the child's chronic anxiety (trait), these scales consist of 37 items, 11 of which compose the Lie scale (Reynolds & Richmond, 1978). The scales reveal three anxiety factors: Physiological Symptoms, Worry and Oversensitivity, and Concentration. This measure has demonstrated validity, and national reliability and normative data are available (Reynolds & Paget, 1982).

THE STATE–TRAIT ANXIETY INVENTORY FOR CHILDREN (STAIC). The STAIC (Spielberger, 1973) includes two 20-item self-report scales that measure both enduring tendencies to experience anxiety (A-Trait) and temporal and situational variations in levels of perceived anxiety (A-State). Normative, reliability, and validity data are available. In factor-analytic studies, the A-State has been found to be bipolar. One pole includes worry, feelings of tension, and nervousness, and the other includes pleasantness, relaxation, and happiness. Two A-Trait factors emerged (Finch, Kendall, & Montgomery, 1974).

FEAR SURVEY SCHEDULE FOR CHILDREN—REVISED (FSSC-R). Ollendick (1978) revised the 80-item, 5-point scale (Scherer & Nakamura, 1968) to create a 3-point scale that assesses specific fears in children. Eight fear content categories are measured. The scale has shown good internal consistency and test–retest reliability. Normative data are available.

CHILDREN'S DEPRESSION INVENTORY (CDI). Developed by Kovacs (1981), the CDI includes 27 items related to the cognitive, affective, and behavioral signs of depression. Each item contains three choices, and children select the one that best characterizes them during the last 2 weeks. The scale has high internal consistency, has moderate test–retest reliability, and correlates in expected directions with measures of related constructs such as self-esteem, negative cognitive attributions, and hopelessness (Kazdin, French, Unis, Esveldt-Dawson, & Sherick, 1983; Kovacs, 1981; Saylor, Finch, Spirito, & Bennett, 1984; see review by Kendall, Cantwell, & Kazdin, 1989). Normative data are available (Finch, Saylor, & Edwards, 1985).

COPING QUESTIONNAIRE—CHILD (CQ-C). The CQ-C was designed to assess changes in children's perceived ability to manage specific anxiety-provoking situations. For the assessment to be relevant, situationally based, and individualized, the diagnostician chose, from the information in the diagnostic interview, three areas of difficulty that were specific to each child. Children rated their ability to cope on a 7-point scale that ranged from *not at all able to help myself* (1) to *completely able to help myself feel comfortable* (7). Test–retest reliability for 20 subjects with anxiety disorders was .46 over a 2-month interval.

Cognitive assessment. The Children's Negative Affectivity Self-Statement Questionnaire (NASSQ) includes self-statements that children endorse on a scale ranging from *not at all* (1) to *all the time* (5), which represents the frequency with which each thought occurred during the past week (Ronan, Kendall, & Rowe, in press). Within the NASSQ, separate versions of anxious self-talk for 7–10 year-olds (11 items) and 11–15 year-olds (31 items) were developed. Scores for the two age groups were converted to a uniform metric and then combined to form a single anxious self-talk score. Test-retest reliability for 20 subjects with anxiety disorders over a 2-month interval was .73.

Parent measures

CHILD BEHAVIOR CHECKLIST (CBCL; ACHENBACH & EDELBROCK, 1983). The CBCL is a 118-item scale that assesses an array of behavioral problems and social competencies. The items are scored on a scale that ranges from not true (0) to *very true* or *often true* (2). The checklist provides scores on several factors or behavior problem areas and identifies internalizing and externalizing problems. Normative data are available. Because of the relevance to the present sample, the CBCL Social scale and a CBCL Health scale (i.e., specific health-related items selected for examination in this study; CBCL Items 24, 30, 56 (a–g), 61, 100, and 108) were scored and analyzed separately.

STATE–TRAIT ANXIETY INVENTORY FOR CHILDREN—MODIFICATION OF TRAIT VERSION FOR PARENTS (STAIC-A-Trait-P). The Strauss (1987) modification of the trait version of the STAIC was used as a parent rating of the child's trait anxiety.

Teacher report. The primary teacher for each child completed the Child Behavior Checklist—Teacher Report Form (Achenbach & Edelbrock,

1983) to provide a picture of the child's classroom functioning. Because children often changed grades over the course of the program, the primary class room teacher often varied across assessments (i.e., from first assessment to 1-year follow-up).

Behavioral observations. Seven observational codes (adapted from Glennon & Weisz, 1978) were used: *gratuitous verbalizations* (e.g., stating a physical complaint, desire to leave, dislike for the task, self-doubt); *gratuitous body movements* (e.g., leg kicking or shaking, rocking body, biting lips, shaking or wiggling foot or hand); *trembling voice* (e.g., shaking speech, stuttering, volume shifts); *avoiding task* (e.g., leaving the room, not talking, sitting down); *absence of eye contact* (e.g., not looking at camera for entire observational interval); *fingers in mouth* (e.g., biting fingernails, moving hand to lips); and *body rigidity* (e.g., holding parts of body unusually stiff, clenching jaw, clasping arms around body, clenching fists, locking knees). Observers rated the subjects on the following three scales: overall anxiety, which ranged from *no signs of anxiety* (no tension, no gratuitous behavior, no avoidance; 1) to *subject appears to be in crisis* (5); fearful facial expression, which ranged from *no tears, tension, or biting of lips* (1) to *tearful, facial tension, clenching of jaws* (5); and problematic performance, which ranged from *a composed, nonavoidant self-description* (1) to *an avoidance of task and/or disjointed and difficult-to-understand self-description* (5).

In-therapy measure. The Child's Perception of Therapeutic Relationship (CPTR), a 7-item, 5-point scale was developed for assessing the child's perception of the therapeutic relationship. Four items relate to the child's liking, feeling close to, feeling comfortable with, talking to, and wanting to spend time with the therapist. The three remaining items refer to the quality and closeness of the therapeutic relationship. The scale ranged from *not at all* (1) to *very* (5). To examine the role of the therapeutic relationship in treatment outcome (Kendall & Morris, 1991; Strupp & Hadley, 1979), this measure was administered by a diagnostician (not the therapist) at posttreatment.

Extra-therapy measure. Pilot data suggested that families vary in the degree to which they are involved (in both helpful and interfering ways) with their child's treatment. At completion of treatment, the therapist rated parental involvement on the basis of the amount of contact with the parent(s), the degree of beneficial parental involvement, and the degree of parental interference.

Procedure

Within a week of referral, clinic staff contacted parents and arranged an intake evaluation. Parents and the child signed informed consent forms, participated in the structured interview, and completed numerous questionnaires, and the child performed the behavioral observation task. Behavioral observations were taken from videotapes of the child's performance at intake. Performance was in response to the request to "Tell us about yourself." Subjects were directed to take the next 5 min and to speak toward the camera. Sample topics (e.g., favorite sport) were provided, and the diagnostician left the room.

Following the intake and the determination of a diagnosis, accepted subjects were randomly assigned to either the 16-week cognitive–behavioral therapy condition or the 8-week wait-list control condition.[1] Treated subjects were randomly assigned to therapists, After the 8-week waiting period, the wait-list control subjects were randomly assigned to therapists. Parents and teachers were required to provide completed measures before therapy began.

During intervention, treated subjects received an average of 17 (16 to 20), 50–60-min sessions, typically meeting once a week. Variations in session schedules were made (e.g., holidays, illness) as needed.

Treatment manual. The 85-page treatment manual (Kendall, Kane, Howard, & Siqueland, 1990) describes the goals and strategies that were used for each treatment session. However, a flexible and clinically sensitive application requires some adjustments (e.g., Dobson & Shaw, 1988; Kendall, Kortlander, Chansky, & Brady, 1992). Several aspects of the standard treatment required honing because of client age, intellectual ability, and family situation. The treatment manual was applied flexibly.

Treatment materials. Treatment materials paralleled those in the *Coping Cat Workbook* (Kendall, 1990). These materials include session-by-session content as well as content-related and therapeutic tasks. In a variety of entertaining formats, the treatment materials facilitate interest and involvement in treatment goals such as recognition of anxious cues, development of coping plans, and the provision of rewards. To help reinforce and generalize the skills, therapists assigned homework tasks (referred to as STIC tasks— Show That I Can). A separate notebook (e.g., *The Coping Cat Notebook*) was used by the child to complete the assignments.

Treatment method: Cognitive–behavioral therapy. Children in the cognitive-behavioral treatment condition received individual therapy that included assisting the child in (a) recognizing anxious feelings and somatic reactions to anxiety, (b) clarifying cognition in anxiety-provoking situations (i.e., unrealistic or negative attributions and expectations), (c) developing a plan to help cope with the situation (i.e., modifying anxious self-talk into coping

---

[1] The methodologically preferred 16-week wait-list control condition was deemed too long to hold diagnosed cases without providing treatment (see the Discussion section).

self-talk as well as determining what coping actions might be effective), and (d) evaluating performance and administering self-reinforcement as appropriate.

Behavioral training strategies with demonstrated efficacy such as modeling, in vivo exposure, role playing, relaxation training, and contingent reinforcement were used. Throughout the sessions, therapists used social reinforcement to encourage and reward the children, and the children were encouraged to verbally reinforce their own successful coping. Also, the children practiced using the coping skills when anxiety-provoking situations arose at home or in school.

The first eight sessions were training sessions in which each of the basic concepts was introduced individually and was followed by practice and reinforcement of the skill. Session 1 consisted of building a rapport with the child and collecting specific information about the kinds of situations and experiences during which the child feels anxious and regarding how the child responds to that anxiety. Session 2 involved teaching the child to identify 2 different types of feelings. Session 3 focused on constructing a hierarchy of anxiety-provoking situations so that the children could distinguish anxious reactions from others and could identify their own particular somatic responses. Session 4 comprised training the children to relax by using a personalized relaxation cassette outside of the sessions. (After Session 3, a parent meeting was held to restate the treatment goals, share impressions and ideas, receive parental input on particular problem areas for each child, and encourage parental cooperation with treatment.) Session 5 consisted of teaching the child to recognize and assess self-talk during anxious situations and to reduce anxiety-provoking self-talk. Session 6 focused on emphasizing coping strategies such as coping self-talk and verbal self-direction, as well as developing appropriate actions to aid in coping with anxious situations. Session 7 involved enabling the child to self-evaluate and self-reward, and Session 8 comprised reviewing concepts and skills.

During the second eight sessions the child practiced the new skills by using both imaginary and in vivo experiences with situations that varied from low stress–low anxiety to high stress–high anxiety and that were specific to each child. For example, in Session 9 the child practiced the newly learned skills (i.e., use of somatic responses as cues to anxious arousal, recognition and modification of anxious self-talk, development of coping strategies, and self-evaluation with reinforcement) in non-stressful and then in low-anxiety situations that began with imaginal experiences and progressed to in vivo exposure. Therapist modeling and role-plays were used. In Sessions 10–13 the child was exposed to imaginal and real situations that caused increasing levels of anxiety. The therapist demonstrated the use of anxious arousal as a cue to apply strategies for coping and encouraged the child to do the same through role play and reinforcement. In Sessions 14 and 15, children practiced in very stressful situations. In addition, children began to prepare a "commercial" or individualized project (i.e., rap song, TV advertisement, radio spot, poem) that was often videotaped or audiotaped and aimed at informing other children about how to cope with distressing anxiety. The last session was used to discuss the therapy experience, to review the skills, and to encourage the child to consider how to apply the skills in everyday life. The child, using available equipment, produced the "commercial" and was given a taped copy to take home.

Wait-list control. Children assigned to the wait-list control condition were given the same measures as those in the treatment condition at the beginning and at the end of the 8-week wait period. All control children and their parents were asked whether they sought alternative treatment during the waiting period, and analyses include only those subjects whose wait-list status had integrity. All wait-list control subjects who continued to meet diagnostic criteria at the post–wait-list assessment received the treatment at the end of the waiting period.

Treatment integrity. The treatment manipulation check involved listening to randomly selected portions of randomly selected cases from all of the audiotaped sessions. A treatment integrity checklist was used. Tapes were chosen at random for each child–therapist combination.

RESULTS

Reliabilities

Initial diagnostic reliabilities (Kappa; Cohen, 1977) were > 85%. During training, diagnosticians resolved disagreements after reobserving the videotape and discussing individual judgments. Analyses of ongoing diagnostic reliabilities demonstrated that, on the basis of six random interviews for four pairs of diagnosticians, there was 100% agreement on all diagnoses for three of the four pairs. For the fourth pair there was 83% agreement for simple phobia and 100% agreement for all other diagnoses.

Behavioral observation codes were assessed as having very good reliability. The following are the Kappa coefficients: gratuitous verbalizations (.91), gratuitous body movements (.93), trembling voice (.79), avoiding task (.89), absence of eye contact (.92), fingers in mouth (.91), and body rigidity

(.89). Interrater agreements for the global rating scales (Pearson *r*s) were .89 (overall anxiety), .84 (fearful facial expression), and .82 (problematic performance).

Group Comparability

Pretreatment differences across conditions were examined by means of one-way analysis of variance (ANOVA) tests or chi-square tests. Variables compared across groups included age, gender, and pretreatment dependent variables. For gender, race, age, and the dependent variables, analyses in which subjects in the treatment condition were compared with those in the wait-list condition resulted in nonsignificant differences, which indicates that the subjects were demographically similar in the two conditions. Similar analyses were conducted for parents' marital status, fathers' level of education, household income, and mothers' and fathers' (separate) levels of depression and anxiety. None of the analyses indicated significant differences.

For the assessment of sample representativeness, ANOVAs and chi squares were used to compare the remainers (n = 47) and the dropouts (n = 13) in terms of age, gender, race, frequency of diagnoses (overanxious disorder, separation anxiety disorder, and avoidant disorder), pretreatment scores on self-report measures, and parents' ratings. Teacher ratings were not used because most dropouts did not provide teacher report form (TRF) data for the CBCL. For all measures, there were no significant differences between remainers and dropouts.

Therapist Comparability

Because therapy was provided by several different therapists, the effectiveness of sessions conducted by the different therapists by comparing both gain scores (pretreatment to posttreatment) and maintenance scores (posttreatment to follow-up) was examined. When comparing individual therapists, it was found that effectiveness did not differ significantly on 27 of the 28 measures. Moreover, analysis of the CPTR scores revealed nonsignificant differences across therapists. Therapist experience (i.e., first clients, second clients) was also found to have nonsignificant relationships (in 23 of 24 instances) with gain and maintenance scores.

Treatment Integrity

The strategies called for in the first eight sessions and the second eight sessions were indeed used in those sessions. There were no instances where other forms of therapeutic intervention were used in place of the treatment manual (although, in rare cases, parents were referred for concurrent couples or marital therapy). The treatment manual was not implemented in a rigid fashion but in a flexible manner that maintained programmatic strategies while permitting individualization on the basis of each child's needs. Accordingly, the independent variable (treatment) was deemed to have integrity.

Treatment Outcome

The effects of treatment were analyzed by means of a 2 (treatment vs. wait-list; between groups) $\times$ 2 (assessment periods; within groups) mixed factorial ANOVA. Because dependent variables were not viewed as multiple measures of a single variable (not interested in the linear combination of dependent measures), MANOVAs were not used.[2] The means and standard deviations of the various measures are presented in Table 1, and changes over time for the two groups are presented in Figures 1, 2, and 3. Where significant main effects and significant interactions were found, only the interaction effects were interpeted.[3]

Analyses of the RCMAS revealed a significant Trial $\times$ Condition interaction, $F(1, 43) = 17.09$, $p < .0001$, a finding similar to that obtained with the STAIC(A-State), $F(1, 45) = 8.55$, $p < .005$, and the STAIC(A-Trait), $F(1, 45) = 9.65$, $p < .003$, and the FSSC–R, $F(1, 42) = 4.68$, $p < .04$ (see Figure 1).

In terms of the children's ability to cope with their most dreaded situations, changes on the CQ–C revealed a significant Conditions $\times$ Trials interaction, $F(1, 40) = 8.52$, $p < .01$. Interaction effects on the NASSQ were significant, $F(1, 42) = 6.05$, $p < .02$. The CDI was consistent with the other dependent measures: Conditions $\times$ Trial interaction, $F(1, 44) = 7.60$, $p < .008$.

---

[2] There are clusters of dependent variables where the linear combination would be of interest (e.g., child self-report measures and parent reports). Accordingly, multiple analyses of variance (MANOVAs) for these clusters of variables were undertaken. As expected, results of MANOVAs for the cluster of children's self-reports and parents' reports indicated significant interactions between Trials and the Treatment Condition (both $ps < .01$).

[3] The present results include some heterogeneity of subjects' diagnoses, a situation that can add to the generalizability of the findings to children with different anxiety disorders. However, one could ask whether the effects of the present treatment were specific to the group of children receiving the overanxious disorder diagnosis. Analyses were conducted to examine the effects for only those subjects whose primary diagnosis was overanxious disorder. The results of 2 (overanxious disorder vs other anxiety disorder) $\times$ 2 (pre- vs. posttreatment) mixed factorial analyses of variance using all of the same dependent variables as in the main study indicated that none of the interactions were significant. Thus, treatment effectivness was neither specific to nor differential for children with overanxious disorder.

TABLE 1
Means and Standard Deviations for the Various Measures

	Treatment			Wait-List Control	
Measures	Pretest	Posttest	Follow-Up[a]	Pretest	Pretest 2
	Child Self-Report				
RCMAS					
M	54.82	41.43	40.92	52.88	51.94
SD	9.25	10.9	10.63	10.59	13.50
STAIC					
A-trait					
M	54.63	36.70	36.29	52.20	46.05
SD	10.39	13.62	11.82	11.65	8.88
A-state					
M	55.19	45.07	45.769	53.85	54.85
SD	10.76	12.61	10.26	10.65	9.01
FSSC–R					
M	138.36	112.92	107.43	132.42	123.37
SD	23.49	28.57	19.00	17.77	25.92
CQ–C					
M	3.68	5.65	5.66	3.69	4.37
SD	1.20	0.88	0.97	1.80	1.20
CDI					
M	11.57	5.50	4.24	10.44	9.28
SD	8.12	5.82	6.50	8.60	7.88
NASSQ					
M	61.18	43.37	41.00	55.57	52.54
SD	23.80	14.69	15.41	25.82	20.06
	Behavioral Observations				
TBO					
M	1.23	0.69	0.80	0.86	0.99
SD	0.10	0.10	0.10	0.12	0.14
	Parent Report				
CBCL					
Internalizing					
M	70.69	58.07	58.78	71.61	69.33
SD	7.03	10.32	9.84	7.74	7.43
Social					
M	40.27	44.11	46.16	43.82	39.52
SD	10.23	9.18	7.19	9.61	10.16
Health					
M	3.79	1.50	2.16	5.25	4.54
SD	2.90	1.73	1.77	2.65	3.08
Externalizing					
M	58.64	51.36	50.19	60.72	60.33
SD	8.78	9.75	10.73	10.10	9.29
STAIC-A-trait–P					
M	65.05	59.00	40.94	69.36	63.55
SD	6.64	9.55	9.50	6.83	12.61

TABLE 1 (*Continued*)

Measures	Treatment			Wait-List Control	
	Pretest	Posttest	Follow-Up[a]	Pretest	Pretest 2
	Teacher Report				
TCBCL					
Internalizing[b]					
M	67.41	59.00	59.53	69.36	63.55
SD	12.68	13.51	12.67	6.83	12.61
Internalizing[c]					
M	74.27	64.36	59.35	69.36	63.54
SD	10.04	13.39	9.45	6.83	12.61
Externalizing					
M	56.06	52.18	51.60	56.27	51.09
SD	6.02	9.24	7.00	8.11	6.38

Note. RCMAS = Revised Children's Manifest Anxiety Scales; STAIC = State–Trait Anxiety Inventory for Children; FSSC-R = Fear Survey Schedule for Children—Revised; CQ–C = Coping Questionnaire for Children; CDI = Children's Depression Inventory; NASSQ = Children's Negative Affectivity Self-Statement Questionnaire; TBO = total behavioral observations; CBCL = Child Behavior Checklist; STAIC-A-TRAIT-P = State–Trait Anxiety Inventory for Children—Parent form; TCBCL = Teacher Report Form of the Child Behavior Checklist. The number of subjects varies because of occasional missing data.
[a] Follow-up data are for 38 of the 47 treated subjects (both those subjects treated directly and those treated after serving as wait-list controls).
[b] These means and standard deviations are for all subjects. These are the data depicted in Figure 2.
[c] These data are for those subjects whose Teacher Report Form Internalizing T scores were >60.

Parent reports, using the CBCL Internalizing T scores, revealed a significant Condition × Trial interaction, $F(1, 44) = 11.36$, $p < .002$. Similarly, the parents' CBCL Social Scale T score revealed a significant interaction, $F(1, 41) = 9.31$, $p < .004$, as did the Health items, $F(1, 44) = 3.04$, $p < .05$. Changes on parents' Externalizing T scores also resulted in a significant interaction, $F(1, 44) = 8.64$, $p < .005$. Parent reports, using the STAIC–P evidenced a significant Condition × Trial interaction, $F(1, 37) = 18.31$, $p < .0001$.

Analyses of the TRF Internalizing ratings revealed a significant trials effect, $F(1, 26) = 12.08$, $p < .01$, and a nonsignificant interaction ($F < 1$; see Figure 2). In addition, because some of the children with anxiety disorders did not display distress in the classroom (TRF Internalizing T scores were in the normal range), analyses of the teacher ratings were conducted for those subjects (both wait-list and treatment) who, at the preassessment period, had an elevated Internalizing T score ($T > 60$). Again, there was a

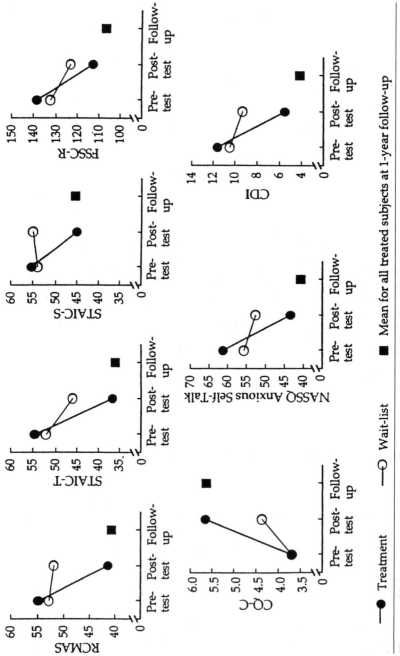

Figure 1. Changes on child self-report measures for treated and wait-list subjects. RCMAS = Revised Children's Manifest Anxiety Scales; STAIC–T = State-Trait Anxiety Inventory for Children—Trait Anxiety; STAIC–S = State-Trait Anxiety Inventory for Children—State Anxiety; FSSC–R = The Fear Survey Schedule for Children—Revised; CQ–C = Coping Questionnaire—Child; NASSQ = Children's Negative Affectivity Self-Statement Questionnaire; CDI = Children's Depression Inventory.

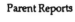

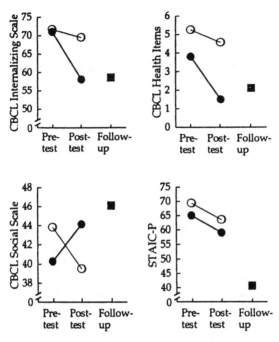

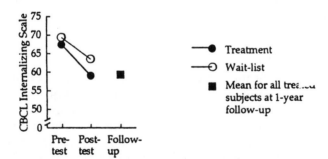

Figure 2. Changes on parent and teacher reports for treated and wait-list subjects. (CBCL = Child Behavior Checklist; STAIC–P = State-Trait Anxiety Inventory for Children—Modification of Trait Version for Parents.)

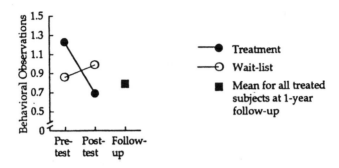

Figure 3. Changes on total behavioral observations for treated and wait-list subjects.

significant trials effect, $F(1, 20) = 10.14$, $p < .005$, and a nonsignificant interaction ($F < 1$). Regarding TRF Externalizing T scores, there was a significant trials effect, $F(1, 26) = 10.93$, $p < .03$, and a nonsignificant interaction. It should be noted, however, that the means for all subjects were well within the normal range (Ts > 50, < 60).

Behavioral observation data were examined for evidence of changes that were due to treatment. Using 2 (treatment vs. wait-list) × 2 (trials) ANOVAs (following arcsine transformation of the observational data), no significant interactions among the separate behavioral codes and ratings (Fs < 1) were found. Because the code frequencies were low, a total behavioral observation score was computed. Analysis of the total behavioral observation data revealed a significant interaction, $F(1, 25) = 7.11$, $p < .01$, which is depicted in Figure 3.

Clinical Significance

Clinically significant improvement, defined as changes that return deviant subjects to within nondeviant limits, can be identified using normative comparisons (Kendall & Grove, 1988). To be considered "clinically significant," improvement had to meet a minimum criterion (e.g., RCMAS T score < 70). It should be noted that the normative mean for an adult sample often covers the various ages of the subjects, whereas for different-aged children the normative mean changes across ages. Accordingly, examinations of whether a specific child met criteria for clinically meaningful change were conducted using the mean appropriate for that specific child's age.

According to parent CBCL Internalizing *T* scores, at the end of treatment 14 of the 17 subjects whose initial *T* scores were above 70 were within the cutoff range. Fully 60% of the treated cases, as evidenced by TRF Internalizing *T* scores, were returned to within nondeviant limits at the end of treatment. The parent structured interview data (diagnoses) showed that 64% of the treated cases did not qualify for a diagnosis at the end of treatment. The child's diagnostic interview data (diagnoses) revealed that 64% of those treated no longer met diagnostic criteria. Of the subjects in the wait-list condition, only 1 did not qualify for an anxiety disorder diagnosis after the wait period.

RCMAS norms (an illustrative anxiety self-report measure) revealed that a significantly greater number of the treated subjects, as compared with wait-list cases, showed clinically significant change, $t(45) = 2.67$, $p < .02$. The CDI (a nonanxiety self-report measure) also revealed a significantly greater number of treated subjects, as compared with wait-list control subjects, who showed clinically significant change, $t(45) = 2.83$, $p < .01$.

It should be noted that in another study (Gosch, Kendall, Panas, & Bross, 1991), the behavioral codes did not discriminate between children diagnosed as having anxiety disorders and children who did not meet criteria for a diagnosis. As a result, it is not meaningful to use the same codes to examine whether treated cases return to a frequency of behavior that is nondisturbed.

Maintenance: 1-Year Follow-Up

Maintenance for 38 of the 47 treated subjects (9 were not available) was examined by means of one way analyses (within subjects) across three assessment periods (pretreatment, posttreatment, and 1-year follow-up). Post hoc analyses of significant *F* ratios used Scheffé tests. The 1-year follow-up means for treated subjects appear in Figures 1–3.

For the RCMAS, STAIC(A-State), STAIC(A-Trait), and FSSC–R, there were significant changes over time, with the present statistical tests for maintenance revealing that the posttreatment and follow-up means did not differ significantly. Similarly, for the NASSQ (anxious self-talk) and the CDI, the reductions that were seen at posttreatment were maintained at 1-year follow-up. With reference to the CQ–C, there were significant improvements in coping that were maintained at follow-up.

Parent CBCL data produced results consistent with the children's self-report data: Group means at follow-up were improved from pretreatment and were not significantly different from posttreatment (i.e., CBCL Inter-

nalizing *T* score, STAIC-A-Trait–P). Similarly, analysis of the total behavioral observation score revealed that treatment-produced gains were
maintained at 1-year follow-up.

Scores for the CPTR and for parental involvement were correlated with
gains (from pre- to posttreatment) and maintenance (posttreatment to
follow-up). In general, the CPTR was not a significant predictor of change
or maintenance. Of the 7 (of 24) significant correlations, 5 were with other
self-report measures. The only multisource significant correlations indicated that the CPTR predicted parent ratings on the STAIC-A-Trait–P,
both gains and maintenance. The higher the CPTR the greater the gains
and maintenance seen by parents on their STAIC-A-Trait–P ratings. The
overall high scores on the CPTR (M = 3.83, SD = 1.14) suggest that the
therapeutic relationships were generally rated as quite positive and that
the high scores may have truncated the range and limited any predictive
relationships.

Although most child clients gave their therapist a high rating for a positive relationship, it was possible to select 7 cases where the relationship
score was approximately one standard deviation below the mean (i.e., <
20). There were no significant differences on any of the parent or teacher
variables when the outcomes for these 7 cases were compared with the
remaining ones for all dependent variables. However, on the child self-
report measures, 3 of 7 measures (i.e., RCMAS, STAIC-A-Trait, and CDI)
showed significantly less improvement (p < .05) for those cases where the
therapeutic relationship was lower: Fs = 4.24, 3.97, and 4.07, respectively.

The therapists' ratings (1–7) of parent involvement were examined for 3
individual items: contact, interference, and beneficial involvement. The
means (Ms = 4.19, 3.44, and 3.16), standard deviations, and ranges indicated that the full range of the rating scale was used. For the amount of contact, only 1 of 24 correlations was significant; for the amount of parental
interference, not one of the correlations was significant. For the amount of
beneficial parental involvement, as rated by therapists, four correlations
were significant. Greater beneficial parental involvement was associated
with greater gains on two children's self-reports (STAIC-A-Trait, r = −.54;
FSSC-R, r = −.41) and the parents' CBCL (r = −.70). There was also a
significant relationship with the maintenance of significant improvement
on self-reported state anxiety (STAIC-A-State, r = .53).

DISCUSSION

Taken together, the present results provide support for the effectiveness
of a cognitive–behavioral intervention for the treatment of anxiety disorders in children. The outcomes of the examination of clinical significance

further buttress the support for the intervention, and the 1-year follow-up data suggest the maintenance of the treatment-produced gains. Given that remainers did not differ significantly from dropouts, that the sample contained male and female as well as African-American and White subjects, and that the child's perception of the therapeutic relationship and the therapists' perception of the parents' involvement were not major predictors of outcome, it seems reasonable to conclude that the primary source of change was the intervention.

The child self-report data and the parent data concur in supporting the beneficial effects of the intervention. However, these respondents were aware of the status (treatment vs. wait-list) of the child and could suggest that expectations of outcome contributed to the reported findings. The fact that the teacher data did not provide outright confirmation of the treatment effects is consistent with an expectational explanation. However teachers often did not view the children with anxiety disorders as having a problem in the classroom initially. In contrast to treatments for externalizing behavior problems, for which teacher reports are an important data source for outcome evaluation, teacher reports for internalizing problems may be less sensitive. It is important that the behavioral observation data, obtained from observers blind to condition, controvert the teacher data and indicate that the positive change reported by both parents and children was accompanied by visible reductions in anxious behavior.

Despite the apparent effectiveness of the overall cognitive-behavioral program, additional research is needed if one wishes to address specific questions. For example, similar to the segments of stress inoculation (Meichenbaum, 1986), the two halves of the treatment were markedly different (e.g., education vs. graduated exposure). Are the positive effects reported herein due to the sequence in which the two halves were provided (education preceding exposure)? Or would the effects from treatments that provide only the educational portion of the treatment be comparable to those from treatments that provide only the exposure portion of the treatment? One could similarly ask about the relative contributions of the cognitive and the behavioral components of the therapy. Nevertheless, the existence of multiple treatment components within the cognitive (e.g., changing self-talk, building coping expectation) and the behavioral (e.g., relaxation in vivo exposure) portions does not permit a determination of the specific treatment components that were active. Although there are data to support the utility of the behavioral components for treating specific fears (cf. King et al., 1988), additional research, designed specifically to address the question of the contributions of the various components of treatment for children diagnosed as having anxiety disorders, is much needed.

The present anxiety-focused treatment had a desirable effect on children's self-reported depressive symptomatology (e.g., the CDI). Given the high incidence of the comorbidity of anxiety and depression in children (Brady & Kendall, 1992), it is likely that alleviating anxious emotional distress had the correlated effect on dysphoric mood. A related question is whether an anxiety-focused intervention can remediate depressive diagnoses. Although the present sample included subjects who were comorbid for depression, the sample size was too small to permit statistical comparisons. Treatments for depressed children (e.g., Stark, Rouse, & Livingston, 1991) might include evaluations of changes in anxiety, and future treatment–outcome research should include an examination of the effects for children with anxiety disorders who are and are not comorbid with depression (see Kendall, Kortlander, et al., 1992).

The therapy was essentially a child-focused intervention. Nevertheless, there were numerous parent contacts: Parents were involved in the assessment and evaluation process, and parent participation in therapy ranged from minimal (e.g., a parents' meeting after three sessions) to somewhat active (e.g., phone calls, many contacts in the waiting room). Although parents were not coclients, as would be the case in systems family therapy, they were active collaborators. The preliminary assessment of parental involvement, based on therapists' ratings, yielded only modest suggestions of a meaningful relationship to outcome. A more rigorous test to unravel the role of parental involvement in the outcome of child therapy (Kendall & Morris, 1991) would require a direct manipulation of varying degrees of parental involvement (e.g., child vs. family treatment). Relatedly, parent training (Fauber & Long, 1991) may be an efficacious ancillary treatment. A study conducted in Australia (Heard, Dadds, & Rapee, 1992) provides some support for this notion: The same cognitive–behavioral treatment provided and evaluated in the present study was found to be effective and, on some measures, enhanced by the inclusion of a parent training component. More generally, there remains the need to study the efficacy of a child- versus a family-focused treatment.

By comparing a specific treatment with a wait-list condition, the present study cannot rule out the potential effects of nonspecific factors, such as the impact of a positive child-therapist relationship. Indeed, therapists in the present study were rated highly by their child clients in terms of the relationship that developed during therapy and, as a result, the primacy of the therapy over the relationship cannot be documented. However, the effects that are due solely to a positive therapeutic relationship may be quite delimited: The analyses of cases with low CPTR scores revealed meaningful influences, but only on the child self-report data—CPTR scores did not influence the parent or teacher measures of treatment gains.

The present study used an 8-week wait-list control. On the basis of discussions of the clinical and research issues, the methodologically preferred 16-week wait-list condition was not used for ethical and clinical reasons. For example, it was deemed inappropriate (e.g., through discussions with a National Institute of Mental Health consultant) to hold children who received an anxiety disorder diagnosis for 16 weeks without treatment. It is important to note, however, that the 8-week wait-list control condition did allow sufficient time for an assessment and evaluation of the transcience of anxiety disorders in children. Indeed, on the basis of the present data, children's anxiety disorders are not transient, with all but 1 case meeting diagnostic criteria at pre- and post–wait-list assessments.

Providing treatment for children, rather than for adult clients, has potential advantages and disadvantages. For example, given the effectiveness of the treatment and the maintenance of gains at 1-year follow-up, it could be argued that treating children may be helpful in preventing a future lifetime of anxiety and distress. The argument here is not that the present treatment eradicated all anxiety, but that this cognitive–behavioral intervention taught children skills that they can use to manage their anxious distress (Kendall, 1989) and that the early intervention will have preventive effects. One potential difficulty is that children ranging in age from 9 to 13 years vary considerably in their social, cognitive, and physical development. Numerous developmental influences must be considered and incorporated into treatment. These results support the intervention for children aged 9–13 years; other developmentally sensitive materials need to be developed for children outside of this age range.

REFERENCES

Achenbach, T. M., & Edelbrock, C. S. (1983). *Manual for the Child Behavior Checklist and Profile.* Burlington: University of Vermont.

American Psychiatric Association. (1987). *Diagnostic and statistical manual of mental disorders* (3rd ed., rev.). Washington, DC: Author.

Barrios, B., Hartman, D., & Shigetomi, C. (1981). Fears and anxieties in children. In E. Mash & L. Terdal (Eds.), *Behavioral assessment of childhood disorders.* New York: Guilford Press.

Beck, A. T., & Emery, G. (1986). *Anxiety disorders and phobias: A cognitive perspective.* New York: Basic Books.

Beutler, L., & Clarkin, J. (1990). *Systematic treatment selection: Toward targeted therapeutic interventions.* New York: Brunner/Mazel.

Brady, E., & Kendall, P. C. (1992). Comorbidity of anxiety and depression in children and adolescents. *Psychological Bulletin, 111,* 244–255.

Clark, D., & Beck, A. T. (1988). Cognitive approaches. In C. Last & M. Hersen (Eds.), *Handbook of anxiety disorders* (pp. 362–385). Elmsford, NY: Pergamon Press.

Cohen, J. (1977). *Statistical power analysis for behavioral sciences.* San Diego, CA: Academic Press.

Costello, E. J. (1990). Child psychiatric epidemiology: Implications for clinical research and practice. In B. B. Lahey & A. E. Kazdin (Eds.), *Advances in clinical child psychology* (Vol. 13, pp. 53–90). New York: Plenum Press.

Dobson, K., & Shaw, B. F. (1988). The use of treatment manuals in cognitive therapy: Experience and issues. *Journal of Consulting and Clinical Psychology, 56,* 673–680.

Dweck, C., & Wortman, C. (1982). Learned helplessness, anxiety, and achievement. In H. Krone & L. Laux (Eds.), *Achievement, stress and anxiety* (pp. 93–125). New York: Hemisphere.

Fauber, R. L., & Long, N. (1991). Children in context: The role of the family in child psychotherapy. *Journal of Consulting and Clinical Psychology, 59,* 813–820.

Finch, A. J., Kendall, P. C., & Montgomery, L. (1974). Multidimensionality of anxiety in children. *Journal of Abnormal Child Psychology, 2,* 311–334.

Finch, A. J., Jr., Saylor, C. F., & Edwards, G. L. (1985). Children's Depression Inventory: Sex and grade norms for normal children. *Journal of Consulting and Clinical Psychology, 53,* 424–425.

Gittelman, R. (1986). *Anxiety disorders of childhood.* New York: Guilford Press.

Glennon, B., & Weisz, J. R. (1978). An observational approach to the assessment of anxiety in young children. *Journal of Consulting and Clinical Psychology, 46,* 1246–1257.

Gosch, E. A., Kendall, P. C., Panas, J., & Bross, L. (1991, November). *Behavioral observations of anxiety disordered children.* Poster presented at the convention of the Association for Advancement of Behavior Therapy, New York, NY.

Hatzenbuehler, L., & Schroeder, H. E. (1978). Desensitization procedures in the treatment of childhood disorders. *Psychological Bulletin, 85,* 831–844.

Heard, P., Dadds, M., & Rapee, R. (1992, July). *The role of family intervention in the treatment of child anxiety disorders.* Paper presented at the World Congress on Behavioural Therapy, Gold Coast, Australia.

Ingram, R., Kendall, P., Smith, T., Donnell, C., & Ronan, K. (1987). Cognitive specificity and emotional distress. *Journal of Personality and Social Psychology, 53,* 734–742.

Institute of Medicine (1989). *Research on children and adolescents with mental, behavioral, and developmental disorders* (IOM-8907). Washington, DC: National Academy Press.

Johnson, S. B. (1979). Children's fears in classroom settings. *School Psychology Digest, 8,* 382–396.

Kane, M., & Kendall, P. (1989). Anxiety disorders in children: Evaluation of a cognitive-behavioral treatment. *Behavior Therapy, 20,* 499–508.

Kanfer, F., Karoly, P., & Newman, P. (1975). Reduction of children's fear of dark by competence-related and situational threat-related verbal cues. *Journal of Consulting and Clinical Psychology, 43,* 251–258.

Kazdin, A. E. (1986). Research designs and methodology. In S. L. Garfield & A. E. Bergin (Eds.), *Handbook of psychotherapy and behavior change* (3rd ed., pp. 23–69). New York: Wiley.

Kazdin, A. E., French, N. H., Unis, A. S., Esveldt-Dawson, K., & Sherick, R. B. (1983). Hopelessness, depression, and suicidal intent among psychiatrically disturbed inpatient children. *Journal of Consulting and Clinical Psychology, 51,* 504–510.

Kendall, P. C. (1989). The generalization and maintenance of behavior change: Comments, consideration, and the "no-cure" criticism. *Behavior Therapy, 20,* 357–364.

Kendall, P. C. (1990). *Coping cat workbook.* (Available from Philip C. Kendall, Department of Psychology, Temple University, Philadelphia, PA 19122.)

Kendall, P. C. (1992). Childhood coping: Avoiding a lifetime of anxiety. *Behavioural Change, 9,* 1–8.

Kendall, P. C., Cantwell, D., & Kazdin, A. E. (1989). Depression in children and adolescents: Assessment issues and recommendations. *Cognitive Therapy and Research, 13,* 109–146.

Kendall, P. C. & Chansky, T. (1991). Considering cognition in anxiety disordered children. *Journal of Anxiety Disorders, 5,* 167–185.

Kendall, P. C., Chansky, T. E., Kane, M., Kim, R., Kortlander, E., Ronan, K., Sessa, F., & Siqueland, L. (1992). *Anxiety disorders in youth: Cognitive-behavioral interventions.* Needham Heights, MA: Allyn & Bacon.

Kendall, P. C., & Grove, W. M. (1988). Normative comparisons in therapy outcome. *Behavioral Assessment, 10,* 147–158.

Kendall, P. C., Howard, B., & Epps, J. (1988). The anxious child: Cognitive-behavioral treatment strategies. *Behavior Modification, 12,* 281–310.

Kendall, P. C., & Ingram, R. (1987). The future for cognitive assessment of anxiety: Let's get specific. In L. Michaelson & M. Ascher (Eds.), *Anxiety and stress disorders: Cognitive-behavioral assessment and treatment* (pp. 89–104). New York: Guilford Press.

Kendall, P. C., Kane, M., Howard, B., & Siqueland, L. (1990). *Cognitive-behavioral therapy for anxious children: Treatment manual.* (Available from Philip C. Kendall, Department of Psychology, Temple University, Philadelphia, PA 19122.)

Kendall, P. C., Kortlander, E., Chansky, T. E., & Brady, E. U. (1992). Comorbidity of anxiety and depression in youth: Treatment implications. *Journal of Consulting and Clinical Psychology, 60,* 869–880.

Kendall, P. C., & Morris, R. (1991). Child therapy: Issues and recommendations. *Journal of Consulting and Clinical Psychology, 59,* 777–784.

Kiesler, D. J. (1971). Experimental designs in psychotherapy research. In A. E. Bergin & S. L. Garfield (Eds.), *Handbook of psychotherapy and behavior change: An empirical analysis* (pp. 36–74) New York: Wiley.

King, N., Hamilton, D. H., & Ollendick, T. (1988). *Children's phobias: A behavioural perspective.* Chichester, England: Wiley.

Kovacs, M. (1981). Rating scales to assess depression in school aged children, *Acta Paedopsychiatrica, 46,* 305–315.

Last, C. G., Hersen, M., Kazdin, A. E., Francis, G., & Grubb, H. J. (1987). Psychiatric illness in mothers of anxious children. *American Journal of Psychiatry, 144,* 1580–1583.

Last, C. G., Phillips, J. E., & Statfeld, A. (1987). Childhood anxiety disorders in mothers and their children. *Child Psychiatry and Human Development, 18,* 103–117.

MacLeod, C., Mathews, A., & Tata, P. (1986). Attentional bias in emotional disorders. *Journal of Abnormal Psychology, 95,* 15–20.

Meichenbaum, D. (1986). *Stress inoculation.* Elmsford, NY: Pergamon Press.

Morris, R. J., & Kratochwill, J. R. (1983). *Treating children's fears and phobias: A behavioral approach.* Elmsford, NY: Pergamon Press.

Ollendick, T. (1978). *Fear Survey Schedule: Revised.* (Available from T. Ollendick, Virginia Polytechnic Institute and State University, Blacksburg, Virginia 24060.)

Ollendick, T. (1986). Behavior therapy with children and adolescents. In S. Garfield & A. Bergin (Eds.), *Handbook of psychotherapy and behavior change* (3rd ed., pp. 525–565). New York: Wiley.

Ollendick, T., & Francis, G. (1988). Behavioral assessment and treatment of childhood phobias. *Behavior Modification, 12,* 165–204.

Orvaschel, H., & Weissman, M. (1986). Epidemiology of anxiety in children. In R. Gittleman (Ed.), *Anxiety disorders of childhood.* New York: Guilford Press.

President's Commission on Mental Health (1978). *Report to the President* (Vol. 1). Washington, DC: U.S. Government Printing Office.

Prins, P. J. M. (1986). Children's self-speech and self-regulation during a fear provoking behavioral test. *Behaviour Research and Therapy, 24,* 181–191.

Reynolds, C. R., & Paget, K. D. (1982, March). *National normative and reliability data for Revised Children's Manifest Anxiety Scale.* Paper presented at the meeting of the National Association of School Psychologists, Toronto, Ontario, Canada.

Reynolds, C. R., & Richmond, B. O. (1978). A revised measure of childr ι's manifest anxiety scale. *Journal of Abnormal Child Psychology, 6,* 271–280.

Ronan, K., Kendall, P. C., & Rowe, M. (in press). Negative affectivity in children: Development and validation of a self-statement questionnaire. *Cognitive Therapy and Research.*

Sarason, I. G. (1975). Anxiety and self-preoccupation. In I. G. Sarason & C. D. Spielberger (Eds.), *Stress and anxiety.* Washington DC: Hemisphere.

ιylor, C. F., Finch, A., Spirito, A., & Bennett, B. (1984). The Children's Depression Inventory: A systematic evaluation of psychometric properties. *Journal of Consulting and Clinical Psychology, 52,* 955–967.

Scherer, M., & Nakamura, C. (1968). Fear Survey Schedule for Children factor analytic comparison. *Behavior Research and Therapy, 6,* 173–182.

Silverman, W. (1987). *Anxiety Disorders Interview Schedule for Children (ADIS).* State University of New York at Albany: Graywind Publications.

Spielberger, C. (1973). *Manual for State-Trait Anxiety Inventory for Children.* Palo Alto, CA: Consulting Psychologists Press.

Stark, K. D., Rouse, L. W., & Livingston, R. (1991). Treatment of depression during childhood and adolescence: Cognitive–behavioral procedures for the individual and family. In P. C. Kendall (Ed.), *Child and adolescent therapy: Cognitive–behavioral procedures* (pp. 165–198). New York: Guilford Press.

Strauss, C. (1987). *Modification of trait portion of State-Trait Anxiety Inventory for Children-parent form.* (Available from the author, Western Psychiatric Institute and Clinic, 3811 O'Hara Street, Pittsburgh, PA 15213.)

Strauss, C., Lease, C., Kazdin, A., Dulcan, M., & Last, C. (1989). Multimethod assessment of the social competence of anxiety disordered children. *Journal of Clinical Child Psychology, 18,* 184–190.

Strauss, C., Lease, C., Last, C., & Francis, G. (1988). Overanxious disorder: An examination of developmental differences. *Journal of Abnormal Child Psychology, 16,* 433–443.

Strupp, H. H., & Hadley, S. (1979). Specific versus non-specific factors in psychotherapy. *Archives of General Psychiatry, 36,* 1125–1137.

Tuma, J. (1989). Mental health services for children: The state of the art. *American Psychologist, 44,* 188–199.

Weissman, M., Leckman, J., Merikangas, K., Gammon, G., & Prusoff, B. (1974). Depression and anxiety disorders in parents and children: Yale Family Study. *Archives of General Psychiatry, 41,* 845–852.

Werry, J. S. (1986). Diagnosis and assessment. In R. Gittelman, (Ed.) *Anxiety disorders of childhood.* New York: Guilford Press.

Wilson, G. (1985). Fear reduction methods and treatment of anxiety disorders. In G. Wilson, C. Franks, K. Brownell, & P. Kendall. *Review of behavior therapy: Theory and practice* (Vol. 8, pp. 82–119). New York: Guilford Press.

Zatz, D., & Chassin, L. (1983). Cognition of test-anxious children. *Journal of Consulting and Clinical Psychology, 51,* 526–535.

Zatz, S., & Chassin, L. (1985). Cognition of test-anxious children under naturalistic test taking conditions. *Journal of Consulting and Clinical Psychology, 53,* 393–402.

Zill, N., & Schoenborn, C. A. (1990). Developmental, learning, and emotional problems: Health of our nation's children, United States, 1988. *Advance data from vital and health statistics* (No. 190). Hyattsville, MD: National Center for Health Statistics.

18

Update on Lithium Carbonate Therapy in Children and Adolescents

Norman Alessi
University of Michigan Medical Center, Ann Arbor

Michael W. Naylor
Northeastern University, Chicago

Mohammad Ghaziuddin
University of Michigan Medical Center

Jon Kar Zubieta
Johns Hopkins University, Baltimore

The use of lithium to treat child and adolescent psychiatric disorders is becoming more common. Since the publication of the report of The Committee on Biological Aspects of Child Psychiatry of the American Academy of Child Psychiatry in 1978, a considerable body of literature has accumulated on the efficacy of lithium in treating adolescent bipolar disorders, childhood aggression, and behavioral disorders associated with mental retardation and developmental disorders. Efforts to understand lithium's mechanism(s) and refinements in psychiatric diagnosis have contributed to its growing use.

Since the introduction of lithium salts for the treatment of manic-depressive illness in adults more than 40 years ago, more than 16,000 articles have been published, with up to 1,000 new articles added annually (Baudhuin et al., 1987; Bunney and Garland-Bunney, 1987; Cade, 1949). In 1978, a review of the published literature on the use of lithium in children and adolescents suggested the efficacy of lithium in adolescent manic-

Reprinted with permission from the *Journal of the American Academy of Child and Adolescent Psychiatry*, 1994, Vol. 33(3), 291–304. Copyright © 1994 by the American Academy of Child and Adolescent Psychiatry.

depressive illness and its possible utility in aggression and hyperactivity, where there was an affective component (Youngerman and Canino, 1978). Also in 1978, The Committee on Biological Aspects of Child Psychiatry of the American Academy of Child Psychiatry offered a report on the status of lithium therapy in children and adolescents (Campbell et al., 1978). Their conclusions were that (1) lithium ". . . should be explored because of its potential therapeutic value . . ." for manic-depressive illness, emotionally unstable character disorders, aggressiveness, and the high-risk offspring of lithium responders; (2) "lithium might be helpful" for childhood depression; and (3) "lithium is probably not helpful" for hyperkinetic syndrome and psychosis (p. 718).

Fifteen years have passed since the publication of these overviews. There have been a number of reports substantiating these earlier conclusions and introducing possible new uses for lithium. With the veritable explosion in the neurosciences, in particular in our understanding of receptor and intracellular mechanisms of functioning, we have gained much greater understanding of not only lithium's mechanism(s) of action but also of its theoretical relationship to specific child and adolescent psychopathology. It is within this context that we review the use of lithium in child and adolescent psychopathology and its purported mechanism(s) of action.

LITERATURE SURVEY

The enthusiasm generated for lithium in the field of adult psychiatry has been paralleled in child and adolescent psychiatry, albeit on a far lesser scale. In fact, only 58 articles on the use of lithium in children and adolescents have been published, and these represent less than 0.5% of the lithium literature. Approximately 55% of the reports have been published since 1978. These reports can be divided into three categories: (1) case reports; (2) case series (reports consisting of two or more than two cases, including open clinical trials); and (3) double-blind, placebo-controlled studies.

Figure 1 shows the breakdown of these reports. Of the 58 reports, the majority, 26 (45%), are case series; 22 (39%) are case reports; and 9 (16%) are double-blind, placebo-controlled studies. A total of 652 patients are represented in these reports. The largest proportion of patients, 483 (74%), were reported in case series; 152 (23%) in double-blind, placebo-controlled studies; and the remaining 24 (3%) in case reports. The diagnostic categories represented in these reports include bipolar disorders, manic-depressive illness, depressive disorders, aggression, conduct disorders, psychotic disorder, attention-deficit hyperactivity disorder (ADHD), emo-

A. Percent of Studies

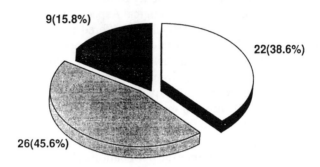

B. Percent of Patients

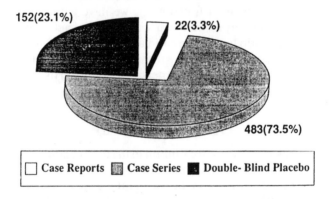

Figure 1. Review of lithium studies. A: Percentage of reports reflecting lithium efficacy. Total of 57 reports; 22 (38%) case reports, 26 (46%) case series, and 9 (16%) double-blind studies. B: Percentage of patients within each group. Total of 657 patients; 22 (3%) case reports, 483 (74%) case series, and 152 (23%) double-blind studies. Cases were included only when the number of either children or adolescents was discernible from the number of adults. Also, these data represent only reports and not instances of chapters or presentations, such as posters in which data may have been presented.

tionally disturbed offspring of lithium-responsive parents, after head trauma, eating disorders, "severe disturbances," and Kleine-Levin syndrome. Despite the increase in the number of reports on the use of lithium carbonate in this age group, most are case reports or case series.

Case reports. Eighteen of the case reports concern the efficacy of lithium in children or adolescents with manic-depressive disorders (Adams et al., 1970; Berg et al., 1974; Carlson and Strober, 1978; Coll and Bland, 1979; Engstrom et al., 1978; Feinstein and Wolpert, 1973; Fisman et al., 1985; Ghadirian and Kusalic, 1990; Hall and Ries, 1983; Joshi et al., 1985; Kelley et al., 1976; Licamelle and Goldberg, 1989; Linter, 1987; Mattsson and Seltzer, 1981; Picker et al., 1990; Potter, 1983; Warneke, 1975; Youngerman and Canino, 1983). The youngest child treated for manic-depression was 5 years old (Feinstein and Wolpert, 1973). In three cases involving adolescents with manic-depressive disorder, the mania was presumed to be medication induced (Ghadirian and Kusalic, 1990; Mattsson and Seltzer, 1981; Shafey, 1986). One case report involved the use of lithium in the treatment of aggression (Lena and O'Brian, 1975). In three single cases of adolescents with Kleine-Levin syndrome, a rare condition restricted almost exclusively to adolescent males and typified by hypersomnolence, behavioral disturbance, and hyperphagia, a reduction in symptoms was noted with lithium (Cawthorne, 1990; Goldberg, 1983; Jeffries and Lefebvre, 1973). The other two cases involved the treatment of children who either were psychotic or had a behavioral disturbance after head trauma (Cohn et al., 1977; Shafey, 1986).

Case series. The 26 case series involved a wide range of psychiatric disturbances, with 16 involving manic-depressive disorders (Annell, 1969; Brumback and Weinberg, 1977; Davis, 1979; DeLong, 1978; DeLong and Aldershof, 1987; Hassanyeh and Davison, 1980; Horowitz 1977; Hsu and Starzynski, 1986b; Kerbeshian and Burd, 1989; Kerbeshian et al., 1987; Rogeness et al., 1982; Steingard and Biederman, 1987; Strober et al., 1988, 1990; Sylvester et al., 1984; Varanka et al., 1988; Weinberg and Brumback, 1976), two depression (Ryan et al., 1988; Strober et al., 1992), four aggression (Siassi, 1982; Somogyi et al., 1988; Vetro et al., 1981, 1985), one ADHD (Whitehead and Clark, 1970), and one Kleine-Levin (Will et al., 1988). There was one case dealing with the response of children with lithium-responsive parents (Dyson and Barcai, 1970). The age ranged from 3 to 19 years old, with several of the youngest children (4 and 5 years old) being mentally retarded or autistic and having bipolar disorders (Kerbeshian and Burd, 1989; Steingard and Biederman, 1987).

Double-blind, placebo-controlled studies. Nine double-blind, placebo-controlled studies involving lithium have been published. Two involve the study of manic-depressive disorders (DeLong and Aldershof, 1987; McKnew et al., 1981), three aggression (Campbell et al., 1972; Campbell et al., 1984b; Sheard, 1975), one psychotic disorders (Gram and Rafaelsen; 1972), one ADHD (Greenhill et al., 1973), and, the most recent, disruptive behavioral disorder and either bipolar or major depressive disorder (Carlson et al., 1992). For an extensive review of the earlier studies see Campbell et al. (1984a).

CLINICAL INDICATIONS

Newer reports, albeit case reports and case series, support earlier observations of the clinical utility of lithium.

Children
Disorders for which lithium should be considered
AGGRESSION. Aggression continues to be the most widely supported clinical diagnostic entity for which lithium is indicated. In a series of studies spanning more than 22 years, Campbell and coworkers demonstrated in two double-blind, placebo-controlled studies that lithium is as efficacious as either chlorpromazine or haloperidol and more so than placebo in the management of impulsive aggression (Campbell et al., 1982; Campbell et al., 1984b). In addition, they observed far fewer side effects in subjects taking lithium. In the psychiatric and neuroscience literature, it is widely noted that lithium affects aggression (Eichelman, 1988; Mattes, 1986).

Although it is obvious that some patients with aggression respond favorably to lithium carbonate pharmacotherapy, it is very difficult to determine which children would benefit. As noted, "the lack of clear guidelines in determining the point at which normal aggression becomes pathological makes the management of childhood aggression very difficult" (Alessi and Wittekindt, 1989, p. 101).

BIPOLAR ILLNESS. Considerable controversy continues as to whether bipolar disorder presents in childhood, its prevalence, and the diagnostic criteria by which to establish the diagnosis. Bowring and Kovacs (1992) suggest that low base rate of occurrence, variable presentation within and across episodes, symptomatic overlap with other more common childhood disorders, and variation of symptomatic expression resulting from the developmental stage of the child account for the difficulties in identifying bipolar illness in children. Despite these obvious difficulties, recent research suggests that scales such as the Mania Rating Scale might be used to differentiate children with bipolar disorders from those with ADHD (Fristad et al., 1992). Although these findings are promising, their replication is needed.

Several diagnostic criteria have been proposed (Anthony and Scott, 1960; Weinberg and Brumback, 1976); however, none have been adequately validated. One possible method is to identify those children or adolescents who have a lithium-responsive parent or parents with cyclical mood disturbances or cyclic psychosis (Dyson and Barcai, 1970). McKnew et al. (1981) studied six children, aged 6 through 12 years, with incapacitating psychopathology whose parents (all of whom had bipolar illness) were lithium responders. Using a double-blind, crossover study of lithium carbonate treatment, the authors reported that two children had a clear-cut response. Those two appeared to have clear evidence of cyclothymia, whereas the four nonresponders did not.

DeLong and Aldershof (1987) described the long-term treatment of children with lithium, using a combination of double-blind placebo-controlled and open designs. They treated 196 children for periods up to 10 years and found that the usefulness of lithium was related to clinical diagnosis. Lithium was most useful in patients with bipolar disorder, in behaviorally disordered offspring of lithium-responsive parents, and in children with "emotionally unstable character disorder." It was not effective in children with attention deficit disorder. Some children with a combination of affective and aggressive symptoms, at times complicated by developmental disorders, also had a favorable response.

Disorders for which lithium might be considered when other medications fail
DEPRESSION. The use of lithium in children as an augmenting agent has been reported only recently (Alessi, 1990). In this case report a 10-year-old girl demonstrated marked improvement after the addition of lithium to an antidepressant.

Adolescents
Disorder(s) for which lithium should be considered
MANIC-DEPRESSIVE ILLNESS. Bipolar affective disorder frequently has its onset during adolescence. Estimates of onset of bipolar affective disorder during adolescence vary widely from 0.075% (one of 1,334) to 20% (Loranger and Levine, 1978; Wiener and del Gaudio, 1976). Joyce (1984) found that 25% of patients with bipolar disorder dated its onset to between the ages of 15 and 19 years. One reason for the wide range of estimated age of onset of bipolar disorder relates to the frequency of misdiagnosis in adolescents

(Carlson and Strober, 1978; Gammon et al., 1983; Hsu and Starzynski, 1986a; Joyce, 1984). Horowitz (1977) found that all eight adolescents in his study eventually diagnosed with manic-depressive illness previously had been diagnosed with schizophrenia.

Several studies demonstrate the effectiveness of lithium carbonate for adolescents with bipolar illness. The response is often dramatic, and remissions have been documented after 5 to 14 days of treatment. Most adolescents, however, may require up to 6 weeks (Hassanyeh and Davison, 1980; Horowitz, 1977; Hsu and Starzynski, 1986a; Strober et al., 1988). In two reports, adolescents relapsed after discontinuation; in one case they responded to restarting of the medication, but in the other they did not.

In an 18-month prospective, naturalistic follow-up study of 37 adolescents with bipolar affective disorder treated with lithium, Strober et al. (1990) found that noncompleters of an 18-month therapeutic trial relapsed nearly three times as often as did completers (92.3% versus 37.5%). Furthermore, completers who had episodes of mania or depression before the index hospitalization had a decreased frequency of affective illnesses while receiving lithium compared with baseline. Although not conclusive, these data suggest that lithium carbonate is an effective prophylactic agent, preventing or decreasing relapses.

Despite the reported efficacy of lithium carbonate in the treatment of adolescent manic-depressive illness, not all adolescents with bipolar affective disorder respond. Factors thought to predict lithium nonresponsiveness include a greater genetic diathesis in younger patients, developmental immaturity, and neurological disorders (Himmelhoch and Garfinkel, 1986; Strober et al., 1988). Lithium resistance is particularly common in adolescents with mixed mania. Himmelhoch and Garfinkel (1986) reported on 46 lithium-resistant bipolar patients, 23 of whom were adolescents. Of these 23, 17 had mixed mania and six had nonmixed mania.

AGGRESSION. Lithium carbonate is frequently effective in the treatment of aggressive adolescents as well as children. In two studies lithium carbonate was administered to institutionalized adolescents. Sheard (1975) found that lithium decreased the frequency and severity of aggression. In the study by Dostal (1972), lithium pharmacotherapy resulted in 65% decrease in the incidence of aggression.

Disorders for which lithium might be considered when other medications fail
REFRACTORY DEPRESSION. Two recent studies have addressed the issue of lithium augmentation of tricyclic antidepressant (TEA) pharmacotherapy in TCA-refractory, depressed adolescents (Ryan et al., 1988; Strober et al., 1992). In Ryan and coworkers' retrospective study of 14 adolescents with unipolar depression unresponsive to antidepressant therapy, augmenta-

tion with lithium carbonate led to a significant improvement in mood and psychosocial functioning in 6 (43%). In Strober and colleagues' group of 24 depressed adolescents who failed to respond to a 6-week open trial of imipramine, two patients (8.3%) had a dramatic response to lithium augmentation and eight patients (33%) had a partial response.

Disorders with limited support for consideration

COMPLICATED BIPOLAR CASES. Lithium carbonate has been effective in the treatment of complicated cases of bipolar disorders in adolescents, especially rapid-cycling bipolar disorder; comorbid Tourette's syndrome and bipolar disorder; organic mood disorder, manic type; and mild mental retardation associated with cyclic mood disturbance (Cohn et al., 1977; Kelly et al., 1976; Kerbeshian and Burd, 1989; Mattsson and Seltzer, 1981).

KLEINE-LEVIN SYNDROME. Several authors have reported that lithium is effective in the acute treatment of Kleine-Levin syndrome, eliminating the attacks or decreasing their frequency and severity (Abe, 1977; Cawthorne, 1990; Goldberg, 1983; Ogura et al., 1976; Will et al., 1988).

EEATING DISORDERS. Very little research has been done on the use of lithium carbonate in the treatment of anorexia nervosa in adolescents (Stein et al., 1982). In a double-blind, placebo-controlled study of 16 hospitalized anorexic patients (aged 12 to 32 years), Gross and coworkers (1981) demonstrated that those receiving active medication showed a significantly greater weight gain than did those receiving placebo.

The use of lithium carbonate for the treatment of bulimia nervosa also has been studied. In the largest study to date, Hsu and associates (1991) found that lithium carbonate was no more effective than placebo in reducing binge/vomit frequency or abnormal eating attitudes. For the depressed bulimic subjects treated with lithium, however, those with higher plasma lithium levels tended to have a lower frequency of vomiting than did those with lower plasma levels.

Extreme caution must be used when treating anorexia nervosa and bulimia nervosa with lithium. Lithium has been implicated in the death of a "normal control" enrolled in a National Institute of Mental Health study who was later found to have an extensive history of anorexia nervosa with self-induced vomiting. Lithium may exacerbate the loss of intracellular potassium in patients who are hypokalemic, thereby enhancing cardiotoxicity of hypokalemia accompanying self-induced vomiting (Kolata, 1980).

MENTAL RETARDATION AND DEVELOPMENTAL DISORDERS. Several reports have described the use of lithium in persons with mental retardation and developmental disorders. Most of these studies have been in adults. Those involving children and adolescents have been mainly in those with bipolar disorder, aggressive behavior, and self-injurious behavior. In some patients, the presence of a family history of bipolar disorder may be an acceptable indication for starting lithium therapy, especially when the behavioral problems show a cyclic tendency (Chandler et al., 1988). In a study of 14 patients with mental retardation, aged 19 to 58 years, Naylor et al. (1974) found that patients with affective symptoms responded to lithium.

There are very few published reports of the use of lithium in children and adolescents with developmental disorders and comorbid bipolar disorder. Undoubtedly this reflects the difficulties inherent in the diagnosis of psychiatric disorders in this population. Nevertheless, several case reports have described the lithium treatment of "short-cycling manic-depressive illness" or "juvenile manic-depressive illness" (Fukuda et al., 1986; Kelly et al., 1976; Linter, 1987). Treatment of autistic children with atypical bipolar symptoms also has been described (Kerbeshian et al., 1987; Steingard and Biederman, 1987).

Lithium pharmacotherapy also has been used to control aggression in persons with developmental disorders. Tyrer and colleagues (1984) studied the effects of lithium on the aggressive behavior of 26 institutionalized patients, aged 14 to 50 years, and found that certain variables differentiated the lithium responders from the nonresponders. These were female gender, overactivity, stereotypy, seizure disorder, and a low frequency of aggressive incidents (< 1/week) before the start of the medication trial. Another study found that rage and aggressivity responded favorably to lithium treatment in behaviorally disordered children with neurological and medical conditions including mental retardation (DeLong and Aldershof, 1987). Campbell et al. (1972) conducted a double-blind study of the comparison of lithium and chlorpromazine in a group of 10 autistic children with a variety of disruptive behaviors. Two patients had an IQ less than 70. In general, neither drug was found to be effective, although in one child a decrease in self-mutilation and violent tantrums was observed with lithium. Self-injurious behavior in persons with mental retardation and developmental disorders may benefit from a trial of lithium carbonate (Winchel and Stanley, 1991).

On the whole, experience with lithium in developmentally disabled populations is limited. Distinction has not often been made in the literature between aggression directed toward others and that directed toward self or between verbal and physical aggression. Apart from its use in some autistic children, there are no reports on its use in the various subtypes of mental retardation, such as Down syndrome and fragile X syndrome.

MECHANISM(S) OF ACTION

Great advances in our understanding of the complexity of lithium's mechanism(s) of action have been made in the past 10 years. Lithium, an alkali metal, now is known to cause profound effects on a number of neurochemical systems including ion channels; neurotransmitters, including serotonin, dopamine, and norepinephrine (NE); and second-messenger systems, such as phosphoinositides (PIs) and cyclic AMP (cAMP). A limited review of the effects of lithium on the second-messenger systems and receptors will be offered, from molecular functioning (second messengers and transduction mechanisms) to receptor number and function (Table 1).

Second-Messenger Systems

Inositol phosphate metabolism. Phosphoinositides act as second messengers in a variety of neurotransmitter systems (for recent reviews see Baraban et al., 1989; Berridge et al., 1989; Hokin, 1985). Stimulation of PI-linked membrane receptors activates a phospholipase C enzyme. This enzyme metabolizes phosphatidylinositol-bis-phosphate to inositol trisphosphate and diacylglycerol. Both compounds act as intracellular second messengers (Figure 2).

Lithium initially was observed to decrease the levels of free myoinositol in the rat brain (Allison and Stewart, 1971). It was also shown that the levels of inositol phosphates were raised after lithium treatment (Allison et al., 1976). Lithium noncompetitively blocks the activity of inositol phosphatase enzymes (inositol polyphosphate 1-phosphatase and inositol monophosphate phosphatase) that are involved in the recycling of free inositol from either the breakdown of inositol triphosphate or inositol monophosphates produced from glucose metabolism. The observation that lithium interferes with the function of PI systems has led to the theory that inositol depletion may underlie the therapeutic effects of lithium by modulating the activity of neurotransmitter systems that use PI as second messengers depending on their overall activity: an overactive cycle would be more inhibited than a less active one by the rapid depletion of the precursor inositol (Berridge et al., 1989). This may partially explain the therapeutic effect of lithium in bipolar disorder or, in general, illnesses that may present with overactivity of PI-linked neurotransmitter systems, without causing decreases in presumably normal, functioning systems.

Adenylate cyclase activity. The actions of lithium within this second-messenger system appear to be complex, involving several steps of the cascade

TABLE 1
Summary of Lithium's Mechanism(s) of Action

Neurosubstrate	Action Effected by Lithium	Result of Lithium's Action	Postulated Psychopathology Effected by Action
Second messengers Inositol phosphate	• Blocks the activity of inositol polyphosphate 1-phosphatase and inositol monophosphate phosphatase	• Leads to the depletion of inositol and dampens the function of the phosphoinositide cycle	• Manic-depressive illness • Aggression?
Adenyl cyclase	• Directly inhibits adenyl cyclase by competing with magnesium • Inhibits G proteins (G$_s$ and G$_i$)	• Reduces or increases adenyl cyclase function depending on proportion of regional G$_s$ and G$_i$ populations	• Manic-depressive illness • Depression? • Aggression?
Receptor functioning Serotonergic	• Down-regulates some serotonergic receptor subtypes • Increases serotonin turnover	• Reduces negative feedback, thereby increasing the release of serotonin	• Aggression? • Depression? • Potentiation of antidepressant effects
Adrenergic β	• Increases the proportion of low-affinity β receptors	• Reduces β receptor function	• Manic-depressive illness • Depression • Potentiation of antidepressant effects
α$_2$	• Induces subsensitivity of α$_2$ receptors	• Increases the release of norepinephrine	
Dopaminergic	• Blocks up-regulation of receptors when given concurrently with neuroleptics • Increases dopamine levels and turnover (regionally specific)	• Prevents D$_2$ up-regulation • Augments the effects of indirect agonists	• Manic-depressive illness

that promotes or inhibits cAP formation (Bunney and Garland-Bunney, 1987). Although lithium directly inhibits adenylate cyclase by competing with magnesium (Mork and Geisler, 1987), it appears its most clinically relevant effects are mediated by inhibition of G proteins that stimulate (G_s) or inhibit (G_i) adenylate cyclase function (Mork and Geisler, 1989a, 1989b). By inhibiting the activity of the G proteins, lithium may cause adenylate cyclase-coupled receptors to remain in a low affinity state for agonists (Risby et al., 1991). Also, by reducing the functional activity of G_i proteins adenylate cyclase will be more activated; the converse will be true for systems in which G_s proteins are predominant.

Receptor Number and Function

Serotonin receptors and function. Long-term treatment with lithium increases 5-hydroxytryptamine (5-HT) turnover and increases CNS tryptophan levels and the concentration of its principal metabolite, 5-hydroxyindole-acetic acid (see Bunney and Garland-Bunney, 1987; Manji et al., 1991). Presynaptic 5-HT receptors are subsensitive after long-term lithium administration, reducing their negative feedback on 5-HT release (Friedman and Wang, 1990). Hippocampal but not cortical 5-HT_{1A} sites have been reported to down-regulate after long-term lithium treatment, without an effect on 5-HT_2 receptors (Odagaki et al., 1990). The long-term administration of lithium induces regionally selective alterations in serotonin release. For example, lithium increases 5-HT release in the hippocampal formation with a concomitant decrease in 5-HT receptors (Treiser et al., 1981). No similar changes have been described in the rat cortex. Similar findings have led to the theory that lithium-induced modifications in receptor number and function are due to increased, regionally selective, synaptic availability of the endogenous transmitter (Hotta et al., 1986), leading to variable enhancements in central 5-HT function.

Adrenergic receptors and function. Adrenergic receptors have been implicated in the pathophysiology of affective and anxiety disorders and aggression. Both presynaptic and postsynaptic adrenergic receptors appear to be affected by lithium administration. The literature yields a complex picture of lithium's effects on both α and β adrenoceptors.

β-Adrenoceptors. Lithium treatment has been reported to decrease total β-receptor binding in rat brain homogenates (Rosenblatt et al., 1979; Treiser and Keller, 1979). However, this finding has not been replicated by other authors (Gross et al., 1988; Maggi and Enna, 1980). Pretreatment with lithium has been shown to prevent the development of reserpine-induced β-receptor supersensitivity (by depletion of NE stores), but this effect was

Adenylate Cyclase System

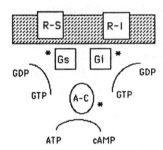

Phosphoinositol Cycle

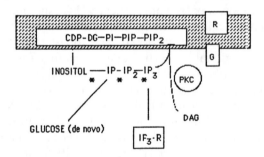

Figure 2. Representation of adenylate cyclase and phosphoinositide (second-messenger) systems. Abbreviations: R = receptor; R-S = stimulatory receptor; R-I = inhibitory receptor; G_s, G_i = stimulatory and inhibitory G-proteins; A-C = adenylate cyclase enzyme; GTP = guanidine triphosphate; GDP = guanidine diphosphate; G = G protein; ATP = adenosine triphosphate; cAMP = cyclic adenosine monophosphate; CDP-DG = cytidine diphosphate: diacylglycerol; PI = phosphatidylinositol; PIP = phosphatidyl-inositol phosphate; PIP_2 = phosphatidylinositol-bis-phosphate; IP = inositol phosphate; IP_2 = inositol-bis-phosphate; IP_3 = inositol triphosphate; PKC = protein kinase C enzyme; IP_3-R = intracellular receptor for IP_3; DAG = diacyglycerol. *Postulated sites of lithium action.

not replicated after destruction of NE neurons with the neurotoxin 6-hydroxydopamine and subsequent lithium administration (see Bunney and Garland-Bunney, 1987). It also appears that lithium does not prevent the down-regulation induced by either direct or indirect agonists (Belmaker, 1981; Rosenblatt et al., 1979). If lithium were to act preferentially by blocking the GTP binding to the G_s protein linked to β receptors (Newman and Belmaker, 1987) it is possible these receptors would be locked in a low affinity state (Risby et al., 1991), preventing the development of supersensitivity but not subsensitivity. Lithium's induction of a low affinity state for the β adrenoceptor may underlie its reported potentiation of antidepressant effects by stabilizing the down-regulation of β receptors induced by these agents.

α-Adrenoceptors. These receptors, possibly located both presynaptically and postsynaptically, are linked, in their presynaptic location, to the modulation of NE release via inhibitory G_i-cAMP mechanisms. Lithium consistently induces subsensitivity of these receptors in both animal (Goodwin et al., 1986; Spengler et al., 1986) and clinical studies (Bambrilla et al., 1988; Garcia-Sevilla et al., 1986) and decreases the high-affinity binding of agonists (^{3}H-clonidine) (Garcia-Sevilla et al., 1986). A decrease in the function of these receptors may in turn reduce their negative feedback over NE release, which indeed is increased after long-term lithium administration (Manji et al., 1991). Increases in the central activity of this system may be partially implicated in lithium's potentiation of antidepressant effects.

$α_1$-Adrenoceptors do not appear to be altered in membrane binding studies (in affinity or number) after long-term lithium treatment. In addition, α-adrenoreceptor up-regulation, induced after reserpine pretreatment, is not prevented by lithium (Gross et al., 1988).

Dopamine receptors and function. Long-term lithium administration has been reported to increase dopamine levels and turnover in tuberoin-fundibular pathways, whereas no changes (increases or decreases) have been reported for striatum, ponsmedulla, and midbrain regions in experimental animals (Bunney and Garland-Bunney, 1987). The concurrent administration of lithium with neuroleptics prevented the supersensitivity and/or upregulation of D_2-dopamine receptors induced by these agents. D_1-receptor-stimulated cAMP formation does not appear to be altered by lithium pretreatment (Whitworth and Kendall, 1989). Although lithium might regionally increase the function of certain dopamine pathways, it again appears to prevent up-regulatory changes in D_2 receptors, which might contribute to its preventive effects on manic-depressive psychosis.

Management Issues

Pharmacokinetics of lithium in children. In one study, nine children, mean age 10.9 years, were given 300 mg of lithium carbonate at 8 A.M. after an overnight fast; blood was drawn at fixed intervals up to 36 hours later (Vitiello et al., 1988). Peak serum lithium level was observed at 2.4 hours, with mean levels of 0.45 mEq/L. The elimination half-life from the body was approximately 17.9 hours, compared with approximately 21 hours in adults (Nielsen-Kudsk and Amdisen, 1979). The elimination rate was significantly higher in children than adults, 40.2 versus 27.6 mL/kg per hour. This 20% difference in half-life may indicate that a child can reach a steady state sooner than an adult and that therapeutic levels can be instituted more quickly. There are no pharmacokinetic studies involving adolescents.

Prediction of lithium dose. There are three methods (but no established standard) for the initiation and achievement of a therapeutic steady-state blood level of lithium (0.6 to 1.2 mEq/L). The first requires the administration of the medication over a period of time with periodic blood draws and appropriate adjustments in the dosage of medication. The second requires the administration of a single test dose of lithium, obtaining a serum level 24 hours later and then using a nomogram to determine the dose to administer. This method has been successful in adults and effective in children (Cooper et al., 1973; Geller and Fetner, 1989). Six subjects received 600 mg of lithium carbonate at 9 A.M. on day 1. Serum lithium level, determined from blood drawn 24 hours later, was between 0.4 and 0.7 mEq/L in all subjects. The Cooper nomogram was used to determine dosage. Although four subjects required increases in dosage from 300 to 600 mg, none had exessive levels.

The third uses a dosage guide with a starting dose of approximately 900/ m^2 (Weller et al., 1986). By this method children would receive approximately 30 mg/kg day. In a study of 15 children, aged 6 to 12 years, the mean steady-state level of lithium, 0.95 ± 0.33 mEq/L, was achieved within 5 days. By this method two children had levels of 1.4 or above.

Monitoring. Given the need to reach therapeutic levels and the absence of a dosage scale, monitoring of lithium level is mandatory. The two methods available are serum and saliva sampling. Despite the claims for the possible use of salivary levels, studies in children suggest that it should be considered only in extreme situations. This hesitancy is based on several factors: (1) there is greater variability in saliva samples than in serum samples; (2) intrasubject variability necessitates the taking of a number of samples from a child to determine an individual ratio; and (3) children may not eat or drink for 12 hours before taking saliva samples (Lena and Bastable,

1978; Perry et al., 1984; Weller et al., 1987). Given these factors, monitoring serum levels is still the technique of choice.

Adverse Effects and Toxicity

For the most part, lithium pharmacotherapy in children and adolescents is well tolerated. Side effects are infrequent and generally mild (Gross et al., 1981; Hsu et al., 1986a; Siassi, 1982; Varanka et al., 1988). Indeed, various investigators state that the frequency and severity of adverse reactions to lithium in children is lower than in adults (Lena, 1989; Siassi, 1982).

Frequently reported side effects in children and adolescents include weight gain, stomach upset, nausea, vomiting, tremor, polydipsia, polyuria, diarrhea, and fatigue (Campbell et al., 1991; Carlson, 1979; Gross et al., 1981; Sheard, 1975; Siassi, 1982; Varanka et al., 1988). Campbell et al. (1991) found that younger children had a greater incidence of side effects than did older children, even after weight, lithium dosage, serum lithium levels, and duration of the optimal dose of lithium carbonate were controlled. Patient diagnosis may also affect the frequency and severity of adverse effects of lithium. In the previously described study, Campbell et al. (1991) reported that autistic children had more side effects than did patients with conduct disorder, even when they accounted for age. Strayhorn and Nash (1977) indict a seizure diathesis and the diagnosis of schizophrenia as conditions that predispose a patient to severe neurotoxicity despite "therapeutic" serum lithium levels. It appears that certain diagnoses and certain types of encephalopathy may place a patient at risk for developing adverse effects, even at "subtherapeutic" dosages.

Central nervous system. Adverse effects involving the CNS are often the most dramatic and serious of all complications resulting from lithium pharmacotherapy. Factors predisposing to neurotoxicity, even in the face of "therapeutic" serum lithium levels, include combination pharmacotherapy (such as haloperidol and lithium), increasing age, seizure diathesis, schizophrenia, intercurrent medical illness, and tissue retention (Strayhorn and Nash, 1977). It is not uncommon for patients treated for an acute bout of mania to develop lithium toxicity after remission. As reviewed by the authors, patients with acute mania tend to sequester more lithium than do normal subjects or patients with well-controlled bipolar disorder. Resolution of the mania leads to "normalization" of lithium metabolism, and toxic lithium levels may result.

Lithium also has been reported to alter EEG patterns in the pediatric age group. Bennett et al. (1983) found that 58% of the patients who had baseline

EEGs subsequently developed EEG abnormalities, including paroxysmal discharges and focal slowing. Brumback and Weinberg (1977) reported that one of their six prepubescent patients with mania developed epileptiform activity on the EEG and four of the six demonstrated EEG slowing with increased δ and θ activity compared with baseline. Contradictory findings have been reported, however.

Other reported CNS abnormalities include increased frequency of migraine headaches (Peatfield and Rose, 1981) and altered cognitive processes. Platt et al. (1981) found that performance in qualitative scores on the Portteus Mazes test decreased, with no change in reaction time or on the Matching Familiar Figures test.

Neuromuscular. Neil et al. (1976) described the case of an 18-year-old woman in whom myasthenia gravis-like symptoms developed during the course of a lithium trial. The symptoms remitted with discontinuation of lithium only to return when the lithium was reinstated. Brust et al. (1979) reported the case of an 18-year-old in whom acute generalized polyneuropathy developed after lithium poisoning. Clinically, the neuropathy resembled the Landry-Guillain-Barré syndrome. In both cases, however, haloperidol was prescribed concurrently, so it is not certain lithium was the offending agent.

Cardiovascular. Rarely, cardiovascular side effects have been reported. Campbell et al. (1972) reported that two 5-year-old boys treated with lithium carbonate developed reversible conduction defects, including mild right ventricular conduction delay, and an atrioventricular nodal rhythm.

Renal. One of the most commonly reported abnormalities is polyuria due to inhibition of the action of antidiuretic hormone on renal adenylate cyclase at the distal tubule and collecting ducts, resulting in decreased renal reabsorption of water (Forrest et al., 1974). Usually reversible, this nephrogenic diabetes insipidus may persist. Few studies have addressed the issue of renal functioning in children receiving long-term lithium treatment. Khandelwal et al. (1984) studied four children who had been treated with lithium carbonate for at least 2 years and reported no change in renal function compared with baseline. There are two separate reports of 14-year-old girls who developed proteinuria during a trial of lithium therapy (Lena et al., 1978; Wood et al., 1989). Although proteinuria typically resolves with discontinuation of the offending agent, sustained proteinuria has been described. Treatment with corticosteroids may be necessary in these cases.

Endocrinological. Perhaps the most widely studied and widely reported adverse effects in adults involve thyroid function. Commonly reported abnormalities include hypothyroidism, goiter formation, the presence of thyroid autoantibodies, and an abnormal thyroid-stimulating hormone response to thyrotropin-releasing hormone. In children and adolescents, biochemical evidence of hypothyroidism (elevated thyroid-stimulating hormone and decreased T4) was reported in two brothers hospitalized for bipolar affective disorder (9 year old) or explosive aggression (7 year old), leading the authors to conclude that the effect of lithium on the thyroid is genetically determined (Picker et al., 1990). In Campbell and coworkers' series (1972), two children demonstrated decreased thyroxine compared with baseline. DeLong and Aldershof (1987) described a case of an 11-year-old boy who developed a goiter and hypothyroidism after 4 years of treatment. Finally, Vetro et al. (1985) reported two cases of lithium-induced goiter out of 17 children treated with lithium.

Miscellaneous. Neutrophilia is such a consistent finding in patients treated with lithium that lithium is often used therapeutically in medical conditions associated with neutropenia. Finally, Cohen and Cohen (1991) published a case report of a 17-year-old boy with Gilbert's disease who developed hyperbilirubinemia in the midst of a lithium trial. The hyperbilirubinemia resolved with discontinuation of the lithium but returned when the patient was rechallenged with lithium.

Lithium in combination with other medications. Lithium in combination with a neuroleptic has been reported to cause somnambulism, seizures, increased incidence of extrapyramidal side effects, and neurotoxicity (Addonizio et al., 1988; Charney et al., 1979; Miller and Menninger, 1987). Development of neurotoxicity was dependent on neuroleptic dosage but was not correlated with serum lithium level (Millet and Menninger, 1987). Parmelee and O'Shanick (1988) published a case series of four adolescents with encephalopathy (three with traumatic brain injury, one with Lennox-Gastault syndrome) who became lethargic, neurotoxic, and aggressive while receiving the combination of lithium carbonate and carbamazepine. Seizure frequency increased. The symptoms resolved within 3 to 8 days of discontinuing the medications.

COMMENT

Lithium has proved to be a useful drug in the management of a variety of psychiatric disorders. Although its use in children and adolescents is not as well documented as in adults and is mainly confined to uncontrolled reports, there is increasing evidence to suggest that it can play an important role in the psychopharmacologic treatment of child and adolescent psychiatric disorders. It has been used mainly in the treatment of mood disorders of adolescents, aggressive and disruptive disorders of childhood, and behavioral disorders coexistent with mental retardation and developmental disabilities. It does not appear to be associated with specific side effects in children and adolescents, nor is there any firm evidence to suggest that its side effects are increased in this population. However, its narrow margin of safety calls for close monitoring and supervision. It is hoped that insights into its basic mechanism of action, coupled with greater sophistication in the assessment of psychopathology, will stimulate controlled and prospective research on its use in children and adolescents.

REFERENCES

Abe K (1977), Lithium prophylaxis of periodic hypersomnia. *Br J Psychiatry* 130:312–316

Adams GL, Kivowitz J, Ziskind E (1970), Manic depressive psychosis, mental retardation, and chromosomal rearrangement. *Arch Gen Psychiatry* 23:305–309

Addonizio G, Roth SD, Stokes PE, Stoll PM (1988), Increased extrapyramidal symptoms with addition of lithium to neuroleptics. *J Nerv Ment Dis* 176:682–685

Alessi NE (1990), Refractory childhood depressive disorders from a pharmacotherapeutic perspective. In: *Refractory Depression: Frontiers in Research & Treatment*, Amsterdam J, ed. New York: Raven Press

Alessi NE, Wittekindt J (1989), Childhood aggressive behavior. *Pediatr Ann* 18:94–101

Allison JH, Blisner ME, Holland WH, Hipps PP, Sherman WR (1976), Increased brain myo-inositol 1-phosphate in lithium-treated rats. *Biochem Biophys Res Commun* 71:664–670

Allison JH, Stewart MA (1971), Reduced brain inositol in lithium treated rats. *Nature New Biol* 233:267–268

Annell A (1969), Manic-depressive illness in children and effect of treatment with lithium carbonate. *Acta Paedopsychiatr* 36:292–301

Anthony J, Scott P (1960), Manic-depressive psychosis in childhood. *J Child Psychol Psychiatry* 1:53–72

Bambrilla F, Catalano M, Lucca A, Smeraldi E (1988), Effect of lithium treatment on the GH-clonidine test in affective disorders. *Eur J Clin Psychopharmacol* 35:601–605

Baraban JM, Worley PF, Snyder SH (1989), Second messenger systems and psychoactive drug action: focus on the phosphoinositide system and lithium. *Am J Psychiatry* 146:1251–1260

Baudhuin MG, Carroll JA, Jefferson JW, Greist JH, Hartley BL (1987), Information and education about lithium: the Lithium Information Center. In: *Depression and Mania: Modern Lithium Therapy*, Johnson FN ed. Washington, DC: IRL Press

Belmaker RH (1981), Receptors, adenylate cyclase, depression and lithium. *Biol Psychiatry* 16:333–350

Bennett WG, Korein J, Kalmijn M, Grega DM, Campbell M (1983), Electroencephalogram and treatment of hospitalized aggressive children with haloperidol and lithium. *Biol Psychiatry* 18:1427–1440

Berg I, Hullin R, Allsopp M, O'Brien P, MacDonald R (1974), Bipolar manic-depressive psychosis in early adolescence: a case report. *Br J Psychiatry* 125:416–417

Berridge MJ, Downes CP, Hanley MR (1989), Neural and developmental actions of lithium: a unifying hypothesis. *Cell* 59:411–419

Bowring MA, Kovacs M (1992), Difficulties in diagnosing manic disorders among children and adolescents. *J Am Acad Child Adolesc Psychiatry* 31:611–614

Brumback RA, Weinberg WA (1977), Mania in childhood, II: therapeutic trial of lithium carbonate and further description of manic-depressive illness in children. *Am J Dis Child* 131:1122–1126

Brust JCM, Hammer JS, Challenor Y, Helaton EB, Lesser RP (1979), Acute generalized polyneuropathy accompany lithium poisoning. *Ann Neurol* 6:360–362

Bunney WE, Garland-Bunney BL (1987), Mechanisms of action of lithium in affective illness: basic and clinical implications. In: *Psychopharmacology: The Third Generation of Progress*, Meltzer HY, ed. New York: Raven Press, pp 553–565

Cade JFJ (1949), Lithium salts in the treatment of psychotic excitement. *Med J Aust* 2:349–352

Campbell M, Cohel IL, Small AM (1982), Drugs in aggressive behavior. *J Am Acad Child Psychiatry* 21:107–117

Campbell M, Fish B, Shapiro T, Collins P, Koh C (1972), Lithium and chlorpromazine: a controlled crossover study of hyperactive severely disturbed children. *J Autism Child Schizophr* 2:234–263

Campbell M, Perry R, Green WH (1984a), Use of lithium in children and adolescent. *Psychosomatics* 25:95–106

Campbell M, Schulman D, Rapport J (1978), The current status of lithium therapy in child and adolescent psychiatry. *J Am Acad Child Psychiatry* 17:717–719

Campbell M, Silva RR, Kafantaris V et al. (1991), Predictors of side effects associated with lithium administration in children. *Psychopharmacol Bull* 27:373–380

Campbell M, Small AM, Green WH, Jennings WG, Anderson L (1984b), Behavioral efficacy of haloperidol and lithium carbonate. *Arch Gen Psychiatry* 41:650–656

Carlson GA (1979), Lithium use in adolescents: clinical indications and management. *Adolesc Psychiatry* 7:410–418

Carlson GA, Rapport MD, Kelly KL, Pataki CS (1992), The effects of methylphenidate and lithium on attention and activity level. *J Am Acad Child Adolesc Psychiatry* 31:262–270

Carlson GA, Strober M (1978), Affective disorders in adolescence: issues in misdiagnosis. *J Clin psychiatry* 39:59–66

Cawthorne P (1990), A disorder unique to adolescence? The Kleine-Levin syndrome. *J Adolesc* 13:401–406

Chandler M, Gualtieri CT, Fahs J (1988), Other psychotropic drugs: stimulants, antidepressants, and lithium carbonate. In: *Psychopharmacology of the Developmental Disabilities.* Aman MG, Singh NN. New York: Springer-Verlag

Charney DS, Kales A, Soldatos CR, Nelson JC (1979), Somnambalistic-like episodes secondary to combined lithium-neuroleptic treatment. *Br J Psychiatry* 135:418–424

Cohen LS, Cohen DE (1991), Lithium-induced hyperbilirubinemia in an adolescent (letter). *J Clin Psychopharmacol* 11:274–275

Cohn CK, DeVaul RA, Wright JR (1977), Post head trauma syndrome in an adolescent treated with lithium carbonate: case report. *Dis Nerv Sys* 38:630–631

Coll P, Bland R (1979), Manic depressive illness in adolescence and childhood: review and case report. *Can J Psychiatry* 24:255–263

Cooper TB, Bergner PE, Simpson GM (1973), The 24-hour lithium level as a prognostication of dosage requirements. *Am J Psychiatry* 130:601–603

Davis RE (1979), Manic-depressive variant syndrome of childhood: a preliminary report. *Am J Psychiatry* 136:702–706

DeLong GR (1978), Lithium treatment of select behavior disorders in children suggesting manic-depressive illness. *J Pediatr* 93:689–694

DeLong GR, Aldershof AL (1987), Long-term experience with lithium treatment in childhood: correlation with clinical diagnosis. *J Am Acad Child Adolesc Psychiatry* 26:389–394

Dostal T (1972), Antiaggressive effect of lithium salts in mentally retarded adolescents. In: *Depressive States in Childhood and Adolescence.* Annell A, ed. Stockholm: Almquist & Wiskell, pp 491–498

Dyson WL, Barcai A (1970), Treatment of children of lithium-responding parents. *Current Therapeutic Research* 12:286–290

Eichelman B (1988), Toward a rational pharmacotherapy for aggressive and violent behavior. *Hosp Community Psychiatry* 39:31–39

Engstrom FW, Robbins DR, May JG (1978), Manic-depressive illness in adolescence. *J Am Acad Child Psychiatry* 17:514–520

Feinstein S, Wolpert E (1973), Juvenile manic-depressive illness. *J Am Acad Child Psychiatry* 12:123–136

Fisman S, Max P, Woodside DB (1985), Affective disorder in an adolescent. *Can J Psychiatry* 30:530–534

Forrest JN, Cohen AD, Torretti J, Himmelhoch JM, Epstein FH (1974), On the mechanism of lithium-induced diabetes insipidus in man and the rat. *J Clin Invest* 53:1115–1123

Friedman E, Wang HY (1990), Effect of chronic lithium treatment on 5-hydroxy-tryptamine autoreceptors and release of 5-[3H] hydroxytryptamine from rat brain cortical, hippocampal, and hypothalamic slices. *J Neurochem* 50:195–201

Fristad MA, Weller EB, Weller RA (1992), The Mania Rating Scale: can it be used in children? A preliminary report. *J Am Acad Child Adolesc Psychiatry* 31:252–257

Fukuda K. Etoh T, Okuma T (1986), Affective disorders in mentally retarded adolescents: report of two cases with lithium treatment. *Jpn J Psychiatry Neurol* 40:551–557

Gammon GD, John K, Rothblum ED, Mullen K, Tischler GL, Weissman MM (1983), Use of structured diagnostic interview to identify bipolar disorder in adolescent inpatients: frequency and manifestations of the disorder. *Am J Psychiatry* 140:543–547

Garcia-Sevilla JA, Guimon J, Garcia-Vallejo P, Fuster MJ (1986), Biochemical and functional evidence of supersensitive platelet alpha-2-adrenoceptors in major affective disorder: effect of long term lithium carbonate treatment. *Arch Gen Psychiatry* 43:51–57

Geller B, Fetner HH (1989), Children's 24-hour serum lithium level after a single dose predicts initial dose at steady-state plasma intervals. *J Clin Psychopharmacol* 9:155

Ghadirian AM, Kusalic M (1990), Rapid cycling following antidepressant in an adolescent. *Biol Psychiatry* 27:1184

Goldberg MA (1983), The treatment of Kleine-Levin syndrome with lithium. *Can J Psychiatry* 28:491–493

Goodwin GM, DeSouza RJ, Wood AJ, Green AR (1986), Lithium decreases 5-HT$_1$ and 5-HT$_2$ receptor and alpha-2-adrenoceptor mediated function in mice. *Psychopharmacology* 90:482–487

Gram LF, Rafaelsen OJ (1972), Lithium treatment of psychotic children and adolescents. *Acta Psychiatr Scand* 48:253–260

Greenhill LL, Rieder RO, Wender PH, Buchsbaum M, Zahn TP (1973), Lithium carbonate in the treatment of hyperactive children. *Arch Gen Psychiatry* 28:636–640

Gross G, Dodt C, Hanft G (1988), Effect of chronic lithium administration on adrenoceptor binding and adrenoceptor regulation in rat cerebral cortex. *Naunyn Schmiedeberg Arch Pharmacol* 337:267–272

Gross HA, Ebert MH, Faden VB, Goldberg SC, Nee LE, Kaye WH (1981), A double-blind controlled trial of lithium carbonate in primary anorexia nervosa. *J Clin Psychopharmacol* 1:376–381

Hall DC, Ries RK (1983), Bipolar illness, catatonia, and the dexamethasone suppression test in adolescence: case report. *J Clin Psychiatry* 44:222–224

Hassanyeh F, Davison K (1980), Bipolar affective psychosis with onset before age 16 years: report of 10 cases. *Br J Psychiatry* 137:530–539

Himmelhoch JM, Garfinkel ME (1986), Mixed mania: diagnosis and treatment. *Psychopharmacol Bull* 22:613–620

Hokin LE (1985), Receptors and phosphoinositide generated second messengers. *Annu Rev Biochem* 54:205–235

Horowitz HA (1977), Lithium and the treatment of adolescent manic depressive illness. *Dis Nerv Syst* 38:480–483

Hotta I, Yamawaki S, Segawa T (1986), Long-term lithium treatment causes serotonin receptor down-regulation via serotonergic presynapses in rat brain. *Neuropsychobiology* 16:19–26

Hsu LKG, Starzynski J (1986a), Mania in adolescence. *J Clin Psychiatry* 47:596–599

Hsu LKG, Starzynski J (1986b), Case reports: lithium-resistant adolescent mania. *J Am Acad Child Adolesc Psychiatry* 25:280–283

Hsu LKG, Starzynski J, Ju ESY (1991), Treatment of bulimia nervosa with lithium carbonate: a controlled study. *J Nerv Ment Dis* 179:351–355

Jeffries JJ, Lefebvre A (1973), Depression and mania associated with Kleine-Levin-Critchley syndrome. *Can Psychiatr Assoc J* 18:439–444

Joshi P, Capozzoli J, Coyle J (1985), Effective management with lithium of a persistent, post-traumatic hypomania in a 10-year-old child. *J Dev Behav Pediatr* 6:352–354

Joyce PR (1984), Age of onset in bipolar affective disorder and misdiagnosis as schizophrenia. *Psychol Med* 14:145–149

Kelly J, Kock M, Buegel D (1976), Lithium carbonate in juvenile manic depressive illness. *Dis Nerv Syst* 37:90–92

Kerbeshian J, Burd L (1989), Tourette disorder and bipolar symptomatology in childhood and adolescence. *Can J Psychiatry* 34:230–233

Kerbeshian J, Burd L, Fisher W (1987), Lithium carbonate in the treatment of two patients with infantile autism and atypical bipolar symptomatology. *J Clin Psychopharmacol* 7:401–405

Khandelwal SK, Varma VK, Murthy RS (1984), Renal function in children receiving long-term lithium prophylaxis. *Am J Psychiatry* 141:278–279

Kolata GB (1980), NIH shaken by death of research volunteer. *Science* 209:475–476, 478–479

Lena B (1979), Lithium in child and adolescent psychiatry. *Arch Gen Psychiatry* 36:854–855

Lena B, Bastable MD (1978), The reliability of salivary lithium estimations in children. *IRCS J Med Sci* 6:208

Lena B, O'Brian EMD (1975), Success with lithium in a disturbed child (letter) *Lancet* 2:1307–1308

Lena B, Surtees SJ, Maggs R (1978), The efficacy of lithium in the treatment of emotional disturbance in children and adolescents. In: *Lithium in Medical Practice*, Johnson FN, Johnson S, eds. Lancaster, England: MTP Press Ltd, pp 79–83

Licamelle WL, Goldberg RL (1989), The concurrent uses of lithium and methylphenidate in a child. *J Am Acad Child Adolesc Psychiatry* 28:785–787

Linter CM (1987), Short-cycle manic-depressive psychosis in a mentally handicapped child without family history: a case report. *Br J Psychiatry* 151:554–555

Loranger AW, Levine PM (1978), Age at onset of bipolar affective illness. *Arch Gen Psychiatry* 35:1345–1348

Maggi A, Enna SJ (1980), Regional alterations in rat brain neurotransmitter systems following chronic lithium treatment. *J Neurochem* 34:888–892

Manji HK, Hsiao JK, Risby ED, Oliver J, Rudorfer MV, Potter WZ (1991), The mechanisms of action of lithium I: effects on serotoninergic and noradrenergic systems in normal subjects. *Arch Gen Psychiatry* 48:505–512

Mattson A, Seltzer RL (1981), MAOI-induced rapid cycling bipolar affective disorder in an adolescent. *Am J Psychiatry* 138:677–679

McKnew DH, Cytryn L, Buchsbaum MS et al. (1981), Lithium in children of lithium responding parents. *Psychiatry Res* 4:171–180

Miller F, Menninger J (1987), Correlation of neuroleptic dose and neurotoxicity in patients given lithium and a neuroleptic. *Hosp Community Psychiatry* 38:1219–1221

Mork A, Geisler A (1987), Mode of action of lithium on the catalytic unit of adenylate cyclase from rat brain. *Pharmacol Toxicol* 60:241–248

Mork A, Geisler A (1989a), Effects of GTP on hormone-stimulated adenylate cyclase activity in cerebral cortex, striatum, and hippocampus from rats treated chronically with lithium. *Biol Psychiatry* 26:279–288

Mork A, Geisler A (1989b), The effects of lithium in vitro and ex vivo on adenylate cyclase in brain are exerted by distinct mechanisms. *Neuropharmacology* 28:307–311

Naylor GJ, Donald JM, Le Poidevin D, Reid AH (1974), A double-blind trial of long-term lithium therapy in mental defectives. *Br J Psychiatry* 124:52–57

Neil JF, Himmelhoch JM, Licata SM (1976), Emergence of myasthenia gravis during treatment with lithium carbonate. *Arch Gen Psychiatry* 33:1090–1092

Newman ME, Belmaker RH (1987), Effects of lithium in vitro and ex vivo on components of the adenylate cyclase system in membranes from the cerebral cortex of the rat. *Neuropharmacology* 26:211–217

Nielsen-Kudsk F, Amdisen A (1979), Analysis of pharmacokinetics of lithium in man. *Eur J Clin Pharmacol* 16:271–277

Odagaki Y, Koyama R, Matsubara S, Matsubara R, Yamashita I (1990), Effects of chronic lithium treatment on serontonin binding sites in rat brain. *J Psychiatry Res* 24:271-277

Ogura C, Okuma T, Nakazawz K, Kishimoto A (1976), Treatment of periodic somnolence with lithium carbonate (letter). *Arch Neurol* 33:143

Parmelee DX, O'Shanick GJ (1988), Carbamazepine-lithium toxicity in brain-damaged adolescents. *Brain Inj* 2:305-308

Peatfield RC, Rose FC (1981), Exacerbation of migraine by treatment with lithium. *Headache* 21:140-142

Perry R, Campbell M, Grega DM, Anderson L (1984), Saliva lithium levels in children: their use in monitoring serum lithium levels and lithium side effects. *J Clin Psychopharmacol* 4:199-202

Picker W, Solomon G, Gertner J (1990), Lithium side effect. *J Am Acad Child Adolesc Psychiatry* 29:489

Platt JE, Camobell M, Green WH, Perry R, Cohen IL (1981), Effects of lithium carbonate and haloperidol on cognition in aggressive hospitalized school-age children. *J Clin Psychopharmacol* 1:8-13

Potter RL (1983), Manic-depressive variant syndrome of childhood: diagnostic and therapeutic considerations. *Clin Pediatr (Phila)* 2:495-499

Risby ED, Hsiao JK, Manji HK et al. (1991), The mechanisms of action of lithium. II. Effects on adenylate cyclase activity and beta-adrenergic receptor binding in normal subjects. *Arch Gen Psychiatry* 48:513-524

Rogeness GA, Reister AE, Wicoff JS (1982), Unusual presentation of manic-depressive disorder in adolescence. *J Clin Psychiatry* 43:37-39

Rosenblatt JE, Pert CB, Tallman JF, Pert A, Bunney WE (1979), The effect of imipramine and lithium on alpha- and beta-receptor binding in rat brain. *Brain Res* 160:186-191

Ryan N, Meyer V, Dachville S, Mazzie D, Puig-Andrich J (1988), Lithium antidepressant augmentation in TCA-refractory depression in adolescents. *J Am Acad Child Adolesc Psychiatry* 27:371-376

Shafey H (1986), Use of lithium and flupenthixol in a patient with pervasive developmental disorder. *Am J Psychiatry* 143:681

Sheard MH (1975), Lithium in the treatment of aggression. *J Nerv Ment Dis* 169:108-118

Siassi I (1982), Lithium treatment of impulsive behavior in children. *J Clin Psychiatry* 43:482-484

Somogyi I, Vetro A, Szentisvanyi I, Szekeley J, Sziland J (1988), Lithium treatment of aggressive children and the EEG. *Acta Paediatr Hung* 29:365-372

Spengler RN, Hollinsworth PJ, Smith CB (1986), Effects of long-term lithium and desipramine treatment upon clonidine-induced inhibition of 3H-norepinephrine release from rat hippocampal slices. *Fed Proc* 45:681

Stein GS, Hartshorn S, Jones J, Steinberg D (1982), Lithium in a case of severe anorexia nervosa. *Br J Psychiatry* 140:526–528

Steingard R, Biederman J (1987), Lithium responsive manic-like symptoms in two individuals with autism and mental retardation. *J Am Acad Child Adolesc Psychiatry* 26:932–935

Strayhorn JM, Nash JL (1977), Severe neurotoxicity despite "therapeutic" serum lithium levels. *Dis Nerv Syst* 32:107–111

Strober M, Freeman R, Rigali J, Schmidt S, Diamond R (1992), The pharmacotherapy of depressive illness in adolescence, II: effects of lithium augmentation in nonresponders to imipramine. *J Am Acad Child Adolesc Psychiatry* 31:16–20

Strober M, Morrell W, Burroughs J, Lampert C, Danforth H, Freenan R (1988), Family study of bipolar I disorder in adolescence. *J Affect Disord* 15:255–268

Strober M, Morrell W, Lampert C, Burroughs J (1990), Relapse following discontinuation of lithium maintenance therapy in adolescents with bipolar illness: a naturalistic study. *Am J Psychiatry* 147:457–461

Sylvester CE, Burke PM, McCauley EA, Christopher J (1984), Manic psychosis in childhood: report of two cases. *J Nerv Ment Dis* 172:12–15

Treiser S, Kellar KJ (1979), Lithium effects on adrenergic receptor supersensitivity in rat brain. *Eur J Pharmacol* 58:85–86

Treiser SL, Cascio CS, O'Donohue TL, Thoa NB, Jacobowitz DM, Kellar KJ (1981), Lithium increases serotonin release and decreses serotonin receptors in the hippocampus. *Science* 213:1529–1531

Tyrer SP, Walsh A, Edwards DE, Berney TP, Stephens DA (1984), Factors associated with a good response to lithium in aggressive mentally handicapped subjects. *Prog Neuropsychopharmacol Biol Psychiatry* 8:751–755

Varanka TM, Weller RA, Weller EB, Fristad M (1988), Lithium treatment of manic episodes with psychotic prepubertal children. *Am J Psychiatry* 145:1557–1559

Vetro A, Pallag P, Szentistvanyi LI, Vargha M, Szilard J (1981), Treatment of childhood aggressivity with lithium. *Aggressologie* 22:27–30

Vetro A, Szentistivanyi LI, Pallag P, Vargha M, Szilard J (1985), Therapeutic experience with lithium in childhood aggressivity. *Neuropsychobiology* 14:121–127

Vitrello B, Behar D, Malone R, Delaney MA, Ryan PJ, Simpson EM (1988), Pharmacokinetics of lithium carbonate in children. *J Clin Psychopharmacol* 8:355–359

Warneke LA (1975), Case of manic-depressive illness in childhood. *Can Psychiatr Assoc J* 20:195–200

Weinberg WA, Brumback RA (1976), Mania in childhood: case studies and literature review. *Am J Dis Child* 130:380–385

Weiner IB, del Gaudio AC (1976), Psychopathology in adolescence. *Arch Gen Psychiatry* 33:187–193

Weller EB, Weller RA, Fristad MA (1986), Lithium dosage guide for prepubertal children: a preliminary report. *J Am Acad Child Adolesc Psychiatry* 25:92–95

Weller EB, Weller RA, Fristad MA, Cartwell M, Tucker S (1987), Saliva lithium monitoring in prepubertal children. *J Am Acad Child Adolesc Psychiatry* 26:173–175

Whitehead PL, Clark LD (1970), Effect of lithium carbonate, placebo, and thioridazine of hyperactive children. *Am J Psychiatry* 127:824–825

Whitworth P, Kendall DA (1989), Effects on lithium on inositol phospholipid hydrolysis and inhibition of dopamine D1 receptor-mediated cyclic AMP formation by carbacol in rat brain slices. *J Neurochem* 53:536–541

Will RG, Young JPR, Thomas DJ (1988), Kleine-Levin syndrome: report of two cases with onset of symptoms precipitated by head trauma. *Br J Psychiatry* 152:410–412

Winchel RM, Stanley M (1991), Self-injurious behavior: a review of the behavior and biology of self-mutilation. *Am J Psychiatry* 148:306–317

Wood IK, Parmelee DX, Foreman JW (1989), Lithium-induced nephrotic syndrome. *Am J Psychiatry* 146:84–87

Youngerman J, Canino IA (1978), Lithium carbonate use in children and adolescents. *Arch Gen Psychiatry* 35:216–224

Youngerman J, Canino IA (1983), Violent kids, violent parents: family pharmacotherapy. *Am J Orthopsychiatry* 53:152–156

19

A Critique of the Application of Sensory Integration Therapy to Children with Learning Disabilities

Theodore P. Hoehn and Alfred A. Baumeister

Vanderbilt University, Nashville

Sensory integration (SI) therapy is a controversial—though popular—treatment for the remediation of motor and academic problems. It has been applied primarily to children with learning disabilities, under the assumption that such children (or at least a subgroup of them) have problems in sensory integration to which some or all of their learning difficulties can be ascribed. The present article critically examines the related issues of whether children with learning disabilities differentially exhibit concomitant problems in sensory integration, and whether such children are helped in any way by means specific to SI therapy. An overview of theoretical contentions and empirical findings pertaining to the first issue is presented, followed by a detailed review of recent studies in the SI therapy research literature, in an effort to resolve the second issue. Results of this critique raise serious doubts as to the validity or utility of SI therapy as an appropriate, indicated treatment for the clinical population in question—and, by extension, for any other groups diagnosed as having "sensory integrative dysfunction." It is concluded that the current fund of research findings may well be sufficient to declare SI therapy not merely an unproven, but a demonstrably ineffective, primary or adjunctive remedial treatment for learning disabilities and other disorders.

Reprinted with permission from the *Journal of Learning Disabilities*, 1994, Vol. 27(6), 338–350. Copyright © 1994 by the American Academy of Child and Adolescent Psychiatry.

Preparation of this article was supported in part by National Institute of Child Health and Human Development Grant No. HD27336, awarded to the John F. Kennedy Center for Research on Human Development at Vanderbilt University.

Sensory integration (SI), as conceived of and advanced by Ayres (e.g., 1972b), has been and remains a subject of considerable controversy in the fields of psychology, education, and medicine (e.g., cf. Lerer, 1981; Price, 1977; Sieben, 1977). According to Ayres (1979), *sensory integration* is defined as "the organization of sensory input for use. The 'use' may be a perception of the body or the world, or an adaptive response, or a learning process, or the development of some neural function" (p. 184). Besides specifying a hypothetical neurological process, the term denotes not only an affiliated theoretical orientation to certain neuropsychological phenomena—encompassing numerous and varied neurological, developmental, and behavioral concepts and constructs—but also its clinical accompaniments. These comprise an original typology of specialized neurobehavioral disorders (collectively referred to as *sensory integrative dysfunction*), as well as associated diagnostic measures and therapeutic practices (see Fisher, Murray, & Bundy, 1991).

The fundamental postulates of sensory integration theory have been well described and discussed in detail (e.g., Ayres, 1972b, 1979; Clark & Shuer, 1978; Fisher & Murray, 1991; Ottenbacher & Short, 1985). The theory, along with its attendant clinical measures and techniques, strongly emphasizes the importance of vestibular, proprioceptive, and tactile stimulation to development and behavior. Provision of these primitive forms of sensation, preferably in combination with and within the context of purposeful motor activity, and the patient's corresponding organization of them (together with concurrent visual, auditory, and/or olfactory sensory inputs) for use, are the aims of SI therapy. Toward this end, occupational therapists typically employ various pieces of equipment, such as textured mitts, carpet squares, scooter boards, ramps, swings, and bounce pads, during treatment.

Sensory integration is seen as requisite to all perceptual–motor activity. Indeed, as Clark and Shuer (1978) noted, SI therapy originally was intended as a treatment for children with cerebral palsy. Its scope of application has since been extended to include many different clinical populations, such as persons with mental retardation (see Arendt, MacLean, & Baumeister, 1988; Clark & Shuer, 1978). However, the therapy has been applied primarily to children with learning disabilities, and its theory directed toward an understanding of this population (e.g., see Clark, Mailloux, & Parham, 1989). Ayres (1972b) hypothesized that such children, or at least a subgroup of them, have problems in sensory integration to which some or all of their learning difficulties can be ascribed. This proposition stems from the complementary notions in Ayres's theory of hierarchical levels of brain function and sequential stages in neurological development (e.g.,

Ayres, 1979). Thus, not only motor acts, but also "higher-level," cognitive abilities, such as reading and writing, are considered dependent on sensory integration. These notions similarly underlie the theory's emphasis on the processing of vestibular, proprioceptive, and tactile sensations, in that such processing is believed to take place chiefly in subcortical areas of the brain (particularly the brain stem), which can be characterized as early-developing, both phylogenetically and ontogenetically.

SI therapy is "theoretically grounded in medical-model logic" in its view of learning disabilities—and motor problems—as representing superficial symptoms that ultimately are attributable to some underlying neurological deficit that is discoverable through diagnostic evaluation, and in its "process" (as opposed to content) approach to treatment and remediation (Ottenbacher & Short, 1985, pp. 289–290). That is, perceptual-motor training programs or academic skills instruction (i.e., tutoring) programs are designed to exercise and directly influence specific motor or academic skills, such as throwing a ball or decoding words, so that they can be acquired and mastered by the child, but the experience is not expected to generalize beyond those particular skills. SI therapy, in contrast, is thought of as acting to remedy (or ameliorate the effects of) certain general sensorimotor disorders responsible for multiple individual motor or academic difficulties, and to lay a sensory processing foundation for the successful development of such skills. Of course, this foundation, as a precursor to learning, is not sufficient in and of itself to result in skillful behavior; traditional teaching methods are still advocated in conjunction with SI therapy (Ayres, 1972b).

An issue central to any analysis of applying SI therapy with children with learning disabilities is whether these children, in addition to their obvious difficulties with respect to academic achievement, legitimately and differentially suffer from problems in sensory integration. A positive resolution of this issue would imply, at least in principle, justification for remedial treatment, in whatever form appropriate. An examination of the arguments and evidence pertaining to SI dysfunction in children with learning disabilities follows.

SI DYSFUNCTION, HYPONYSTAGMUS, AND LEARNING DISABILITIES

Ayres's theory of sensory integration and concepts of SI dysfunction were developed and operationalized within the context of a series of factor-analytic studies that she conducted in the 1960s and 1970s (Ayres, 1965,

1966a, 1966b, 1969, 1972d, 1977). The studies used a variety of perceptual–motor (and other) measures and involved as subjects 4- to 10-year-old children both with and without learning disabilities. On the basis of the results of these psychometric tests and factor analyses, Ayres claimed to have identified certain characteristic factors that emerge from the scores of children with learning disabilities and serve to differentiate them from their nondisabled peers. Among various other classificatory schemes and designations (see Cummins, 1991), which commonly involve five categories of dysfunction, these perceptual–motor factors, or syndromes, have been termed (a) disorder in postural, ocular, and bilateral integration; (b) apraxia (or disorder in praxis, the ability to plan and execute motor acts); (c) disorder in form and space perception; (d) auditory–language problems; and (e) tactile defensiveness (Ayres, 1972b).

Numerous clinical measures (e.g., the Southern California Sensory Integration Tests [SCSIT, Ayres, 1972c, 1980]; the Southern California Postrotary Nystagmus Test [SCPNT, Ayres, 1975]; and the Sensory Integration and Praxis Tests [Ayres, 1989]) designed to evaluate one's status in terms of these syndromes have subsequently been developed. Although the syndromes, subsumed under the general conceptual rubric of SI dysfunction, ostensibly owe their discovery and content to basic, overall performance differences existing between children with learning disabilities and those without, these clinical measures customarily are used to distinguish, *among* children with learning disabilities, those who purportedly have SI dysfunction from those who do not. It is only with respect to the former subgroup that remediation via SI therapy is advocated and claimed to be effective (e.g., Ayres, 1972a). As to the estimated prevalence of SI dysfunction within the population of children with learning disabilities, it was reported in a recent SI therapy outcome study (Carte, Morrison, Sublett, Uemura, & Setrakian, 1984; see also Morrison & Sublett, 1986) that 70% of the potential subjects designated by public schools as learning disabled were diagnosed in preexperimental screening as having SI dysfunction.

The results of an early, controlled—but flawed (e.g., see Schaffer, 1984)—study of SI treatment and academic achievement led Ayres (1978) to further refine her diagnostic and prognostic criteria by proposing that children with learning disabilities and SI dysfunction who exhibit hyporeactive postrotary nystagmus, or *hyponystagmus*, are particularly likely to benefit from SI therapy. Postrotary nystagmus is an involuntary lateral oscillation of the eyes, characterized by fast forward motions (i.e., in the same direction as the stimulus) and slow returns, that follows rapid rotational deceleration. It is a reflexive response to stimulation of the semicircular canals in the inner ear and, as such, is considered a major, objective sign of vestibular-system functioning. In SI research and clinical practice, postrotary nystagmus, measured quantitatively in terms of duration, is routinely assessed by means of the SCPNT. Hyponystagmus is defined as a total duration (post-clockwise and counterclockwise rotation) standardized score of less than −1 *SD* (Ayres, 1975, 1978). Several diagnostic and outcome studies have reported an approximate 50% incidence of hyponystagmus in their samples of children with learning disabilities (Ayres, 1978; Ottenbacher, 1978, 1980; the latter two studies involving the same subjects) or children with learning disabilities and SI dysfunction (Carte et al., 1984; Ottenbacher, Short, & Watson, 1979; Ottenbacher, Watson, Short, & Biderman, 1979; the latter two studies involving the same subjects).

Although in her 1978 article Ayres referred to "duration of postrotary nystagmus" as a separate "domain of sensorimotor and language functions" (or SI factor), this variable has been identified elsewhere with a more general syndrome concerning disorders in "postural and bilateral integration" (e.g., Ottenbacher, 1978), or "vestibular–bilateral integration" (Ottenbacher & Short, 1985). Both hypo- and hypernystagmus (i.e., an SCPNT total score greater than 1 *SD*) are interpreted as abnormal and as evidence of probably different types of vestibular dysfunction (Ayres, 1975, 1978); hypernystagmus, though comparatively rare among children with learning disabilities, is considered a sign of greater neuropsychological impairment (Ayres, 1978; Ottenbacher, 1980). Prone extension posture, equilibrium reactions (specifically, standing balance), and muscle tone have been found to share significant variance with (normal vs. abnormal) SCPNT scores in children with learning disabilities (Ottenbacher, 1978; see also Ayres, 1978). Poor performance in terms of these informal neurobehavioral measures, or *clinical observations* (Ayres, 1976), are considered supplemental, "soft" signs of dysfunction (e.g., Ottenbacher, 1978). Similar claims regarding disorders in the vestibular–proprioceptive system of children with learning disabilities—and attendant arguments concerning the proper focus of intervention—have been made by investigators outside the SI paradigm (e.g., deQuiros, 1976; deQuiros & Schrager, 1979).

As intimated previously, an impressive collection of clinical constructs, assessment tools, and treatment procedures has been developed on the basis of hypothesized differences in sensory integration between children with and without learning disabilities, particularly with respect to vestibular-system functioning and hyponystagmus. The findings of several recent studies, however, have called into question certain fundamental empirical assertions and theoretical assumptions that underlie this enterprise.

Within the context of a larger research project (see Carte et al., 1984; Morrison & Sublett, 1986), Morrison and Sublett (1983) examined reliability of the SCPNT for a sample of 89 children, ages 6 years to 11 years, with learning disabilities and SI dysfunction. As expected, in comparison to nondisabled children in a similar age range (Punwar, 1982), the children in this sample evidenced significantly depressed SCPNT scores. (Almost no children demonstrated hypernystagmus during screening, and none was included in the sample for analysis.) The variance of these scores was significantly greater than that reported for the normative data, however. More important, even though estimates of both intrascorer and test-retest reliability were statistically significant in the Morrison and Sublett (1983) study, they were lower than those found with nondisabled children (e.g., Ayres, 1975; Punwar, 1982). Thus, based on the results of a separate analysis for reliability of duration scores that fell into the clinically deviant category of hyponystagmus, the authors stated that

> a child could have a total duration score of 12 seconds during one evaluation with a high probability of having a score of 16 seconds and, therefore, of being in the normal range in a later evaluation. The reverse of this is also true. A child's score may move into the deviant range from one evaluation to the next. (Morrison & Sublett, 1983, p. 697)

In addition to such concerns regarding the reliability of the SCPNT (see also Ayres, 1989), various investigators have questioned the validity of this test, and of measures of postrotary nystagmus in general. Polatajko (1983) and, more recently, Cohen (1989) cited numerous problems with the SCPNT, most notably that the test is administered in the light, with the subject's eyes open, thereby affording visual as well as vestibular stimulation during rotation. This can lead to optokinetic nystagmus, owing to the rapidly moving, repetitive nature of the visual field, and a consequent reduction in postrotary nystagmus duration as compared to that elicited in the dark. Testing in the light also permits fixation of the stationary surround once rotation has stopped, which can serve to reduce nystagmus durations by means of visual suppression. Regarding this latter confound, as Polatajko (1985) has suggested, if it can be expected that children with learning disabilities will tend to follow directions less well than will children without learning disabilities, then failure to follow the SCPNT instruction "Do not fixate" would predict and explain findings of lower postrotary nystagmus durations and higher incidences of hyponystagmus among the former group of children. Various other extravestibular factors, such as arousal level, attentional state, and behavioral disturbances—applicable to all measures of postrotary nystagmus—likewise are known to influence durations, and certain of these factors may be especially relevant to the validity and reliability of assessment in children with learning disabilities (see Morrison & Sublett, 1983).

Polatajko (1983), in blind testing, failed to find any significant correlations between SCPNT total duration scores and several pure measures of vestibular function during rotation for a sample of 40 boys, ages 8 years to 12 years, half of whom had learning disabilities. Results of the validity study further indicated no significant differences between groups in the incidence of abnormal scores on or responses to the SCPNT. She concluded that "the SCPNT should not be considered a test of vestibular function and all conclusions based on SCPNT results should be carefully reviewed" (p. 122).

In a subsequent investigation of the *vestibular dysfunction hypothesis* regarding children with learning disabilities (i.e., that disorders in vestibular functioning are related to academic problems), a postulate shared by SI theory and other, similar, perspectives (e.g., deQuiros & Schrager, 1979), Polatajko (1985) likewise employed an electronystagmograph to record vestibular nystagmus (i.e., compensatory eye movements) produced by subjects during rotational acceleration and deceleration in the dark. Forty children with learning disabilities and 40 nondisabled children, all between 8 years and 12 years of age, were tested using blind procedures. The Peabody Individual Achievement Test (PIAT) (Dunn & Markwardt, 1970) and the Slosson Intelligence Test (SIT) (Slosson, 1963) were also administered to the subjects.

The results of the study belied all three empirical predictions that Polatajko (1985) derived from the vestibular dysfunction hypothesis. These predictions were (a) that children with learning disabilities would differ from those without on measures of vestibular-system functioning: No significant differences were found between groups either in the intensity of their vestibular responses or in the relative incidence of vestibular dysfunction (i.e., hypo- or hyperresponsivity, using the results for the nondisabled children as normative data); (b) the corollary of *a*, that children with hypo-, average, or hyperresponsivity would differ on measures of academic functioning: No significant differences were observed among the vestibular responsivity groups on the PIAT or the SIT; and (c) as a complement to *b*, that there would be a direct relationship between performance on measures of vestibular functioning and measures of academic abilities: No significant correlations were obtained between vestibular intensity variables and IQ or academic achievement scores, either for all subjects combined, or separately for the group with learning disabilities and the group without. These findings led Polatajko to propose

that the vestibular dysfunction hypothesis be rejected. The rejection of that hypothesis for learning disabilities has a number of implications. The practical implications are that vestibular dysfunction should be abandoned as a meaningful type of learning disorder, and that the fairly common practice of sensory integrative therapy for such children should be re-evaluated. (p. 291)

Finally, Cummins (1991) conducted a reexamination of the results of Ayres's factor-analytic studies in combination, also including a multiple-regression study (Ayres, 1971) and a recent factor analysis (Ayres, Mailloux, & Wendler, 1987) for appraisal. Cummins's analysis revealed a lack of consistency between Ayres's factor labels and the content of these purported factors, with no core groups of component variables existing across studies with which to reliably identify similarly named factors or distinguish them from other factors. Even more troubling was the finding that none of the putative factors possessed a content such that the scores produced by children with learning disabilities could reliably be distinguished from those produced by children without learning disabilities. It was concluded that "the body of data that has been examined provides no validity for either the diagnostic procedures or the remedial programs for children with LD that have been derived from Ayres' multivariate studies" (p. 168). Other problems with Ayres's factor-analytic studies (e.g., too many tests having been administered to too few subjects), and with the validity of her syndromes of SI dysfunction and related SCSIT diagnostic measures, in general, have been noted elsewhere (e.g., Reed, 1978; Westman, 1978).

Aside from the general concerns raised regarding theoretic and diagnostic issues involved in an adequate understanding of the possible relationships among SI dysfunction, hyponystagmus, and learning disabilities, there stands the practical, empirical matter of whether children with learning disabilities actually benefit from SI therapy in any specific and unique way. This topic, crucial as it is to the future of SI theory and practice, will next be addressed by means of a detailed review of the relevant research literature.

REVIEW OF SI THERAPY RESEARCH

Ottenbacher (1982b) conducted an early, comprehensive literature review. He performed a meta-analysis of 8 studies, culled from an initial corpus of 49, that met a minimal set of criteria regarding methodological/design adequacy. Each study (a) utilized SI therapy (judged in light of an operational definition adapted from Ayres, 1979) as the independent variable; (b) involved a comparison between at least two groups or conditions: the SI treatment and a no-treatment control; (c) included measures of motor or reflex functioning, academic abilities, and/or language skills as dependent variables; and (d) reported results in a quantitative form. The majority of subjects were children with learning disabilities, although two of the studies involved children or adults with mental retardation, and children with various other handicapping conditions were included in the research, as well.

Based on the outcomes of both effect-site and combined-probability analyses of 47 statistical hypothesis tests generated by the eight studies, Ottenbacher (1982b) concluded, "The effect of sensory integration therapy applied to the representative population appears to have empirical support" (p. 577). Effects were found to be greatest for measures of motor/reflex functioning and least (though still considerable) for language measures. Furthermore, children with learning disabilities appeared to benefit from treatment more than did subjects with mental retardation. However, diagnostic category was confounded not only with type of dependent measure, but also with chronological age, rendering interpretation problematic.

Although Ottenbacher's (1982b) quantitative review was generally supportive as to the efficacy of SI therapy, the studies reviewed, as well as the form of the review itself, are open to numerous criticisms. Many of the studies, as indicated in the review, suffered from possible inadequacies in subject sampling and group assignment. Similar flaws in method and/or design, such as failure to ensure blind evaluation of subjects, have been cited elsewhere (e.g., see Densem, Nuthall, Bushnell, & Horn, 1989). Regarding the form of the review, it should be noted that although some studies involved more than two groups (i.e., an alternative treatment group in addition to the SI treatment and control groups), only data from SI treatment groups and no-treatment control groups were included in the analyses. Results concerning alternative treatment groups were ignored. The possibility exists, therefore, that factors not specific to treatment, such as placebo or Hawthorne effects, could mistakenly have been taken as evidence uniquely favoring SI therapy, thus biasing the outcome of the review. Also, as Ottenbacher observed, his use of individual hypothesis tests as the units of analysis, with multiple results being derived from any one study, leads to problems regarding nonindependence of the primary data. Indeed, Ottenbacher and Short (1985), in citing certain limitations of the meta-analysis, later characterized it as merely providing "suggestive support for the effects of sensory integration therapy in the eight studies reviewed" (pp. 319–320). At any rate, sufficient time has passed and, one hopes, enough good research has been conducted since 1982 to warrant a more current review of the SI therapy literature.

Research Description

A search was initiated for experimental reports assessing the effectiveness of SI therapy that have been published since Ottenbacher's (1982b) review. The same basic criteria as employed by Ottenbacher were used for the selection of studies, except that in consideration of the relative paucity of applicable research, the stipulation was dropped that one of the groups be a no-treatment control, which on ethical and/or practical grounds was sometimes not included in an experiment. However, the present qualitative review was restricted to only those studies that utilized children with learning disabilities as subjects (see Arendt et al., 1988, for a recent review of research involving subjects with mental retardation).

A total of seven studies were found that met all the inclusion criteria. Of these studies, two were closely related in that they pertained to a single, common experiment. Specifically, Morrison and Sublett (1986) reported results of certain measures for a subset of subjects who had participated in an experiment originally described by Carte et al. (1984). However, with the exception of one measure for which the data overlapped, different outcome areas were addressed in the two reports. For this reason, both papers were retained in the final review. Table 1 contains a brief synopsis of each of the seven constituent studies.

Samples. Subjects were early school-age children, about 5 to 11 years old, with males far outnumbering females in every study. All samples were described as having both learning disabilities (nonspecific as to subtype) and SI dysfunction. Diagnoses regarding learning disabilities, which could be in terms of reading, spelling, or arithmetic, were based on identification by school personnel and/or results of preexperimental psychoeducational assessments. Diagnoses regarding SI dysfunction were based on clinical observations (see Ayres, 1976, 1980) and results of preexperimental administration of the SCSIT and the SCPNT. With the exception of the Ottenbacher (1982a), Carte et al. (1984), and Morrison and Sublett (1986) investigations, the studies relied on clinically referred subject populations, with the children primarily exhibiting problems in motor coordination. All subjects in the above-named studies, and about half of those in the Wilson, Kaplan, Fellowes, Gruchy, and Faris (1992) study, were receiving some degree of special education assistance in public schools during the course of the experimental examination. Subjects in the Humphries, Wright, McDougall, and Vertes (1990) study, on the other hand, did not receive special education assistance; it was not reported whether subjects in the Humphries, Wright, Snider, and McDougall (1992) study or the Polatajko, Law, Miller, Schaffer, and Macnab (1991) study were receiving such assistance.

TABLE 1
Characteristics of the Reviewed SI Therapy Outcome Studies

Study	N	Design	Treatment	Outcome Areas
Carte et al. (1984)	87	Two groups: SI treatment and no-treatment control; pre/posttests	Two or three 45-min sessions per week over 9-month period (66 sessions total)	PRN; perceptual processing; academic abilities
Humphries et al. (1990)	30	Three groups: SI treatment, PM treatment, and no-treatment control; pre/posttests	One 1-hr sessions per week for 24 weeks	Sensorimotor functioning (including PRN); cognitive, language, and academic abilities
Humphries et al. (1992)	103	Three groups: SI treatment, PM treatment, and no-treatment control; pre/posttests	Three 1-hr sessions per week for approximately 8 months (72 sessions total)	Sensorimotor functioning (including PRN); cognitive, language, and academic abilities; attention; self-concept
Morrison & Sublett (1986)	47	Same experiment as in Carte et al. (1984)	Same experiment as in Carte et al. (1984)	Vestibular functioning (including PRN)
Ottenbacher (1982a)	3	Single-subject methodology: 5 weeks of baseline, followed by 20 weeks of SI treatment intervention	Three 50-min sessions per week	PRN
Polatajko et al. (1991)	67	Two groups: SI treatment and PM treatment (no-treatment control dropped midway); pretest, 6- and 9-month posttests	One 1-hr session per week for 6 months	Motor skills; academic abilities; self-esteem
Wilson et al. (1992)	29[a]	Two groups: SI treatment and tutoring treatment; pretest, 6-month midtest, 12-month posttest	Two 50-min sessions per week for approximately 12 months (75–80 sessions total)	PRN; motor skills; academic abilities; self-esteem; behavior

Note. SI = sensory integration; PRN = postrotary nystagmus; PM = perceptual–motor.
[a] Four discontinued treatment after midtest.

In recognition of the theoretical and presumed clinical significance of vestibular functioning in regard to sensory integration and learning disorders, four of the seven studies either restricted their samples entirely to children with hyponystagmus or isolated a hyponystagmus subsample for particular analysis. Every subject in the Wilson et al. (1992) study was characterized as having hyponystagmus. Approximately half of the sample tested by Carte et al. (1984) were so identified, resulting in a hyponystagmus subsample of 45 children. These same subjects constituted essentially the entire hyponystagmus sample reported on later by Morrison and Sublett (1986). Finally, 2 of the 3 subjects in the Ottenbacher (1982a) study had initial hyponystagmus.

Designs and methodologies. All of the studies examined the effects of therapy over multiple treatment sessions on certain outcome measures, rather than any immediate response changes that might occur during the moment of treatment delivery. The research focused on the fundamental question of whether SI therapy is effective, as opposed to concomitant, more sophisticated issues regarding how and why the therapy operates. Within the classification scheme for SI therapy research proposed and discussed by Tickle-Degnen (1988), such investigations of basic effectiveness over multiple sessions are characterized as *Diachronic Model 1* research.

Six of the seven studies employed a mixed-factor design, with group (SI treatment, alternative treatment, and/or no-treatment control) as a between-subjects factor and time of test (pretest, midtest, and/or posttest) as a repeated-measures, or within-subjects, factor. Subjects were randomly assigned to SI treatment or comparison conditions, following stratification or matching on the basis of such variables as sex, age, and entry-level ability. Analyses in each of these studies revealed no significant differences among groups on psychometric variables, type and degree of SI dysfunction, or overall pretest measures.

In contrast to the other studies, Ottenbacher's (1982a) employed single-subject methodology. It included baseline and intervention components but did not involve multiple baselines across subjects. Furthermore, although all his subjects were male and of a similar age, they were not equated on IQ or SCSIT subtest scores.

In every study, SI treatment was reportedly confined to the use of specific SI therapy principles and techniques, designed to provide "vestibular, proprioceptive, and tactile stimulation within a meaningful, self-directed activity in order to elicit an adaptive motor response" (Wilson et al., 1992, p. 12), and was conducted over a relatively long period of time and considerable number of sessions. SI and comparison treatment programs were administered by trained, experienced occupational therapists (or other appropriate professionals) in all cases. Although in the Ottenbacher (1982a) study a single therapist provided SI treatment to all 3 subjects during common sessions of intervention, in all of the group studies, individualized treatment programs were implemented on a one-to-one basis. Four studies involved a comparison between SI and an alternative treatment condition, the temporal parameters of therapy being equated across conditions. Within the Humphries et al. (1990) and Humphries et al. (1992) studies, the same therapists administered both the SI and the perceptual-motor (PM) treatments, with subjects randomly assigned to a therapist within a treatment condition. In contrast, Polatajko et al. (1991) utilized multiple therapists across both their SI and PM treatment conditions. Finally, in the Wilson et al. (1992) study, occupational therapists provided SI therapy, whereas special education teachers conducted the academic skills tutoring.

Assessments in the Humphries et al. (1990), Humphries et al. (1992), Wilson et al. (1992), and Polatajko et al. (1991) studies were all reported to have been conducted by personnel who were unaware of the subjects' group assignments. In the latter study, furthermore, the tester also was naive as to the experimental hypotheses. Whether the Ottenbacher (1982a), Carte et al. (1984), and Morrison and Sublett (1986) investigations involved blind evaluation is unclear from the reports.

Data analyses. In cases in which an initial difference between groups on a specific dependent variable approached or reached statistical significance, pretest score was included as a covariate when evaluating treatment effects in the Humphries et al. (1990) and Humphries et al. (1992) studies. In the Polatajko et al. (1991) study, age, IQ, and pretest score were used as covariates when analyzing all motor and academic variables, and pretest score was used when analyzing self-esteem measures. To control their Type I error rates in view of the large number of dependent variables each involved, all of the group studies except for Humphries et al. (1990) and Polatajko et al. (1991) tested effects via multivariate analyses of variance (MANOVAs) or multivariate analyses of covariance (MANCOVAs) followed by individual ANOVAs or ANCOVAs.

Both graphic and statistical analyses of the data were performed in the Ottenbacher (1982a) study, the only investigation to utilize single-subject methodology. The Polatajko et al. (1991) research was alone among the group studies in not employing repeated-measures statistical procedures within the primary analysis. Instead, data for the two treatment groups were compared at the 6-month posttest, and again, independently, at the 9-

month (follow-up) posttest. (Results pertaining to changes in performance over time were reported only in a cursory form, with no specifics provided as to statistical method or outcomes of the analyses.)

The remaining group studies varied somewhat as to inclusiveness of the results provided in their reports. In the Carte et al. (1984) and Morrison and Sublett (1986) investigations, main effects for group and time of test, as well as their interaction, were reported for all dependent variables. Only inter-action, or treatment, effects were reported in the Humphries et al. (1990) and Humphries et al. (1992) studies. Wilson et al. (1992) reported Group × Time of Test interactions within both a midtest (i.e., pretest vs. midtest) and a posttest (i.e., pretest vs. midtest vs. posttest) analysis, and time-of-test main effects within the posttest analysis only.

Findings

With regard to the Carte et al. (1984) study, results for the total sample and for the hyponystagmus subsample were the same on all dependent variables. In addition, no significant Age (i.e., groups divided into older and younger subgroups) × Group × Time of Test interaction effects were found in the total sample.

Postrotary nystagmus. All of the studies except for Polatajko et al. (1991) included postrotary nystagmus (assessed by means of the SCPNT and intended as a comparatively direct index of vestibular-system functioning) as an outcome measure. In fact, it represented the sole dependent variable in the Ottenbacher (1982a) study, the results of which were mixed. The single subject with initially normal nystagmus durations (mean baseline duration = 18.8 s) exhibited a significant decline with SI treatment (mean duration for final week of intervention = 11.5 s), as predicted based on evi-dence of gradual habituation or adaptation through repeated exposure to vestibular stimulation in persons with normal vestibulo-ocular reflexes (e.g., Crampton, 1964). However, outcomes for the other 2 subjects were inconsistent. Although both children evidenced initially low nystagmus durations (mean baseline durations = 3.5 s and 8.6 s, respectively), they dif-fered considerably in terms of changes in duration over the course of the study (mean durations for final week of intervention = 12.0 s and 10.0s, re-spectively). Thus, although SI treatment apparently resulted in a significant increase in postrotary nystagmus duration (as hypothesized) one subject with hyponystagmus, it had no such effect for another.

Results concerning postrotary nystagmus in the remaining studies were uniformly negative as to the existence of facilitative effects specific to SI therapy. In the Carte et al. (1984) study—and for essentially the same data reported by Morrison and Sublett (1986)—significant main effects of group, with nystagmus durations overall being longer for the SI treatment group than for the no-treatment control group, and time of test, with durations for both groups being longer at posttest than at pretest, were observed, but there was no significant interaction. (At posttest, the SI treatment group's mean duration was significantly higher than that of the control group. However, the former group's mean duration has also been higher at pretest; though not significantly so.) The Group × Time of Test interaction effect was not significant in either the Humphries et al. (1990) or the Humphries et al. (1992) study. Likewise, Wilson et al. (1992) found no significant interaction effects in their 6-month midtest and 12-month posttest analyses. The time-of-test main effect in the posttest analysis was significant, with nystagmus durations for both the SI treatment group and the tutoring treatment group being longer at mid- and posttest than at pretest.

Sensorimotor, perceptual, and motor measures. All of the group studies included some combination of dependent variables that assessed sensorimotor, perceptual, or motor functioning. (Results concerning postrotary nystagmus were isolated for discussion in the previous section.) In those studies in which certain subtests of the SCSIT were used as both screening tools and dependent measures, the subtests were restricted to those judged to have acceptable levels of test–retest reliability.

In the Carte et al. (1984) study, significant effects were found only for time of test, with performance improving from pretest to posttest for both the SI treatment group and the no-treatment control group, on (a) the Target Test (Reitan & Davison, 1974), a measure of visual tracking, attention, and immediate memory, and (b) six subtests of the Underlining Test (Rourke & Orr, 1977), a measure of rapid visual–perceptual analysis. Within that same overall experiment, Morrison and Sublett (1986) found no significant effects on two measures, other than postrotary nystagmus, of vestibular (and proprioceptive) functioning: (a) equilibrium reactions, tested using the Primitive Reflex and Postural Adjustment Assessment procedure (Pothier, Friedlander, Morrison, & Herman, 1983), with protective extension added, and (b) visual–motor integration, assessed by means of the Developmental Test of Visual-Motor Integration (VMI) (Beery, 1982).

Similarly, although both groups improved from pretest, Polatajko et al. (1991) found no significant differences between their SI treatment group and PM treatment group at either the 6-month posttest or the 9-month follow-up on scores for the Battery Composite or the Fine Motor and Gross Motor subtests of the Bruiniks-Oseretsky Test of Motor Proficiency

(BOTMP) (Bruininks, 1978). No significant Group × Time of Test interaction effects were observed by Wilson et al. (1992) in either the 6-month midtest or the 9-month posttest analysis for (a) fine motor skills, assessed via the Fine Motor subtests of the BOTMP and the SCSIT Motor Accuracy Test-Revised; (b) visual–motor skills, assessed via the VMI, the Design Copying subtest of the SCSIT, and a handwriting scale; or (c) gross motor skills, assessed via the Gross Motor and Upper Limb Coordination subtests of the BOTMP and the Clinical Observations of Motor and Postural Skills test (Wilson, Pollock, Kaplan, & Law, 1991). The time-of-test main effects in the posttest analysis were significant for all three measurement groupings, with performance for both the SI treatment group and the tutoring treatment group increasing over the course of the study.

A few positive, although inconsistent, results regarding the efficacy of SI therapy were obtained on a subset of sensorimotor measures in the two remaining studies. In the Humphries et al. (1990) study, significant Group × Time of Test interactions were found (a) for the Gross Motor Composite and Battery Composite scores on the BOTMP, with the SI treatment group improving significantly more from pretest to posttest than did the no-treatment control group (the PM treatment group being intermediate in improvement) on the former measure, and (b) on the Motor Accuracy Right subtest of the SCSIT, with the SI treatment group improving significantly more than did either the PM treatment group or the control group. No significant interactions were found for the Fine Motor Composite score on the BOTMP, other selected subtests of the SCSIT, the VMI, or Vestibular Functioning and Praxis categories of clinical observations.

In like manner, Humphries et al. (1992) reported a significant Group × Time of Test interaction for their Motor Planning category of clinical observations, with the SI treatment group improving significantly more from pretest to posttest than did either the PM treatment group or the no-treatment control group. On the other hand, significant interaction effects also were found (a) for the Gross Motor Composite and Battery Composite scores on the BOTMP—as in the Humphries et al. (1990) study—except that the PM treatment group improved significantly more than did either the SI treatment group or the control group, and (b) on the Design Copying subtest of the SCSIT, with the PM treatment group improving significantly more than did the SI treatment group (the control group being intermediate in improvement). No significant interactions were found for a Vestibular Functioning category of clinical observations, the Fine Motor Composite score on the BOTMP, other selected subtests of the SCSIT, or the VMI.

Cognitive, language, and academic measures. All of the group studies except for Morrison and Sublett (1986) included some combination of dependent variables that assessed cognitive, language, and/or academic abilities. Results concerning these measures were uniformly negative as to the existence of facilitative effects specific to SI therapy.

Carte et al. (1984) found no significant main or interaction effects on scores for the Comprehension subtest of the Gates-MacGinitie Reading Tests, Levels R through D (MacGinitie, 1978), and the Reading (decoding), Spelling, and Arithmetic subscales of the Wide Range Achievement Test (WRAT) (Jastak & Jastak, 1978). Likewise, in the Humphries et al. (1990) study, Group × Time of Test interactions were not significant regarding Wechsler Intelligence Scale for Children–Revised (WISC–R) (Wechsler, 1974) Verbal, Performance, and Full Scale IQs; the Test of Language Development–Primary (Newcomer & Hammill, 1982) Spoken Language Quotient; or scores for the Reading, Spelling, and Arithmetic subscales of the WRAT.

Cognitive measures in the Humphries et al. (1992) study comprised the WISC–R and Wechsler Preschool and Primary Scale of Intelligence (Wechsler, 1967), the Test of Visual–Perceptual Skills (Gardner, 1982), and the Gestalt Closure and Number Recall subtests from the Kaufman Assessment Battery for Children (Kaufman & Kaufman, 1983). Language measures comprised the Grammatic Closure subtest from the Illinois Test of Psycholinguistic Abilities (Kirk, McCarthy, & Kirk, 1968), the Sentence Repetition subtest from the Clinical Evaluation of Language Functions (Semel & Wiig, 1980), the Listening Comprehension subtest from the Durrell Analysis of Reading Difficulty (Durrell & Catterson, 1980), and the Test of Auditory Analysis Skills (Rosner, 1975). Measures relating to academic abilities consisted of the Reading, Spelling, and Arithmetic subscales of the WRAT, copying quality and rate indices from the Zaner-Bloser Handwriting Evaluation Scale (Zaner-Bloser, 1975), and a 10-point rating of printing readiness from the Basic School Skills Inventory (Goodman & Hammill, 1975). A MANCOVA testing the treatment (i.e., interaction) effect for all these psychoeducational variables was not significant.

The Reading Cluster, Mathematics Cluster, and Written Language Cluster of the Woodcock-Johnson Psycho-Educational Battery (WJPEB) (Woodcock & Johnson, 1977) constituted the academic measures utilized by Polatajko et al. (1991). Although both groups improved from pretest on all three measures, no significant differences between the SI treatment group and PM treatment group at either the 6-month posttest or the 9-month follow-up were observed on any of them.

Finally, the Group × Time of Test interaction effect on academic measures, represented by the Broad Cognitive Index, Reading Cluster, Perceptual Speed Cluster, and Preschool Cluster of the WJPEB, was also not significant in the Wilson et al. (1992) study. The time-of-test main effect in the posttest analysis was significant, with performance for both the SI treatment group and the tutoring treatment group increasing over the course of the study.

Self-esteem/self-concept, attention, and behavioral measures. Three of the group studies included some combination of dependent variables that assessed self-esteem or self-concept, attention, and/or behavior. Again, results concerning these measures were uniformly negative as to the existence of facilitative effects specific to SI therapy.

The Humphries et al. (1992) study included measures of (a) attention, represented by an informal continuous-performance task, the Matching Familiar Figures test (Kagan, Rosman, Day, Albert, & Phillips, 1964), the 10-item short form of the Conners Parent and Teacher Questionnaire (Conners, 1973), and informal ratings of subjects' organizational skills by parents and teachers, and (b) self-concept, assessed by means of the North York Self-Concept Scale (North York School Board, 1980). The Group × Time of Test interaction was not significant in a MANCOVA that included these psychoeducational variables.

Polatajko et al. (1991) found no significant differences between their SI treatment group and PM treatment group at either the 6-month posttest or the 9-month follow-up on Behavioral Academic Self-Esteem (BASE) (Coopersmith & Gilberts, 1982) ratings or on scores for the Cognitive Development factor scale of the Personality Inventory for Children (Part I)–Revised (Wirt, Lachar, Klinedinst, & Seat, 1984). Improvement from pretest was evident only with regard to the BASE standard scores for the SI treatment group.

Likewise, in the Wilson et al. (1992) study, no significant interactions were observed on (a) the Pictorial Scale of Perceived Competence and Social Acceptance for Young Children (Harter & Pike, 1983), a measure of self-esteem; (b) the Abbreviated Symptom Questionnaire (Goyette, Conners, & Ulrich, 1978), a behavioral measure; (c) the Hyperactivity Index of said questionnaire; or (d) the Behavioral Observation Forms of the Miller Assessment for Preschoolers (Miller, 1982), scored so as to assess both hyperreactivity and hyporeactivity. The time-of-test main effects in the posttest analysis were significant for the various behavioral measures, with performance for both the SI treatment group and the tutoring treatment group increasing over the course of the study, but not for the measure of self-esteem.

SUMMARY AND DISCUSSION

The related issues of whether children with learning disabilities differentially exhibit concomitant problems in sensory integration—if sensory integration and SI dysfunction as defined and interpreted by Ayres and her disciples exist at all—and whether such children are helped in any way by means specific to SI therapy have been addressed in the present article. An overview of theoretical contentions and empirical findings pertaining to the first issue was presented, followed by a detailed review of recent studies in the SI therapy research literature, in an effort to resolve the second issue. Results of this critique raise serious doubts as to the validity or utility of SI therapy as an appropriate, indicated treatment for the clinical population in question—and, by extension, for any other groups diagnosed as having "sensory integrative dysfunction."

Cummins (1991) determined that, at least within the scope of Ayres's factor-analytic data, there is no factual basis for her typology of SI dysfunction (e.g., Ayres, 1972b), and that the alleged syndromes do not distinguish between or adequately describe the sensorimotor capabilities of children with and without learning disabilities. Furthermore, with respect to the conceptually and clinically emphasized putative disorders involving vestibular processing, the investigation by Polatajko (1985) failed to find any empirical support for the vestibular dysfunction hypothesis regarding children with learning disabilities (see also Brown et al., 1983). In a similar vein, Polatajko (1983) and Cohen (1989) have argued against the validity of the SCPNT as a measure of postrotary nystagmus and vestibular-system functioning, with the commonly reported finding of decreased nystagmus duration in children with learning disabilities perhaps being attributable to certain peculiarities and deficiencies in the testing procedure (e.g., see Polatajko, 1985). In fact, Cohen contended that

> no evidence in the oculomotor literature, either with human or with animal subjects, supports the notion that after stimulation the time constant becomes longer than the subject's initial time constant. If vestibular function were to improve, the time constant would be expected to become shorter, not longer. Thus, the premise of the SCPNT, that decreased nystagmus duration indicates impaired vestibular function, is incorrect. (p. 476)

Finally, in the group-design outcome studies reviewed herein, (the lack of) effects of SI treatment did not vary within a study between subjects with learning disabilities and SI dysfunction who had hyponystagmus and those who did not (Carte et al., 1984; see also Law, Polatajko, Schaffer, Miller, & Macnab, 1991), nor did such outcomes differ between studies that included only the former children as subjects (i.e., Morrison & Sublett, 1986; Wilson et al., 1992) and studies that did not discriminate on this basis (i.e., Humphries et al., 1990; Humphries et al., 1992; Polatajko et al., 1991).

These theoretical and empirical considerations, taken in toto, decidedly undermine any case for applying SI therapy to children with learning disabilities, whether that application is restricted to those diagnosed as having SI dysfunction or as having hyponystagmus.

The present critique focused on the efficacy of SI therapy as a treatment intervention for children with learning disabilities. Seven research studies, published since Ottenbacher's (1982b) review, that met certain minimal criteria were examined. With the possible exception of the Ottenbacher (1982a) experiment, these studies, unlike some previous efforts in this area (e.g., Ayres, 1972a, 1978), have arguably avoided any major shortcomings in design, methodology, or data analysis. One might suppose, furthermore, that any such potential inadequacies would likely tend to bias results in favor of SI treatment (cf. Schaffer, 1984). Even so, the findings of the studies, as cited above, reveal no convincing evidence for the existence of facilitative effects specific to SI therapy.

As has been indicated, postrotary nystagmus, assessed by means of the SCPNT, is presumed in SI research and clinical practice to represent a relatively direct index of vestibular-system functioning, and vestibular function enjoys a position of singular importance with respect to SI theory and therapy. Yet, of the six studies that included postrotary nystagmus as an outcome measure, only the experiment conducted by Ottenbacher (1982a) produced results that could in any way be construed as supporting the efficacy of SI therapy. Even in that case, the results were inconsistent. Although the lone subject with initially normal nystagmus durations exhibited a significant decline with SI treatment, and 1 of the 2 subjects with initially low nystagmus durations exhibited a significant increase, the other did not.

Ottenbacher's (1982a) findings can perhaps be put in proper perspective by noting that in the Wilson et al. (1992), Carte et al. (1984), and Morrison and Sublett (1986) investigations, significant time-of-test main effects, but no significant Group × Time of Test interactions, were obtained. This suggests that tutoring and no treatment, respectively, were as effective as SI therapy in increasing nystagmus durations. An obvious interpretation of all these findings, and of past reports concerning positive effects of SI therapy on postrotary nystagmus (e.g., Ottenbacher, Short, & Watson, 1979), is that the observed changes in nystagmus duration were due to changes in extravestibular variables (e.g., see Cohen, 1989; Morrison & Sublett, 1983); to maturation; and/or to non-specific treatment effects (e.g., placebo or Hawthorne effects)—or, most likely, represent artifacts of regression toward the mean, especially in light of the considerable test-retest variability in SCPNT scores for children with learning disabilities and SI dysfunction found by Morrison and Sublett (1983). Consistent with this interpretation is the fact that Morrison and Sublett (1986) observed no significant corresponding changes over the course of their study in equilibrium reactions or visual-motor integration, two measures also believed to at least indirectly assess vestibular function.

SI therapy is claimed to alter sensorimotor neural organization. Therefore, one might reasonably expect effects of the therapy, if any, to have their greatest impact on measures of sensorimotor, perceptual, and/or motor functioning. It could perhaps be argued that this expectation was borne out by the results of two of the reviewed studies. The study conducted by Humphries et al. (1992) was basically a replication of the Humphries et al. (1990) study, but with a larger sample size and more-intensive programs of treatment intervention (along with an increase in the number and type of outcome variables). In both studies, significant Group × Time of Test interaction effects were found for various sensorimotor measures, and in the initial study, these effects, as predicted, all favored the SI treatment group over the PM treatment group and the no-treatment control group. In the replication study, however, the significant interaction effects were more often due to improvement in the PM treatment group exceeding that in the SI treatment group than the opposite. Moreover, with respect to Gross Motor Composite and Battery Composite scores on the BOTMP, the patterns of results for the two treatment groups actually reversed themselves between studies. Thus, these findings, circumscribed and inconsistent as they are, in reality can hardly be taken as evidence for any special efficacy of SI therapy.

Only time-of-test main effects, and not interactions, were significant in the Polatajko et al. (1991), Wilson et al. (1992), and Carte et al. (1984) studies, indicating that perceptual–motor training, academic skills tutoring, and no treatment, respectively, were as effective as SI therapy in improving perceptual processing and motor skills. Together, the above results clearly signify that maturation and/or nonspecific treatment effects—or even the possibility (as suggested by Polatajko et al., 1991) that although their rationales may differ, "the distinction made between SI and PM tasks is artificial" (p. 171)—were responsible for any improvements in performance seen among subjects in these studies, as well as in the Humphries et al. (1990) and Humphries et al. (1992) investigations.

Enhanced academic functioning, along with more general cognitive and language functioning, in children with learning disabilities can be regarded as the raison d'être of SI therapy. As Carte et al. (1984) noted,

> the hypothesized interrelationship between the vestibular somatosensory systems and learning would imply: (1) a causal role of SI dysfunction for learning disabilities and/or (2) a

strong disruptive influence of brain stem and vestibular dysfunction on higher cognitive functions. Subsequently these dysfunctions would preclude (or greatly retard) remediation of learning disabilities, unless a specific therapy directed at correcting these deficits were provided. (p. 194)

No significant Group × Time of Test interaction effects were obtained on cognitive, language, or academic measures in any of the reviewed studies, however. Time-of-test main effects were significant for those content area clusters of the WJPEB measured in the Polatajko et al. (1991) and Wilson et al. (1992) studies, but the fact that performance for the SI treatment groups and the PM and tutoring comparison treatment groups in these studies improved over time on such measures is not particularly surprising or interesting. Thus, contrary to postulation, SI therapy appears to have no discernible, and certainly no unique, effect on academic-related abilities within this subject population, just as it has no apparent effects on theoretically prerequisite sensorimotor, perceptual, and motor functions.

Humphries et al. (1992) have acknowledged that "putting the present findings into perspective also requires dispelling the notion that occupational therapists may claim to directly improve higher level academic, language, and cognitive performance through their treatments" (p. 39). Although this would surely seem an accurate assessment, the question naturally arises: What, then, is the purpose, if any, of SI therapy? In view of the findings of the Humphries et al. (1992), Polatajko et al. (1991), and Wilson et al. (1992) studies, it definitely is not collateral enhancement of self-esteem or self-concept, or improvements in attention and/or behavior.

In short, although the investigators, who were predominantly affiliated with the profession of occupational therapy, often endeavored to explain away their null results (e.g., see Wilson et al., 1992), the findings of the recently conducted outcome studies reviewed in this article speak for themselves. Simply put, and to reiterate: They reveal absolutely no unique benefits, regarding any of the tested outcome areas, conveyed by SI therapy to the children with learning disabilities (and purported SI dysfunction) who served as subjects in these studies.

CONCLUSION

The Committee on Children with Disabilities (1985) of the American Academy of Pediatrics has stated that "neurophysiologic retraining programs such as patterning, optometic exercises, and *sensory integration thera-*

pies [italics added], although reported by some to have beneficial results in selected cases, lack value" (p. 648). Consistent with this appraisal, Arendt et al. (1988), based on their empirical review of SI therapy research involving persons with mental retardation and on a critical examination of theoretical issues regarding said therapy, recently concluded that "until the therapeutic effectiveness of sensory integration therapy with mentally retarded persons is demonstrated, there exists no convincing empirical or theoretical support for the continued use of this therapy with that population outside of a research context" (p. 409). The present critique of the application of SI therapy to children with learning disabilities leads us to concur with the above position with respect to this, and SI theory and therapy's core target population as well. Our only addendum is that the current fund of research findings may well be sufficient to declare SI therapy not merely an unproven, but a demonstrably ineffective, primary or adjunctive remedial treatment for learning disabilities and other disorders.

REFERENCES

Arendt, R. E., MacLean, W. E., Jr., & Baumeister, A. A. (1988). Critique of sensory integration therapy and its application in mental retardation. *American Journal on Mental Retardation, 92*, 401–411.

Ayres, A. J. (1965). Patterns of perceptual–motor dysfunction in children: A factor analytic study. *Perceptual and Motor Skills, 20*, 335–368.

Ayres, A. J. (1966a). Interrelations among perceptual–motor abilities in a group of normal children. *American Journal of Occupational Therapy, 20*, 288–292.

Ayres, A. J. (1966b). Interrelationship among perceptual–motor functions in children. *American Journal of Occupational Therapy, 20*, 68–71.

Ayres, A. J. (1969). Deficits in sensory integration in educationally handicapped children. *Journal of Learning Disabilities, 2*, 160–168.

Ayres, A. J. (1971). Characteristics of types of sensory integrative dysfunction. *American Journal of Occupational Therapy, 25*, 329–334.

Ayres, A. J. (1972a). Improving academic scores through sensory integration. *Journal of Learning Disabilities, 5*, 338–343.

Ayres, A. J. (1972b). *Sensory integration and learning disorders.* Los Angeles: Western Psychological Services.

Ayres, A. J. (1972c). *Southern California sensory integration tests–Manual.* Los Angeles: Western Psychological Services.

Ayres, A. J. (1972d). Types of sensory integrative dysfunction among disabled learners. *American Journal of Occupational Therapy, 26*, 13–18.

Ayres, A. J. (1975). *Southern California postrotary nystagmus test–Manual.* Los Angeles: Western Psychological Services.

Ayres, A. J. (1976). *Interpreting the Southern California Sensory Integration Tests.* Los Angeles: Western Psychological Services.

Ayres, A. J. (1977). Cluster analyses of measures of sensory integration. *American Journal of Occupational Therapy, 31,* 362–366.

Ayres, A. J. (1978). Learning disabilities and the vestibular system. *Journal of Learning Disabilities, 11,* 18–29.

Ayres, A. J. (1979). *Sensory integration and the child.* Los Angeles: Western Psychological Services.

Ayres, A. J. (1980). *Southern California sensory integration tests–Manual* (rev. ed.). Los Angeles: Western Psychological Services.

Ayres, A. J. (1989). *Sensory integration and praxis tests–Manual.* Los Angeles: Western Psychological Services.

Ayres, A. J., Mailloux, Z. K., & Wendler, C. L. W. (1987). Developmental dyspraxia: Is it a unitary function? *Occupational Therapy Journal of Research, 7,* 93–110.

Beery, K. E. (1982). *Revised administration, scoring, and teaching manual for the Developmental Test of Visual–Motor Integration.* Cleveland: Modern Curriculum Press.

Brown, B., Haegerstrom-Portnoy, G., Yingling, C. D., Herron, J., Gallin, D., & Marcus, M. (1983). Dyslexic children have normal vestibular responses to rotation. *Archives of Neurology, 40,* 370–373.

Bruininks, R. H. (1978). *Bruininks-Oseretsky test of motor proficiency–Examiner's manual.* Circle Pines, MN: American Guidance Service.

Carte, E., Morrison, D., Sublett, J., Uemura, A., & Setrakian, W. (1984). Sensory integration therapy: A trial of a specific neurodevelopmental therapy for the remediation of learning disabilities. *Journal of Developmental and Behavioral Pediatrics, 5,* 189–194.

Clark, F., Mailloux, Z., & Parham, D. (1989). Sensory integration and children with learning disabilities. In P. N. Pratt & A. S. Allen (Eds.), *Occupational therapy for children* (2nd ed., pp. 457–509). St. Louis: C. V. Mosby.

Clark, F. A., & Shuer, J. (1978). A clarification of sensory integrative therapy and its application to programming with retarded people. *Mental Retardation, 16,* 227–232.

Cohen, H. (1989). Testing vestibular function: Problems with the Southern California Postrotary Nystagmus Test. *American Journal of Occupational Therapy, 43,* 475–477.

Committee on Children with Disabilities. (1985). School-aged children with motor disabilities. *Pediatrics, 76,* 648–649.

Conners, C. K. (1973). Rating scales for use in drug studies with children [Special issue]. *Psychopharmacology Bulletin,* pp. 24–84.

Coopersmith, S., & Gilberts, R. (1982). *Behavioral academic self-esteem.* Palo Alto, CA: Consulting Psychologists Press.

Crampton, G. H. (1964). Habituation of ocular nystagmus of vestibular origin. In M. B. Bender (Ed.), *The oculomotor system* (pp. 332–346). New York: Harper & Row.

Cummins, R. A. (1991). Sensory integration and learning disabilities: Ayres' factor analyses reappraised. *Journal of Learning Disabilities, 24,* 160–168.

Densem, J. F., Nuthall, G. A., Bushnell, J., & Horn, J. (1989). Effectiveness of a sensory integrative therapy program for children with perceptual–motor deficits. *Journal of Learning Disabilities, 22,* 221–229.

deQuiros, J. B. (1976). Diagnosis of vestibular disorders in the learning disabled. *Journal of Learning Disabilities, 9,* 39–47.

deQuiros, J. B., & Schrager, O. L. (1979). *Neuropsychological fundamentals in learning disabilities* (rev. ed.). Novato, CA: Academic Therapy.

Dunn, L. M., & Markwardt, F. C., Jr. (1970). *Peabody individual achievement test–Manual.* Circle Pines, MN: American Guidance Service.

Durrell, D. D., & Catterson, J. H. (1980). *Durrell analysis of reading difficulty* (3rd ed.). San Antonio, TX: Psychological Corp.

Fisher, A. G., & Murray, E. A. (1991). Introduction to sensory integration theory. In A. G. Fisher, E. A. Murray, & A. C. Bundy (Eds.), *Sensory integration: Theory and practice* (pp. 3–26). Philadelphia: F. A. Davis.

Fisher, A. G., Murray, E. A., & Bundy, A. C. (Eds.). (1991). *Sensory integration: Theory and practice.* Philadelphia: F. A. Davis.

Gardner, M. F. (1982). *Test of visual–perceptual skills (non-motor).* Seattle: Special Child Publications.

Goodman, L., & Hammill, D. D. (1975). *Basic school skills inventory.* Chicago: Follett.

Goyette, C. H., Conners, C. K., & Ulrich, R. F. (1978). Normative data on revised Conners Parent and Teacher Rating Scales. *Journal of Abnormal Child Psychology, 6,* 221–236.

Harter, S., & Pike, R. (1983). *Procedural manual to accompany the Pictorial Scale of Perceived Competence and Social Acceptance for Young Children.* Denver: University of Denver Press.

Humphries, T., Wright, M., McDougall, B., & Vertes, J. (1990). The efficacy of sensory integration therapy for children with learning disability. *Physical & Occupational Therapy in Pediatrics, 10*(3), 1–17.

Humphries, T., Wright, M., Snider, L., & McDougall, B. (1992). A comparison of the effectiveness of sensory integrative therapy perceptual–motor training in treating children with learning disabilities. *Journal of Developmental and Behavioral Pediatrics, 13,* 31–40.

Jastak, J. F., & Jastak, S. (1978). *The wide range achievement test–Manual* (rev. ed.). Wilmington, DE: Jastak Associates.

Kagan, J., Rosman, B. L., Day, D., Albert, J., & Phillips, W. (1964). Information processing in the child: Significance of analytic and reflective attitudes. *Psychological Monographs, 78*(1), 1–37.

Kaufman, A. S., & Kaufman, N. L. (1983). *Kaufman assessment battery for children.* Circle Pines, MN: American Guidance Service.

Kirk, S. A., McCarthy, J. J., & Kirk, W. D. (1968). *Examiner's manual: Illinois test of psycholinguistic abilities* (rev. ed.). Urbana: University of Illinois Press.

Law, M., Polatajko, H. J., Schaffer, R., Miller, J., & Macnab, J. (1991). The impact of heterogeneity in a clinical trial: Motor outcomes after sensory integration therapy. *Occupational Therapy Journal of Research, 11*, 177–189.

Lerer, R. J. (1981). An open letter to an occupational therapist. *Journal of Learning Disabilities, 14*, 3–4.

MacGinitie, W. H. (1978). *Gates-MacGinitie reading tests* (2nd ed.). Chicago: Riverside.

Miller, L. J. (1982). *Miller assessment for preschoolers–Manual.* Littleton, CO: Foundation for Knowledge in Development.

Morrison, D., & Sublett, J. (1983). Reliability of the Southern California Postrotary Nystagmus Test with learning-disabled children. *American Journal of Occupational Therapy, 37*, 694–698.

Morrison, D., & Sublett, J. (1986). The effects of sensory integration therapy on nystagmus duration, equilibrium reactions and visual–motor integration in reading retarded children. *Child: Care, Health and Development, 12*, 99–110.

Newcomer, P. L., & Hammill, D. D. (1982). *Test of language development–Primary.* Austin, TX: PRO-ED.

North York School Board. (1980). *North York self-concept scale.* Toronto: Author.

Ottenbacher, K. (1978). Identifying vestibular processing dysfunction in learning-disabled children. *American Journal of Occupational Therapy, 32*, 217–221.

Ottenbacher, K. (1980). Excessive postrotary nystagmus duration in learning-disabled children. *American Journal of Occupational Therapy, 34*, 40–44.

Ottenbacher, K. (1982a). Patterns of postrotary nystagmus in three learning-disabled children. *American Journal of Occupational Therapy, 36*, 657–663.

Ottenbacher, K. (1982b). Sensory integration therapy: Affect or effect. *American Journal of Occupational Therapy, 36*, 571–578.

Ottenbacher, K., & Short, M. A. (1985). Sensory integrative dysfunction in children: A review of theory and treatment. In M. Wolraich & D. K. Routh (Eds.), *Advances in developmental and behavioral pediatrics* (Vol. 6, pp. 287–329). Greenwich, CT: JAI.

Ottenbacher, K., Short, M. A., & Watson, P. J. (1979). Nystagmus duration changes of learning disabled children during sensory integrative therapy. *Perceptual and Motor Skills, 48*, 1159–1164.

Ottenbacher, K., Watson, P. J., Short, M. A., & Biderman, M. D. (1979). Nystagmus and ocular fixation difficulties in learning-disabled children. *American Journal of Occupational Therapy, 33*, 717–721.

Polatajko, H. J. (1983). The Southern California Postrotary Nystagmus Test: A validity study. *Canadian Journal of Occupational Therapy, 50,* 119–123.

Polatajko, H. J. (1985). A critical look at vestibular dysfunction in learning-disabled children. *Developmental Medicine & Child Neurology, 27,* 283–292.

Polatajko, H. J., Law, M., Miller, J., Schaffer, R., & Macnab, J. (1991). The effect of a sensory integration program on academic achievement, motor performance, and self-esteem in children identified as learning disabled: Results of a clinical trial. *Occupational Therapy Journal of Research, 11,* 155–176.

Pothier, P. C., Friedlander, S., Morrison, D. C., & Herman, L. (1983). Procedure for assessment of neurodevelopmental delay in young children: Preliminary report. *Child: Care, Health and Development, 9,* 73–83.

Price, A. (1977). Sensory integration in occupational therapy. *American Journal of Occupational Therapy, 31,* 287–289.

Punwar, A. (1982). Expanded normative data: Southern California Postrotary Nystagmus Test. *American Journal of Occupational Therapy, 36,* 183–187.

Reed, H. B. C., Jr. (1978). Review of Southern California Sensory Integration Tests. In O. K. Buros (Ed.), *The eighth mental measurements yearbook* (pp. 1407–1408). Highland Park, NJ: Gryphon.

Reitan, R. M., & Davison, L. A. (Eds.). (1974). *Clinical neuropsychology: Current status and applications.* Washington, DC: Winston.

Rosner, J. (1975). *Helping children overcome learning difficulties: A step-by-step guide for parents and teachers.* New York: Walker.

Rourke, B. P., & Orr, R. R. (1977). Prediction of the reading and spelling performances of normal and retarded readers: A four-year follow-up. *Journal of Abnormal Child Psychology, 5,* 9–20.

Schaffer, R. (1984). Sensory integration therapy with learning disabled children: A critical review. *Canadian Journal of Occupational Therapy, 51,* 73–77.

Semel, E. M., & Wiig, E. H. (1980). *Clinical evaluation of language functions–Diagnostic battery.* Columbus OH: Merrill.

Sieben, R. L. (1977). Controversial medical treatments of learning disabilities. *Academic Therapy, 13,* 133–147.

Slosson, R. L. (1963). *Slosson Intelligence Test (SIT) for children and adults.* East Aurora, NY: Slosson.

Tickle-Degnen, L. (1988). Perspectives on the status of sensory integration theory. *American Journal of Occupational Therapy, 42,* 427–433.

Wechsler, D. (1967). *Manual for the Wechsler preschool and primary scale of intelligence.* San Antonio, TX: Psychological Corp.

Wechsler, D. (1974). *Manual for the Wechsler intelligence scale for children–Revised.* San Antonio, TX: Psychological Corp.

Westman, A. S. (1978). Review of Southern California Sensory Integration Tests. In O. K. Buros (Ed.), *The eighth mental measurements yearbook* (pp. 1408–1409). Highland Park, NJ: Gryphon.

Wilson, B. N., Kaplan, B. J., Fellowes, S., Gruchy, C., & Faris, P. (1992). The efficacy of sensory integration treatment compared to tutoring. *Physical & Occupational Therapy in Pediatrics, 12*(1), 1–36.

Wilson, B. N., Pollock, N., Kaplan, B., & Law, M. (1991). *The development of a valid, reliable measure of motor and postural skills.* Unpublished manuscript.

Wirt, R. D., Lachar, D., Klinedinst, J. K., & Seat, P. D. (1984). *Multidimensional description of child personality: A manual for the Personality Inventory for Children* (rev. ed.). Los Angeles: Western Psychological Services.

Woodcock, R. W., & Johnson, M. B. (1977). *Woodcock-Johnson psycho-educational battery.* Hingham, MA: Teaching Resources.

Zaner-Bloser. (1975). *Handwriting evaluation scale.* Columbus, OH: Author.

20

Effects of a Preschool Plus Follow-On Intervention for Children at Risk

Arthur J. Reynolds
Pennsylvania State University, University Park

The effects of the Chicago Child Parent Center and Expansion Program were investigated for 6 social competence outcomes up to 2 years postprogram. A total of 1,106 low-income Black children were differentially exposed to school-based, comprehensive-service components for up to 5 or 6 years of intervention (preschool to Grade 3). Results indicated that the duration of intervention was significantly associated, in the expected direction, with reading and mathematics achievement, teacher ratings of school adjustment, parental involvement in school activities, grade retention, and special education placement. Analysis of 7 intervention and comparison groups revealed that participation in the follow-on intervention for 2 or 3 years significantly contributed to children's adjustment above and beyond preschool intervention and background factors. Both preschool and follow-on intervention meaningfully contributed to the cumulative effect of intervention.

The purpose of this study was to investigate the effects of a federally funded extended early intervention for economically disadvantaged children—the Chicago Child Parent Center and Expansion Program. Three

Reprinted with permission from *Developmental Psychology*, 1994, Vol. 30(6), 787–804. Copyright © 1994 by the American Psychological Association, Inc.

This study was partially supported by grants from the A. L. Mailman Family Foundation and the Center for the Study of Child and Adolescent Development, Pennsylvania State University, I gratefully acknowledge the Department of Research, Evaluation and Planning of the Chicago Public Schools for cooperation in data collection. I also thank Nick Bezruczko, Jeanne Borger, Mavis Hagemann, Nancy Mavrogenes, and Bill Rice for assistance in data collection and organization. I am further grateful to Ann Crouter, Tony D'Augelli, Robert Slavin, and Edward Zigler for valuable comments on previous drafts of this article.

major questions were addressed: (a) Is the duration of program participation associated with better academic and social outcomes? (b) Does participation in follow-on intervention improve children's adjustment above and beyond participation in preschool and kindergarten? and (c) Are the effects of intervention stable at the 2-year follow-up assessment? The answers to these questions are needed for two reasons. First, the number of children at risk as a result of poverty and associated factors has been increasing. The poverty rate for young children is 25%, and this rate is expected to increase in the future (Natriello, McDill, & Pallas, 1990). Also increasing in recent years has been the number of children with mental health and academic problems, which now afflict nearly one third of all children (Tuma, 1989). Systematic identification and implementation of effective early intervention programs may help prevent these problems. Second, the effects of preschool intervention plus follow-on intervention into the primary grades are largely unknown. In a time of limited financial resources and significant need, the appropriate timing and duration of such programs are important considerations in identifying the best available means of improving children's adjustment.

RESEARCH CONTEXT

Early childhood interventions are designed to provide cognitive and social enrichment during a sensitive period of development. Their goal is to promote children's healthy development to successfully negotiate the transition to school (Schweinhart & Weikart, 1988; Wachs & Gruen, 1982) and, in the long run, to contribute to the prevention of poor adjustment outcomes such as school failure and poverty. Studies of intensive experimental programs (Consortium for Longitudinal Studies, 1983; Lazar, Darlington, Murray, & Snipper, 1982), Head Start (Hubbell, 1983; McKey et al., 1985), and many other programs (White, 1985) have shown that 1 or 2 years of preschool can improve children's school readiness, early academic achievement, and school competence such as lower grade retention and special education placement. Some evidence indicates that preschool participation contributes to longer term outcomes such as reduced school dropout and delinquency as well as increased employment (Berrueta-Clement, Schweinhart, Barnett, Epstein, & Weikart, 1984; Schweinhart, Barnes, & Weikart, 1993).

During the transition to formal schooling in kindergarten and Grade 1, however, the direct effects of intervention on scholastic and intellectual outcomes begin to dissipate so that by Grade 3 there often are no differences found between participants and nonparticipants (McKey et al., 1985; White, 1985; see Barnett, 1992, for additional interpretations). Although the lack of long-term effects on scholastic achievement initially was interpreted to mean that preschool is ineffective, it is now widely acknowledged that it is unrealistic to expect preschool or any short-term intervention by itself to permanently alter children's cognitive and social development, especially without taking into account the environments children enter after preschool (Woodhead, 1988; Zigler & Berman, 1983).

In response to concerns about the fading effects of preschool interventions as well as the desire to optimize children's success in school, many investigators have recommended that early interventions should last longer to be most effective (National Head Start Association, 1990; Zigler & Styfco, 1993). Presumably, such programs may improve children's transition from preschool to formal schooling by providing continued comprehensive services to reinforce preschool learning, maintain or improve parent involvement, and coordinate academic and social services (Brim & Phillips, 1988; Ramey & Ramey, 1992). Research has demonstrated that the transition to full-time schooling is an important process in children's lives (Alexander & Entwisle, 1988; Entwisle & Hayduk, 1982; Reynolds, 1991) and may be facilitated by interventions that seek to encourage positive transactions among children, teachers, and parents. However, there is little empirical support for the efficacy of such extended programs. Although Project Follow Through was originally designed for this purpose, an 87% reduction in expected funding and changes in objectives have limited determinations of its success as a follow-on program (House, Glass, McLean, & Walker, 1978; Zigler & Styfco, 1993).

In one of the few studies of its effects as a follow-on program, Abelson, Zigler, and DeBlasi (1974) found that 35 children who participated in Follow Through from kindergarten to third grade after enrolling in Head Start preschool scored significantly higher in cognitive performance than 26 children who did not attend preschool or Follow Through. The 4-year program did not, however, raise children's performance to the level of non-disadvantaged children's. Nevertheless, Abelson et al. (1974) concluded that "a one year Head Start experience, if not followed by a subsequent compensatory effort, has little lasting effect on children's performance" (p. 766). Continuing effects of Follow Through versus no intervention were found in math achievement and general knowledge for boys and girls in one of two waves of cohorts (Seitz, Apfel, Rosenbaum, & Zigler, 1983). Other studies of government-funded programs generally support the viability of extended childhood interventions (Madden, Slavin, Karweit, Dolan, & Wasik, 1993; Meyer, 1984), including analyses of early 1970s cohorts of the Chicago Child Parent Centers (Conrad & Eash, 1983; Fuerst & Fuerst, 1993). However, the relative contributions of preschool and follow-on intervention have not been investigated.

Of nongovernment-funded model programs, only one study has directly addressed the differential effects of preschool and follow-on intervention. Horacek, Ramey, Campbell, Hoffmann, and Fletcher (1987) evaluated the Carolina Abecedarian Project, a university-based preschool (lasting 5 years) and school-age (lasting 3 years) intervention program enrolling 54 and 53 children randomly assigned to experimental and control groups. End-of-program results at second grade indicated significant associations between the extent of intervention and reading achievement, math achievement, and grade retention. As expected, children participating in preschool and the school-age intervention had the lowest rate of retention and the highest level of academic achievement. The school-age intervention, however, had no independent effect on grade retention or achievement beyond that of the preschool intervention. Follow-up analyses through age 15 (Campbell & Ramey, 1993) largely supported those of the previous study. Only the preschool intervention significantly contributed to child outcomes at ages 12 and 15. It is interesting to note that the school-age component was effective (for reading achievement) only when paired with preschool intervention. This finding suggests that follow-on intervention may be most effective as a continuation of earlier intervention.

ISSUES OUTSTANDING ON EFFECTIVENESS

Although these studies are suggestive of positive effects of interventions beyond preschool, much further investigation is warranted before firm conclusions can be drawn about their efficacy. Neither Abelson et al. (1974) nor Horacek et al. (1987), for example, found significant effects of the follow-on intervention controlling for the effects of preschool and child background factors. One reason may have been the small sample sizes used, which substantially reduced the statistical power to detect differences between groups. Not only would studies of larger samples provide more statistically powerful tests, but they would also yield more stable and robust estimates of effects. Several other issues also are apparent from previous studies.

Duration and Timing

The appropriate duration and timing of intervention programs also is unclear from previous studies. Although it is apparent that 3 or 4 years of intervention yield stronger and more lasting effects than 1 year of preschool, more uncertain is the optimal number of years necessary to ensure long-lasting effects. Will 2 or 3 years of good-quality intervention produce the same effects as 4 years, or should programs run beyond 4 years? Of equal importance is the timing of such interventions. Does it matter if the intervention begins at preschool or kindergarten as long as children get continuous intervention beyond a year or two? Previous studies (Abelson et al., 1974; Fuerst & Fuerst, 1993; Jordon, Grallo, Deutsch, & Deutsch, 1985) suggest that preschool may not be as important as receiving a continuous intervention from preschool to at least Grade 2. To the contrary, Horacek et al. (1987) found no independent effects of follow-on intervention indicating, along with other studies of early intervention (e.g., Andrews et al., 1982; Consortium of Longitudinal Studies, 1983), that timing may be most important. Most studies, however, confound timing and duration of intervention exposure. Studies testing a wide range of intervention conditions for different lengths of time are necessary. Of course, longitudinal effects of these levels of intervention are essential.

Large-Scale, Established Programs

Besides additional studies with larger samples and varied intervention exposure, more studies are needed of large-scale government-funded programs. Most of the evidence of mid- to long-term effects of early interventions comes from experimental or model programs that are initiated by researchers and program developers. These programs are often tested at only one or two sites, they have substantial financial and human resources for training and implementation, and they have very low child-to-staff ratios (i.e., 5 to 1). These conditions are at variance with more typical large-scale and financially restricted programs conducted in low-income communities and sponsored by federal and state governments (Zigler & Muenchow, 1992). Consequently, generalization of findings of long-term effects to Head Start-type programs is unclear and may require a leap of faith (Woodhead, 1988). Although experimental programs indicate the effects of interventions that are possible, policy makers want to know the actual effects of government-funded programs and what exactly taxpayers are getting for their money. As Haskins (1989) indicated, "it is surprising that after 20 years, we still do not have good long-term studies of Head Start. The American public spends more than $1 [now 4] billion per year on Head Start, and yet we have little credible evidence of the positive outcomes that we know . . . are possible" (p. 280). Of course, model programs have and will continue to inform program and policy development. However, more direct evidence is needed, especially on longer term effectiveness.

Multiple Domains

Finally, future studies of the effects of interventions would benefit from the use of a wider range of outcomes. Given the inherently multiple objectives of intervention programs, a focus on one or two outcomes (e.g., intelligence and cognitive achievement) restricts a comprehensive understanding of program effectiveness. Recent shifts toward the use of such measures as grade retention and special education placement have been important in broadening conceptions of program outcomes (Berrueta-Clement et al., 1984; Consortium for Longitudinal Studies, 1983; Zigler & Trickett, 1978). For large-scale, government-funded programs, however, evidence across multiple domains remains limited. The National Head Start Association (1990) recommended social competence as the most appropriate outcome of early childhood interventions. It also includes parent involvement because Head Start and similarly designed intervention programs often require parent involvement in school activities. Increased parent involvement has been hypothesized to be a mechanism by which interventions transmit long-term effects (Bronfenbrenner, 1975; Seitz, 1990; Wachs & Gruen, 1982). Reynolds (1992c) provided empirical support for this proposition.

THE PRESENT STUDY

This study investigates the effects of the federally funded Child Parent Center and Expansion Program, a large-scale comprehensive preschool-to-Grade 3 intervention for economically and educationally disadvantaged children in the Chicago Public Schools. This school-based program is designed to improve children's school readiness through structured instructional support services, parental involvement, and a focus on reading and language development. A panel of 1,106 Black children were differentially exposed to preschool, kindergarten, and follow-on components, thus allowing for detailed assessments of up to 5 or 6 years of intervention. Finally, the large sample and prospective longitudinal data allow for assessment of the program across multiple outcomes up to 2 years following the intervention. This study addressed the following questions: (a) Is the duration of program participation associated with better academic and social outcomes? (b) Does participation in the primary-grade component improve children's adjustment above and beyond participation in preschool and kindergarten? and (c) Are the effects of intervention stable up to 2 years post-program?

METHOD

Sample

Children are part of the Longitudinal Study of Children at Risk (LSCAR; Reynolds, 1991, 1992b; Reynolds & Bezruczko, 1993), a comprehensive and prospective investigation of the Elementary and Secondary Education Act Title I Child Parent Center and Expansion Program (hereinafter referred to as CPC). Funds for Title I (or Chapter I) are dispersed by the U.S. Department of Education to school districts with large proportions of educationally needy low-income children. The original sample included 1,539 low-income, minority children (95% Black and 5% Hispanic) in 26 schools who graduated from Chicago's government-funded kindergarten programs in 1986. The sample included 1,150 children in all 20 CPCs with kindergartens and a minimum-intervention comparison group of 389 children in six randomly selected schools participating in a locally funded kindergarten program for low-income children. Children entered the programs in either preschool (1983–1985) or kindergarten (1985–1986). For both the CPC and local kindergarten program, enrollment requires residency in school neighborhoods eligible for Chapter I services, and applicants were accepted on a most-in-need basis. All families that were eligible voluntarily enrolled their children in a preschool or kindergarten program, although in many cases they were recruited by schools and social service agencies. Groups were similar on many family and child variables (see Table 1). The sample, by definition, fairly well represents a large percentage of children at risk as a result of poverty in Chicago and probably other large metropolitan school districts. Moreover, children were at multiple risk of school difficulties. The school poverty rate for children in the study sample was 66%, compared with 42% for the total school system.

By the end of their fifth-grade year in the spring of 1991 (Grade 5 for continuously promoted children), 1,245 (81%) children remained active in the school system. This group was similar to the original kindergarten sample on several background characteristics, including gender, race, age at school entry, school socioeconomic status, and kindergarten achievement.[1] This

---

[1] For example, 51% of the original sample were girls compared with 52% in Grade 5; 68% of the original sample enrolled in preschool compared with 70% of the Grade 5 sample. Mean reading readiness scores (Iowa Tests of Basic Skills) also were comparable. To be included in the Grade 5 sample, children had to satisfy several conditions, among them being active in the school system in Grade 5 and in either Grade 3 or Grade 4. The test scores of some children were imputed (<30 per year). (See Reynolds [1992b] and Reynolds and Bezruczko [1993] for addition information on the sample and instrumentation.)

TABLE 1
Description of Child and Family Sociodemographic Factors for Intervention Groups

| Intervention Group | n | Percentage | | | | School Poverty[c] | Mean | |
		Girls	High School Graduate	Lunch Subsidy[a]	Expect College[b]		Kindergarten Age	No. of Siblings
With follow-on								
1. PS + KG + PG-3	160	56	68	95	52	62.1	63.8	2.2
2. No PS + KG + PG-3	76	49	66	95	51	62.1	63.8	2.3
3. PS + KG + PG-2	302	52	60	90	58	67.4	63.3	2.3
4. No PS + KG + PG-1/2	36	31	67	100	42	65.8	63.9	2.8
5. PS + KG + PG-1	80	53	55	97	54	63.7	62.6	2.3
Without follow-on								
6. PS + KG only	207	56	56	94	48	65.8	62.9	2.4
7. Non-CPC comparison group	191	53	55	90	44	63.0	63.8	2.8

Note. All percentages were not significantly different from one another on the basis of chi-square tests ($p > .05$, $df = 6$). Differences among means were based on analysis of variance. A significant difference was found for age, $F(6, 1033) = 2.4$, $p < .026$. Total $N = 1,052$. For parent education and lunch subsidy, $n = 758$; for parent expectations, $n = 751$. The percentage of children missing data on these parent variables did not differ among groups and ranged from 23% to 33%. PS = preschool, KG = kindergarten, PG = primary grade, CPC = Child Parent Center.

[a] Lunch subsidy = full or reduced.
[b] Expect college = parent expects child to graduate from college (coded from 1 to 4 in analyses).
[c] School poverty is averaged at the school level rather than at the individual level.

total sample recovery rate is substantially higher than the typical rate of 50% for longitudinal studies (Kessler & Greenberg, 1981). The study sample included 1,106 Black children. Because they constituted only 5% of the sample, 60 Hispanic children were excluded from the study sample. Also excluded were 79 children who participated in Head Start or Follow Through programs. These exclusions had no effect on the findings of the study and allow for a well-defined study sample of children affected by the program.[2] Consequently, this is a study of inner-city, Black children exposed to the CPC intervention program for different lengths of time.

CPC Program

In 1967, the federal government provided Title I (now Chapter I) funds for the establishment of several Child Parent Centers in the Chicago Public Schools for economically and educationally disadvantaged children. The program is currently implemented in 25 centers throughout the city. This study reports on the 20 centers that have both preschool and kindergarten components. In 1978, a CPC expansion program was added to the CPCs to provide program services into the primary grades. Funded by the State of Illinois, 14 centers provide services up to Grade 2, and 6 centers provide services up to Grade 3. Consequently, the total program includes preschool, kindergarten, and primary-grade services up to Grade 3. The preschool and kindergartens are in separate buildings or in wings of the main elementary schools. In the primary grades, the program is incorporated in the neighborhood elementary schools.

Like Head Start and other multifaceted interventions for children at risk, the program provides comprehensive health, social, academic, and school support services to promote reading readiness and affective development for school entry and beyond. There is no uniform curriculum as the CPCs tailor the program to their needs. Unlike Head Start, the CPC program provides services from preschool to Grade 3 for up to 6 years of intervention. The preschool component is a structured half-day program for 3- and 4-year-olds and is designed to promote children's reading-language skills and affective development through reduced class size, parent involvement, staff training, and structured learning activities. Similarly, the kindergarten

---

[2]Inclusion of Head Start and Follow Through children was beyond the scope of the present study. Neither group was representatively sampled. Head Start and Follow Through children were less academically and socially adjusted than the non-CPC comparison group, of which they would have been a part. Including them as part of the comparison group would have increased rather than decreased the estimated effects of the program. Hispanic children had, on average, higher scores on adjustment outcomes than Black children.

component provides all-day services (6 hr at most sites) to promote reading readiness and affective development. The primary-grade (follow-on) component provides extended intervention services for increased learning opportunities through reduced class sizes, parental involvement activities, and instructional coordination (see Chicago Public Schools, 1974, 1987a, for additional information). All of the components run 5 days per week for the 9-month school year. Children were enrolled for the following number of years: 0 years, $n = 191$ (comparison group), 1 year, $n = 25$, 2 years, $n = 135$, 3 years, $n = 169$, 4 years, $n = 253$, 5 years, $n = 254$, and 6 years, $n = 79$.

The CPCs emphasize a core philosophy that includes the provision of comprehensive services, parent involvement, and a child-centered focus on the acquisition of reading-language skills. All are believed to be strongly associated with program quality (Chafel, 1992; Schweinhart & Weikart, 1988; Zigler & Muenchow, 1992). See the Appendix for a description of implementation effectiveness.

Comprehensive services. The comprehensive services include (a) attending to children's nutritional and health needs (i.e., free breakfasts and lunches, and health screening), (b) coordinated adult supervision including a CPC head teacher, parent resource teacher, school-community representative as well as a teacher aide for each class, (c) funds for in-service teacher training in child development as well as instructional supplies, and (d) emphasis on reading readiness, frequent reading activities, reinforcement, and feedback. The parent resource teacher organizes the parent-resource room, which is designed to initiate education activities for parents as well as to foster parent-child interactions. The school community representative monitors parental as well as child school involvement and, if necessary, visits families in their home. The average class size of the preschool component was 17 with an adult-to-child ratio of approximately 1 to 8. For the kindergarten and primary-grade components, average class sizes were 25 with an adult-to-child ratio of approximately 1 to 12. The per-pupil annual expenditure for the preschool and kindergarten programs is $3,800 and $3,300, respectively, for the follow-on intervention (1992 dollars; Chicago Public Schools, 1992).

Unlike CPC children, children in the comparison group received no continuous and systematic intervention from preschool through Grade 3. Average class sizes were 30 in kindergarten and 30 in the primary grades. Comprehensive school support services, additional staff (i.e., head teacher and parent resource teacher), and extra instructional supplies were not provided. Besides basic funding for the kindergarten program, teacher assistants and in-service teacher training in child development were provided.

Instruction was whole class rather than small group or individualized. Extra instructional supplies were not provided.

Parent involvement. As implied in the program's title, a central philosophy of the program is that parent involvement is the critical socializing force in children's development. Because of the stresses associated with poverty and economic hardship, low-income families often are disconnected from schools and other community support systems that are important for healthy development (McLoyd, 1990). Direct parent involvement in the CPCs is expected to enhance parent-child interactions as well as attachment to school, thus promoting school readiness and social adjustment (Baumrind, 1971; Bronfenbrenner, 1975). At least one-half day per week of parent involvement in the center is required. To meet the different needs of families, parent involvement includes a wide range of activities such as serving as classroom aides, tutoring children, performing clerical tasks, accompanying classes on field trips, interacting with other parents in the center's parent resource room, participating in reading groups with other parents, attending school meetings and programs, participating in educational workshops, doing craft projects for use in the school or at home, and taking trips to the library with teachers or their children. Schools also frequently sponsor night courses for parents to obtain additional education, including their high school certificates. Besides class sizes, the major difference between program components was that in the primary grades, parent involvement is encouraged rather than required, and both parent involvement and curriculum coordination are conducted by a single teacher.

Child-centered focus on reading and literacy development. The smaller class sizes and greater number of adult supervisors allow more individualized and child-centered attention to develop reading comprehension and writing skills. This focus is based on the philosophy that failure to learn to read is a major cause of school maladjustment of children at risk (Chall, Jacobs, & Baldwin, 1990). Through a broad spectrum of activities in small groups, whole classes and independent study, children learn cognitive and social skills. Teachers provide frequent feedback and positive reinforcement as well as emphasize task accomplishment, all of which are associated with successful school performance and adjustment (Stallings, 1975). They frequently read stories to the class to develop the idea that reading is fun and to demonstrate "book language." Moreover, classes go on field trips to such places as the Museum of Science and Industry and the zoo. In-service teacher training sessions conducted by the Bureau of Early Childhood reinforce the emphasis on child-centered activities.

Intervention Groups

Six intervention groups (plus the comparison group) were formed to directly assess the effects of the CPC program (preschool to Grade 3). To receive program services, children must have been present in the sites that have program services. For several reasons, all children did not stay in the sites through Grade 3. For example, some parents preferred to send their children to regular school programs, some families moved out of the school neighborhood, and administrative requirements limited follow-on support to Grade 2 in several schools. Entry in kindergarten rather than in preschool was due to many factors, including parents' work schedules and length of residence in the school neighborhood. Nonresidence in an intervention neighborhood rather than low parental interest prevented the non-CPC comparison group from participating in the CPCs. Groups are listed in order of their extent of follow-on intervention during the primary grades (PG; 1 to 3 years) as well as the preschool (PS) and kindergarten (KG) interventions. They included 1,052 children instead of 1,106; the remaining 54 children did not fit into the groups.

With follow-on intervention. 1. Full intervention group (PS + KG + PG-3) included children who received all components of the program. They had at least 1 year of CPC preschool, all-day kindergarten, and 3 years of the primary-grade intervention ($n = 160$).

2. Kindergarten and primary-grade intervention group through Grade 3 (no PS + KG + PG-3) included children with no CPC preschool experience but who participated in all-day kindergarten with some support services from the CPC, and all 3 years of the primary-grade component ($n = 76$).

3. Preschool, kindergarten, and Grade 2 intervention group (PS + KG + PG-2) included children who participated in at least 1 year of preschool, kindergarten but 2 years of the primary-grade component ($n = 302$).

4. Kindergarten and primary-grade intervention group through Grade 2 (no PS + KG + PG-1/2) included children with no CPC preschool experience but who participated in all-day kindergarten with some support services from the CPC, and 1 or 2 years of the primary-grade component ($n = 36$).

5. Preschool, kindergarten, and Grade 1 intervention group (PS + KG + PG-1) included children who participated in at least 1 year of preschool, kindergarten, and only 1 year of the primary-grade component ($n = 80$).

Without follow-on intervention. 6. Preschool and kindergarten intervention group (PS + KG) participated in both CPC preschool and kindergarten but not the primary-grade component ($n = 207$).

7. The non-CPC comparison group did not participate in preschool, kindergarten, or primary-grade intervention programs but did enroll in the locally developed all-day kindergarten program for children at risk (n = 191). Like CPC children, children in the comparison group were eligible for Chapter I services and had educational need as a result of economic disadvantage. Because of their participation in the alternative kindergarten program (i.e., minimum-treatment comparison group), the analysis may be a conservative test of the effects of the CPC program. Because most children in the United States enroll in kindergarten, this test is more ecologically valid.

Group Comparability

The study design has two major advantages that rendered comparisons among groups valid. First, all of the children were eligible for intervention services as a result of economic and educational disadvantage. Parents voluntarily enrolled their children in a preschool or kindergarten program, and schools made significant efforts to recruit needy children. A second, more unique strength of the study was the use of multiple intervention groups that varied considerably in the duration or strength of intervention. Data on the duration of intervention enhances the capacity to determine program effectiveness (Rossi & Freeman, 1989; Yeaton & Sechrest, 1981). The variation in exposure to intervention provided several contrasts among groups with similar educational needs and degrees of self-selection. For example, self-selection is unlikely to be a significant factor in adjustment differences between the PS + KG and PS + KG + PG-3 groups because both enrolled in preschool. Consequently, comparisons among the CPC intervention groups were emphasized in the analyses. To control for potential selection effects into the follow-on intervention, kindergarten achievement as well as several child background factors were used as covariates.

The major disadvantage of the design is that because the intervention groups were formed naturally in large part, group equivalence cannot be determined with certainty, at least as well as a design based on random assignment to groups. Consequently, results of the study must be interpreted with caution as well as cross-validated with additional studies. Schweinhart et al. (1993) recommended that intensive studies, which tend to be higher in internal validity, and extensive studies, which tend to be higher in external validity, complement each other well.

Group differences. Table 1 shows that the intervention groups were comparable on several sociodemographic factors, including sex, parent education (i.e., high school graduate or not), eligibility for free lunch (full, reduced, or none), the process measure of parent expectations for children's educational attainment (i.e., "How far in school will the child get?"), school poverty (percentage of children in poor families within school area), age at kindergarten entry (school records), and number of siblings (child report). Only for age at kindergarten entry were group differences significant, and these were less than 1 month (e.g., for the PS + KG + PG-1 group). The overall pattern of results slightly favored the full intervention groups. Groups also were equivalent on single-parent family status, $\chi^2(6, N = 405)$ = 8.11, p = .23, and employment status, $\chi^2(6, N = 405)$ = 5.84, p = .44. For example, 72% of the PS + KG + PG-3 group, 76% of the PS + KG group, and 72% of the non-CPC comparison groups lived with single parents.

Moreover, the intervention groups were similar on reading and math achievement at the end of kindergarten, which suggested that differential selection into the follow-on component was minimal. Following the order in Table 1, group means for kindergarten reading achievement (Iowa Tests of Basic Skills) were, respectively, 42, 38, 43, 34, 35, 39, and 37 standard scores. Significant differences (because of preschool participation) occurred only for the PS + KG + PG-3 and the non-CPC comparison group and the PS + KG + PG-2 and the non-CPC comparison group (Scheffés method at the .05 level). More important, there were only small differences among groups in cognitive-achievement growth rates from the beginning to the end of kindergarten (before follow-on intervention), indicating that significant changes in growth rates that occur during the program are likely to be attributable to the intervention.[3]

Nevertheless, the sociodemographic variables were used as control variables in the analyses. The inclusion of parent education, eligibility for lunch subsidy, and the process measure of parent expectations, which were collected after the end of the intervention (Grades 2 and 4), may result in conservative estimates of intervention effects. Because the CPC program is designed, in part, to enhance parent skills and attitudes toward education, these three factors have almost certainly been affected by the intervention. Consequently, their inclusion in the analysis would tend to reduce estimates of effects. Even though the covariates were unrelated to program participation, they were included to increase the precision of estimates (Rossi & Freeman, 1989).

---

[3] Data on pretreatment growth rates are important determinants of group comparability (Moffitt, 1991). Group differences in growth rates in reading achievement before follow-on intervention were as follows (all relative to the PS + KG + PG-3 group): PS + KG + PG-2 (−1.9), PS + KG + PG-1 (+1.2), no PS + KG + PG-3 group (−0.6), PS + KG group (−1.9), and non-CPC comparison group (−3.8 standard-score points). Only the growth rates between the PS + KG + PG-3 and the non-CPC comparison group (because of preschool participation) were significantly different (based on covariance-adjusted scores).

Intervention by attrition analyses. To further investigate the comparability of groups, I conducted an attrition analysis. It could be argued, for example, that differential attrition among the intervention groups may explain any observed effects, independent of intervention exposure. Sample recovery for the CPC group was 82% for those entering in preschool, 74% for those entering in kindergarten, and 80% for those entering the non-CPC comparison group schools in kindergarten.[4] The difference between the CPC preschool group and the kindergarten group was significant. Following Jurs and Glass (1971), a two-way analysis of variance for kindergarten reading achievement was conducted to determine whether children who left were fundamentally different than those who stayed. Results indicated significant main effects for intervention group (three levels), $F(2, 1524) = 37.1$, $p < .001$, but nonsignificant effects for attrition (two levels), $F(1, 1524) = 0.8$, $p > .371$, and for the Intervention $\times$ Attrition interaction, $F(2, 1524) = 0.62$, $p > .541$. These findings indicate that attrition among groups was unlikely to influence the observed effects of the intervention.

Outcome Measures

Six outcomes, measured in Grades 3 through 5, were used to evaluate the effects of the CPC intervention program. With the exception of parental involvement, they have been frequently used in previous studies.

Reading achievement and mathematics achievement. Reading comprehension and mathematics total subtest scores on the Iowa Tests of Basic Skills (ITBS; Hieronymus & Hoover, 1990; Hieronymus, Lindquist, & Hoover, 1980) were used as measures of cognitive achievement. Both nationally standardized subtest scares have demonstrated high reliability (internal consistency reliabilities $> .90$) and predictive validity (Hieronymus & Hoover, 1990). The reading comprehension subtest included 47, 49, and 54 items, respectively, in Grades 3 through 5; the mathematics total subtest had, respectively, 88, 95, and 101 items. Norm-referenced in 1988, the ITBS is group-administered each year in April. Developmental standard scores were used for all analyses, and they are comparable across test levels. The Grade 3 scores are based on the 1978 norm-referenced test (Form 7 Level 9) but were converted to 1988 scores.

Tests were administered under standardized procedures by school personnel other than the classroom teacher. Staff from the central offices of the

---

[4] Sample recovery (Grade 5) for children entering at ages 3 and 4 were, respectively, 83% (413 of 499 children) and 81% (384 of 475 children) of the original sample of 1,539. Sample recovery rates for the CPC kindergarten and non-CPC comparison groups were, respectively, 74% (130 of 176 children) and 80% (313 of 389 children).

school district as well as school counselors and other teachers conducted testing under the supervision of a school testing coordinator. Consequently, test administration was independent of the intervention experiences received.

Teacher ratings of school adjustment. Teachers rated children's school adjustment on the following six-item composite rating scale with each item rated from *poor/not at all* (1) to *excellent/much* (5): (a) concentrates on work, (b) follows directions, (c) is self-confident, (d) participates in group discussions, (e) gets along well with others, and (f) takes responsibility for actions. On the basis of principal-components analysis, this reliable scale (α = .94) has been used successfully in previous studies with this sample (Reynolds, 1989, 1991) and correlates .85 with the total teacher rating scale from which it was derived. Moreover, the scale's moderate correlations with Grade 4 reading and mathematics achievement (rs = .48 and .54, respectively) suggest adequate construct distinction. Although teacher ratings may have some degree of bias and subjectivity, they are essential in providing a well-rounded view of children's school adjustment. Because children were rated in Grades 3 to 5, teachers were largely unaware of children's intervention history.

Parental involvement in school. Teachers rated parents' behavioral involvement in school from the item, parents' involvement in school activities. It was rated on a scale from *poor/not at all* (1) to *excellent/much* (5). Although teacher reports have a subjective component, the focus on general school relations is clearly an area about which teachers have knowledge (Reynolds, 1991; Stevenson & Baker, 1987). The use of teacher report was supported by principal-components analysis, which suggested its relative independence from measures of school progress. Also, previous research with this sample has indicated a moderate and significant relationship between parent and teacher reports of parent involvement in school (Reynolds, 1992a). Nevertheless, because of the use of a single item, the effects of intervention on parental involvement are likely to be conservative.

Special education placement. Any child assigned to special education classrooms (self-contained or otherwise) through Grade 3, Grade 4, and Grade 5 were coded 1; all others were coded 0. This defined a cumulative classification of placement. Major categories of assignment included mildly mentally retarded, behavioral disorder, and learning disabled.

Grade retention. Children on record as repeating a grade at least once between kindergarten and Grade 5 were coded 1 (retained); all other children were coded 0 (promoted or not retained). Data on retention was obtained from a grade-by-grade analysis of the school system's computerized records. A child was coded as retained if he or she had identical grade codes in consecutive school years. Retainees were included in the analysis with their age-level peers.

RESULTS

Findings are reported in three sections: (a) preliminary analysis of children with and without intervention experience and by duration of experience, (b) primary analysis of mean differences among the intervention groups, mainly between the full intervention and preschool and kindergarten groups, and (c) additional analyses of group differences by school mobility and across sites.

Preliminary Analysis of Participation in Intervention

Before the association between the duration of intervention and child outcomes is determined, a summary analysis of intervention and comparison groups was conducted. Table 2 presents end-of-program adjusted means and proportions of children with any CPC experience and non-CPC participants. Results are based on multiple regression analysis with CPC intervention status binary coded. The covariates were the variables in Table 1. As expected, children with any CPC intervention experience significantly outperformed the non-CPC comparison group on four of six outcomes at the end of the follow-on program. These included reading achievement, mathematics achievement, parent involvement, and cumulative grade retention. Group differences were negligible for teacher ratings of school adjustment and cumulative special education placement. These differences remained in Grade 4. In Grade 5, only for reading and mathematics achievement did children with any CPC experience significantly (at the .025 level) outperform children with no experience, but by smaller margins (2.5 and 3.0 points, respectively). The difference for grade retention was notable (5.5%, $p < .08$). The covariates were effective in removing variance in adjustment due to individual and family factors.[5] Their inclusion generally reduced the magnitude of group differences as would be

---

[5] Valid sample sizes for kindergarten age, number of siblings, parent education, eligibility for lunch subsidy, and parent expectations were, respectively, 1,040, 895, 758, 758, and 751. The percentage of missing data across the intervention groups ranged from 23% to 33%. These proportions were not significantly different from one another, $\chi^2(6, N = 1052) = 7.44$, $p > .28$. To determine if missing data influenced the results, a dummy variable was created for the parent variables (1 = missing, 0 = complete) and was entered as a covariate in the analysis. Coefficient estimates were in most cases nonsignificant. Because the analyses were based on pairwise present cases, children with valid values for any combination of variables were included.

TABLE 2

Adjusted Means of Child Parent Center (CPC) Intervention and Comparison Groups for Six Outcomes at the End of the Program (Grade 3) with Sociodemographic Factors Controlled

Group	Reading Achievement	Math Achievement	Teacher Ratings	Parent Involvement	Grade Retention	Special Education
CPC intervention (all)	94.6*	99.9*	18.8	2.5*	19.2*	7.8
Comparison	90.6	96.5	18.5	2.2	26.2	8.9

Note. $n = 915$ for CPC group. $n = 191$ for comparison group. Differences for grade retention and special education placement were cumulative percentages and were based on logistic regression analysis. Sociodemographic control factors = sex, parent education, eligibility for lunch subsidy, parent expectations, school socioeconomic status in kindergarten, kindergarten age, and number of siblings.
*$p < .025$.

expected given the descriptive pattern in Table 1. Overall, these findings support the positive influence of participation in early childhood intervention found in previous studies of the LSCAR (Reynolds, 1992c; Reynolds & Bezruczko, 1993) and in many others (Consortium of Longitudinal Studies, 1983; Lazar et al., 1982). However, results suggest that duration of intervention should be taken into account.

To examine the relationship between duration of intervention (0 to 6 years) and program outcomes, I computed correlations using Joreskog and Sorbom's (1988) method for ordinal variables. Number of years of intervention was significantly associated, in the expected direction, with all six outcomes. At Grade 3, correlations were as follows: for grade retention ($r = -.27$), reading achievement ($r = .26$), mathematics achievement ($r = .25$), parent involvement in school ($r = .24$), teacher ratings ($r = .14$), and special education placement ($r = -.08$). By Grade 5, correlations between intervention exposure and the outcomes were generally smaller, but they remained statistically significant. The largest correlations were for grade retention ($r = -.22$) and reading and math achievement ($rs = .21$).

As illustrated in Figure 1, however, the associations were not completely linear; rather, a threshold was evident at 4 or 5 years of intervention for reading achievement, math achievement, and grade retention (the small sample receiving 1 year warrants cautious interpretation). Planned comparisons were conducted to test the hypothesis of a threshold effect, contrasting the groups that had 4 or more years of intervention with those having less than 4 years of intervention. Results indicated significant differences favoring the 4-year threshold interpretation. Both at the end of the program and at the 2-year follow-up, 4- to 6-year participants performed significantly higher in reading achievement and math achievement and had a significantly lower rate of grade retention than those with less than 4 years of intervention. For example, Grade 5 reading achievement (adjusted for covariates) for the 4- to 6-year group was 115.6 compared with 109.7 for counterparts in the comparison group ($p < .0001$). Grade 5 cumulative grade retention rates were, respectively, 19.7% and 31.5% ($p < .0001$). Adjustment outcomes of the latter group also were not statistically different from the non-CPC comparison group.

Four- through 6-year participants scored above the Chicago average in reading and mathematics achievement; 5- and 6-year participants were retained at or below the national retention rate at third grade (Meisels & Liaw, 1991). Six-year participants performed best across all outcomes. This threshold pattern may partly explain the modest correlations between intervention exposure and program outcomes. This pattern of findings remained after the influence of the sociodemographic factors in Table 1

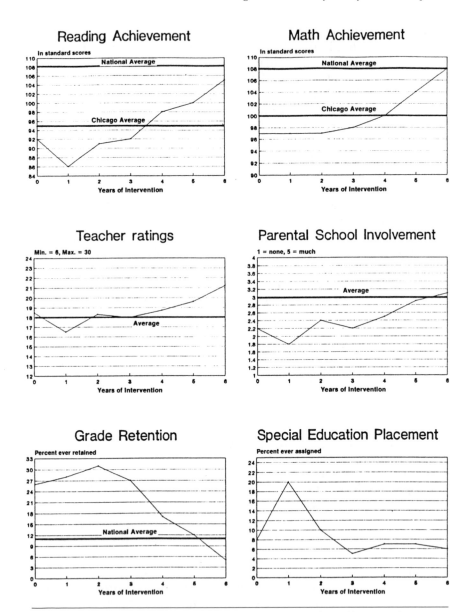

Figure 1. End-of-program outcomes (Grade 3) by duration of intervention.

were controlled. Results suggest the advantage of early and continuous participation in intervention.

Primary Analysis 1: Mean Comparisons Among Intervention Groups

Tables 3 and 4 present unadjusted means for five intervention groups and the minimum-treatment non-CPC comparison group over the 3-year period of study. For parsimony, means for the no PS + KG + PG-1/2 group are not shown. Their adjustment was similar to the non-CPC comparison group and the PG + KG group for all outcomes. Adjusted means were based on an analysis of covariance by means of multiple regression (Cohen & Cohen, 1983) with the sociodemographic factors as covariates and kindergarten achievement for comparisons among the CPC intervention groups.[6] Analyses proceeded after the determination of significant multivariate differences (repeated measures multivariate analysis of variance) across the four continuous and ordinal outcomes for intervention group, $F(24, 1586) = 3.21$, $p < .0001$; time, $F(8, 394) = 146.68$, $p < .0001$; and Group $\times$ Time, $F(48, 2354) = 1.76$, $p < .001$. Also affirmed was the critical covariance assumption of parallel regression slopes between intervention and comparison groups. No differential effects of the intervention were detected by gender, parent education, and grade retention and for 1 year versus 2 years of preschool participation (see Reynolds, 1993).

As with the preliminary analysis, the full intervention group through Grade 3 performed significantly better than the non-CPC comparison group and the PS + KG group. At the end of the program (with unadjusted standard scores), the PS + KG + PG-3 group had the highest achievement in reading ($M = 103.1$, percentile rank = 41%) and mathematics ($M = 106.6$; percentile rank = 47%), teacher ratings ($M = 20.6$ out of 30), and parent involvement ($M = 3.0$ out of 5) as well as the lowest incidence of retention (6.3% ever retained). The non-CPC comparison group performed, on average, significantly lower on five of six outcomes at the end of the program: reading ($M = 90.8$, percentile rank = 19%), math ($M = 96.6$, percentile rank 19%), teacher ratings ($M = 18.7$ out of 30), parent involvement ($M = 2.3$ out of 5), and grade retention (26% ever retained). This retention rate is over four times greater than the full intervention group.

---

[6] Variances explained by the model (including kindergarten achievement) for continuous and ordinal outcomes in Grade 3 were as follows: 37% (reading and math achievement), 21% (teacher ratings), and 12% (parent involvement). Also, following the recommendations of Cook and Shadish (1994) and Moffitt (1991), entering kindergarten achievement test scores were added to model as a second pretest. Results supported those in Tables 3 and 4. Entering kindergarten scores contributed less than 0.5 points to program effects on achievement and nothing to effects on the other outcomes.

TABLE 3
Unadjusted Means and Adjusted (Adj.) Means for Four Outcomes by Intervention Group

Intervention Group	n	End of Program		1-Year Follow-Up		2-Year Follow-Up	
		M	Adj. M	M	Adj. M	M	Adj. M
Reading Achievement							
With follow-on							
PS + KG + PG-3	160	103.1	102.2[a,b,d]	108.5	107.7[a,b,c,d]	117.8	116.8[a,b,c]
No PS + KG + PG-3	76	100.1	100.3[a,b,d]	102.4	102.6[a]	111.7	112.0
PS + KG + PG-2	302	95.9	95.1[a]	104.2	103.2[a]	115.7	114.7[a,b]
PS + KG + PG-1	80	91.7	92.0	102.0	102.1	109.2	109.5
Without follow-on							
PS + KG only	207	90.7	91.4	100.7	101.1	109.0	109.7
Non-CPC comparison group	191	90.6	90.8	99.4	99.6	109.8	109.9
Mathematics Achievement							
With follow-on							
PS + KG + PG-3	160	106.6	106.1[a,b,d]	111.8	111.5[a,b]	123.0	122.4[a,b]
No PS + KG + PG-3	76	102.8	102.9[a,b,d]	109.6	109.7	118.9	119.0
PS + KG + PG-2	302	100.8	100.0[a]	110.4	109.4[a]	120.5	119.5[a]
PS + KG + PG-1	80	97.2	97.7	106.7	107.1	115.7	116.1
Without follow-on							
PS + KG only	207	97.1	97.8	106.8	107.2	116.6	117.2
Non-CPC comparison group	191	96.5	96.6	105.3	105.3	115.2	115.4

Teacher Ratings of Adjustment

	N						
With follow-on							
PS + KG + PG-3	151	20.6	20.3[a,b]	20.0	20.1[a,b,c]	19.8	19.3[a,c]
No PS + KG + PG-3	65	19.2	19.2	18.4	18.6	17.9	17.9
PS + KG + PG-2	276	19.0	18.8	19.7	19.5	19.6	19.3[b,c]
PS + KG + PG-1	64	18.8	18.9	18.0	18.3	18.6	18.5
Without follow-on							
PS + KG only	178	18.2	18.3	18.6	18.7	18.1	18.1
Non-CPC comparison group	171	18.5	18.7	18.5	18.4	18.5	18.3

Parental School Involvement

	N						
With follow-on							
PS + KG + PG-3	145	3.0	3.0[a,b,c]	2.6	2.6	2.6	2.5
No PS + KG + PG-3	62	2.3	2.3	2.3	2.3	2.3	2.2
PS + KG + PG-2	266	2.7	2.7[a,b,c]	3.0	2.9[a,b,c]	2.8	2.7[b,c,]
PS + KG + PG-1	62	2.5	2.5	2.4	2.4	2.6	2.6
Without follow-on							
PS + KG only	172	2.4	2.4	2.4	2.4	2.3	2.3
Non-CPC comparison group	159	2.2	2.4	2.4	2.4	2.5	2.5

Note. Covariates included the child and family variables in Table 1. Kindergarten achievement was added for comparisons among groups with preschool intervention. PS = preschool, KG = kindergarten, PG = primary grade, CPC = Child Parent Center.

[a] Significantly different from non-CPC comparison group at the .025 level.
[b] Significantly different from PS + KG group or PS + KG + PG-1 group at the .025 level.
[c] Significantly different from no-PS + KG + PG-3 group at the .025 level.
[d] Significantly different from PS + KG + PS-2 group at the .025 level.

TABLE 4
Unadjusted Means and Adjusted (Adj.) Rates for Grade Retention
and Special Education Placement by Intervention Group

Intervention Group	n	End of Program		1-Year Follow-Up		2-Year Follow-Up	
		%	Adj. %	%	Adj. %	%	Adj. %
Grade Retention							
With follow-on							
PS + KG + PG-3	160	6.3	6.6[a,b,c,d]	12.5	11.8[a,b,c]	13.8	15.3[a,b,c]
No PS + KG + PG-3	76	13.2	12.3[a,b]	21.1	18.7[a]	27.6	27.3
PS + KG + PG-2	302	15.0	16.9[a,b]	16.9	17.3[a]	20.9	22.8[a,b]
PS + KG + PG-1	80	23.8	22.0	27.5	24.9	31.3	30.6
Without follow-on							
PS + KG only	207	27.5	25.7	27.5	25.0	32.4	31.8
Non-CPC comparison group	191	26.2	26.0	27.8	25.9	31.4	31.3
Special Education Placement							
With follow-on							
PS + KG + PG-3	160	10.0	10.9[b]	10.0	10.5	11.9	12.5
No PS + KG + PG-3	76	6.6	6.8	14.5	14.4	14.5	14.4
PS + KG + PG-2	302	5.3	5.3	5.6	5.7[c]	6.3	6.3[c]
PS + KG + PG-1	80	8.8	9.0	11.3	11.2	13.8	13.8
Without follow-on							
PS + KG only	207	4.4	4.2	8.7	8.4	10.6	10.6
Non-CPC comparison group	191	8.9	8.3	11.0	10.5	11.5	10.9

Note. Covariates included the child and family variables in Table 1. Kindergarten achievement was added for comparisons among groups with preschool intervention. PS = preschool, KG = kindergarten, PG = primary grade.
[a]Significantly different from non-CPC comparison group at the .025 level.
[b]Significantly different from PS + KG group or PS + KG + PG-1 group at the .025 level.
[c]Significantly different from no-PS + KG + PG-3 group at the .025 level.
[d]Significantly different from PS + KG + PS-2 group at the .025 level.

In the remainder of this section, comparisons between the full intervention groups (PS + KG + PG-3 and PS + KG + PG-2) and the preschool-kindergarten group (PS + KG) are highlighted to determine the contribution of the follow-on intervention independent of preschool intervention. For comparisons among groups with preschool and kindergarten intervention experience, means were adjusted for both reading and math achievement at the end of kindergarten, before participation in the follow-on intervention. Because of the number of contrasts analyzed, statistical significance was set at the .025 level. Results are reported by outcome.

Reading and math achievement. At the end of the program (Grade 3), the full intervention groups performed significantly higher than the non-CPC comparison group in reading and math achievement. Only the PS + KG + PG-3 group, however, had significantly higher scores than the PS + KG group (adjusted for covariates and kindergarten achievement). These differences were maintained up to the 2-year follow-up assessment.[7] Notably, the gap between the full intervention and comparison groups narrowed over time (i.e., from 11 to 7 points) as a result of the comparison groups catching up rather than the full intervention group falling back. The PS + KG + PG-2 full intervention group did overtake the PS + KG group by Grade 5 in reading achievement but not in math achievement.

Of additional interest was the significantly better performance of the no PS + KG + PG-3 group over the PS + KG and the PS + KG + PG-2 groups at the end of the program (Grade 3). These results show the strong immediate effect of the follow-on intervention. However, these observed differences were short-lived as no differences were found among these groups by Grade 5. Only the PS + KG + PG-3 group significantly surpassed the no PS + KG + PG-3 group's performance by the 2-year follow-up. This result was probably due to the added value of preschool intervention, which suggests that while intervention in kindergarten and primary grades has an immediate effect, this effect may not last without prior preschool experience. Nevertheless, the equivalent performance over time of the no PS + KG + PG-3 and PS + KG + PG-2 groups—despite their equal duration of intervention—indicates that age of entry into intervention was unrelated to reading and math achievement. Duration of intervention of exposure was important, especially beyond 3 years.

---

[7]These differences for achievement were independent of grade retention. For example, after grade retention was entered as a covariate, the PS + KG + PG-3 full intervention group scored 6 points higher in reading achievement and 4 points higher in math achievement than the PS + KG group at the 2-year follow-up compared with 7 and 5 points, respectively, as reported in Table 3. Of course, this is a restrictive test because grade retention is a proven outcome of early childhood intervention rather than a predictor. Separate estimation of intervention effects on achievement for retained and promoted children yielded no significant differences.

All intervention groups performed, on average, substantially below the national mean in Grade 5. For example, the average score of the non-retained full intervention group was at the 28th percentile, 1 year below the national mean for fifth graders. As with reading achievement, math achievement scores were considerably below the national mean for fifth graders (i.e., 29th percentile).

Teacher ratings. At the end of the program, only the PS + KG + PG-3 intervention group had significantly higher ratings than the PS + KG and non-CPC comparison groups. This difference was maintained in Grade 4 but was somewhat reduced in Grade 5. To the contrary, ratings of the PS + KG + PG-2 group increased over time. In Grade 5, they were rated significantly higher than the PS + KG group and the no PS + KG + PG-3 group despite their equal years of intervention. This finding indicates that the age of entry into intervention influences social adjustment in the classroom rather than cognitive school achievement. Indeed, improving socioemotional adjustment is a major goal of the CPC preschool program.

Parental school involvement. Although both full intervention groups had significantly higher teacher ratings of parental school involvement than three other groups at the end of the program, only the involvement of the PS + KG + PG-2 group was significantly higher by Grade 5. The PS + KG + PG-2 group also was significantly higher in parent involvement than the no PS + KG + PG-3 group at the 2-year follow-up. This provides additional evidence that early entry into intervention affects nonachievement outcomes more than achievement outcomes. The general decline in parent involvement over time may reflect the shift from family-child relations to peer relations as children begin to enter early adolescence. As with achievement and teacher ratings, the PS + KG group had no better ratings on parent involvement than the non-CPC comparison group.

Grade retention. At the end of the program, the PS + KG + PG-3 full intervention group had a significantly lower cumulative rate of grade retention than all other intervention groups, and the PS + KG + PG-2 group had a lower rate of grade retention than the PS + KG group and the non-CPC comparison group. Groups maintained most of their advantages through the 2-year follow-up assessment. By Grade 5, 15.3% of the PS + KG + PG-3 group was retained in grade, which translates to a 52% reduction over the PS + KG group. The PS + KG + PG-2 group had a retention rate of 22.8% by Grade 5, which translates to a 28% reduction over the PS + KG group. The full intervention groups outperformed the non-CPC comparison group by similar margins.

At the end of the program, the no PS + KG + PG-3 group had a significantly lower rate of grade retention than both the PS + KG and non-

CPC comparison groups. However, by Grade 5 their rate was not significantly different from these groups plus the PS + KG + PG-1 and PS + KG + PG-2 groups. For the latter comparison, the trend favored the PS + KG + PG-2 group. These results support the value of preschool plus follow-on intervention.

Special education placement. There was no consistent evidence of intervention effects on special education placement at the end of the program or at Grade 5. Only the PS + KG + PG-2 group had substantially lower placement rates than the other groups, and these were significant in relation to the no PS + KG + PG-3 group only. It is surprising that the comparison groups without follow-on intervention had slightly lower rates of special education placement than those with follow-on intervention. These overall findings suggest that differential exposure to intervention is unrelated to placement in special education. Of course, the assumption that all children who needed services received them may be tenuous, which would explain why children with less intervention were as likely as children with more intervention to receive services.

Primary Analysis 2: Effect Sizes of Intervention Components

So far the analyses reveal that the follow-on intervention significantly contributes to adjustment outcomes above and beyond the preschool and kindergarten intervention up to 2 years postprogram. Moreover, children participating in the full intervention from preschool to Grade 2 or 3 had consistently better adjustment than most of the other groups, especially the PS + KG and non-CPC comparison groups. Figure 2 summarizes the effect size (ES) of the preschool and primary-grade components as well as the full intervention (preschool to Grade 3) at the end of the program and at the 2-year follow-up. The effects of the kindergarten component are not reported because all of the children received kindergarten services, thus these effects are not meaningful. ESs are proportions of standard deviations and are comparable across outcomes regardless of the metric used. They are calculated by dividing the mean difference (adjusted) between intervention and comparison groups by the pooled standard deviation of each respective outcome (Hedges & Olkin, 1985).[8] Values of .20 and above in absolute value were interpreted as educationally meaningful. This is equivalent to a

---

[8] Pooled standard deviations for Grades 3, 4, and 5, respectively, were as follows: reading achievement (15.83, 15.45, and 16.84), math achievement (12.90, 12.94, and 15.03), teacher ratings (5.31, 5.36, and 5.38), grade retention (0.39, 0.41, and 0.43), parental school involvement (1.19, 1.17, and 1.28), and special education placement (0.26, 0.29, and 0.31). Effect sizes for grade retention and special education placement were adjusted for their binary-coded properties through the probit method (Glass, McGaw, & Smith, 1981).

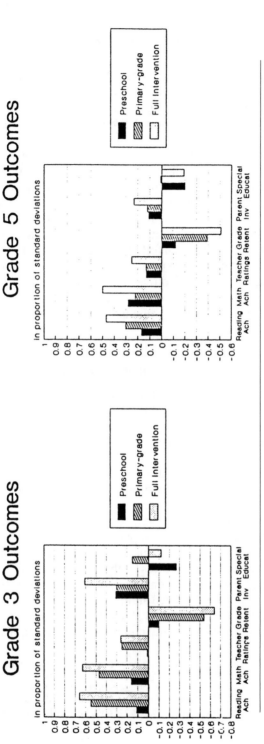

Figure 2. Effect sizes of intervention at end of program and at 2-year follow-up. Reading Ach = reading achievement; Math Ach = math achievement; Grade Retent = grade retention; Parent Inv = parental school involvement; Special Educat = special education.

10-point difference (i.e., 55% to 45%) in success rates between groups (Cohen, 1988; Rosenthal, 1991).

The effect of the full intervention was estimated as the difference in adjusted means between the full intervention group and the non-CPC comparison group. The primary-grade intervention effect was based on analysis of covariance by means of multiple regression with years of primary-grade intervention as the independent variable and the sociodemographic variables in Table 1 and end-of-kindergarten reading achievement and mathematics achievement as covariates. Only children participating in the CPC intervention were included in the analysis to determine the ESs of the primary-grade component. The effect of preschool was estimated as the difference between the ESs of the total intervention and the primary-grade component (i.e., [PS + PG] − PG).

At the end of the program, the effects of the full intervention were educationally meaningful for five of six outcomes (no effects for special education placement). In order of magnitude, they were as follows: reading achievement, ES = .66; grade retention, ES = −.64; mathematics achievement, ES = .63; parent involvement in school, ES = .61; teacher ratings, ES = .26; and special education placement, ES = −.12. Effects of the full intervention remained moderately educationally meaningful up to 2 years following the program for reading achievement (ES = .47), mathematics achievement (ES = .50), and grade retention (ES = −.51). The ES for grade retention is equivalent to a 62.5%–37.5% success-rate advantage for the intervention group. Alternatively, the mean rate of grade retention in the intervention group was lower than the rate of 69% of children in the non-CPC intervention group. Effects on teacher ratings, parent involvement in school, and special education placement were smaller but in the meaningful range (ESs = .20–.25).

Both preschool and follow-on components contributed substantially to the full intervention effect, indicating that participation in the full intervention is more effective than participation in either the preschool or primary-grade component alone. For example, Grade 5 ESs of the preschool component were, respectively, .18, .28, .12, −.12, .11, and −.20 for reading achievement, math achievement, teacher ratings, grade retention, parental school involvement, and special education placement. ESs for the follow-on component were, respectively, .29, .22, .11, −.39, .11, and .00. This overall pattern illustrates the cumulative effect of intervention exposure. The better performance of the PS + KG + PG-3 group compared with the preschool-kindergarten only and primary-grade only groups indicates a possible synergistic effect of preschool plus follow-on intervention.

Additional Analyses

Intervention effect versus school-stability effect. Because participation in the full intervention required staying in an intervention school during the primary grades, an alternative explanation to the observed differences between intervention and comparison groups is that the absence of school mobility caused such differences. To address this issue, the full intervention group (PS + KG + PG-3) was compared with two groups of school-stable children (through Grade 3). Full intervention participants significantly and meaningfully outperformed school-stable non-CPC participants on reading achievement, mathematics achievement, and grade retention up to 2 years following the intervention. For reading achievement, the 9.6-point advantage of the full intervention group at the end of the program was 5.3 points at Grade 5. Also, the full intervention group had a 38% lower rate of retention (adjusted) than the school-stable comparison group in Grade 5 (15% vs. 24%).

Similar findings were obtained when children in the full intervention group were compared with children in the PS + KG group who did not change schools from Grade 1 to 3. For example, the full intervention group had a 7-point advantage over their school-stable no follow-on peers in Grade 5 reading achievement. These results disconfirm the hypothesis that the observed intervention effects are due to school stability.

Intervention effects by site. The earlier findings concerned effects of the CPC intervention averaged across all sites (or schools) that implemented the intervention. Because the sites differed, to some degree, in their school characteristics and the extent of parent involvement, analyses of site differences were undertaken.[9] Table 5 presents children's performance at the six sites that implemented the full intervention through Grade 3. Also shown are each school's poverty index (school socioeconomic status in 1986) and mean parental school involvement. Values for parent involvement are the schoolwide averages of teacher ratings of parent participation in school activities in Grade 1: the time when the maximum amount of parent data were available. Parent involvement and school poverty had the most variability across sites. Differences in teacher training and experiences, amount of resources, and provision of comprehensive services were similar across sites (Chicago Public Schools, 1986, 1987a).

Only at School 5 were adjustment outcomes consistently below that of the non-CPC comparison group and the PS + KG group. Not surprisingly, School 5 had a relatively high rate of poverty (68% of families) and low parental school involvement (M = 2.5), the combination of which may have reduced the effectiveness of the program. Schools with higher rates of parental involvement had the best-adjusted children (Schools 1, 2, and 3).

---

[9] See page 594.

TABLE 5
Mean Performance of Children Participating in the Full Intervention to Grade 3 by School

| | School Factor | | Grade 5 Outcome | | | | |
School	Poverty Index[a]	Parent Involvement[b]	Reading Achievement	Math Achievement	Teacher Ratings	Grade Retention[c]	Special Education[c]
School 1	61.8	3.6	123.2	125.8	17.2	4.8	19.1
School 2	72.1	3.5	119.5	124.6	20.3	5.6	13.9
School 3	56.1	3.1	117.5	123.5	21.5	33.3	7.4
School 4	55.0	2.8	114.8	121.0	22.8	25.0	4.2
School 5	68.0	2.5	107.1	117.8	17.1	16.7	16.7
School 6	59.8	2.4	113.2	119.1	19.8	5.3	5.3

[a] Percentage of poor families in school region.
[b] Parental school involvement is reported as average of teacher ratings for all study children.
[c] Values are in percentages.

School poverty rates were unrelated to reading and math achievement but were associated, in the expected direction, with teacher ratings, grade retention, and special education placement (rs = .54 to .68 in absolute value). School parent involvement was positively and significantly associated with school reading and math achievement (rs = .90, .97), although magnitudes should be interpreted cautiously because of the small number of observations. These latter findings suggest that fidelity to parental involvement is a major ingredient in program success.

Analyses of the sites that implemented the intervention through Grade 2 also revealed that a majority of centers performed at or above the overall average for the 14 sites. For Grade 5 reading achievement, 8 of 14 sites performed at or above the overall average. Ten of 14 sites had lower rates of grade retention than the overall average. Smaller relationships were found, however, among school poverty, parent involvement, and the adjustment outcomes across these sites. School poverty was most associated with special education placement (r = .33); school parent involvement was most associated with grade retention (r = −.42).

Within-group multiple regression analyses at the individual level supported parental school involvement as a predictor of adjustment. For both full intervention groups, parental school involvement was significantly associated with Grade 5 school achievement and grade retention above and beyond the influence of the covariates (betas in .20 range). For other intervention groups (i.e., PS + KG and non-CPC comparison), parent involvement marginally contributed to adjustment differences (betas in .10 range). These findings suggest that parent involvement in school may be a mechanism through which the intervention affects adjustment outcomes.

DISCUSSION

This study investigated the effects of differential participation in a federally funded early childhood intervention program on the development of inner-city Black children. In response to the three research questions, results indicated that (a) duration of exposure to the intervention was significantly related to adjustment outcomes after the influence of potentially confounding variables was controlled, (b) follow-on intervention significantly contributed to children's school adjustment above and beyond preschool intervention, and (c) both follow-on and total intervention effects were significant and stable up to 2 years following the program. Although both preschool and follow-on participation contributed to positive adjustment, full participation in the CPC program yielded the largest effects over time.

Effects of Government-Funded, Follow-On Intervention

Most important, the present study uniquely contributes to knowledge based on early childhood interventions by providing empirical support for the independent effects of follow-on intervention. As indicated in the introduction, previous studies have rarely separated the effects of preschool from those of follow-on intervention, and none have reported effects for large-scale, government-funded programs. By using multiple intervention and comparison groups, several longitudinal outcomes, and different methods of investigating potential confounding factors, the present study is a more rigorous test than most previous studies of extended childhood intervention.

Along with previous studies of government-funded programs (Fuerst & Fuerst, 1993; Madden et al., 1993; Seitz et al., 1983), the present findings provide substantial empirical support for childhood interventions that extend into the primary grades as originally proposed in Follow Through and more recently (National Head Start Association, 1990; Zigler & Styfco, 1993). Study findings differ somewhat from those of the Carolina Abecedarian Project (Campbell & Ramey, 1993; Horacek et al., 1987), which indicated that school-age intervention did not significantly contribute to adjustment outcomes independent of preschool intervention. These results may have been due to several factors, including the low statistical power of the research design and the longer duration and intensity of the preschool intervention (year round for 5 years) in relation to the school-age intervention. Nevertheless, as in the present study, these researchers found a positive relationship between the extent of intervention and adjustment outcomes.

In adding significantly to the effect of preschool and kindergarten intervention, participation in the CPC follow-on intervention bolstered children's scholastic achievement above the levels that were observed for participation in only preschool and kindergarten intervention. Thus, follow-on intervention reversed the declining effects of earlier intervention. Of course, extended intervention may just delay the onset of fading effects by a few years. Follow-up data beyond 2 years postprogram, however, are necessary to answer this question. Even a delay in the onset of declining effects, however, is a meaningful improvement given the documented relationship between early childhood adjustment and later outcomes such as educational attainment and social responsibility (Brooks-Gunn, Guo, & Furstenberg, 1993; Lloyd, 1978; Schweinhart et al., 1993). But study results also indicate that fading effects of intervention are not inevitable. Although the effects of the follow-on and total interventions declined over time, they remained sizable at the 2-year follow-up, especially for school achievement and grade retention (see Figure 2). Consistent with Reynolds (1993), effects of the preschool intervention increased from Grades 3 to 5.

Longer lasting interventions, which provide an array of services such as smaller class sizes, teacher training, and parent involvement activities, allow children greater opportunities to develop scholastic and social skills necessary for sustained effects. Several studies (Alexander & Entwisle, 1988; Entwisle & Hayduk, 1988; Reynolds, 1991) support the value of intervening school-based and family support factors in promoting successful adjustment to the primary grades. This suggests that interventions designed to enhance adult-child relationships as well as cognitive skills may foster successful school transitions compared with unassisted transitions. Because children at risk in inner cities experience more stressful and persistent negative life events than their more advantaged peers, such cognitive and social support programs may encourage the development of adaptive skills. The linkage between preschool and primary-grade intervention is a source of continuity for many children.

Timing and Duration of Intervention

The results indicate no particular advantage of preschool intervention over primary-grade intervention. Both early participation in and longer duration of intervention contributed to group differences in adjustment. Children with the highest achievement test scores, highest teacher ratings, and the lowest incidence of grade retention were those who participated in both preschool and follow-on intervention. One conclusion of these findings is that duration of intervention exposure is just as important a factor in intervention theory and design as age of participation. A longer period of intervention exposure was necessary to enhance children's adjustment over time. Also, duration of intervention was more associated with reading and math achievement than age of entry. Children who participated in only the preschool and kindergarten components did no better in achievement than children who participated in just the follow-on component. Moreover, the PS + KG + PG-2 and no PS + KG + PG-3 groups—which participated for an equal number of years but entered the program at different times— performed similarly in reading and math achievement at the 2-year follow-up.

A second conclusion is that the effect of timing of intervention may vary by domain. Early entry into intervention did not substantially influence school achievement and, to a lesser extent, grade retention, but children who participated in preschool intervention were more likely to perform better in social adjustment, including teacher ratings of classroom adjustment, parent involvement in school activities, and special education placement. For example, the PS + KG + PG-2 had significantly higher ratings of classroom adjustment and parental school involvement and a significantly lower rate of special education placement at the 2-year follow-up than children who entered in kindergarten but who also had the same number of years of intervention. These differences are consistent with the theory of the program. Preschool intervention is more focused on social development and parent involvement than the primary-grade intervention. The primary-grade intervention is more academically oriented, and parent involvement is encouraged rather than required.

Overall, these findings support the principle of developmental continuity rather than of critical periods. For more lasting effects, early childhood interventions must provide substantial support services through two sensitive periods development: at the beginning of preschool and during and after the transition to formal schooling. This contiguity of services enables each successive year of intervention to build on earlier ones until a threshold is reached (see Figure 1). Of course, evidence for the appropriate timing of interventions is limited in this study to ages 3 to 8. Evidence of the timing of interventions outside this age range awaits further study.

Domains of Effects

The strongest and most stable effects of the total intervention were on reading achievement, mathematics achievement, and grade retention. These outcomes represent mastery of basic skills and social expectations, which predict educational success (Natriello et al., 1990). This result is not surprising given that scholastic and school competence are primary goals of the program. These effects of extended intervention are more developmentally significant than might be anticipated because both low school achievement and grade retention are risk factors for poor adjustment outcomes such as school dropout, delinquency, and unemployment (Berrueta-Clement et al., 1984; Lloyd, 1978; Schweinhart et al., 1993). Present findings reinforce previous analyses indicating that the greatest and most stable effects of early childhood interventions are on scholastic competence rather than on intellectual aptitude (Consortium for Longitudinal Studies, 1983; Haskins, 1989; Woodhead, 1988).

The study also found intervention effects on parent involvement in school and teacher ratings of adjustment, but these effects were not consistent over time and were smaller in magnitude than effects on school achievement and grade retention. Although participants in the full intervention consistently had higher ratings than the non-CPC comparison group, the follow-on intervention did not have major effects on these outcomes. Only the PS + KG + PG-2 group consistently and significantly outperformed the other CPC groups on teacher ratings and parent involvement in school. The observed effects, however, are indications that the intervention worked as predicted by the program theory. Short-term effects on classroom adjustment and parent involvement may lead to longer term effects on scholastic competence.

There are two likely explanations for smaller effects on teacher ratings and parent involvement. Both parental involvement and teacher ratings were narrowly defined. Parent involvement was assessed by a single item; teacher ratings were assessed with six items of positive social and school adjustment. More comprehensive and refined measures may have yielded larger and more robust effects. Second, regarding parent involvement in school, continuous effects would not be expected throughout the schooling process because parents tend to become less involved in school as children grow older. The relative lack of significant intervention effects for special education placement, if not a true reflection of the intervention, may be caused by the low incidence of placement across the sample or by the lack of referral of children to services who needed them (e.g., non-CPC comparison group).

Which aspects of the intervention contributed to effectiveness? Although the design of the study does not allow for precise identification of the critical components, parent involvement is one likely ingredient. School parental involvement was directly and positively related to differential performance across sites and was a predictor of adjustment within each of the full intervention groups. Previous studies in this longitudinal study indicate that parent involvement is a mechanism through which interventions exert their effectiveness (Reynolds, 1991, 1992c). Like Head Start, a central theory behind the CPC program is enhancing family functioning, especially the family-school relationship. Of course, the provision of comprehensive services and a child-centered focus on cognitive enrichment also are characteristic of successful early intervention programs (Chafel, 1992; Schweinhart & Weikart, 1988) and may have contributed to the present findings. Future studies of programs that vary in the provision of services and staff resources will be important in identifying each factor's specific influence.

National Comparisons

Although children participating in the full interventions performed significantly better than comparison-group and preschool–kindergarten-group children on several outcomes, their adjustment was still below the level of the typical child nationally. Children who enrolled in the full intervention through Grade 3, for example, were on average 1 year behind the national average in reading comprehension and 6 months behind in mathematics in Grade 5. This finding is consistent with previous studies (Abelson et al., 1974; Horacek et al., 1987; Lee, Brooks-Gunn, & Schnur, 1988). But children participating in the full intervention did score 1 month above the average child in the Chicago Public Schools in reading and mathematics. This is notable because of the substantially higher rate of school poverty of children in this study (66%) as compared with the city-wide average (42%). Moreover, the rate of retention for the full intervention group was below the national public school average in Grades 3 and 5 (see Figure 1; Meisels & Liaw, 1991). Thus, although early childhood interventions should not be expected to bring most disadvantaged children's academic performance up to the level of their more advantaged peers, the results for grade retention show that meaningful differences in children's school adjustment can be achieved.

Study Strengths and Limitations

Among the methodological strengths of the present findings were (a) the variation in duration of intervention exposure, (b) the relatively large sample sizes of the groups participating in the intervention, (c) tracing children up to 2 years following the intervention, and (d) the simultaneous consideration of multiple adjustment outcomes, including the rarely considered construct of parental school involvement. As a consequence of these features, generalizability of results to children in typical inner-city schools is enhanced, thus providing direct evidence of what may be expected from Head Start-type interventions with different lengths (Haskins, 1989).

A major limitation of the study is the possibility that self-selection into the intervention rather than the intervention caused the observed differences in children's adjustment. Consequently, results should be interpreted with caution and cross-validated with other samples and programs. Several design features and results appear to limit the plausibility of the self-selection interpretation, however. First, the groups were well matched on several sociodemographic factors, such as parent education, eligibility for free lunch, school poverty rates, parent expectations for educational attainment, age, and family size. If self-selection was present, differences on some of these factors would have been expected. Because parent expectations, parent education, and eligibility for free lunch were collected during the program—and thus may have been affected by it—their inclusion in the analysis may have corrected, to some extent, the effects of selection. Also, achievement scores at the end of kindergarten were similar among the CPC intervention groups, and these scores were included in the analyses of follow-on effects. Furthermore, growth rates in achievement from the beginning to the end of kindergarten were similar among groups. Consequently, the significantly better adjustment at the 2-year follow-up of children participating in the preschool plus follow-on intervention is unlikely to be explained by selection and maturational factors.

A second factor that reduces the plausibility of the self-selection interpretation was that school stability was ruled out as an explanation of intervention effects. The full intervention group through Grade 3 significantly outperformed the more advantaged, school-stable non-CPC comparison group as well as the school-stable preschool–kindergarten group on reading achievement, mathematics achievement, and grade retention. This finding increases the likelihood that group differences were the result of participation in the intervention. Moreover, analyzing data from many children in the present sample by latent-variable structural modeling, Reynolds (1992c) found no evidence that unmeasured variables such as school mobility biased the effect of preschool intervention on cognitive readiness or later school adjustment.

A third factor limiting the self-selection hypothesis was that entry into the CPC program is based on educational and economic need, and schools often recruited families. Enrolled children were most likely to be in greatest need of the program. Consequently, the observed effects of the program may be underestimates rather than overestimates of true effects. The early studies of Head Start, for example, may have underestimated program effects because comparison groups were drawn from less disadvantaged samples (Campbell & Erlebacher, 1970; Lee et al., 1988). An advantage of the present study is that comparisons were made among groups that already had been exposed to components of the intervention, thus would tend to be more equivalent than traditional treatment and control comparisons.

Finally, the pattern of findings is inconsistent with the pattern expected if the self-selection hypothesis was true. If self-selection were present, program effects would be relatively consistent over time, albeit inflated. To the contrary, the pattern of observed intervention effects varied substantially over time and by outcome. For example, effects on cognitive achievement in reading and math declined somewhat by Grade 5. Effects on teacher ratings and parental school involvement declined substantially over time. Group differences in special education placement were minimal. Selection into preschool or follow-on components does not easily explain these varied findings.

Nevertheless, confirmation of these results awaits follow-up analyses with this and other samples. Of course, even if self-selection is not a plausible explanation for the findings of this study, results are not necessarily generalizable to the total population of young children or to other programs that differ in philosophy and scope. For example, like Head Start, the CPCs have had over 25 years of experience implementing the program that ensures a minimum level of program quality. Consequently, generalizability of findings is limited to relatively established programs that serve large proportions of low-income and minority populations. Yet the present investigation of a large-scale government-funded program is a substantial improvement over many previous studies of relatively small-scale demonstration programs.

Conclusion and Implications

The major finding of this study is the significant and independent contribution to children's school adjustment of follow-on intervention for economically disadvantaged children. This demonstration indicates that established, government-funded programs can be successful when they continue to Grades 2 and 3. Consequently, the implementation of preschool plus follow-on programs may be an effective way to bolster children's school adjustment. One, 2, and even 3 years of intervention had limited influence on adjustment outcomes at the end of the program or up to 2 years afterward. Of course, this study does not indicate that preschool intervention is ineffective in improving children's adjustment. Indeed, preschool intervention significantly contributed to child outcomes (see Figure 2). Rather, extended programs add significantly to the effect of preschool intervention, especially for children who need greater support than can be provided in a 1- or 2-year program. Given the relatively modest expenditure of approximately $4,000 (1992 dollars) annually per pupil for Head Start-type early childhood programs such as the CPCs, the potential benefit may be significant over the long term.

A second conclusion is that duration of intervention exposure may be just as important, and in some cases, more important to children's adjustment than the timing of intervention. Group differences in school achievement, for example, were largely influenced by duration rather than by earlier enrollment. An implication of this study is that duration of intervention should be a major focus of theory and research on early childhood intervention. A question for future research is to determine the optimal combination of timing and duration of intervention. Although it appears that 1 or 2 years of preschool is insufficient by itself to ensure lasting effects for many children, continued investigation of the effects of different combinations of earlier and later intervention would be helpful, especially beyond the age range tested in this study. Consequently, the present movement toward downward expansion of intervention programs from birth to age 3 must be matched with equal concern for upward expansion to formal schooling and beyond implied by the principle of developmental continuity. Present findings that earlier intervention influenced social outcomes more than school achievement also warrant further investigation.

Continued follow-up of this sample will determine the stability of the intervention's effects. Evidence on long-term effectiveness across a range of outcomes is necessary to better understand what can be expected of preschool and follow-on intervention programs for children at risk. But studying the effectiveness of interventions should not come at the cost of paying less attention to other family and school influences on adjustment, especially those that may contribute to long-term effects of intervention. Contemporary studies are increasingly finding that successful adjustment is the result of a complex array of factors working in concert rather than one or two factors working in isolation. Early childhood is only the beginning of the process of adjustment, and this process must be supported continuously.

REFERENCES

Abelson, W. D., Zigler, E. F., & DeBlasi, C. L. (1974). Effects of a four-year Follow Through program on economically disadvantaged children. *Journal of Educational Psychology, 66*, 756–771.

Alexander, K. L., & Entwisle, D. R. (1988). Achievement in the first 2 years of school: Patterns and processes. *Monographs of the Society for Research in Child Development, 53*(2, Serial No. 218).

Andrews, S. R., Blumenthal, J. B., Johnson, D. L., Kahn, A. J., Ferguson, C. J., Lasater, T. M., Malone, P. E., & Wallace, D. B. (1982). The skills of mothering: A study of Parent Child Development Centers. *Monographs of the Society for Research in Child Development, 47*(6, Serial No. 198).

Barnett, W. S. (1992). Benefits of compensatory preschool education. *Journal of Human Resources, 27*, 279–312.

Baumrind, D. (1971). Current patterns of parental authority. *Developmental Psychology Monograph, 4*(No. 1, Part 2), 1–103.

Berrueta-Clement, J. R., Schweinhart, L. J., Barnett, W. S., Epstein, A. S., & Weikart, D. P. (1984). *Changed lives: The effects of the Perry Preschool Program on youths through age 19.* Ypsilanti, MI: High/Scope.

Brim, O. G., & Phillips, D. A. (1988). The life-span intervention cube. In E. M. Hetherington, R. M. Lerner, & M. Perlmutter (Eds.), *Child development in life-span perspective* (pp. 277–299). Hillsdale, NJ: Erlbaum.

Bronfenbrenner, U. (1975). Is early intervention effective? In M. Guttentag & E. Struening (Eds.), *Handbook of evaluation research* (Vol. 2, pp. 519–603). Beverly Hills, CA: Sage.

Brooks-Gunn, J., Guo, G., & Furstenberg, F. F. (1993). Who drops out and who continues beyond high school? A 20-year follow-up of Black urban youth. *Journal of Research on Adolescence, 3,* 271–294.

Campbell, D. T., & Erlebacher, A. (1970). How regression artifacts in quasi-experimental evaluations can mistakenly make compensatory education look harmful. In J. Helmuth (Ed.), *Compensatory education: A national debate: Vol. 3. Disadvantaged child* (pp. 321–342). New York: Brunner/Mazel.

Campbell, F. A., & Ramey, C. T. (1993, March). *Mid-adolescent outcomes for high risk children: An examination of the continuing effects of early intervention.* Paper presented at the biennial meeting of the Society for Research in Child Development, New Orleans, LA.

Chafel, J. A. (1992). Funding Head Start: What are the issues? *American Journal of Orthopsychiatry, 62,* 9–21.

Chall, J. S., Jacobs, V. A., & Baldwin, L. E. (1990). *The reading crisis: Why poor children fall behind.* Cambridge, MA: Harvard University Press.

Chicago Public Schools. (1974). *Child Parent Centers.* Washington, DC: Office of Education. (ERIC Document Reproduction Service No. ED108145).

Chicago Public Schools. (1985). *Meeting the mandate: Chicago's government funded kindergarten programs.* Chicago: Department of Research and Evaluation.

Chicago Public Schools. (1986). *Chapter 2 all-day kindergarten program final evaluation report: Fiscal 1985.* Chicago: Department of Research and Evaluation.

Chicago Public Schools. (1987a). *Chapter 2 all-day kindergarten program final evaluation report: Fiscal 1986.* Chicago: Department of Research and Evaluation.

Chicago Public Schools. (1987b). *1985–1986 test scores and selected school characteristics: Elementary schools.* Chicago: Department of Research and Evaluation.

Chicago Public Schools. (1992). *ECIA Chapter I Application: Fiscal 1991.* Chicago: Author.

Cohen, J. (1988). *Statistical power anlaysis for the behavioral sciences* (Rev. ed.). New York: Academic Press.

Cohen, J., & Cohen, P. (1983). *Applied multiple regression/correlation analysis for the behavioral sciences* (2nd ed.). Hillsdale, NJ: Erlbaum.

Conrad, K. J., & Eash, M. J. (1983). Measuring implementation and multiple outcomes in a Child Parent Center compensatory education program. *American Educational Research Journal, 20,* 221–236.

Consortium for Longitudinal Studies. (1983). *As the twig is bent: Lasting effects of preschool programs.* Hillsdale, NJ: Erlbaum.

Cook, T. D., & Shadish, W. R. (1994). Social experiments: Some developments over the past fifteen years. *Annual Review of Psychology, 45,* 545–580.

Entwisle, D. R., & Hayduk, L. A. (1982). *Early schooling: Cognitive and affective outcomes.* Baltimore: Johns Hopkins University Press.

Entwisle, D. R., & Hayduk, L. A. (1988). Lasting effects of elementary school. *Sociology of Education, 61,* 147–159.

Fuerst, J. S., & Fuerst, D. (1993). Chicago experience with an early childhood program: The special case of the Child Parent Center program. *Urban Education, 28,* 69–96.

Glass, G. V., McGaw, B., & Smith, M. L. (1981). *Meta-analysis in social research.* Beverly Hills, CA: Sage.

Haskins, R. (1989). Beyond metaphor: The efficacy of early childhood education. *American Psychologist, 44,* 274–282.

Hedges, L. V., & Olkin, I. (1985). *Statistical methods for meta-analysis.* New York: Academic Press.

Hieronymus, A. N., & Hoover, H. D. (1990). *Iowa Tests of Basic Skills: Manual for school administrators* (Suppl.). Chicago: Riverside.

Hieronymus, A. N., Lindquist, E. F., & Hoover, H. D. (1980). *Iowa Tests of Basic Skills: Primary battery.* Chicago: Riverside.

Horacek, H. J., Ramey, C. T., Campbell, F. A., Hoffman, K. P., & Fletcher, R. H. (1987). Predicting school failure and assessing early intervention with high-risk children. *Journal of the American Academy of Child and Adolescent Psychiatry, 26,* 758–763.

House, E. R., Glass, G. V., McLean, L. D., & Walker, D. F. (1978). No simple answer: Critique of the Follow Through evaluation. *Harvard Educational Review, 48,* 128–160.

Hubbell, R. (1983). *A review of Head Start since 1970.* Washington, DC: U.S. Department of Health and Human Services.

Joreskog, K. G., & Sorbom, D. (1988). *PRELIS: A Program for multivariate data screening and data summarization. A preprocessor for LISREL.* Mooresville, IN: Scientific Software.

Jordon, T. J., Grallo, R., Deutsch, M., & Deutsch, C. P. (1985). Long-term effects of early enrichment: A 20-year perspective on persistence and change. *American Journal of Community Psychology, 13,* 393–415.

Jurs, S. G., & Glass, G. V. (1971). The effect of experimental morality on the internal and external validity of the randomized comparative experiment. *Journal of Experimental Education, 40,* 62–66.

Kessler, R. C., & Greenberg, D. L. (1981). *Linear panel analysis: Methods of quantitative change.* New York: Academic Press.

Lazar, I., Darlington, R. B., Murray, H. W., & Snipper, A. S. (1982). Lasting effects of early education: A report from the consortium for longitudinal studies. *Monographs of the Society for Research in Child Development, 47* (2/3, Serial No. 195).

Lee, V. E., Brooks-Gunn, J., & Schnur, E. (1988). Does Head Start work? A 1-year follow-up comparison of disadvantaged children attending Head Start, no preschool, and other preschool programs. *Developmental Psychology, 24,* 210–222.

Lloyd, D. N. (1978). Prediction of school failure from third-grade data. *Educational and Psychological Measurement, 38,* 1193–1200.

Madden, N. A., Slavin, R. E., Karweit, N. L., Dolan, L. J., & Wasik, B. A. (1993). Success for all: Longitudinal effects of a restructuring program for inner-city elementary schools. *American Educational Research Journal, 30,* 123–148.

McKey, R. H., Condelli, L., Ganson, H., Barrett, B. J., McConkey, C., & Plantz, M. C. (1985). *The impact of Head Start on children, families, and communities* (DHHS Publication No. OHDS 85-31193). Washington, DC: U.S. Government Printing Office.

McLoyd, V. (1990). The impact of economic hardship on Black families and children: Psychological distress, parenting, and socioemotional development. *Child Development, 61,* 311–346.

Meisels, S. J., & Liaw, F. (1991, April). *Does early retention in grade reduce the risk of later academic failure?* Paper presented at the annual meeting of the American Educational Research Association, Chicago.

Meyer, L. (1984). Long-term academic effects of the direct instructional Project Follow Thru. *Elementary School Journal, 84,* 380–392.

Moffitt, R. (1991). Program evaluation with nonexperimental data. *Evaluation Review, 15,* 291–314.

Natriello, G., McDill, E. L., & Pallas, A. M. (1990). *Schooling disadvantaged children: Racing against catastrophe.* New York: Teachers College Press.

National Head Start Association. (1990). *Head Start: The nation's pride, a nation's challenge.* Alexandria, VA: Author.

Ramey, S. L., & Ramey, C. T. (1992). Early educational intervention with disadvantaged children—to what effect? *Applied and Preventive Psychology, 1,* 131–140.

Reynolds, A. J. (1989). A structural model of first-grade outcomes for an urban, low socioeconomic status, minority population. *Journal of Educational Psychology, 81,* 594–603.

Reynolds, A. J. (1991). Early schooling of children at risk. *American Educational Research Journal, 28,* 392–422.

Reynolds, A. J. (1992a). Comparing measures of parental involvement and their effects on academic achievement. *Early Childhood Research Quarterly, 7,* 441–462.

Reynolds, A. J. (1992b). Grade retention and school adjustment: An explanatory analysis. *Educational Evaluation and Policy Analysis, 14*, 101–121.

Reynolds, A. J. (1992c). Mediated effects of preschool intervention. *Early Education and Development, 3*, 139–164.

Reynolds, A. J. (1993, November). *One year of preschool intervention or two: Does it matter for low-income black children from the inner city?* Paper presented at the Second National Head Start Research Conference, Washington, DC.

Reynolds, A. J., & Bezruczko, N. (1993). School adjustment of children at risk through fourth grade. *Merrill-Palmer Quarterly, 39*, 457–480.

Rosenthal, R. (1991). *Meta-analytic procedures for social research* (Rev. ed.). Newbury Park, CA: Sage.

Rossi, P. H., & Freeman, H. E. (1989). *Evaluation: A systematic approach* (4th ed.). Newbury Park, CA: Sage.

Schweinhart, L. J., Barnes, H. V., & Weikart, D. P. (1993). *Significant benefits: The High/Scope Perry Preschool study through age 27.* Ypsilanti, MI: High/Scope.

Schweinhart, L. J., & Weikart, D. P. (1988). The High/Scope Perry Preschool Program. In R. H. Price, E. L. Cowen, R. P. Lorion, & J. Ramos-McKay (Eds.), *14 ounces of prevention: A casebook for practitioners* (pp. 53–65). Washington, DC: American Psychological Association.

Seitz, V. (1990). Intervention programs for impoverished children: A comparison of educational and family support models. *Annals of Child Development, 7*, 73–103.

Seitz, V., Apfel, N., Rosenbaum, L., & Zigler, E. (1983). Long-term effects of Projects Head Start and Follow Through: The New Haven Project. In Consortium for Longitudinal Studies (Eds.), *As the twig is bent: Lasting effects of preschool programs* (pp. 299–332). Hillsdale, NJ: Erlbaum.

Stallings, J. (1975). Implementation and child effects of teaching practices on Follow-Through classrooms. *Monographs of the Society for Research in Child Development, 40* (Serial No. 163).

Stenner, A. J., & Mueller, S. G. (1973, December). A successful compensatory education model. *Phi Delta Kappan,* 246–248.

Stevenson, D. L., & Baker, D. P. (1987). The family-school relation and the child's school performance. *Child Development, 58*, 1348–1357.

Tuma, J. M. (1989). Mental health services for children: The state of the art. *American Psychologist, 44*, 188–199.

Wachs, T. D., & Gruen, G. E. (1982). *Early experience & human development.* New York: Plenum.

White, K. R. (1985). Efficacy of early intervention. *Journal of Special Education, 19*, 401–416.

Woodhead, M. (1988). When psychology informs public policy: The case of early childhood. *American Psychologist, 43*, 443–454.

Yeaton, W. H., & Sechrest, L. (1981). Critical dimensions in the choice and maintenance of successful treatments: Strength, integrity, and effectiveness. *Journal of Consulting and Clinical Psychology, 49,* 156–167.

Zigler, E., & Berman, W. (1983). Discerning the future of early childhood intervention. *American Psychologist, 38,* 894–906.

Zigler, E., & Muenchow, S. (1992). *Head Start: The inside story of America's most successful educational experiment.* New York: Basic Books.

Zigler, E., & Styfco, S. (Eds.). (1993). *Head Start and beyond: A national plan for extended childhood intervention.* New Haven, CT: Yale University Press.

Zigler, E., & Trickett, P. K. (1978). IQ, social competence, and evaluation of early childhood intervention programs. *American Psychologist, 33,* 789–798.

APPENDIX

Implementation

The Child Parent Center and Expansion (CPC) program has been consistently implemented with success on the basis of classroom observations, interviews, and school records (Chicago Public Schools, 1986, 1987a). For example, the average child attendance rate across centers in preschool (1984–1985) was 94%, and 93% in kindergarten and the primary grades (1986–1988; Chicago Public Schools, 1987b). Detailed observation of the kindergarten component found that all centers provided comprehensive services, parent involvement activities, and child-centered services (Chicago Public Schools, 1985, 1987a). Only the amount of parent involvement in school varied substantially by site. School-level parent involvement ranged from 2.2 to 3.9 across sites, based on a 5-point teacher rating scale measured in Grade 1 (1 = *poor/not at all* to 5 = *excellent/much*). Nevertheless, overall parent involvement in the CPCs remained consistently higher than in non-CPC sites (Chicago Public Schools, 1986, 1987a). The amount of parent involvement also was similar between centers implementing the program through Grade 3 and centers implementing the program through Grade 2 (*M*s = 3.0). The primary modes of involvement were participation in school activities and in parent-resource rooms.

By extension, the preschool and primary-grade components, which are implemented in the same sites and have many of the same personnel as the kindergarten component, also were implemented successfully. Previous evaluations have reported sucessful implementation of the program from preschool to Grade 3 (Conrad & Eash, 1983; Stenner & Mueller, 1973). Conrad and Eash, for example, found that the CPCs were rated higher than regular school programs in child centeredness (e.g., work independently in small groups), evaluation of child activities, and parent involvement in school activities. These findings are consistent with the program's 25 years of implementation since 1967 (15 years for the primary-grade component). Consequently, the program is included in the U.S. Department of Education's National Diffusion Network, a compository of high-quality educational programs.

Teacher questionnaire reports indicated that teachers had an average of 12.5 years of experience. Approximately 50% had bachelor's degrees and 50% had master's degrees (Chicago Public Schools, 1987a). Of the kindergarten teachers surveyed, 86% had kindergarten or primary grade certificates. These experiences were similar across centers and schools.

---

[9] Because comparison-group children resided in different schools than intervention-group children, a nested design with unit as an additional factor was not possible. Analyses of the six schools that did have a balanced, nested design (children within program within school) yielded results that were consistent with those reported. For example, the PS + KG + PG-3 group scored 6 points higher in reading achievement than the PS + KG group in the balanced design compared with 7 points as reported in Table 3. Adding site dummy variables to the model also did not alter the interpretation of results.

21

Ameliorating Early Reading Failure by Integrating the Teaching of Reading and Phonological Skills: The Phonological Linkage Hypothesis

Peter J. Hatcher

Cumbria Education Authority and University of York, York, England

Charles Hulme and Andrew W. Ellis

University of York

We present a longitudinal intervention study of children experiencing difficulties in the early stages of learning to read. Our subjects, 7-year-old poor readers, were divided into 4 matched groups and assigned to 1 of 3 experimental teaching conditions: Reading with Phonology, Reading Alone, Phonology Alone, and a Control. Although the Phonology Alone group showed most improvement on phonological tasks, the Reading with Phonology group made most progress in

Reprinted with permission from *Child Development*, 1994, Vol. 65, 41–57. Copyright © 1994 by the Society for Research in Child Development, Inc.

We gratefully acknowledge the help given to us by the teachers and other colleagues (Joan Armstrong, Judith Botham, Deborah Catlett, Pam Chaldecott, Gill Dicken, Janet Hatcher, Penny Kennedy, Mary Kirk [speech therapist], Judith Lord, Cynthia McKerr, Margaret Munn, Joyce Rogers, and Mary Savage) who helped construct the teaching programs, the teachers who participated in the study (Joan Baxter, Richard Burford, Barbara Corbishley, Gill Dicken, Suzanne Edmundson, Claire Ellis, Carol Feeney, Geraldine Gaizely, Mary Gill, Elma Hardy, Anne Harrison, Janet Hatcher, Christine Johnson, Joan Kendall, Anne McGraw, Catherine Rafferty, Ros Rankine, Mary Rice, Joyce Rogers, Ruth Simpson, Gill Slessor, Joyce Smith, and Gordon Wealleans) and the psychologists (Kathryn Aspinall, Debra Brewer, Peter Crompton, Mike Dawson, Charlie Haigh, Alix Grabham, Nigel Harbron, John Heath, Colin McGuinness, Janet Pinney, Don Sinclair, Douglas Thomson, and Michael Watmough), who carried out the greater part of the testing of the children involved. We gratefully acknowledge the willing participation of the children and their parents, the schools and class teachers, and Cumbria Education Authority, without whose support this study would not have been possible. We thank Maggie Snowling for her invaluable help. We also thank three anonymous referees for very helpful comments on an earlier version of this article.

*reading. These results show that interventions to boost phonological
skills need to be integrated with the teaching of reading if they are to be
maximally effective in improving literacy skills.*

There is now a massive body of evidence linking the development of
reading skills in children to their underlying phonological skills. This
evidence has come from a variety of sources, including studies of children
with specific reading difficulties (or dyslexia) and correlational studies of
normal children (see Adams, 1990; Goswami & Bryant, 1990; Hulme &
Snowling, 1991; and Wagner & Torgesen, 1987, for recent reviews).

The dominant approach to studying the relationship between phonological skills and learning to read has come from studies of phonological
awareness. Phonological awareness refers to the ability to reflect explicitly
on the sound structure of spoken words. Phonological awareness tasks are
among the best predictors of reading skill and, typically, these relationships
can be shown to account for significant amounts of variance in reading
skill, even after the effects of intelligence have been partialed out (see, e.g.,
Goswami & Bryant, 1990; and Wagner & Torgesen, 1987, for reviews).

One of the most influential studies of these relationships is that of
Bradley and Bryant (1983), who set out to test whether difficulties on one
measure of phonological awareness (sound categorization) were causally
related to the development of reading skills. At the beginning of their longitudinal study, the sound categorization ability of over 409 4- and 5-year-
old children was assessed before the children started to learn to read. Over 3
years later, their reading and spelling ability and verbal intelligence were
assessed. Performance on the sound categorization task was predictive of
later reading scores, even when measures of intelligence and memory were
taken into account.

In an effort to check that this correlation between early sound categorization skills and reading reflected a causal influence, Bradley and Bryant
included a training study. Sixty-five children who initially were poor at
sound categorization were split into four groups. One group was trained in
sound categorization, and a second group in addition to this was taught
letter-sound correspondences (and received exercises relating the sound
structure of words to their spelling patterns using plastic letters). There were
also two control groups: one was taught to group words according to semantic categories while the other received no training. After training, which was
spread over 2 years, the group that had been taught both sound categorization and letter-sound correspondences was some 8–10 months ahead of the
semantic categorization control group in reading scores. The group that

had only been taught to categorize sounds was about 4 months ahead of the semantic categorization control group in reading, but this difference was not statistically significant. At a later follow-up, 4 years after the first, the same pattern of results was still in evidence, with the group taught sound categorization and letter-sound correspondences still ahead in reading and spelling; though at this point neither trained group was significantly ahead of the taught control group, and interpretation of the data was clouded by ceiling effects (Bradley, 1987). However, given the small numbers of children in this intervention study, these null results must be interpreted with caution: the 4-month difference at first follow-up might well have proved significant given larger numbers of children.

These results are extremely impressive, but they fail to clinch the argument for a causal role of sound categorization ability in learning to read. To prove this would require evidence that the group taught to categorize words only on the basis of their sound was significantly ahead of the group taught to categorize on the basis of meaning. Although there was a tendency for this to happen, the crucial comparison was not statistically reliable.

The difference between the group trained in sound categorization alone and the group who also received training in letter-sound correspondences is notable, however. The exercises that the latter children received involved relating sounds in words to their spelling patterns, in combination with sound categorization training, and led to substantial improvements in reading and spelling skills. A natural implication of this result is that the integration of training in phonological skills with letter-sound training (or more broadly with phonically based reading instruction) may be particularly effective as a way of improving reading skills. According to this view, training in phonological skills in isolation from reading and spelling skills may be much less effective than training that forms explicit links between children's underlying phonological skills and their experiences in learning to read. We will term this the "phonological linkage hypothesis."

There are three other important training studies that are consistent with this hypothesis. Lundberg, Frost, and Peterson (1988) trained a large group of Danish kindergarten children in phonological awareness before formal reading instruction began. The trained children were better than a control group at reading in grade 2, though the difference in grade 1 was not quite significant. The size of the effects on literacy skills obtained in this study is small, though such effects may be important, especially if they provide a foundation for further development as children get older. In line with our phonological linkage hypothesis this study does suggest, however, that training on phonological skills alone is not a very powerful way of affecting reading development.

In the study of Cunningham (1990), two groups of kindergarten and first-grade children were given different forms of phonemic awareness training. A "skill and drill" group received training in phoneme segmentation and blending, while a "metalevel" group received training that in addition explicitly emphasized the link between the phonemic awareness training and reading. This latter training involved exercises in which the applications of segmentation and blending in reading were demonstrated and practiced. A control group listened to stories and discussed them with a teacher.

Cunningham found that the trained groups made more progress with reading than the control group and that, among the older children, the "metalevel" training had more effect than "skill and drill" training. This result fits nicely with our phonological linkage hypothesis. However, as in the case of Bradley and Bryant's sound categorization and letter-sound group, the "metalevel" group really received both teaching in reading and phonemic awareness training. Without a group simply given reading instruction alone, it is hard to be sure that it really is the integration of phonological training and reading instruction that is crucial to this group's success.

The third training study is that of Ball and Blachman (1988, 1991). Their study involved two groups of kindergarten children. A "phoneme awareness" training group received training in word segmentation, letter names and sounds, sound categorization (as in Bradley and Bryant's study), and DISTAR spell-by-sounds training. A "language activities" group received training in letter names and letter sounds and general language activities. There was also an unseen control group. The results showed that reading and spelling scores improved most in the "phoneme awareness" group. In line with our phonological linkage hypothesis, this study shows that phonological training combined with the teaching of letter names, letter sounds, and spelling skills is effective.

As well as these training studies, there is evidence from a number of experimental studies that is consistent with our phonological linkage hypothesis. For example, Tunmer, Herriman, and Nesdale (1988) looked at the relation between phonemic awareness and nonword reading (a relatively pure measure of decoding skill). They found that, although all the children who performed well on the nonword decoding task had good phonemic awareness skills, there were some children who had good phonemic awareness but read nonwords poorly. They conclude that "phonological awareness is necessary but not sufficient for acquiring phonological recoding skill." A similar conclusion was drawn by Byrne and Fielding-Barnsley (1989). They looked at young, preliterate children's ability to understand the alphabetic principle; that is, to demonstrate an understanding that particular phonemes in words are represented systematically by particular letters. To examine this they first taught 3–5-year-old children to read the words "mat" and "sat." The children were then simply asked to decide whether the printed word "MOW" was pronounced as "mow" or "sow." Above-chance performance on this task requires an understanding of the alphabetic principle while placing minimal extra cognitive demands on very young children. Byrne and Fielding-Barnsley found that reliable performance on this task was achieved only by children who could perform phonemic segmentation, understood that the initial sound segments of different words shared the same identity (that /s/ in SAT is the same as /s/ in SOW, e.g.), and had also learned the letters corresponding to the sounds 'm' and 's'. Thus both phoneme awareness and knowledge of letter identity were needed for children to grasp the alphabetic principle which is one component of a phonic decoding reading strategy: neither phoneme awareness nor letter identity knowledge alone was sufficient.

The phonological linkage hypothesis has important implications for our understanding of the way children learn to read and also has important educational implications. The main aim of the present study is to test this hypothesis in the context of an educationally realistic longitudinal intervention study with children who are showing significant difficulties in the early stages of learning to read.

In the present study we chose to look at the effectiveness of structured interventions in alleviating the reading problems of a large sample of poor readers. We chose to study 7-year-olds because by this age it is possible to identify with some certainty those children who are experiencing difficulties in learning to read. Following from the phonological linkage hypothesis, we wished to test whether an intervention that involved a combination of phonological training and reading instruction would be more effective than an intervention involving either reading instruction alone or phonological training alone.

This design allows us to assess whether simply training phonological skills is enough to improve the reading skills of poor readers: in this case the reading of both groups given phonological training should improve. In contrast, our phonological linkage hypothesis makes the specific prediction that the children given an integrated combination of reading and phonological training should make more progress than any of the other groups. Support for our hypothesis would have obvious practical implications for the design of teaching programs for children experiencing difficulties in the early stages of learning to read.

METHOD

In the present study we examine the effectiveness of three different structured methods of teaching with children who are having difficulties in the early stages of learning to read. We also relate progress made by these children to measures of their phonological skills taken before teaching began. The children were assessed before teaching began ($t1$, in September 1989) and after teaching was completed ($t2$, April–May 1990) some 7 months later. The 20 weeks of teaching were spread over a 25-week period between mid-October and early April. To assess the durability of any effects on reading and spelling, all children were reassessed 9 months after the interventions had ceased ($t3$, January 1991). All assessments were carried out "blind" as to the group membership of the child.

Subjects

The starting point for the present study was a county-wide reading survey of 6- and 7-year-olds in their third year of infant schooling in Cumbria Education Authority, United Kingdom. This screening used the Carver (1970) test, a group-administered, single word reading test, where children have to underline one of a group of words to match the word that has been spoken by the examiner. Following the survey, 188 children were identified as having reading quotients of less than 86. These children were then screened for severe general learning difficulties using the Raven's Coloured Progressive Matrices (Raven, 1965). Twenty children with a percentile rank on the matrices of less than 25 and a Carver reading quotient of less than 71 were excluded. Other children were excluded for a wide variety of reasons including failure to obtain parental consent to participate (six), changes in school (nine), and children being given Statements of Special Educational Need which give them a legal entitlement to special educational provision (seven). From the remaining children, 128 were selected and divided into four groups of 32, matched on IQ, reading ability, and age. Subsequently, however, three children were lost from the study, as they moved out of the area, reducing the total sample to 125. The children included in the study showed a wide range of IQs (68–122) and can be considered representative of 7-year-old children experiencing reading problems.

For the purposes of matching subject groups, two verbal (similarities and vocabulary) and two performance (object assembly and block design) subtests of the WISC–R (Wechsler, 1974) were used to estimate IQ. Scaled scores were converted to short-form IQ scores (with a mean of 100 and a standard deviation of 15) according to the procedure proposed by Tellegen and Briggs (1967; see also Sattler, 1982). Matching on reading ability was achieved using the British Ability Scales (BAS) Word Reading Test (Elliott, Murray, & Pearson, 1983). On the basis of these scores the four groups were closely matched for sex, age, IQ, and reading age. The distribution of children between groups was balanced within and across schools. There were 18 boys and 14 girls in each group. The four groups were assigned to one of three experimental teaching conditions and a control condition. These were Reading with Phonology (R + P), Reading Alone (R), Phonology Alone (P), and a Control (C). The details of the four groups are shown in Table 1.

Procedure

Cognitive measures. At the beginning of the project, all children received a large battery of 19 tests measuring general intellectual, reading, spelling, arithmetic, memory, and phonological skills. These tests were administered in a fixed order in three sessions. We describe here only the subset of 12 measures analyzed in the present paper.

READING. Progress in reading was assessed by tests of word and nonword pronunciation and text reading accuracy and comprehension.

EARLY WORD RECOGNITION TEST. An Early Word Recognition Test was constructed to differentiate between the progress of children who were at a very early stage of acquiring a "sight vocabulary." Forty-two words found at the first book stage of seven different reading schemes used in the schools participating in the study were used. Scoring was based upon the total number of words read aloud correctly.

TABLE 1

Means (and Standard Deviations) for Age, BAS Word Reading Ages, and Prorated WISC-R Full-Scale IQ for the Four Groups ($N = 124$)

Group	Age	Reading Age	IQ
Reading with Phonology ($N = 32$)	7.47	5.85	93.56
	(.30)	(.53)	(12.00)
Reading Alone ($N = 31$)	7.45	5.90	93.06
	(.31)	(.47)	(12.30)
Phonology Alone ($N = 30$)	7.47	5.90	94.57
	(.32)	(.57)	(12.12)
Control ($N = 31$)	7.56	5.95	93.16
	(.29)	(.53)	(11.71)
$F(3, 120)$ ratio	<1.00	<1.00	<1.00

BRITISH ABILITY SCALES (BAS) WORD READING TEST A. This test (Elliott et al., 1983) was used as a standardized measure of context-free word recognition. The test consists of a graded list of 90 words and was administered before matching groups and again after the intervention was completed.

NEALE ANALYSIS OF READING ABILITY (REVISED, FORM 1). This test (Neale, 1989) was used as a measure of reading accuracy in context and of reading comprehension. The test comprises a graded sequence of passages, each of which has an accompanying list of comprehension questions.

NONWORD READING TEST. This test was included as a relatively pure measure of phonic decoding skill. A list of 70 phonotactically legal nonwords was presented to each child to pronounce. The test was graded in difficulty from simple one-syllable CVC (consonant, vowel, consonant) nonwords to complex multisyllabic forms. It was explained to the child that the test consisted of "pretend" words that they would not know and that they should attempt to say as many of the "pretend" words as they could. Testing was discontinued when the child had failed on five consecutive items. Scoring was based on the number of nonwords read correctly with a phonically regular pronunciation.

SPELLING. The Schonell (Schonell & Schonell, 1956) Graded Word Spelling Test: List B was used to measure spelling ability. This test consists of 100 words (mostly phonically regular) which range from CVC to multisyllabic word forms.

ARITHMETIC. The BAS Basic Number Skills Test: Test A (Elliott et al., 1983) was used to measure arithmetic skills. The test consists of 34 orally presented items relating to a booklet of pictures and 34 paper and pencil problems of graded difficulty.

PHONOLOGICAL SKILLS—SOUND DELETION. A modified version of Bruce's (1964) Word Analysis Test was used to measure the ability to delete sounds from spoken words. There were 24 items, six in each section of the test. Before presenting the test, the examiner introduced the concept of sounds in words by using examples such as detecting the sound /k/ in 'cat'. Each of the first three test sections was preceded by two practice items which were presented according to a similar format. When introducing the first section (deletion of beginning sounds), the examiner said, "Say the word 'seat' . . . What word is left if the /s/ sound is taken away from the beginning of 'seat'?" Where children could not do that they were told, "If we take the /s/ sound away from 'seat' we are left with the word 'eat'." The examiner presented the second example for section 1 by asking, "What word is left if the /p/ sound is taken away from the beginning of 'pin'?" Where necessary help was given. The same format was used when presenting examples for sections 2 (deletion of final sounds) and 3 (deletion of middle sounds). The examiner presented the questions for sections 1–3 by using the stem, "What word is left if . . . ?" The first two items in each section continued with reference to the sound and position of elision, for example, ". . . the /j/ sound is taken away from the beginning of 'jam'?" The next two items continued with reference to just the sound to be deleted, for example, ". . . the /s/ sound is taken away from 'spin'." The last two items continued without reference to either the concept "sound" or to the position of elision, for example, ". . . the /h/ is taken away from 'hill'."

Section 4 was preceded by the examiner's remarking, "The sounds that I want you to listen to now will be in different positions in the words." Section 4 items were presented using the stem, "What word is left if . . .?" and without reference to either the concept "sound" or to the position of elision which varied from item to item.

Section 1 was discontinued at the point where children made five consecutive errors. The entire test was discontinued at the point where children made five consecutive errors beyond the first item of section 2. Scoring was based upon the overall number of correct responses.

SOUND BLENDING. A Sound Blending Test was constructed and used to measure the ability to blend a sequence of sounds into nonwords. The test stimuli consisted of 30 sets of two to seven sounds that could be blended to produce nonwords. In the order of presentation there were five sets of two-sound (VC or CV), six sets of three-sound (CVC), eight sets of four-sound (CVCC or CCVC forming final and initial blends), five sets of five-sound (VCVCC or VCCVC), and five sets of six-sound combinations (CVCCVC or VCCCVC) and one seven-sound combination (CVCCCVC).

Each set of sounds was read by the examiner at the rate of two sounds per second. The sounds were either consonants or short vowels. When presenting consonant sounds, the examiner tried to ensure that the vowel following each consonant was reduced to a minimum. The test was discontinued after children had made five consecutive errors. Scoring was based upon the number of correct responses.

NONWORD SEGMENTATION. The test stimuli consisted of 30 sets of nonwords, each of which consisted of from two to seven phonemes. In the order of presentation there were five items with two sounds (VC or CV), seven with three sounds (CVC), seven with four sounds (CVCC or CCVC), five with five sounds (VCVCC or VCCVC), four with six sounds (VCCVCC, CCVCCV, or CVCCVC), and two with seven sounds (CVCCCVC and (VCCCVC).

The examiner introduced the task by saying, "A nonword is a word like 'ot' or 'ip'. It sounds a bit like a real word but it doesn't make sense. It is a pretend word. 'Uk' and 'af' are also nonwords." Two coins were put on the table, and the examiner introduced the first of three examples by saying, "I am going to say a nonword. I will then use these coins to break it up into separate sounds." After saying 'ot' the examiner pronounced the sounds /o/–/t/ and simultaneously with each sound pushed a coin forward. The examiner then said, "Did you see how I left a gap between each sound? Now I want you to say nonword 'ip' and to break it up into separate sounds just like I did. Use the coins and leave a gap between each sound." If necessary, the task was demonstrated and children asked to copy what they had been shown. Two more examples were given following the same format. In the examples used to introduce the test, the examiner pronounced the separate sounds at the rate of two per second. The vowel sound after each consonant was minimized; all vowels were short. The examiner introduced test items by saying, "Now I am going to say some more nonwords. Use the coins to break them up into separate sounds. Only say the sounds that you hear. Leave a gap between each sound." For each successive item the number of coins corresponding to its constituent sounds was put on the table and the nonword pronounced.

Children's responses were accepted as correct when they produced the appropriate sounds, each of them separated in time from other sounds and accompanied by the simultaneous pushing forward of a coin. The test was discontinued after children had made five consecutive errors. Scoring was based on the number of correct responses.

SOUND CATEGORIZATION. A modified version of Bradley's (1984) sound categorization test was used to measure the ability to recognize rhyme and alliteration in spoken words. The experimental stimuli were 30 sets of four words. Within each set three words contained a common sound that the fourth lacked. The first 20 sets were rhyme oddity tasks, with the distinctive sound being the last consonant in the first 10 sets and the medial vowel in the second 10. The final 10 sets of words constituted an alliteration oddity task. Each set of tasks was preceded by two examples or practice items. Scoring was based upon the total number of correct responses.

Teaching procedures. Our aim was to contrast the effectiveness, in boosting our subjects' reading skills, of an integrated program of reading with phonological training (R + P), with training in phonology alone (P), or with reading instruction alone (R). Each program involved the children being taught individually for 40 30-min sessions spread over 20 weeks. The children in the three experimental groups were taught by a total of 23 teachers; each teacher worked individually with a total of between two and nine children. Since most of the teachers were involved with sets of three children (one from each experimental condition), the times of the day that the children were taught was varied. The minimum period of time between any one child's teaching sessions was 42 hours. All teachers received 3 days' training in how to use the teaching materials prepared for each of the interventions. The teachers involved in the research project comprised eight learning-support teachers who visited the schools, seven school-based special-needs teachers, seven class teachers, and one head teacher. The teachers were granted relief from their normal duties in order to carry out the research interventions. Adherence to the teaching protocols was monitored via regular meetings with the principal investigator and the completion of written records for each teaching session.

For reasons of space we give here only brief details of the teaching procedures used. (Further details of the procedures, together with samples of the materials used, are available from the first author.)

PHONOLOGICAL TRAINING ALONE (P). This training package (which was purely phonological, involving no reading) consisted of nine sections of phonological tasks based broadly on the "levels of difficulty" and activities referred to by Lewkowicz (1980), Lundberg et al. (1988), Rosner (1975), Stanovich, Cunningham, and Cramer (1984), and Yopp (1988). The sections covered the identification and supply of rhyming words, the identification of words as units within sentences, the identification and manipulation of syllables, the identification and discrimination of sounds within words, sound synthesis (into words), word segmentation (into sounds), the omission of sounds from words, sound substitution within words, and the transposition of sounds within words. Some of the activities (sound deletion, word segmentation, and sound synthesis) were equivalent to those used in the phonological portions of the assessment battery, in that they involved the same tasks but different stimuli. Each section consisted of a number of activities (68 in the package) which varied in terms of teaching mode, cognitive task and level of stimulus difficulty. The package was ordered, in terms of progressing from easier to more difficult activities.

The activities were presented as sequenced in the package and at a rate commensurate with children's success with the materials. Teachers were provided with record sheets with which to monitor children's progress. At the end of each 30-min session teachers entered the child's score on the record sheet appropriate for each of the activities covered in the session. A criterion of at least 80% success was used to determine when a child moved from one activity to the next or from one section to the next.

READING WITH PHONOLOGY (R + P). This package was modeled on the work of Clay (1985) but included the addition of phonological activities from the phonology (P) condition described above. Several changes were made in the way that Clay's (1985) teaching strategies and diagnostic tests were presented. The individual tests and teaching strategies were set out in sections covering reading and writing in context, reading and writing words, and looking at and writing letters. Each of the sections had a common format with the aims, materials needed, and instructions specified. Each of the teaching strategies also had specified criteria for their use and discontinuation. Identified areas of weakness were linked to specific teaching strategies by a chart.

The first four teaching sessions were taken up with the assessment of each child's responses to easy and to hard text, words, and letters. Sessions 5–40 followed the teaching format outlined by Clay (1985). This included re-reading a book that could be read with greater than 94% accuracy, reading the book introduced at the end of the previous session with the teacher taking a running record, letter identification (where necessary), writing a story (linked to phonological activities), cutting up the story (where necessary), and introducing a new book and attempting to read it. The criterion for moving up to the next level of difficulty was greater than 94% reading accuracy, over three sessions. A common set of 73 books, split into 20 levels (graded in difficulty according to the list provided by the New Zealand Department of Education, 1987) was used by all teachers. There were three or four books at each difficulty level.

Some comparisons between the amount of time spent on phonological training in the P and R + P groups can be made. The P group obviously spent more time on the phonological activities and completed on average 66.97 of the 68 phonology activities. In the R + P group the children completed a minimum of 31.21 of the phonological activities. In addition, however, the children in the R + P group carried out activities to link reading and phonology that were not included in the P group's activities. These linking activities included practicing letter-sound associations, relating spellings to sounds using plastic letters (as advocated by Bradley & Bryant, 1983), and writing words while paying attention to letter-sound relationships. The phonological and phonological linkage activities were carried out in the middle part of each session and lasted approximately 10 min. The phonological linkage exercises were linked to points arising from the children's writing (writing a story) and their reading during the first part of each session.

READING ALONE (R). The Reading Alone package was identical to that used with group R + P except for the omission of any explicit reference to phonology and all of the teaching strategies explicitly concerned with phonological linkage activities. In the early stages of the intervention period, teachers were frequently reminded of the importance of not referring to phonology or letter-sound relationships when working in this condition. Where children already exhibited such skills, teachers accepted them but made neither positive nor negative comments about them.

Some comparisons between the amount of time spent on reading instruction, and the form it took, in the R and R + P groups can be made. In the R group more time was spent on reading books of appropriate difficulty and building up reading and writing vocabularies through the use of structured multisensory teaching techniques (as advocated by Bryant & Bradley, 1985) in place of the phonological and phonological linkage activities undertaken by the R + P group. Through these children were not taught letter-sound associations, they were taught letter names. In addition, their reading instruction devoted more time to teaching the usefulness of context and meaning in reading and the use of self-checking and correction for attempts at reading unknown words. In short, this program involved individualized, highly structured teaching, embodying many current recommendations for good practice (Pumfrey & Elliott, 1990), but it lacked the explicit phonological linkage instruction given to the R + P group. It should be noted, however, that questionnaires completed by the children's classroom teachers indicated that virtually all the children in the study were receiving phonic reading instructions at school. The extent of this instruction showed no systematic differences between the different groups in the study. In no cases did such phonic teaching involve exercises in phonological awareness of the sort used for the P and R + P groups.

CONTROL (C). These children received their regular classroom teaching without any special form of additional provision from our study. Some of these children, however, like those in the other groups, were receiving additional remedial teaching that was independent of that provided by our study. Fifteen children in the control group received such help compared to five in the R + P group, seven in the R group, and six in the P group. Clearly, these differences in the amount of independent help given tend to operate against our hypothesis, since the largest number of children receiving help was in the control group and the smallest number was in the R + P group.

RESULTS

Our aim in this study was to assess the differential effectiveness of three teaching methods in helping children who are experiencing difficulties in the early stages of learning to read. Our primary data, therefore, come from the changes in reading (and also spelling) between the pre- and post-tests. The inclusion of arithmetic provides an important control capable of showing that any gains are specific to the domain of literacy rather than reflecting general, nonspecific improvements. We present the data on attainments first before going on to deal with the results from the phonological tasks.

Attainment in Reading, Spelling, and Arithmetic

The means (and standard deviations) for the reading, spelling, and arithmetic measures on the pre- and posttests for the four groups are shown in Table 2 below. The results of the standardized tests are presented in terms of attainment ages since these are easy to interpret, though in all cases analyses were conducted on the raw scores.

The children in the four groups were matched for reading ability using the BAS Word Reading Test only. As can be seen from Table 2, although the groups are closely matched on BAS reading age, they are not as closely matched as we would have hoped on the other measures of literacy skill.

TABLE 2

Means (and Standard Deviations) for the Pre- and Postintervention Attainment Measures of Reading, Spelling, and Arithmetic in the Four Groups

	Group						
	Reading with Phonology ($N = 32$)		Reading Alone ($N = 31$)		Phonology Alone ($N = 30$)		Control ($N = 31$)	
Early Word Identification:[a]								
$t1$	20.22	(10.08)	20.10	(9.49)	21.03	(11.63)	20.90	(9.59)
$t2$	32.72	(10.55)	32.32	(7.68)	29.73	(10.54)	29.32	(9.05)
BAS Word Reading:[b]								
$t1$	5.85	(.53)	5.90	(.47)	5.90	(.57)	5.96	(.53)
$t2$	6.73	(.85)	6.56	(.43)	6.55	(.69)	6.60	(.67)
Neale Accuracy:[b]								
$t1$	5.10	(.21)	5.04	(.19)	5.18	(.43)	5.11	(.30)
$t2$	6.13	(1.00)	5.78	(.54)	5.81	(.90)	5.66	(.80)
$t3$	6.77	(1.58)	6.22	(.82)	6.31	(1.03)	6.25	(1.15)
Neale Comprehension:[b]								
$t1$	5.29	(.30)	5.32	(.34)	5.43	(.50)	5.41	(.49)
$t2$	6.39	(.92)	6.00	(.97)	5.94	(.80)	5.88	(.73)
$t3$	6.99	(1.28)	6.47	(.94)	6.46	(1.11)	6.35	(.97)
Nonword Reading:[c]								
$t1$	4.34	(4.53)	3.55	(3.71)	6.00	(7.28)	3.65	(5.51)
$t2$	15.59	(14.16)	10.77	(8.14)	15.53	(10.28)	11.87	(10.97)
Schonell Spelling:[b]								
$t1$	5.78	(.59)	5.83	(.50)	5.93	(.56)	5.77	(.55)
$t2$	6.77	(.93)	6.54	(.55)	6.66	(.63)	6.49	(.74)
$t3$	7.19	(1.02)	6.90	(.62)	6.99	(.82)	6.92	(.78)
BAS Arithmetic:[b]								
$t1$	6.64	(.61)	6.83	(.64)	6.76	(.57)	6.69	(.66)
$t2$	7.39	(.59)	7.50	(.51)	7.37	(.63)	7.44	(.57)

[a] Maximum score = 42.
[b] Attainment ages expressed in years.
[c] Maximum score = 70.

The main issue of interest is the extent to which the four groups have made differential progress on these attainment measures. Analyses to address this question need to take account of the fact that the groups are not perfectly matched for their levels of literacy attainment at $t1$. The $t1$ literacy scores (Early Word Recognition, BAS Word Reading, Neale Accuracy, Neale Comprehension, Nonword Reading, and Spelling) for all subjects were subjected to a principal components analysis. This yielded a single factor (literacy skill) accounting for 70.1% of the variance. In subsequent analyses, the $t1$ literacy skill factor scores were used as a covariate when examining differences between groups at $t2$ on the different measures of literacy attainment. In each analysis, planned contrasts were used to test whether each of the trained groups differed from the control group. The use of planned contrasts does not require a significant overall effect for groups, and we therefore present only the results of the contrasts. Our prediction was that the R + P group would be consistently ahead of the control group in literacy skills at $t2$.

We chose to present separate analyses of our different measures of literacy skill (rather than a single multivariate analysis of covariance) because these measures were chosen to give an assessment of partially independent components of literacy skill. The Early Word Recognition and BAS tests provide a measure of context-free word recognition skill. The Neale Analysis of Reading Ability measures word recognition ability in context and the ability to comprehend what has been read. The Nonword Reading Test provides a relatively pure measure of children's ability to apply phonic decoding strategies to unfamiliar words out of context. The Schonell spelling test provides a measure of spelling ability. We wished to assess the extent to which our interventions had affected each of these measures; these measures are, however, correlated, and there is a degree of redundancy in these separate analyses (Huberty & Morris, 1989).

The use of analysis of covariance requires that the covariate is correlated with the dependent variable and that there is homogeneity of regression between the covariate and the dependent variable in the different groups considered (Tabachnick & Fidell, 1989). Both of these assumptions were met by our data for the literacy and arithmetic measures. Prior to conducting analyses, the data were also screened for outliers (Tabachnick & Fidell, 1989). One child in Group R was clearly an outlier as his scores on two of the $t2$ literacy measures (BAS and Neale Accuracy) were more than 3.5 SD above the group mean. This child was therefore excluded from all analyses of the data, reducing the total sample to 124.

Reading. As can be seen from Table 2, the improvements in reading following the intervention, at $t2$, tend to be consistently larger in the Reading with Phonology (R + P) group.

For the Early Word Recognition test, Group R + P differed significantly from the Control group, $F(1, 119) = 7.90$, $p < .01$, as did Group R, $F(1, 119) = 7.17$, $p < .01$, though Group P, $F(1, 119) = 0.23$, N.S., did not differ significantly from the Control.

For the BAS word recognition test, Group R + P differed significantly from the Control group, $F(1, 119) = 5.60$, $p < .02$, but neither Group R, $F(1, 119) = 0.26$, N.S., nor Group P, $F(1, 119) = 1.21$, N.S., differed significantly from the Control.

For the Neale Analysis of Reading Ability Accuracy scores, Group R + P differed significantly from the Control group, $F(1, 119) = 15.97$, $p < .001$, but neither Group R, $F(1, 119) = 2.96$, N.S., nor Group P, $F(1, 119) = 0.09$, N.S., differed significantly from the Control.

For the Neale Analysis of Reading Ability Comprehension scores, Group R + P differed significantly from the Control group, $F(1, 119) = 11.95$, $p < .001$, but neither Group R, $F(1, 119) = 1.33$, N.S., nor Group P, $F(1, 119) = 0.06$, N.S., differed significantly from the Control.

For the Nonword Reading scores, Group R + P differed significantly from the Control group, $F(1, 119) = 4.00$, $p < .05$, but neither Group R, $F(1, 119) = 0.02$, N.S., nor Group P, $F(1, 119) = 1.45$, N.S., differed significantly from the Control.

Thus, for every one of our reading measures, the R + P group has made significantly more progress than the control group, and in every case apart from one, the other treated groups have failed to make significantly more progress than the control group.

Spelling. As in the case of reading, it appears that Group R + P has made more progress in spelling than the other treated groups. The spelling scores were analyzed in the same way as the reading scores; Group R + P differed significantly from the Control group, $F(1, 119) = 5.88$, $p < .02$, but neither Group R, $F(1, 119) = 0.68$, N.S., nor Group P, $F(1, 119) = 0.49$, N.S., differed significantly from the Control.

Arithmetic. In contrast to the results for reading, the changes in arithmetic skills seem similar in all four groups. An analysis of covariance was conducted on the $t2$ arithmetic scores with the $t1$ scores as the covariate, followed by planned contrasts, as for the reading and spelling measures. This showed that in no case did any of the treatment groups differ from the control (Group R + P, $F(1, 119) = 0.04$, N.S., Group R, $F(1, 119) = 0.12$, N.S., Group P, $F(1, 119) = 0.83$, N.S.). This pattern confirms that the previous differential effects observed for reading and spelling are not a consequence of any general, artifactual improvement in Group R + P.

Long-term Effects of Intervention: Reading and Spelling Scores 9 Months Later
Reading. Reading was assessed using the Neale Analysis, and spelling with

the Schonell test, 9 months after the intervention had ceased. Table 2 shows that the larger improvements in reading on the Neale in the R + P group appear to be maintained at $t3$, 9 months after teaching finished. An analysis of the $t3$ scores, using the $t1$ literacy skill factor scores as a covariate, followed by planned contrasts, was conducted.

For the Neale Analysis of Reading Ability accuracy scores, Group R + P differed significantly from the Control group, $F(1, 119) = 8.48$, $p < .01$, but neither Group R, $F(1, 119) = 0.29$, N.S., nor Group P, $F(1, 119) = 0.15$, N.S., differed significantly from the Control. An identical pattern emerged for the Neale Analysis of Reading Ability comprehension scores, where Group R + P differed significantly from the Control group, $F(1, 119) = 12.38$, $p < .001$, but neither Group R, $F(1, 119) = 1.06$, N.S., nor Group P, $F(1, 119) = 0.01$, N.S., differed significantly from the Control.

Thus the improvements in reading skill shown by the group given the integrated phonological and reading package were maintained 9 months after our intervention had ceased.

Spelling. It appears from Table 2 that the differential on spelling at $t2$ has become weaker by $t3$. An analysis of the $t3$ spelling scores using the $t1$ literacy skill factor scores as a covariate followed by planned contrasts showed that in no case did any of the treatment groups differ from the control, Group R + P, $F(1, 119) = 2.46$, N.S., Group R, $F(1, 119) = 0.06$, N.S., Group P, $F(1, 119) = 0.01$, N.S.

Changes in Phonological Skills

Our phonological linkage theory holds that in order to be effective in boosting reading skills the training of phonological and reading skills needs to be integrated. Our results support this position insofar as the group given integrated reading and phonological training (R + P) improved more in reading skills than did the other groups who were given equal amounts of teaching concentrated solely on reading (R) or on phonological training (P). Moreover, the improvements seen were selective to reading, since a similar pattern of gains was not seen in arithmetic. The gains in reading were also shown to be durable.

One possible objection however, would be that the integration of reading and phonological training was more effective because (contrary to a naive view) this package was actually more effective in improving phonological skills than was the phonological training alone. According to this argument there might be something uniquely effective for improving phonological skills in combining phonological exercises with explicit reference to the printed word as happened in the R + P group. Such a view is quite plausible. Given the highly abstract nature of the phoneme as a unit of speech (see, e.g., Liberman, Shankweiler, Fischer, & Carter, 1974) it could be that children would benefit greatly in learning to perform tasks involving phoneme manipulation from the availability of visual letter symbols which stand in a direct correspondence to them. On this view, the greater improvements in literacy skills seen in the R + P group may, in reality, be a simple product of the better training of phonological skills in this group. There is an obvious way in which to test this idea: since we have independent measures of phonological ability taken before and after the teaching interventions we can compare the groups on these measures.

The means (and standard deviations) for the four phonological measures on the pre- and posttests for each of the four groups are shown in Table 3. As can be seen, there are substantial improvements in phonological skills in all of the groups, but the size of these improvements is consistently larger in the Phonology (P) group. To examine the reliability of any differential improvement an analysis of variance was carried out on the post- ($t2$) minus pre-intervention ($t1$) difference scores followed by planned contrasts comparing each of the treatment groups with the control. (In this case we were unable to use analyses of covariance, analogous to the ones used for reading and spelling, because tests revealed heterogeneity of regression

TABLE 3

Means (and Standard Deviations) for the Pre- and Postintervention Raw Scores on Measures of Phonological Ability for the Four Groups

	Group			
	Reading with Phonology (N = 32)	Reading Alone (N = 31)	Phonology Alone (N = 30)	Control (N = 31)
Sound Deletion:[a]				
$t1$	2.88 (3.08)	2.94 (3.80)	3.80 (4.27)	2.39 (3.05)
$t2$	9.91 (7.41)	6.19 (4.56)	13.70 (6.17)	7.39 (6.20)
Nonword Segmentation:[b]				
$t1$	9.31 (8.04)	10.29 (6.89)	11.40 (7.19)	8.32 (7.31)
$t2$	15.81 (8.60)	16.10 (6.88)	18.63 (6.09)	14.94 (7.66)
Sound Blending:[b]				
$t1$	6.91 (4.94)	5.97 (4.67)	7.57 (5.81)	7.13 (6.12)
$t2$	12.09 (5.52)	10.71 (5.29)	14.43 (5.16)	11.03 (7.11)
Sound Categorization:[b]				
$t1$	14.31 (6.06)	13.81 (5.64)	14.60 (5.61)	13.29 (4.71)
$t2$	17.56 (5.77)	16.90 (5.85)	18.27 (5.85)	15.65 (5.42)

[a]Maximum score = 24.
[b]Maximum score = 30.

across groups between two of the phonological measures [sound deletion and nonword segmentation] and phonological ability factor scores derived from a principal components analysis.)

For the Sound Deletion test, Group P, $F(1, 120) = 11.14$, $p < .001$, differed significantly from the Control group, but neither Group R, $F(1, 120) = 1.43$, N.S., nor Group R + P, $F(1, 120) = 1.98$, N.S., differed significantly from the Control. Similarly, for the Sound Blending test, Group P differed significantly from the Control group, $F(1, 120) = 6.61$, $p < .01$, but neither Group R, $F(120) = 0.54$, N.S., nor Group R + P, $F(1, 120) = 1.28$, N.S., differed significantly from the Control. However, for Sound Categorization in no case did a treatment group differ from the control, Group P, $F(1, 120) = 0.92$, N.S., Group R, $F(1, 120) = 0.30$, N.S., Group R + P, $F(1, 120) = 0.44$, N.S., and the same was true for Nonword Segmentation, Group P, $F(1, 120) = 0.20$, N.S., Group R, $F(1, 120) = 0.34$, N.S., Group R + P, $F(1, 120) = 0.01$, N.S.

There is a clear trend for Group P to make more progress on the phonological measures than the other groups, although in only two cases is this group's progress significantly better than that of the Control group. Given this pattern, it seemed possible that by looking at the joint effects of these measures in a single analysis we would find an overall superiority of Group P to the Control group. In some cases although individual analyses of variance are not significant, a multivariate analysis that takes account of the joint effect of a number of related variables can produce a significant effect (Tabachnick & Fidell, 1989). To explore this possibility, the difference scores ($t2 - t1$) for the four phonological measures were entered into a multivariate analysis of variance followed by planned contrasts. These revealed that, on a composite measure of phonological skill, Group P had made significantly more progress than the Control group, $F(4, 117) = 4.20$, $p < .005$, but neither Group R, $F(4, 117) = 0.74$, N.S., nor Group R + P, $F(4, 117) = 0.86$, N.S., differed significantly from the Control. Overall, therefore, Group P has made significantly more progress in phonological skills than the Control group while neither of the other two treated groups has.

These results show clearly that the differences in literacy scores between the P and R + P groups cannot simply be attributed to differences in the extent of improvements in phonological skills. Only Group P made significant progress in phonological skills, but this was not matched by comparable improvements in their literacy skills. In contrast, the R + P group did not make significant improvements in phonological skills, but they were the only group to make significant progress in learning to read and to spell. These results also suggest that it is relatively difficult to improve phonological skills in poor readers. Although the R + P group spent an appreciable amount of time being trained on phonological tasks, this apparently was not sufficient to bring about a significant improvement in their phonological skills.

DISCUSSION

This longitudinal intervention study of children with difficulties mastering early reading skills has produced a number of findings of both practical and theoretical significance. Before discussing our results it is important to emphasize that the intervention we conducted did not involve total control of the children's experience in learning to read. Rather our intervention involved just a small supplement of individualized tuition that was additional to the teaching that these children were otherwise receiving.

Our most notable result is that we have been able to demonstrate selective effects on these children's reading skills. In line with the phonological linkage hypothesis, we have shown that an effective way of improving reading skills involves a joint approach that integrates the training of phonological skills with the teaching of reading. Spending an equivalent amount of time concentrating on either component in isolation (reading or phonology) is less effective. Although the individual teaching of reading received by the Reading Alone group did produce some gains, they were not as large as in the group given both reading and phonological training. This is an important, and not at all obvious, result. Generally the most effective way to teach a given skill is to teach it directly. Our children given the reading and phonology package actually received less time being directly taught reading skills than did the Reading Alone group. The fact that they nevertheless made significantly more progress in reading is quite surprising and impressive.

According to our phonological linkage hypothesis, it is crucial that in the R + P group explicit links were formed between reading activities and phonological knowledge. To this end the children in this group undertook linkage activities such as relating spellings to sounds using plastic letters and writing words while paying attention to letter-sound relationships. In addition, of course, the R + P group received instruction in reading (comparable to the R group) and phonological training (comparable to the P group). A skeptic might argue that the explicit linkage activities are not crucial to the success of the R + P group and that instead children in this group might abstract the relationship between print and sound once they have some level of exposure to both phonological and reading exercises. This is certainly a possibility that our data cannot refute. We would, however, expect separate training in reading and phonological skills to be less effective than the explicit linkage given to the R + P group. The study of Byrne and Fielding-Barnsley (1989), described in the introduction, supports this idea. They looked at young children's understanding of the alphabetic principle, the concept that particular phonemes in words are represented systematically by particular letters. As we noted earlier, Byrne and Fielding-Barnsley found that such understanding was achieved only by children who could perform phonemic segmentation, understood phoneme identity, and had also been taught explicitly the critical phoneme-symbol relations (that S says /s/ and M says /m/, e.g.). This training of phoneme-symbol relations is an example of what we have termed a phonological linkage exercise in that it forces children to relate their awareness of phonemes to the process of reading words. Byrne and Fielding-Barnsley found that such training was necessary for their young children to come to understand the alphabetic principle. To test the critical role of our phonological linkage exercises more directly in the context of our own study would require a further study in which children received both reading and phonological instruction, but without explicit linkage exercises.

Leaving these details aside, our results certainly provide support for the view that phonological training alone is not a powerful way of improving children's reading skills. As we discussed earlier, Bradley and Bryant (1983) trained children in sound categorization and found that the gains in reading that resulted were not significantly greater than in a control group trained in semantic categorization. Similarly, Lundberg et al. (1988) found that training phonological skills in kindergarten children produced small effects on their later progress in learning to read. Our own results from older children with quite marked reading difficulties provide further evidence that improvements in phonological skills in isolation do not translate directly into improvements in reading skill. These findings therefore cast doubt on the simple theory that there is a direct causal path from phonological skills to reading skills. Our data support the more subtle position that adequate phonological skills may be necessary, but not sufficient, for learning to read effectively.

The phonological linkage hypothesis, and the support we have obtained for it, fits in well with a recent study concerned with the effectiveness of Clay's (1985) reading recovery program (Iversen & Tunmer, in press; Tunmer, in press). In Iversen and Tunmer's study a reading recovery program was compared with a modified program in which children also received systematic phonological training. The modified program was found to be more effective than the reading recovery program alone, just as our results would lead us to expect.

Intervention studies are notoriously difficult to conduct. We should like to stress a number of aspects of the design of the present study that help to strengthen the conclusions that can be drawn from it. One central point concerns the specificity of the effects obtained. The effects have been shown to be specific in two ways. First, we have shown that the improvements obtained are not completely general: there was not an equivalent pattern of improvement in arithmetic. This rules out nonspecific factors, such as motivation or teachers' expectations, as explanations of the results obtained. Second, we have shown that the beneficial effects on literacy development derived from an integrated approach to teaching reading and phonology are not purely mediated by changes in phonological skill. We produced larger effects on phonological skills in the Phonology Alone group without having any significant effect on literacy skills. This is not to say that improving phonological skills in children with reading difficulties is unimportant. Our results do show quite clearly, however, that working on phonological skills in isolation is not an optimal method for improving literacy skills. This, of course, is exactly the pattern of results predicted by the phonological linkage hypothesis: teaching both phonological and reading skills and their interrelationship is far more effective than working on either in isolation.

Though our primary focus in this study has been on reading, we have also looked at spelling. Theoretically it has sometimes been argued that reading and spelling develop partially independently and that phonological strategies are more important for the development of spelling than the development of reading (Goswami & Bryant, 1990; Snowling & Hulme, 1991). If this were the case, we might expect slightly different effects of our interventions on progress in spelling than on progress in reading. In particular, if phonological skills are more intimately involved in learning to spell than in learning to read, it might be expected that phonological training alone would be of more benefit to spelling than reading. Our results obviously do not support this position. The P group did not make significant progress in learning to spell, while the R + P group made significant progress in spelling as they did in reading. Our results cannot refute the idea that learning to read and learning to spell are partially separate processes, but they do suggest that there is a strong association between the learning of these two skills. For children having difficulties in the early stages of learning to read and to spell it appears that an integrated package of reading and phonological training can be expected to improve both their reading and spelling skills, though gains in spelling appear rather smaller and less durable than those for reading.

Our main focus in this paper has been to demonstrate the effectiveness of one particular approach to teaching children with reading difficulties. One obvious question that arises, however, is the extent to which the effects obtained in our study will generalize across subjects. The children in our study were a representative group of poor readers corresponding, roughly, to the bottom 25% of reading skill. These 7-year-olds were struggling with the earliest stages of learning to read. It seems likely to us that the effects obtained would show wide generality. We know, for example, that children of high IQ with highly specific reading difficulties commonly experience underlying phonological difficulties (see Hulme & Snowling, 1991, for a review of this evidence). There seems every likelihood that such children with more specific reading difficulties would show an equivalent pattern of benefit from an integrated approach to teaching reading and phonological skills. It would, nevertheless, be useful to confirm this empirically. It is certainly possible, however, that a minority of children has such severe phonological difficulties that training in these skills will be relatively ineffective for them (see Hulme & Snowling, 1992; Snowling & Hulme, 1989; and Stackhouse & Snowling, 1992, for a discussion of some examples of such cases). This is an important issue for future intervention studies to address. Lovett, Warren-Chaplin, Ransby, and Borden (1990) failed to find a differential effect of letter-sound versus whole-word teaching methods with a group of dyslexic children. They did not, however, include any measures to improve these children's phonological skills of the sort used with the R + P group in the present study.

Although we believe our results will show considerable generality, it is possible, indeed likely, that individual differences among children will interact with the effects of teaching that they are given. We have data pertaining to this which are too complex to present in full. In a principal components factor analysis with VARIMAX rotation of all the 19 measures obtained at $t1$, we found six factors, the first three of which were Reading Ability, Phonological Ability, and Verbal Ability. We computed a composite measure of progress in reading between $t1$ and $t2$ based on scores from three of our reading measures (BAS, Neale accuracy, and Neale comprehension). The predictors of reading progress differed across the groups in an interesting way. For Group R the best predictor ($r(29) = .72$) was phonological ability at $t1$ (neither pre-intervention reading ability nor verbal ability were significant predictors: r's$(29) = .14$ and $.20$, respectively). For Group P, on the other hand, the best predictor ($r(28) = .54$) was reading ability at $t1$ (neither pre-intervention phonological ability nor verbal ability were significant predictors: r's(28) = .30 and −.02, respectively). For Group R + P the best predictor (r(30) = .54) was again phonological ability at $t1$ (neither pre-intervention reading ability nor verbal ability were significant predictors, r's(30) = .33 and .14, respectively). These results indicate that for children given only help with reading their preexisting level of phonological ability is an important determinant of their success in learning to read. On the other hand, for children only given help to develop their phonological skills, their pre-existing level of reading skill will exert a powerful effect on whether this intervention is effective in improving their reading skills. These results complement our phonological linkage hypothesis in indicating that phonological and reading skills need to be united if interventions to help poor readers are to be effective.

Another issue concerns generality across ages. Our children were on average 7½ years old and in the early stages of mastering reading and spelling skills. It is possible that training phonological skills will be more important for young children than older children. This is an important developmental issue for future studies to address.

We hope that the educational implications of our findings will be obvious. We have evidence from a controlled study showing the effectiveness of a structured teaching procedure that unites the teaching of phonological and reading skills. The amount of extra teaching received by the children in our study, although not at all trivial (40 30-min sessions over 20 weeks), is at a level that makes our intervention educationally realistic. The magnitude of the gains achieved also makes them educationally (as well as statistically!) significant. One slightly disappointing aspect of our results, however is that the scores at the final follow-up ($t3$) suggest that the gains made by the R + P group, although still significant in reading accuracy and comprehension, tend to diminish. It may be that poor readers such as the children in our study require continuing support to recover fully from their early reading problems.

The results of our study also relate quite directly to a very large number of educational studies that have been concerned with the importance of phonics in the teaching of reading. In such studies, comparisons have typically been made between teaching methods that concentrate on reading for meaning and exclude phonics and those that make heavy use of phonics. It is obviously hard to exert rigorous control over irrelevant factors in such studies. However, the outcomes of a number of such studies (for reviews, see Adams, 1990; Chall, 1983) are impressively consistent in suggesting that phonic-based methods are more effective than meaning-based methods (though no one, we hope, would wish to belittle the importance of children learning to read for meaning). Our small-scale experimental study might be seen as providing evidence that complements these educational studies. In our study, poor readers in the R + P group certainly benefited from a remedial program that included many elements of phonic-based methods together with explicit training in phonological skills. In contrast, the R group, who received a highly structured approach that emphasized the use of context and meaning but omitted direct phonic teaching, was less successful.

One issue concerning the educational implications of our study is raised by the fact that all teaching was carried out on an individual basis. This is likely to maximize the effectiveness of any intervention but may also place constraints on how widely the methods could be used. Some of the procedures used in our intervention clearly need to be conducted on an individual basis (e.g., children reading and having their errors corrected by the teacher). However, some of the key elements of the R + P program, such as relating letters to sounds, making explicit links between the sounds of words and their spelling patterns, and certain phonological training exercises could be modified for use in small groups: this would be a useful extension of the present research.

Theoretically, the finding of support for the phonological linkage hypothesis raises a number of issues relevant to the normal development of reading skills and how best to facilitate them. Most obviously it raises the question of to what extent links between phonology and reading need to be made explicit in the teaching of reading. It also raises the question of the extent to which children may differ in the ease with which they bring to bear the phonological skills that they possess in the task of learning to read and spell. As well as differing in the degree of phonological competence they possess, children may also differ in their ability and propensity to access this competence. This may represent another dimension of individual differences that contributes to differences in learning to read. If this is so, an important and parallel educational question is how children's access to underlying phonological skills can be facilitated in the teaching of reading.

REFERENCES

Adams, M. J. (1900). *Beginning to read: Learning and thinking about print.* Cambridge, MA: MIT Press.

Ball, E. W., & Blachman, B. A. (1988). Phoneme segmentation training: Effect on reading readiness. *Annals of Dyslexia, 38,* 208–225.

Ball, E. W., & Blachman, B. A. (1991). Does phoneme awareness training in kindergarten make a difference in early word recognition and developmental spelling? *Reading Research Quarterly*, **26**, 49–66.

Bradley, L. (1984). *Assessing reading difficulties: A diagnostic and remedial approach* (2d ed.), London: Macmillan Education.

Bradley, L. (1987, December). *Categorising sounds, early intervention and learning to read: A follow-up study.* Paper presented at the British Psychological Society conference, London.

Bradley, L., & Bryant, P. E. (1983). Categorising sounds and learning to read: A causal connexion. *Nature*, **301**, 419–421.

Bryant, P. E., & Bradley, L. (1985). *Children's reading difficulties.* Oxford: Blackwell.

Bruce, D. J. (1964). The analysis of word sounds by young children. *British Journal of Educational Psychology*, **34**, 158–170.

Byrne, B., Fielding-Barnsley, R. (1989). Phonemic awareness and letter knowledge in the child's acquisition of the alphabetic principle. *Journal of Educational Psychology*, **81**, 313–321.

Carver, C. (1970). *Word recognition test.* London: Hodder & Stoughton.

Chall, J. S. (1983). *Learning to read: The great debate* (2d ed.). New York: McGraw-Hill.

Clay, M. (1985). *The early detection of reading difficulties* (3d ed.). Tadworth, Surrey: Heinemann.

Cunningham, A. E. (1990). Explicit versus implicit instruction in phonemic awareness. *Journal of Experimental Child Psychology*, **50**, 429–444.

Elliott, C. D., Murray, D. J., & Pearson, L. S. (1983). *British Ability Scales.* Windsor: NFER-Nelson.

Goswami, U., & Bryant, P. (1990). *Phonological skills and learning to read.* London: Erlbaum.

Huberty, C. J., & Morris, J. D. (1989). Multivariate analysis versus multiple univariate analyses. *Psychological Bulletin*, **105**, 302–308.

Hulme, C., & Snowling, M. (1991). Phonological deficits in dyslexia: A "sound" reappraisal of the verbal deficit hypothesis? In N. Singh & I. Beale (Eds.), *Progress in learning disabilities* (pp. 260–283). New York: Springer-Verlag.

Hulme, C., & Snowling, M. (1992). Deficits in output phonology: A cause of reading failure? *Cognitive Neuropsychology*, **9**, 47–72.

Iversen, S., & Tunmer, W. E. (in press). Phonological processing and the reading recovery program. *Journal of Educational Psychology.*

Lewkowicz, N. K. (1980). Phonemic awareness training: What to teach and how to teach it. *Journal of Educational Psychology*, **72**, 686–700.

Liberman, I. Y., Shankweiler, D., Fischer, F. W., & Carter, B. (1974). Explicit phoneme and syllable segmentation in the young child. *Journal of Experimental Child Psychology*, **18**, 201–212.

Lovett, M. W., Warren-Chaplin, P. M., Ransby, M. J., & Borden, S. L. (1990). Training the word recognition skills of reading disabled children: Treatment and transfer effects, *Journal of Educational Psychology*, **82**, 769–780.

Lundberg, I., Frost, J., & Peterson, O. (1988). Effects of an extensive program for stimulating phonological awareness in pre-school children. *Reading Research Quarterly*, **23**, 263–284.

Neale, M. D. (1989). *Neale Analysis of Reading Ability: Revised British edition*. Windsor: NFER-Nelson.

New Zealand Department of Education. (1987). *Classified guide of complementary reading materials—books for junior classes: A classified guide for teachers*. Wellington: Department of Education.

Pumfrey, P. D., & Elliott, C. D. (Eds.). (1990). *Children's difficulties in reading, writing and spelling*. Basingstoke, Hants: Falmer.

Raven, J. C. (1965). *The Coloured Progressive Matrices Test*. London: Lewis.

Rosner, J. (1975). *Helping children overcome learning difficulties: A step-by-step guide for parents and teachers*. New York: Walker.

Sattler, J. M. (1982). *Assessment of children's intelligence and special abilities* (2d ed.). London: Allyn & Bacon.

Schonell, F. J., & Schonell, F. E. (1956). *Diagnostic and attainment testing: Including a manual of tests, their nature, use, recording and interpretation*. London: Oliver & Boyd.

Snowling, M., & Hulme, C. (1989). A longitudinal case study of developmental phonological dyslexia. *Cognitive Neuropsychology*, **6**, 379–401.

Snowling, M., & Hulme, C. (1991). Speech processing and learning to spell. In R. Ellis & R. Bowler (Eds.), *Language and the creation of literacy* (pp. 33–39). Baltimore: Orton Dyslexia Society.

Stackhouse, J., & Snowling, M. (1992). Barriers to literacy development in two cases of developmental verbal dyspraxia. *Cognitive Neuropsychology*, **9**, 273–300.

Stanovich, K. E., Cunningham, A. E., & Cramer, B. B. (1984). Assessing phonological skills in kindergarten children: Issues of task comparability. *Journal of Experimental Child Psychology*, **38**, 175–190.

Tabachnick, B. G., & Fidell, L. S. (1989). *Using multivariate statistics* (2d ed.). New York: Harper & Row.

Tellegen, A., & Briggs, P. F. (1967). Old wine in new skins: Grouping Wechsler subtests into new scales. *Journal of Consulting Psychology*, **31**, 499–506.

Tunmer, W. E. (in press). Phonological processing and reading recovery: A reply to Clay. *New Zealand Journal of Educational Studies*.

Tunmer, W. E., Herrimen, M. L., & Nesdale, A. R. (1988). Metalinguistic awareness abilities and beginning reading. *Reading Research Quarterly*, **23**, 134–158.

Wagner, R., & Torgesen, J. (1987). The nature of phonological processing and its causal role in the acquisition of reading skill. *Psychological Bulletin*, **101**, 192–212.

Wechsler, D. (1974). *Wechsler Intelligence Scale for Children: Revised*. New York: Psychological Corp.

Yopp, H. K. (1988). The validity and reliability of phonemic awareness tests. *Reading Research Quarterly*, **23**, 159–177.